Oxford Handbook of Human Action

Oxford Handbook of Human Action

Edited by

Ezequiel Morsella

John A. Bargh

Peter M. Gollwitzer

OXFORD
UNIVERSITY PRESS

2009

OXFORD
UNIVERSITY PRESS

Oxford University Press, Inc., publishes works that further
Oxford University's objective of excellence
in research, scholarship, and education.

Oxford   New York
Auckland   Cape Town   Dar es Salaam   Hong Kong   Karachi
Kuala Lumpur   Madrid   Melbourne   Mexico City   Nairobi
New Delhi   Shanghai   Taipei   Toronto

With offices in
Argentina   Austria   Brazil   Chile   Czech Republic   France   Greece
Guatemala   Hungary   Italy   Japan   Poland   Portugal   Singapore
South Korea   Switzerland   Thailand   Turkey   Ukraine   Vietnam

Copyright © 2009 by Oxford University Press

Published by Oxford University Press, Inc.
198 Madison Avenue, New York, New York 10016

www.oup.com

Oxford is a registered trademark of Oxford University Press

Library of Congress Cataloging-in-Publication Data
Oxford handbook of human action / edited by Ezequiel Morsella, John A.
Bargh, Peter Gollwitzer.
p. cm.—(Oxford Series in Social Cognition and Social
Neuroscience; 2)
Includes bibliographical references and index.
ISBN: 978-0-19-530998-0
1. Intentionalism.   I. Morsella, Ezequiel.   II. Bargh, John A.
III. Gollwitzer, Peter M.
BF619.5.O94 2008
150—dc22   2008004997

ACKNOWLEDGMENTS

First and foremost, we would like to thank the chapter contributors for sharing their wonderful insights and findings regarding the fascinating topic of the science of human action. We also acknowledge the advice and assistance of Ran Hassin, Jeremy Gray, Robert Krauss, Andy Poehlman, John Paul Russo, Robert B. Tallarico, Lawrence Williams, the Department of Psychology at Yale University, and the editorial team at Oxford University Press.

We wish also to acknowledge the tremendous debt all of us who study the psychology of action have to Professor Wolfgang Prinz and his laboratory at the Max Planck Institute for Human Cognitive and Brain Sciences, Germany. His research on action representations and on the "common coding" between perceptual and actional representations paved the way for the many of us interested in the basic mechanisms of action.

Ezequiel Morsella would like to dedicate this book to the memory of Ines Morsella, who, with the gift of two turtles for his eighth birthday, piqued his lifelong love for natural science. Peter Gollwitzer would like to dedicate this book to Gabriele, Jakob, and Anton. John Bargh thanks his two fellow editors for sharing with him over the years their exceptional scholarship and insights: PMG in the domain of motivational theory and research and EM in the domains of action and consciousness. To each, he would like to express his personal as well as professional debt of gratitude.

CONTENTS

CONTRIBUTORS

Henk Aarts
Department of Psychology
Utrecht University
Utrecht, The Netherlands

Karen E. Adolph
Department of Psychology
New York University
New York, NY

J. Wayne Aldridge
Department of Neurology and
Department of Psychology
University of Michigan
Ann Arbor, MI

Gisa Aschersleben
AE Entwicklungspsychologie
Saarland University
Saarbrücken, Germany

John A. Bargh
Department of Psychology
Yale University
New Haven, CT

Roy F. Baumeister
Department of Psychology
Florida State University
Tallahassee, FL

Kent C. Berridge
Department of Psychology
University of Michigan
Ann Arbor, MI

Karin C. A. Bongers
Social Psychology Program
Radboud University
Nijmegen, The Netherlands

C. Miguel Brendl
Department of Faculty and Research
INSEAD
Boulevard de Constance
Fontainebleau, France

Charles S. Carver
Department of Psychology
University of Miami
Coral Gables, FL

Tanya L. Chartrand
The Fuqua School
of Business and
Department of Psychology and
Neuroscience
Duke University
Durham, NC

Jonathan D. Cohen
Department of Psychology and
Center for the Study of Brain, Mind and
Behavior
Princeton University
Princeton, NJ

Rajal G. Cohen
Department of Psychology
Pennsylvania State University
University Park, PA

Clayton E. Curtis
New York University
Department of Psychology and
Center for Neural Science
New York, NY

Ruud Custers
Department of Psychology
Utrecht University
Utrecht, The Netherlands

Rick Dale
Department of Psychology
Cornell University
Ithaca, NY

Amy N. Dalton
The Fuqua School of Business
Duke University
Durham, NC

Jean Decety
Department of Psychology and
Center for Social and Cognitive
Neuroscience
University of Chicago
Chicago, IL

Gary S. Dell
Beckman Institute
University of Illinois, Urbana–Champaign
Urbana, IL

Mark D'Esposito
University of California, Berkeley
Helen Wills Neuroscience Institute,
Department of Psychology, and
Henry H. Wheeler Jr. Brain Imaging Center
Berkeley, CA

Roland Deutsch
Universität Würzburg
LS Psychologie II
Würzburg, Germany

Ap Dijksterhuis
Social Psychology Program
Radboud University
Nijmegen, The Netherlands

Baruch Eitam
Department of Psychology
The Hebrew University
Jerusalem, Israel

Rob Ellis
School of Psychology
University of Plymouth
Plymouth, United Kingdom

Birgit Elsner
Institute of Psychology
University of Potsdam
Potsdam, Germany

Jens Förster
Department of Social Psychology
University of Amsterdam
Amsterdam, The Netherlands

John M. Franchak
Department of Psychology
New York University
New York, NY

Ronald S. Friedman
Department of Psychology
University at Albany
State University of New York
Albany, NY

Matthew T. Gailliot
Department of Psychology
Florida State University
Tallahassee, FL

Simone V. Gill
Department of Psychology
New York University
New York, NY

Georg Goldenberg
Neuropsychological Department
Krankenhaus Munchen-Bogenhausen
Munchen, Germany

Peter M. Gollwitzer
Department of Psychology
New York University and Universität
Konstanz
New York, NY

Jordan Grafman
Chief, Cognitive Neuroscience Section
National Institute of Neurological
Disorders and Stroke
National Institutes of Health
Bethesda, MD

Jeremy R. Gray
Department of Psychology
Yale University
New Haven, CT

Ran R. Hassin
Department of Psychology
The Hebrew University
Jerusalem, Israel

Philip Holmes
Program in Applied and Computational
Mathematics
Department of Mechanical and Aerospace
Engineering
Princeton University
Princeton, NJ

Bernhard Hommel
Leiden Institute for Brain and Cognition
Leiden University
Leiden, The Netherlands

Shaziela Ishak
Department of Psychology
New York University
New York, NY

Steven Jax
Moss Rehabilitation Research Institute
Philadelphia, PA

Amy S. Joh
Department of Psychology and
Neuroscience
Duke University
Durham, NC

Kyungil Kim
Department of Psychology
Ajou University
Suwon, Korea

Tali Kleiman
Department of Psychology
The Hebrew University
Jerusalem, Israel

Iring Koch
Max Planck Institute for Human Cognitive
and Brain Sciences and
Institut für Psychologie
RWTH Aachen University
Aachen, Germany

Catalina Kopetz
Department of Psychology
University of Maryland, College Park
College Park, MD

Stephen C. Krieger
Department of Neurology
Mount Sinai Medical Center
New York, NY

Regina Krieglmeyer
Universität Würzburg
LS Psychologie II
Würzburg, Germany

Frank Krueger
Cognitive Neuroscience Section
National Institute of Neurological
Disorders and Stroke
National Institutes of Health
Bethesda, MD

Arie W. Kruglanski
Department of Psychology
University of Maryland,
College Park
College Park, MD

Nira Liberman
Tel Aviv University
Tel Aviv, Israel

Gordon D. Logan
Department of Psychology
Vanderbilt University
Nashville, TN

Arthur B. Markman
Department of Psychology
University of Texas
Austin, TX

Ruud G. J. Meulenbroek
Nijmegen Institute for Cognition and
Information
Radboud University Nijmegen
Nijmegen, The Netherlands

Ezequiel Morsella
Department of Psychology (SFSU) and
Department of Neurology (UCSF)
San Francisco State University and
University of California, San Francisco
San Francisco, CA

David T. Neal
Department of Psychology and
Neuroscience
Duke University
Durham, NC

Gabriele Oettingen
Department of Psychology
New York University and Universität
Hamburg
New York, NY

Elizabeth J. Parks-Stamm
Department of Psychology
New York University
New York, NY

Jesse Preston
Psychology Department
University of Illinois, Urbana–Champaign
Champaign, IL

Wolfgang Prinz
Max Planck Institute for Human
Cognitive and Brain Sciences
Leipzig, and
AE Entwicklungspsychologie
Saarland University
Saarbrücken, Germany

Deidre L. Reis
Department of Psychology
Yale University
New Haven, CT

Daniel Richardson
Department of Psychology
University of California, Santa Cruz
Santa Cruz, CA

David A. Rosenbaum
Department of Psychology
Pennsylvania State University
University Park, PA

Michael F. Scheier
Department of Psychology
Carnegie Mellon University
Pittsburgh, PA

Patrick Simen
Program in Applied and Computational
Mathematics
Department of Psychology and Center for
the Study of Brain, Mind and Behavior
Princeton University
Princeton, NJ

Jessica A. Sommerville
Department of Psychology and Institute for
Learning and Brain Sciences
University of Washington
Seattle, WA

Michael Spivey
Department of Psychology
Cornell University
Ithaca, NY

Fritz Strack
Universität Würzburg
LS Psychologie II
Würzburg, Germany

Dianne M. Tice
Department of Psychology
Florida State University
Tallahassee, FL

Jonathan Vaughan
Department of Psychology
Hamilton College
Clinton, NY

Jill A. Warker
Beckman Institute
University of Illinois, Urbana–Champaign
Urbana, IL

Daniel M. Wegner
Harvard University
Cambridge, MA

David A. Westwood
School of Health and
Human Performance
Dalhousie University
Halifax, Canada

Christine A. Whalen
Department of Psychology
University of Wisconsin
Madison, WI

Wendy Wood
Department of Psychology and Neuroscience
Duke University
Durham, NC

The Mechanisms of Human Action: Introduction and Background

Ezequiel Morsella

Abstract

This chapter prepares the reader for the journey provided by the in-depth chapters of the *Oxford Handbook of Human Action*. In this primer, following a historical survey of the study of human action and discussion of the particular challenges encountered when 'reverse engineering' human action, the basic questions about human action are reviewed in six sections. The sections cover how actions are: [1] mentally represented (e.g., embodied, propositional, and ideomotor theories), [2] encoded neurally (e.g., neural systems, population vectors, and mirror neurons), [3] controlled (e.g., hierarchical control, distributed control, and conflict), [4] acquired (e.g., instrumental learning and automaticity), [5] activated and selected (e.g., priming, action production, volition, and ethological approaches), and [6] the nature of action in the social world (e.g., mimicry). The chapter concludes with a discussion of the future of the study of human action.

Keywords: actions, conditioning, instrumental learning, reverse engineering, mental representation, action plans

A few minutes at a local café allow one to appreciate the wide array of actions that humans are capable of expressing—reading the newspaper, waiting for a friend, shaking hands, grabbing the waiter's attention with a "cappuccino, please." Some actions at the café may be reflexive, automatic, voluntary, social, communicative, or reflect that hidden resource called "will power." As ordinary as these actions are, they remain exceedingly difficult to understand from a scientific point of view. What are the neural and cognitive mechanisms by which actions are learned, mentally stored, and expressed? What is the difference between actions that are mediated consciously and those that are mediated unconsciously? How does an idea such as a mental image of a tree lead to the movements of a pen or paintbrush?

These are exciting times because such questions are beginning to be answered scientifically. It is our hope that this book will address most if not all questions regarding the nuts and bolts of human action, questions that have been surprisingly neglected in the history of experimental psychology (Nattkemper & Ziessler, 2004). Oversight of this important topic stemmed in part from the rigid, nonrepresentational stance of the behaviorist era and from psychology's overall preference of the problem of knowledge representation, as in perception and memory, over that of action (Rosenbaum, 2005).

Beyond Stimulus and Response

Building on Pavlov's (1927) classic investigations on conditioned reflexes, behaviorism (about 1919 through 1948) discouraged discussion of the inner workings of the "black box" (the mind and brain; Watson, 1919). Instead, it construed human action as the product of simple, observable stimulus–response contingencies in which all learning depended on events such as "reinforcement" or "punishment" (Skinner, 1953). But clever experimentalists soon demonstrated that instrumental learning (e.g., maze learning) could occur incidentally, that is, without any form of reward or other contingency (*latent learning*; Bindra, 1976; Tolman & Honzik, 1930) and that mental representations such as "cognitive maps" and "grammar trees" were necessary to explain behaviors that can occur independently of external cues, as in the case of language production (Chomsky, 1959), fast serial actions such as typing or piano playing (Lashley, 1951), and maze learning (Tolman, 1948). For example, it was demonstrated that laboratory animals could still solve mazes and reach goal boxes while navigating in the dark, through opaque substances (e.g., murky water), or while negotiating a maze that had been rotated (Eichenbaum & Cohen, 2001). It was clear that animals could solve such feats only because of something not in the external world but "in their head." (See Chapter 2 for a treatment of the limitations of other *sensorimotor* accounts.) In short, sophisticated experimental techniques (sometimes requiring rats to swim through mazes filled with murky water) were necessary to prove that *ideas can influence action,* an obvious fact outside the psychology laboratory. After the fall of behaviorism,[1] action began to be construed as a function of internal, mental representations (Miller, Galanter, & Pribram, 1960).

In this way, the stimulus of explanatory value moved from the external world into the internal, conceptual world but perhaps too far therein. Following behaviorism, the Zeitgeist of the "cognitive revolution" seemed to forget William James's (1890/1950) famous adage that *thinking is for doing* and placed cognition in a lofty "information-processing" realm far removed from physical action (Barsalou, 2003; Eimer, Hommel, & Prinz, 1995; Glenberg, 1997), leading to the *symbol grounding problem* (Harnad, 1990; see the discussion later in this chapter). Thus, the study of action ironically fell victim to one paradigm and then also to the reactionary movement against it.

The Challenge of Reverse Engineering

Independent of scientific trends, the study of human action has continuously suffered from the inherent problems that are encountered when undertaking the *reverse engineering* of action (Pinker, 1997), problems not encountered with the actions of everyday artifacts such as toasters, automatic doors, and computers, which are designed and engineered according to clear-cut plans (originating in human minds). Knowledge regarding the workings of artifacts—clocks, hydraulic systems, telephone switchboards, and transistor circuits—have historically influenced the ways we think about human action (Schultz & Schultz, 1996). But just as artificial modes of transportation such as wheels, tank tracks, and jet engines are not suitable models of biological locomotion, artificial cognition, as in the standard von Neumann serial computer, is not suitable for understanding biological cognition (Arkin, 1998; von Neumann, 1958).

Unlike artificial actions, biological actions have been crafted during the happenstance and tinkering process of evolution (Gould, 1977). Referring to evolutionary products, the ethologist Lorenz (1963) states, "To the biologist who knows the ways in which selection works and who is also aware of its limitations it is no way surprising to find, in its constructions, some details which are unnecessary or even detrimental to survival" (p. 260). Regarding robot design, a roboticist cautions, "Biological systems bring a large amount of evolutionary baggage unnecessary to support intelligent behavior in their silicon based counterparts" (Arkin, 1998, p. 32).

Even within the same organism, the same kind of action can be implemented by vastly different mechanisms (Marr, 1982), some of which may be more elegant and efficient than others. Thus, the mechanisms underlying human action may employ strategies that are inconsistent, suboptimal, inefficient, or deeply counterintuitive (de Waal, 2002; Lorenz, 1963; Simpson, 1949; see review in Marcus, 2008). When, for example, one carries out the simple action of bringing a utensil toward the mouth, one intuits that a point located near the hand is causing the upward motion when in fact it is the contraction of the bicep muscle, closer to the trunk, that is largely responsible for the action. If such simple acts are difficult to comprehend intuitively, it is not surprising that it is a great challenge to decipher the more complex actions at the café, which may involve language, behavioral suppression, and the curiosities of social interaction, where a simple smile can emerge from multiple, distinct cognitive and neural mechanisms, depending on whether it is natural or forced (Wild et al., 2006).[2]

For all these reasons, at the time of the *Psychology of Action* (1996), the precursor to this book, there was little relevant empirical research on action itself, so the book focused mainly on forward-looking proposals, that is, on how might action be expected to unfold, given the assumptions of the major cognitive, social, and motivational models of the time. Since that time, there has been a surge of research on the mechanisms of human action, and so the time is now ripe for a new bible on human action, one that collects this new knowledge in a single, concise source. With an emphasis on underlying mechanisms, the chapters making up this book provide up-to-date summaries of the published research on focal topics and bring together findings from eminent researchers of motor control, neurology, cognitive neuroscience, and psycholinguistics as well as of cognitive, developmental, social, and motivational psychology.

The New Study of Action

The study of human action has benefited from diverse areas of investigation that tend to be descriptive (reflecting how things actually are) rather than normative (reflecting how things should be). No longer constrained by avoiding taboo subjects such as neural circuits, ideas, volition, and consciousness, the study of action is now tackled from a naturalistic point of view in which *anything* is open to investigation provided it be constrained by behavioral and neuroscientific evidence. For instance, it is now common to study the role of affect, goals, and consciousness in human action (see Chapters 14, 15, 16, 27, 28, and 30). Thus, current approaches address different aspects of human action in a complementary fashion. In the following sections, the reader is prepared for the wonderful journey provided by the in-depth chapters of the *Oxford Handbook of Human Action*. In this primer, the basic research questions about human action are reviewed in six sections. The sections cover how actions are (a) mentally represented, (b) encoded neurally, (c) controlled, (d) acquired, and (e) activated and selected and (f) the nature of action in the social world.

Representations: How Are Actions Mentally Represented?
Ideomotor Approaches

Since the fall of behaviorism, the notion of *mental representation* has influenced our understanding of the mechanisms of human action. Contemporary *ideomotor* approaches (Greenwald, 1970; Hommel,

Müsseler, Aschersleben, & Prinz, 2001; cf. Chapters 2 and 18), for example, have resuscitated classic, prebehaviorist notions regarding the nature of the link between mental representation (perceptual or memorial) and action (Carpenter, 1874; Harleß, 1861; James, 1890/1950; Lotze, 1852). Again, according to James, *thinking is for doing*, meaning that mere thoughts of actions produce impulses that, if not curbed or controlled by "acts of express fiat," result in the performance of those actions (James, 1890/1950, pp. 520–524). He added that this was how voluntary actions are learned and generated: The image of the sensorial effects of an action leads to the corresponding action—effortlessly and without any knowledge of the motor programs involved. In such a "forward-looking" arrangement, the capacity to predict the consequence of motor acts is paramount (Berthoz, 2002; O'Regan & Noë, 2001). (For a treatment of why motor programs are unconscious, see Chapters 2 and 6; Gray, 1995; Grossberg, 1999; Prinz, 2003.)

Unlike traditional approaches, which divorce input from output processes and envisage representations as consisting primarily of sensory-like traces rather than action-like ones, contemporary ideomotor approaches propose that perceptual and action codes activate each other by sharing the same representational format (Hommel et al., 2001). In this way, these "single-code" models explain stimulus–response compatibility effects (Chapters 2 and 18) and, more generally, how perception leads to action.

A recurrent theme in the study of action is that *goal-based representations* rather than *means representations* are critical in the execution of many human actions, whether for simple acts such as voluntarily flexing a finger or more complex acts (Chapters 2, 15, and 18). Goal representations are also featured in cybernetic models of voluntary action (Carver & Scheier, 1990), which focus on the interplay between goal pursuit and affect (Chapter 16). The view that perception and memory are primarily in the service of action[3] is also consonant with contemporary *embodied*[4] approaches toward the nature of mental representation and action (Chapters 7 and 13; Barsalou, 1999; Glenberg, 1997; Pulvermuller, 2005; Smith & Semin, 2004). (For a proposal regarding the important influence of episodic memory on future action, see Schacter & Addis, 2007.)

Embodied Versus Classical Approaches

Following the cognitive revolution, theorists from diverse disciplines (e.g., cognitive psychology, computer science, philosophy, robotics, and social psychology) have challenged "classical" theories of representation in which meaning is represented by amodal and arbitrary symbols. These classical theories (cf. Markman & Dietrich, 2000) were inspired by developments in computer science, artificial intelligence, logic, and information theory (Arkin, 1998; Barsalou, 1999). The symbols in these amodal theories do not retain any of the properties of the sensorimotor states that gave rise to them (Barsalou, 1999; Kosslyn, Ganis, & Thompson, 2003): Things of all kinds could be represented by binary digits, truth tables, feature lists, frames, schemata, semantic nets, and the like (e.g., Burgess & Lund, 1997; Landauer & Dumais, 1997). For instance, the perceptual data of a table are transformed into a set of arbitrary symbols whose "meaning" is captured only by the functional consequences of the propositions they form (Lakoff & Johnson, 1999). Much as a particular string of ones and zeros can stand for different things depending on whether the computer program is a text editor, a graphics program, and so on, the form these propositions take matters only in terms of the outcome of the operations that will be performed on them;

apart from their functional consequences, the symbols themselves remain meaningless (Glenberg, 1997).

From the classical standpoint, human action is seen as an "output" of a high-level, centralized system that is much like a serial processor and is heavily involved in forming an accurate internal model of the world. To function adaptively within unpredictable environments, such centralized systems require tremendous computational power in order to continually update their internal, amodal model of the world. This error-prone and time-consuming translational process is not required in embodied systems (Arkin, 1998), for information is already residing either in the environment or in mental representations that maintain properties of the sensorimotor states that gave rise to them (Barsalou, 1999). Another strength of embodied models is that they do not suffer from the symbol grounding problem (Harnad, 1990) of classical theories because the meaning of mental representations is grounded—redeemed or "cashed in," in a sense—in interactions with the world.[5]

Resembling pre–20th-century ideas in which semantic representations are image-like traces of the experiences that produced them,[6] a number of embodied theories have been proposed (Barsalou, 1999; Glenberg, 1997; Hauk, Davis, Kherif, & Pulvermuller, 2008; Paivio, 1979). These approaches are consistent with behavioral evidence showing that perceptual symbols such as the shape of an object are activated during language comprehension (Zwaan, Stanfield, & Yaxley, 2002) and with neuroimaging and neuropsychological evidence demonstrating that semantic knowledge is distributed throughout different regions of the brain in a principled fashion (Martin & Caramazza, 2003; Hauk et al., 2008), including areas subserving motor functions (Damasio, Tranel, Grabowski, Adolphs, &

Damasio, 2004; Gainotti, Silveri, Daniele, & Giustolisi, 1995; Martin, 2001; Oliveri et al., 2004; Pulvermuller, 2005; Tranel, Damasio, & Damasio, 1997; Warrington, 1975).

For instance, visual-semantic areas of the brain are activated during the processing of concrete semantics (Kan, Barsalou, Solomon, Minor, Thompson-Schill, 2003; Kellenbach, Wijers, & Mulder, 2000), and listening to action-related sentences activates frontoparietal motor circuits (Tettamanti et al., 2005). Most strikingly, reading the words "garlic," "cinnamon," and "jasmine" elicits activation in the primary olfactory cortex, but neutral words such as "glasses" and "door" do not (González et al., 2006). In short, it seems that the specific area in which a particular bit of semantic knowledge is stored is related to the regions involved in the acquisition or processing of the relevant information (Nyberg, Habib, McIntosh, & Tulving, 2000; Thompson-Schill, Aguirre, D'Esposito, & Farah, 1999).[7]

Current, "nonclassical" approaches are also consonant with historical notions of situated action and cognition (e.g., Vygotsky, 1962), in which concepts can be created from the "internalization" of overt behavior (Chapter 7). Consistent with this standpoint, covert mental training improves performance on overt tasks (Nyberg, Eriksson, Larsson, & Marklund, 2006), and neuroimaging evidence demonstrates that similar areas of the brain are activated for real, observed, and imagined actions (Chapter 13; Brown & Martinez, 2007; Decety 1996a, 1996b; Grafton, Fadiga, Arbib, & Rizzolatti, 1997). In addition, in a PET experiment, Parsons et al. (1995) found that motor areas of the brain are activated while participants judge whether pictures of hands, in various orientations, depicted the left or the right hand. Parsons et al. (1995) suggested that, in order to perform the task, participants had to mentally rotate their own hands; thus, the answer was gleaned through embodied knowledge. Similarly, Wexler, Kosslyn, and Berthoz (1998) found evidence supporting the hypothesis that transformations of mental images are mediated in part by motor processes. What is more, it seems that not only can cognitive processes influence action, but action can influence cognition,[8] as in the vocal rehearsal exhibited during the phonological loop (Baddeley, 1986) or in the movements of the eye, hand, and arm that are expressed during other working memory tasks (Chapters 7 and 12; Morsella & Krauss, 2004; Postle, Idzikowski, Della Sala, Logie, & Baddeley, 2006).

Embodied approaches have been used to explain how bodily activity and actions interact with memory function (Dijkstra, Kaschak, & Zwaan, 2007), affect (Beilock & Holt, 2007; Flack, 2006), and attitudes. Chen and Bargh (1999) showed that participants are faster to make approach movements of the arm (pulling a lever toward oneself) when responding to positive attitude objects and faster to make avoidance movements (pushing the lever away) when responding to negative attitude objects. This was true even though participants' conscious, explicit task in the experiment was not to evaluate the objects at all but merely to "knock off the screen" the names of these objects as soon as they appeared. Similar results have been found with clenching the fist in the presence of pleasant words; such a power grip is believed to activate positive affect (Tops & de Jong, 2006).

Conversely, Cacioppo, Priester, and Berntson (1993) show that motor expressions (arm flexion versus extension) can influence attitude formation. In their experiment, participants viewed neutral stimuli (ideographs) while flexing (i.e., pulling toward them) or extending (i.e., pushing away) their arms. Cacioppo et al. (1993) predicted that, as an approach behavior, arm flexion would activate positive attitudes and that extension, as an avoidance behavior, would activate negative attitudes. In support of the hypothesis, it was found that participants liked stimuli more if they appeared during flexion than extension. The idea is that the bodily response—flexion or extension—automatically and unwittingly activates its corresponding attitude or affect (for related findings, see Neumann, Förster, & Strack, 2003; Neumann & Strack, 2000; Solarz, 1960).

James (1950) proposed a similar idea—that bodily expressions occur reflexively, brought about by situational forces, and that the perception of these events constitutes the *feeling* (or conscious representation) of the emotional experience:

> The other day I was standing at a railroad station with a little child, when an express train went thundering by. The child, who was near the edge of the platform, started, winked, had his breathing convulsed, turned pale, burst out crying, and ran frantically towards me and hid his face. I have no doubt that this youngster was almost as much astonished by his own behavior as he was by the train. (p. 487)

It is not our purpose here to treat the well-known merits and weaknesses of the James–Lange theory of emotions (for a excellent treatment of the topic, see Lang, 1994).

An a priori weakness of embodied approaches is that it remains unclear how abstract concepts could be represented in an analogical, embodied format (but see Barsalou, 1999; Boroditsky & Ramscar, 2002) and how disparate forms of information could be combined, manipulated, or transformed from one format into another. Empirically, it is not clear whether lesions of action-related regions of the brain do in fact lead to impairments regarding the semantic knowledge of action (cf. Daprati & Sirigu, 2006; Grafton & Ivry, 2004; Heilman,

Rothi, & Valenstein, 1982). For example, Mahon and Caramazza (2008) point out that patients suffering from cognitive deficits due to brain lesions can show impairments in the way they use certain objects but can nonetheless name those objects, or even recognize the pantomimes associated with those objects, without difficulty. In addition, Mahon and Caramazza (in press) highlight a potential fallacy of embodied approaches—the incorrect assumption that the consistent activation of circuit or region *x* (e.g., a motor region) during process *y* (e.g., object naming) implies that region *x* constitutes process *y*. For these reasons, Mahon and Caramazza (in press) present *grounding by interaction*, a theoretical approach that serves as a compromise of embodied and classical approaches. (For a review of additional strengths and weaknesses of embodied and classical theories, see Markman & Dietrich, 2000; for a treatment against embodied or analogical representations, see Pylyshyn, 2002.)

Neural Substrates: How Are Actions Encoded Neurally?

Population Vectors

Hubel and Wiesel's (1968) pioneering research on feature detector cells in the visual cortex of the cat led to conceptual advances regarding the neural basis of perception in general. Similarly, the psychophysiological research of Georgopoulos and colleagues (Bagrat & Georgopoulos, 1999; Georgopoulos, Caminiti, Kalaska, & Massey, 1983) on the motor cells of the monkey illuminated how coherent actions (e.g., moving the arm leftward) could be encoded by a population of cells. This line of research revealed that, just as a given neuron in the visual cortex is tuned to fire most to the visual presence of one feature (e.g., a horizontal line) but less to another (e.g., a vertical line), each cell in the motor cortex of the monkey fires most when an arm movement is made in a particular, "preferred" direction (e.g., 180 degrees) and fires less when movements are made in another, "nonpreferred" direction (e.g., 45 degrees). (In this arrangement, 45 degrees would be the preferred direction of another motor cell.)

In this way, during any given movement, each cell of the motor cortex fires to a different degree, depending on how close the direction of the overt movement is to its preferred direction. In a very democratic manner, the direction of a given movement is thus encoded neurally by the summed activity (the *population vector*) of all the cells. These cells form part of the motor "homunculus" identified by Wilder Penfield (Penfield & Rasmussen, 1950). Today, it is known that the brain is replete with such somatotopic maps (cf. Aflalo & Graziano, 2006) and population vectors (Pellionisz & Llinas, 1980).

Population vectors have been found in the basal ganglia, cerebellum, and premotor areas. They even exist in the spinal cord of the frog (Bizzi, Mussa-Ivaldi, & Giszter, 1991). In the motor cortex of the monkey, they are related to action *planning* rather than action *expression,* as a change in the vector can occur as long as 300 milliseconds before the onset of a corresponding change in overt behavior. In other cases, the population vector can change without any change in emergent behavior, for behavioral expression of the vector requires an additional downstream process. (Regarding *how* the efference from these motor cells influence action, see Kakei, Hoffman, & Strick, 1999.) When overt action does unfold, electromyographic activity in the corresponding muscles occurs 50 milliseconds following the discharge of cortical motor cells, and movement follows this electromyographic activity by 70 milliseconds (Bindra, 1976). Kinesthetic feedback from this muscular activation reaches the somatosensory cortex 80 milliseconds after the initial cortical motor discharge.

Falling under the rubrics of "proprioception," "reafference," "efference copy," "corollary discharge," and "exafference," feedback from efferent central processes in the brain or from the muscles has been proposed to serve important roles in perception and consciousness (see footnote 3). For a recent account regarding the neural correlates of feedback from the premotor to the somatosensory cortex, see Christensen et al. (2007).

Mirror Neurons

Importantly, for the cells of the primary motor cortex (Figure 1.1), it is the direction of the movement and not its end point that tends to be encoded. This suggests that this level of processing is lower in the hierarchy than the kinds of representations treated in ideomotor views and in theories of high-level motor control (Chapters 2, 6, and 18). Indeed, processing at higher levels of the motor hierarchy (e.g., in premotor, parietal, and association cortical areas) has been found to be essential in the planning of actions based on mental representations, whether they be based on immediate perceptual information, past experience, or future goals (Gazzaniga, Ivry, & Mangun, 2002).

Mirror neurons (Rizzolatti et al., 1990; see review in Rizzolatti, Sinigaglia, & Anderson, 2008), for example, become active both when you perceive a given type of action and when you engage in that action yourself (Frith & Wolpert, 2003; Meltzoff & Prinz, 2002). At this high level of encoding, neurons fire with respect to motor acts rather than with respect to the movements that form them.[9] According to Rizzolatti, Fogassi, and Gallese (2004), "The cortical motor system, in addition to its role in action organization, is also involved in action understanding and imitation" (p. 427). Thus, these neural events seem to be more related to encoding the kinds of end-state representations proposed by several theories (see also Ashe et al., 1993; Iacoboni & Dapretto, 2006) that may form part of a "vocabulary" of action representations (Rizzolatti et al., 2004). (Bizzi and colleagues, too, propose a componential approach in which expressed actions are understood as stemming from an inventory of "motor primitives"; cf. Bizzi & Mussa-Ivaldi, 2004.)

In humans, the mirror system encompasses large segments of the premotor cortex and the inferior parietal lobule (Rizzolatti et al., 2004). Mirror neurons are particularly relevant to "common code" theories of speech perception (e.g., Liberman & Mattingley, 1985) in which perception relies in part on the motor codes used to produce speech— *sounds perceived as alike are produced as*

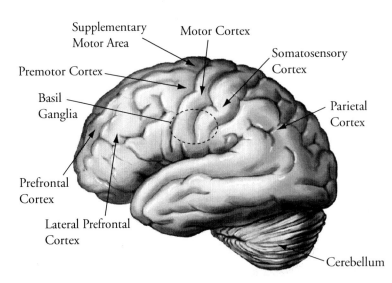

Fig. 1.1 Major brain areas involved in human action.

alike (see review in Galantucci, Fowler, & Turvey, 2006; see also Pickering & Garrod, 2006).

Control: How Are Actions Controlled?

Hierarchical Control

In general, higher levels in the control hierarchy encode overarching goals and provide more specific subgoals for lower levels. The actual execution of the action is controlled at lower levels of the motor hierarchy that have more defined goals because of more spatial and temporal constraints (Chapter 6; Arkin, 1998; Gazzaniga et al., 2002).

During everyday actions such as grasping a cup or blocking a soccer ball, highly flexible "online" adjustments are made unconsciously (Goodale & Milner, 2004; Rosenbaum, 2002). Because the physical spatial relationship between the objects of the world and one's body is seldom unchanging (e.g., a cup is sometimes at left or right), each time an action is performed, new motor programs are generated online in order to deal with peculiarities of each setting (Chapters 6 and 21). But our conscious mind tends to be concerned with the *invariant* aspects of action—the stable goals of having coffee each morning ("somehow") or blocking penalty kicks (again, "somehow"). High-level action planning may be concerned with achieving a final end state (e.g., flicking a switch or relating good news), which can be met in multiple ways (Chapter 6), as in the case of *motor equivalence* (Lashley, 1942), in which several different behaviors can lead to the same end state: Without training, one can successfully perform the act of writing *hello* by manipulating a pencil with one's mouth, even though this novel act requires a manner of motor control very different from that occurring during manual writing.

Even reflexive responses (and conditioned reflexes) are quite flexible and contextually sensitive (Chapter 21). This was most dramatically demonstrated by Wickens (1938), who employed a variation of the Watson–Lashley finger withdrawal response. In this task, subjects rest their hands palm downward on an electrode and remove their hands as quickly as possible in response to electric shock. To determine whether subjects learned a specific motor plan (as proposed by Watson) or a more general avoidance response toward the stimulus (as proposed by Tolman), Wickens cleverly turned the subject's hand over so that the electrode was still touching the palm but the palm was now facing upward. Compared to the classic, palm-downward manipulation, withdrawing in this scenario requires an anatomically "antagonistic" muscle group. Watson would predict a lack of a transfer learning, for a new muscular reflex must be learned: Exhibiting the original response would actually drive the finger toward the electrode. Tolman's position, however, predicted that the subject will nonetheless immediately avoid the shock since he or she has already learned a global (i.e., molar) shock-avoidance response and not a specific muscular reflex. Wickens's study and subsequent research has decisively supported Tolman's view.

At the highest level of the hierarchy are the representations that are most abstract and enduring. These representations are believed to be encoded in the prefrontal cortex (Chapter 10; Miller & Cohen, 2001), in which the representation of a goal (e.g., to pick up the laundry) can be sustained independent of environmental stimulation because of several possible cellular and circuit-based properties of this large region. Encoded in the prefrontal cortex, these representations have been characterized as "active memory in the service of control" (Miller & Cohen, 2001, p. 173). Without the prefrontal cortex, monkeys are incapable of performing actions requiring information beyond that which is furnished by the environment. Thus, monkeys with lesions of the lateral prefrontal cortex cannot perform *delayed response tasks,* in which responding correctly depends on holding certain cues (e.g., "open the door on the left") in mind for extended periods of time (Goldman-Rakic, 1992).

Lower levels in the control hierarchy (e.g., motor cortex and brain stem) translate high-level goal representations into movement with the help of the cerebellum and basal ganglia. With respect to action, the cerebellum seems to be concerned primarily with its fluidity, timing, and accuracy (see review in Ghez & Thach, 2000) and with the formation, storage, and retrieval of highly skilled movement representations (Puttemans, Wenderoth, & Swinnen, 2005). The many regions forming the basal ganglia (see review in DeLong, 2000) seem to be dedicated primarily to the initiation and force (or "gain" control) of action (Keele & Ivry, 1991; Kolb & Wishaw, 2006) and to the resolution of response competition (Gazzaniga et al., 2002), leading some to construe it as essential for action selection: "[There are] many competitors vying for control of the body's effector mechanisms . . . the basal ganglia [complex is] the key arbiter" (Prescott & Humphries, 2007, p. 104). (For treatments of higher-level, cognitive functions of the cerebellum and basal ganglia, consult Schmahmann, 1998; Strick, 2004; Utter & Basso, 2008; for a review of the role of the thalamus in human action, see Tan, Temel, Blokland, Steinbusch, & Visser-Vandewalle, 2006.)

However, as mentioned previously, the human nervous system is far from a system having only hierarchical control. Instead, it is best characterized as a *hybrid* system (Arkin, 1998) that has both hierarchical, deliberative control system(s) and quasi-independent decentralized control systems (Gazzaniga et al., 2002; Norman & Shallice, 1980).

Distributed Control

In *Evolving Brains,* the neurobiologist John Allman (2000) likens the human nervous system to a power generation plant he had visited in the 1970s. As expected, the plant profited from contemporary computer technology, but he was surprised to see that, aside from the contemporary technology, the plant continued to use obsolete, vacuum and pneumatic technologies. When he queried about the reasons for this strange mix, he was told that the demand for power had always been too great for the plant to ever be shut down:

> The brain has evolved in the same manner as the control systems in this power plant. The brain, like the power plant, can never be shut down and fundamentally reconfigured, even between generations. All the old control systems must remain in place, and new ones with additional capacities are added and integrated in such a way as to enhance survival. (Allman, 2000, p. 41)

Contemporary approaches thus speak of the mind as being composed of multiple, agentic information-processing structures having different phylogenetic origins, mind-sets, operating principles, and agendas (e.g., homeostatic concerns such as nutrition and hydration; Gallistel, 1980; Metcalfe & Mischel, 1999; Minsky, 1985; Öhman & Mineka, 2001; Tetlock, 2002). Dennett (1991) pointed out that primate brains are "based on millennia of earlier nervous systems; they were regularly flooded with multimodal information, and this gave them a new problem, one of higher-level control. There wasn't a convenient captain already on board, so these conflicts had to sort themselves out without any higher executive" (p. 188). The evolutionary trend toward increased compartmentalization of function in the nervous system introduced various integrative solutions, including reflexes, neural convergence, and perhaps the state identified as consciousness, which seems to be necessary to integrate high-level systems that are vying for (specifically) skeletal muscle control (Chapter 30; Morsella, 2005).

Far from the simplistic, idealized reflexes envisioned by behaviorists, observed human action results from many forms of action control systems, with each system possibly having different phylogenetic origins, operating principles, and distributed anatomical structures (Chapter 7). At macrolevels of analysis, there is the neuropsychological discovery of the "two visual paths" (Ungerleider & Mishkin, 1982), in which one path seems to be dedicated for knowledge representation and the other for action and behavior (Chapter 4; Milner & Goodale, 1995). These dual-path systems cast doubt on the old stage models that still implicitly guide research in many areas of psychology, models in which conscious perception guides behavioral choices, which then guide action. Dissociations are also reported to exist between instrumental action and affective states. For example, though resembling "wanting" because of their repetitive and persistent nature, some addiction-related behaviors are actually unaccompanied by "liking," that is, by the congruent subjective drives (Chapter 24; Baker, Piper, McCarthy, Majeskie, & Fiore, 2004; Berridge & Robinson, 1995).

Multiple, simultaneous information pathways are also evident in fear conditioning (Öhman, Carlsson, Lundqvist, & Ingvar, 2007). This form of learning is believed to be mediated in part by modularized nuclei in the amygdala of the midbrain that receive polysensory information from afferent pathways that are different from those feeding cortical loci, such as visual area 1 of the occipital lobe (Lavond, Kim, & Thompson, 1993; LeDoux, 1996; Olsson & Phelps, 2004). For example, nuclei in the amygdala process polysensory information to evaluate emotional aspects of a situation, while the visual cortex and other structures do so to evaluate different aspects. This process occurs roughly in parallel (for adaptive reasons, the amygdalar pathway is slightly faster; LeDoux, 1996; Öhman et al., 2007).

In conditions such as prosopagnosia, patients are impaired in identifying faces but can still demonstrate affective learning toward these stimuli. For example, though claiming to "not know" a given face, a patient suffering from this condition can nonetheless exhibit a galvanic skin response to the face if that face was previously associated with an unpleasant experience (Tranel & Damasio, 1985). This line of research has shown that even normals can have inexplicable "gut feelings" (or "somatic markers"; Damasio, Tranel, & Damasio, 1991) reflecting the inclinations (or response tendencies) of systems whose inner workings and learning histories are opaque to awareness (LeDoux, 2000; Öhman & Mineka, 2001; Olsson & Phelps, 2004). Together, these findings support the view that the mind is composed of quasi-autonomous, agentic systems that evolved independently and are modularized in the brain with partially independent learning histories.

Therefore, more often than not, emergent human action reflects an unravelable combination of various processes. Some aspects of action may result from reflexive spinal mechanisms, central pattern generators in the spinal cord or brain stem (e.g., for locomotion), species-specific affective motor programs (e.g., fear-related motor programs involving the periaqueductal gray matter; Eichenbaum & Cohen, 2001), or one of the five descending tracts (corticospinal, rubrospinal, tectospinal, vestibulospinal, and recticulospinal) by which the brain innervates the spinal cord and influences emergent behavior. To complicate matters further, it is known that both motor and sensory areas of the brain can influence action control (Jeannerod, 2003). For example, corticospinal fibers (once characterized as forming the voluntary, *pyramidal* tract) are found in somatosensory cortex, and movement-related cellular signals are found in the traditionally "perceptual" posterior parietal cortex (Andersen et al., 2004).[10] During a given

action, different cortical regions participate in different ways, in parallel. For example, the supplementary motor area, a region anterior to the premotor area, seems to reflect internal goals and motivations, whereas the lateral premotor area is concerned more by externally based sources of information, such as action-related objects and proprioceptive feedback (Figure 1.2; Gazzaniga et al., 2002).[11]

Acquisition: How Are Actions Acquired?

Notions of acquired action—in contrast to that of the inborn, Cartesian reflex— go back at least to Carpenter (1874) and to James's (1890/1950) conceptualization of the

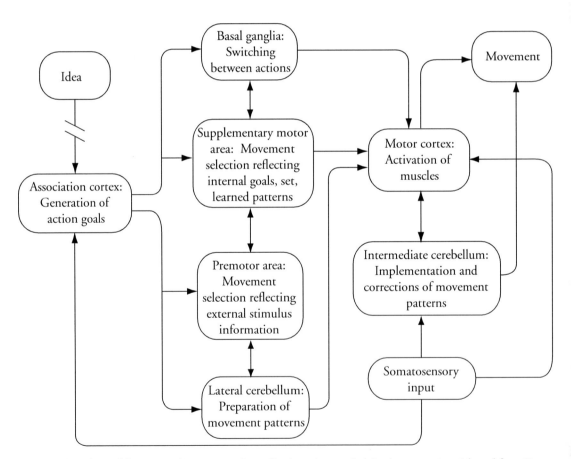

Fig. 1.2 Hypothesized function and interconnections of brain regions underlying human action. Adapted from Figure 11.47, from *Cognitive Neuroscience: The Biology of the Mind, Second Edition* by Michael S. Gazzaniga, Richard B. Ivry, and George R. Mangun. Copyright © 2002 by W. W. Norton & Company, Inc. Used by permission of W. W. Norton & Company, Inc.

unconscious "habit" (James, 1890/1950, pp. 520–524), which James held to be the causal force behind most behaviors, a claim that is now corroborated by substantial research (Chapters 5, 10, 11, 20, and 21).

Instrumental Learning

Regarding instrumental (or "operant") learning, behaviorists spoke of a "three-term contingency" in which a particular stimulus (e.g., a button) is associated with a response (e.g., pressing the button) that leads to an outcome (e.g., food; Skinner, 1953). The three "term contingency" was schematized as $S \rightarrow R \rightarrow O$. In a simple case, if O happens to be rewarding (or *reinforcing*), the connection between $S \rightarrow R$ was strengthened such that R was more likely to occur in the future in the presence of S. Similarly, in neural network models of operant conditioning (cf. Breiter & Gasic, 2004; Carlson, 1994; Rolls & Treves, 1998; Shepherd, 1994), connections are strengthened between whichever perceptual-related and motor-related representations (as neural patterns) happened to be activated within some temporal window following reward. This occurs by the "blind" *potentiating* of the often arbitrary (Rolls, 2007) connections between both kinds of representation. It seems that different brain regions mediate the five elements of the $S \rightarrow R \rightarrow O$ process, with the dopaminergic system, frontal cortex, and basal ganglia being heavily involved in the process (Breiter & Gasic, 2004; Carlson, 1994).

It is important to appreciate that, because learning is based not on *neurotaxis* (i.e., the moving and relocation of neuronal structures) but rather on the strengthening of neural connections that already exist (Kandel & Hawkins, 1992; Sherrington, 1906), such a system for operant learning requires incredibly vast connectivity between all potential input and output patterns. In other words, in lieu of neurotaxis, stimuli of all kinds should be "linkable" to motor outputs of all kinds. (For the limitations of such arbitrary links, see Seligman & Hager, 1972; for the shortcomings of any *associationistic* approach, see Gallistel & Gibbon, 2001.) In addition, as a "coincidence" detector, the outcome-based component of the process responsible for strengthening or weakening the connections between the relevant Ss and Rs must be capable of influencing only those representations that have been recently activated.

Neuroscientific evidence reveals that, in nonhuman primates, the learning of arbitrary mappings between stimuli and responses (e.g., green light $\rightarrow$ finger movement) is mediated by neurons in the dorsal premotor cortex; lesions of this region in humans lead to deficits in visuomotor learning (Grafton & Ivry, 2004; Halsband & Freund, 1990). Lesions of high-level cortical areas (especially the supplementary motor area) tend to lead to deficits in *action selection* (i.e., generating the wrong response), whereas lesions of the basal ganglia and cerebellum tend to lead to deficits in the expression of actions, that is, generating the correct response but expressing it poorly (Gazzaniga et al., 2002).

Automaticity

Regarding skill learning and automaticity, it is known that the neural correlates of novel actions are distinct from those of actions that are overlearned, such as driving or tying one's shoes (Chapter 20). Regions primarily responsible for the control of movements during the early stages of skill acquisition are different from the regions that are activated by overlearned actions. In essence, when an action becomes automatized, there is a "gradual shift from cortical to subcortical involvement, associated with a decreasing necessity to inhibit preexisting response tendencies and the development of an internally, feedforward-driven execution mode" in which the anterior cerebellum and putamen play a critical role (Puttemans et al., 2005, p. 4277). In addition, significant changes from practice can occur within a single region (e.g., primary motor cortex; Karni et al., 1998; Padoa-Schioppa & Bizzi, 2003).

Activation Dynamics: How Are Action Plans Activated and Selected?

Several theoretical approaches shed light on the "which" and "when" of human action. These theories on the mechanisms underlying the *activation* and *selection* of action plans have benefited enormously from research on language production (Chapter 8). For example, speaking too fast or too slow leads to errors that are qualitatively similar to those that occur when typing, playing a musical instrument, or performing other serial actions at nonoptimal speeds (Dell, Burger, & Svec, 1997; Lashley, 1951).

Language Production

Although a seemingly effortless task that occurs in a fraction of a second, uttering a word is actually a quite sophisticated act of great precision, involving multiple kinds of representations. From the tens of thousands of words stored in the mental lexicon, the speech system must select the one word that best captures the intended meaning. We are seldom aware of the exact words that we will utter when formulating a new sentence, yet speaking occurs without difficulty. It is action selection at its finest.

There is a consensus in psycholinguistics that at least two levels of representation are in play during word retrieval (Chapter 8; Dell, 1986; Levelt, Roelofs, & Meyer, 1999). One level, the word representation, corresponds to the meaning and syntactic properties of a word (e.g., that *cat* is an animal), and another level, the phonological representation, pertains to the phonological properties of a word (e.g., that *cat* is composed of the phonemes /k/, /ae/, and /t/). Accordingly, evidence from diverse sources demonstrates that word retrieval involves two distinct stages: one is devoted to the selection of a word's representation and its syntactic features, and the other, occurring on the order of 40 milliseconds later (van Turennout, Hagoort, & Brown, 1998), is aimed at retrieving word phonology (Caramazza, 1997; Levelt, 1989). In addition, there is little disagreement that, at first, the semantic system activates a cohort of related lexical nodes. If the speaker wants to say "cat," for instance, the word nodes for TIGER, DOG, and WHISKER may receive activation along with "cat." (This sometimes leads to a *semantic error,* the most common of speech errors; see Dell, 1986.) In normal circumstances, the target lexical node—cat, in our example—is selected because it reaches the highest level of activation.

Speech production is mediated primarily by areas of the frontal lobes, including Broca's area (the inferior frontal gyrus; Broadmann's areas 44 and 45), a premotor region that has been traditionally thought of as devoted to language production but is now proposed to play a more general and less defined role in cognition and action production (Novick, Trueswell, & Thompson-Schill, 2005). In *Broca's Region*, Grodzinsky and Amunts (2006) conclude that there is "no general agreement on how the functions related to Broca's region should be characterized" (p. xiv).

Inspired by fundamental properties of neurons, parallel-distributed processing approaches (Dell, 1986; Rumelhart, McClelland, & the PDP Research Group, 1986) introduced the notion of *cascade* processing (McClelland, 1979) to illuminate how information flows from one stage of processing to the next in cognitive tasks such as identifying a printed word. Cascade processing was later used to illuminate the nature of speech production (Dell, 1986). According to cascade approaches, activation flows in a manner such that the phonological representations of words can be activated even though those words are not "selected" for speech production. *Serial models,* on the other hand, propose that only the word selected to be produced can activate phonology (Butterworth, 1992; Levelt et al., 1999). Consistent with cascade but not serial models, it has been shown that naming an object is facilitated if the name of the object happens to sound like the color in which the object is presented (e.g., a bowl presented in blue versus in red; Navarrete & Costa, 2004), suggesting that the color name of the object was activated incidentally.[12] (For evidence that activation can cascade even onto articulatory processes, see Goldrick & Blumstein, 2006.) Assessing the limitations of such activation is a current object of substantial research (see reviews by Goldrick, 2006; Rapp & Goldrick, 2000).

The Flow of Activation

Consistent with the cascade approach and the basic neurophysiological characteristics of perceptual processing (Ganz, 1975), *continuous flow* (Eriksen & Schultz, 1979) describes how incidental objects can activate action plans. For example, in interference tasks such as the classic Eriksen flanker task (Eriksen & Eriksen, 1974), participants are first trained to press one button with one finger when presented with the letter "S" or "M" and to press another button with another finger when presented with the letter "P" or "H." After training, participants are instructed to respond to targets that are flanked by distracters. For example, they are instructed to respond to the letter presented in the center of an array (e.g., SS*P*SS [targets italicized]) and to disregard the flanking letters (the distracters). In terms of response time and errors, the least interference is found when the distracters are identical to the target (e.g., SSSSS). Interference is greatest when the distracters are associated

with responses that are different from those associated with targets and is less when they are different in appearance (stimulus interference) but associated with the same or a similar response. The strong and reliable effect of response interference, reflecting conflict at the response rather than the stimulus identification level (van Veen, Cohen, Botvinick, Stenger, & Carter, 2001), suggests that flanking letters can activate response codes to some extent (cf. Starreveld, Theeuwes, & Mortier, 2004). In support of continuous flow and cascade models, psychophysiological research shows that, in such response-interference tasks, competition involves simultaneous activation of the brain areas associated with the target- *and* distracter-related responses (DeSoto, Fabiani, Geary, & Gratton, 2001).

In a neuroimaging study, van Veen et al. (2001) demonstrated that, although both response and stimulus interference are associated with differences in performance, it is the former that most activates the anterior cingulate cortex, a brain region located on the medial surface of the frontal lobe that is interconnected with many motor areas and is believed to play a role in cognitive control (Chapters 3 and 26; Botvinick, Braver, Carter, Barch, & Cohen, 2001; Brown & Braver, 2005). Specifically, it has been proposed that this region detects conflicts in the information-processing stream. Following conflict detection, the dorsolateral prefrontal cortex resolves the conflict by activating the "requirements of the task at hand" and "biasing information processing in favor of appropriate responses" (van Veen & Carter, 2006, p. 237). Damage to this region in humans has been shown to impair the ability to inhibit task-irrelevant information and internal representations during performance on a range of tasks (Knight, Staines, Swick, & Chao, 1999). Moreover, using a variety of task paradigms, neuroimaging and animal lesion studies have strongly implicated the dorsolateral prefrontal cortex in inhibitory processing and the implementation of cognitive control (MacDonald, Cohen, Stenger, & Carter, 2000). Thus, cognitive control can be dissociated into evaluative and executive components, which rely on distinct brain regions (van Veen & Carter, 2006).

Ethological Approaches

The idea of action plans becoming activated automatically and then competing for behavioral expression is also featured in the ethological tradition, another approach that opposed the basic tenets of behaviorism. From the ethological standpoint, action plans are more likely to be incorrectly selected for expression, or "breakthrough," under conditions of high response competition and cognitive load, for inhibition is presumably harder to maintain under these circumstances. Such breaking through seems to occur in an intriguing phenomenon observed by ethologists known as "displacement activity" (Tinbergen, 1952), in which an animal, when torn between two competing response tendencies (as in an approach–avoidance conflict), expresses a third, bizarre and unrelated response tendency, such as hopping or grooming.

In addition to displacement, ethologists introduced to the student of action the exciting concepts of *fixed-action pattern* (e.g., egg-retrieving behavior of the goose), *taxis* (e.g., the phototaxis of moths toward light or chemotaxis of ants toward scent trails), and *innate releasing mechanism,* whereby a particular stimulus or configuration of stimuli activate complex patterns of behavior (e.g., sexual or aggressive display behavior) in a particular circumstance (Arkin, 1998; Gould, 1982). Ethologists proposed that animals have an intrinsic need to express certain motor patterns regardless of whether the actions are functional in the current context. For example, a caged squir-

rel seems "sated" after expressing digging behaviors toward a nut even though the nut remains unburied and in plain view (Thorpe, 1964). If unexpressed, motor energies are then damned up, building pressure such that the slightest provocation, including inappropriate stimuli, can elicit the expression of the corresponding action. Thorpe (1964) observes that during the extreme case of "vacuum activity" (Lorenz, 1963), "the tension may accumulate to the point at which the action pattern goes off without any external stimulus at all" (p. 22). Today, these notions are important for the study of addiction, in which *pharmacological withdrawal,* due to falling levels of the drug in the blood, is distinct from the longer-lasting *behavioral withdrawal,* the intrinsic urge to express the actions that compose the drug-ingesting ritual, regardless of whether such acts lead to drug delivery (see review in Baker, Japuntich, Hogle, McCarthy, & Curtin, 2006).

The ethological idea of fixed-action patterns is consonant with the notion of learning behavioral *scripts* (Schank & Abelson, 1977)—complex sequential behavioral repertoires that are stereotypic and defined by certain situations (e.g., how to behave at a restaurant). Similar notions are captured by the terms *frames* (Minsky, 1975) and *schema* (Arbib, 1981; Neisser, 1967; Piaget, 1971). According to Arkin (1998), "A schema is the basic unit of behavior from which complex actions can be constructed; it consists of the knowledge of how to act and perceive as well as the computational process by which it is enacted" (p. 43).

Priming

Beyond the issue of language production, language research more generally has had an important influence on our understanding of activation dynamics. For example, the idea of temporary concept activation or "priming" was first introduced by Lashley

(1951) to account for the nature of the nonsequential mechanisms (e.g., hierarchical grammar trees) underlying serial actions such as speaking, typing, and piano playing, and was based on his observations of slips in language production (Dell et al., 1997). The highly influential and generative idea of temporary construct priming (Chapter 9) in social psychology was based on Lashley's (1951) original insight (Bargh & Chartrand, 2000). In addition, the pioneering work of Meyer and Schvaneveldt (1971) on word associations (e.g., ocean–water) introduced the "sequential priming" paradigm, which made tests of automatic attitude activation (Fazio, Sanbonmatsu, Powell, & Kardes, 1986) and goal activation (Bargh, Raymond, Pryor, & Strack, 1995) possible. And it was from LaBerge and Samuels's (1974) pioneering work on the cognition of reading that the notion of immediate, automatic activation of concepts by their corresponding environmental stimuli came. Perhaps it's fair to say that what vision research has done for the study of perception, language research has done for the study of action (Remez, personal communication, 2004).

Activation Before Selection

One can readily imagine scenarios that illustrate the evolutionary advantage of having responses potentiated regardless of an actor's present intentions (see Bargh, 1997). Note, however, that the adaptive value of multiply active action plans, though it helps us prepare for all possible near futures in our environment, must still be reconciled with the temporal limitations of the skeletomotor system, in which words and actions can be expressed only one at a time (Lashley, 1951; Wundt, 1900).

Activation before selection is a feature of simple motor acts, wherein a given action goal activates all movement representations that could lead to the desired end state (Rosenbaum, Slotta, Vaughan, &

Plamondon, 1991). For example, there is substantial evidence that when, say, reaching for a cup of coffee, at first the premotor regions of both hemispheres are activated, but soon thereafter "activation eventually becomes lateralized over the contralateral motor cortex—the presumed outcome of a competition for one hand over the other" (Gazzaniga et al., 2002, p. 484). According to Cisek and Kalaska (2005), "The motor system could begin to specify the metrics of several potential actions based on sensory information, while at the same time weighing the likelihood, costs, and benefits of each, before arriving at a decision. . . . Decision-making underlying voluntary behavior can then be viewed at least in part as the process of selecting from [a] pragmatic representation of motor options the one that will be released" (p. 801) (see Chapter 25).

Activation before selection is also evident in the classic "time of intention" studies by Benjamin Libet (cf. Libet, 2004). In these experiments, participants are free to make a button-press or other response whenever they choose (simulating the state of free will) and are asked only to note when (by reference to a sweep-hand clock in front of them) they had made the intention to respond. Libet at the same time was measuring brain activation potentials associated with the instigation of action. The "surprising" finding was that the action potential consistently came 200 to 500 milliseconds before the participant's conscious awareness of intending to make the response (Libet, 1999). (For a related finding involving an even greater span of time, see Soon, Brass, Heinze, & Haynes, 2008.) Current research suggests that the judgment of conscious intention is associated with activity in the presupplementary motor area and the intraparietal sulcus (Berti & Pia, 2006).

Consistent with this standpoint, findings suggest that incidental stimuli (e.g., hammers) can automatically set us to physically interact with the world (e.g., to perform a power grip;

Chapter 11; Chen & Bargh, 1999; Tucker & Ellis, 2001, 2004; see neuroimaging evidence in Grézes & Decety, 2002; Longcamp, Anton, Roth, & Velay, 2005). Beyond such motor acts, actions can be unconsciously influenced by covert stimuli—when primed with the concept "old," people walk slower; when primed with "library," they make less noise; and when primed with "hostility," they become more aggressive (Aarts & Dijksterhuis, 2003; Bargh, Chen, & Burrows, 1996; Carver, Ganellen, Froming, & Chambers, 1983). In everyday life, evidence of activation before selection is obvious in action slips (Botvinick & Bylsma, 2005; Heckhausen & Beckmann, 1990) and is most dramatic in some neuropsychological conditions. Some lesions result in actions that are "stimulus driven" and are often perceived as impulsive, situationally inappropriate, and uncooperative (Chan & Ross, 1997).

Caused by damage to the frontal lobes (especially the supplementary motor area), the syndrome *utilization behavior* induces a state of disinhibition in which patients are incapable of suppressing actions that are elicited by environmental, action-related objects (Lhermitte, 1983). For example, a patient afflicted with this syndrome will manipulate an object (e.g., a hammer) even when instructed not to do so (Rossetti & Pisella, 2003). Patients describe such actions as foreign and dissociated from their conscious will. In *alien hand syndrome* (Bryon & Jedynak, 1972) and *anarchic hand syndrome* (Marchetti & Della Sala, 1998), brain damage causes hands and arms to function autonomously, carrying out relatively complex goal-directed behavior (e.g., the manipulation of tools; Yamadori, 1997) that are maladaptive and, in some cases, at odds with a patient's reported intentions.

These approaches suggest that multiple action plans are activated in parallel,[13] and action production is driven by some form of selective disinhibition (Rumelhart et al., 1986), such that competitor plans

are somehow inhibited or counteracted (regarding the role of consciousness in these processes, see Chapter 30; Libet, 1999; Morsella, 2005; Shallice, 1972).

Conflict

Distributed control, together with activation before selection, naturally leads to action conflicts.[14] Regarding conflict, as outlined by Curtis and D'Esposito (Chapter 3), there is an important conceptual distinction between *inhibition* (e.g., of an efferent signal in the central nervous system) and *counteraction* (Lorenz, 1963), as when micturition and the patellar reflex are counteracted by contracting the external urethral sphincter and leg muscles, respectively. It is important to appreciate that there is no homunculus in charge of suppressing one action in order to express another action: "no single area of the brain is specialized for inhibiting all unwanted actions" (Chapter 3, p. 72). Interestingly, ideomotor approaches have arrived at a similar conclusion, for Lotze and James's "acts of express fiat" referred not to a homunculus reigning action in but rather to the actions of an incompatible idea (i.e., a competing action plan):

> According to Lotze, in order to carry out a voluntary action, two conditions must be fulfilled. First, there must be an idea or mental image of what is being willed (*Vorstellung des Gewollten*). Second, all conflicting ideas or images must be absent or removed (*Hinwegräumung aller Hemmungen*). When these two conditions are met, the mental image acquires the power to guide the movements required to realize the intention, thus converting ideas in the mind into facts in the world (Prinz, Aschersleben, & Koch, this volume, p. 38)

Internal ("intrapsychic") strife from action conflict, although inherently unpleasant (Lewin, 1935; Morsella, 2005), is acceptable because it is *expressed* action that matters most from an evolutionary standpoint.

Unlike activations, urges, propensities, or beliefs, actions are significant because they are the cognitive products that natural selection operates on directly (Roe & Simpson, 1958): "The main way in which brains actually contribute to the success of survival machines is by controlling and coordinating the contraction of muscles" (Dawkins, 1976, p. 49), or, as put forth by T. H. Huxley, "The great end of life is not knowledge, but action." Moreover, such conflict is not only unavoidable but adaptive given biological constraints (cf. Livnat & Pippenger, 2006).

The cognitive apparatus appears to be an *affinity-based* system that "prefers" conflict-free over conflict-ridden situations, perhaps in part because the latter is energy inefficient, requiring energy to do both x and to counteract doing x (Chapter 27): Of two plans leading to the same goal, the plan associated with the least strife (e.g., blinking instead of enduring breathlessness for the same end) is selected. Because conflict is inherently unpleasant, even *approach–approach* conflicts are avoided if possible (Lewin, 1935). Thus, by "blindly" avoiding the strife from action conflict, a form of internal harmony is achieved, and the organism becomes more adaptable and suffers less deprivations and tissue damage (Dempsey, 1951).

The Stream of Action

Research on activation dynamics suggest that there is no such thing as a pure state of inaction (Skinner, 1953). Although factors such as fatigue, illness, and circadian rhythms modulate the degree of overall behavioral output, there is a stream of action just as there is a stream of consciousness (cf. Chapter 21; James, 1890/1950). The stream of action is driven by a continuous series of activations stemming from various sources. Tremendous endurance is required to curb this continuous outpouring of actions. (According to the Guinness World

Records, 2005, the record time for remaining motionless is around 20 hours, still a negligible fraction of the span of waking life.)

Strongly echoing James's (1890/1950) notion that thinking is for doing and Sechenov's (1863) provocative idea that conscious thoughts should be regarded as inhibited actions, action selection has been regarded as driven by disinhibition of competing alternatives (see Libet, 1999; Luria, 1932). (Related to Sechenov's idea is the case of the patient who, suffering from lesions of the parietal lobe, was incapable of suppressing the expression of imagined actions; Schwoebel, Boronat, & Coslett, 2002.) Somehow, although there are many contenders, one action plan at a time is selected for production. From this point of view, perceptions always lead to actions automatically, and all that can be done in the process of selection is to inhibit the execution of undesired plans. Given the nature of activation dynamics, perhaps one can go further and propose that, at the end of a day, one is tired not only from what one has done but also from all of what one could have done but never did.

Consciousness and Volition

Together, research on activation dynamics and action control suggest that, contrary to our intuitions, consciousness is not required for many forms of human action. In addition to the unconscious "online" motor adjustments mentioned previously, actions such as licking, chewing, and swallowing can occur unconsciously, given the appropriate stimulation (Bindra, 1976). In addition, one must consider the complexity, sophistication, and controlled nature of unconscious reflexes such as the pupillary reflex and peristalsis (Gallistel, 1980; Shepherd, 1994). Moreover, behaviors of notable complexity occur during unconscious states, such as coma, seizures, and persistent vegetative states, in which patients can behave as if awake but possess no consciousness (Laurey, 2005). Following brain injuries in which a general awareness is spared, complex actions can be decoupled from consciousness. For example, in *blindsight* (Weiskrantz, 1992), patients report to be blind but still exhibit visually guided behaviors (see also Goodale & Milner, 2004). One must also consider the intricacy of the actions expressed in alien hand syndrome, anarchic hand syndrome, and utilization behavior (see the previous discussion).

In normal circumstances, ideas can pop into mind without conscious invitation, and actions such as spoonerisms, action slips, and peristalsis can occur without one's consent. These phenomena challenge our intuition that the conscious mind is *the* primary agent controlling what one does (Wegner, 2002) and are critically important for longstanding basic philosophical issues such as the nature of free will (Chapter 23), the self, self-regulation (Chapters 15, 16, 23, 24, and 27), and the subjective experience of will.

Action in the Social World

Renewed focus on mechanisms of human social action has stemmed from diverse areas of research, including "theory of mind" (Leslie, 1994), the neural correlates of self-referential processing (e.g., medial prefrontal cortex; Jenkins, Macrae, & Mitchell, 2008; Macrae, Heatherton, & Kelley, 2004), and the social implications of mirror neurons. These areas of research strongly suggest that at least some of the neural machinery needed to produce action is involved in the perception of the action of others. Thus, the study of action directly impacts and informs the study of development (Chapter 19), social cognition, and social perception like it never did before.

Mimicry

People have default tendencies to act in the same way as those around them.

Mimicry is operating soon after birth; Meltzoff (2002) concluded that the imitative abilities of infants represent a "primordial connection between infant and caretaker" (p. 19). This tendency—and its unconscious and unintentional nature—has also been demonstrated in human adults in the "chameleon effect" research of Chartrand and colleagues (Chapter 22). People tend to adopt the speaking styles (Giles, Coupland, & Coupland, 1991), posture, facial gestures, and arm and hand movements of strangers with whom they interact, without intending to or being aware that they are doing so (Chartrand & Bargh, 1999; Chartrand, Maddux, & Lakin, 2005). Moreover, this unconscious imitation also tends to increase liking and bonding between the individuals—serving as a kind of natural "social glue" between new acquaintances. In neuropsychological populations, imitative response tendencies are displayed dramatically in patients with frontal brain lesions (Brass, Derffuss, Mattes-von Cramon, & von Cramon, 2004).

Thus, our perceptions of how other people are acting around us are the basis for a major unconscious guidance system as to how we ourselves should act in that situation. In the absence of any other information, the best behavioral strategy in a given situation (from the point of view of evolution and adaptation) is what most others are already doing (Campbell, 1974; Dawkins, 1976; Maynard Smith, 1982). Thus, as a default option or starting point for your own behavior—especially in new situations and with strangers—"blindly" or unconsciously adopting what others around you are doing makes good adaptive sense.

The Future of the Study of Human Action

Many fields are now "starting from scratch," reinterpreting what human action actually is. The everyday actions witnessed at a café remain a mystery, but at least today we learn about them from an all-inclusive standpoint and appreciate *what they are not.* They are not the products of a simple input–output reflex arc devoid of ideas, nor are they the function of a strictly hierarchical, serial processor that uses only amodal symbols. In addition, no homunculus resides in the cognitive apparatus and takes charge of suppressing this or that action (Chapters 3 and 30). And it is clear that in order to understand the human action, one must "open the hood" and examine the hardware at hand (e.g., neural circuits) while taking into account the functional role of enigmatic physical states such as consciousness.

Future research may extend the study of action to include experimentally overlooked ways by which we interact on the world. For instance, many of our goals are reached indirectly by influencing the behaviors of others, as in indirect speech acts (e.g., asking someone, "Could you please pass the salt"; Austin, 1962). In addition, just as flicking a light switch with one's index finger is obviously an action, so is the directed activity of "locked-in" patients, who are fully paralyzed and control their environment without muscles but via a brain–computer interface (electrodes implanted in brains that, via remote control, guide a computer cursor; cf. Andersen, Essick, & Siegel, 1987). Do these kinds of actions obey ideomotor principles? How are they encoded neurally in the control hierarchy? Moreover, many aspects of normal action may be illuminated by analyzing the nature of *dream action,* that is, the actions we express and somehow believe to be our own while dreaming (Hobson, 1999; Muzur, Pace-Schott, & Hobson, 2002). Interestingly, during the (somewhat) motionless dream state, we are still capable of vividly experiencing many aspects of normal action,

such as response conflict, action selection, and the systematic attribution of action to the self and to others.

The "brain mapping" of human action has not yet caught up to that of, say, the visual system (though there is still controversy about the function of several of its subregions, such as the fusiform cortex; Grill-Spector, Sayres, & Ress, 2006). Yet such a map seems within reach given the precision of today's neuropsychological analyses and batteries, and the fruitful union between sophisticated behavioral paradigms and developments in psychophysiology (e.g., transcranial magnetic stimulation, functional magnetic resonance imaging, and diffusion tensor imaging). Moreover, research has begun to identify, not only the networks of neuroanatomical regions that constitute the mechanisms underlying human action, but the ways in which these regions must interact in order to instantiate these mechanisms. More generally, for a given mental process, it seems that the *mode* of interaction among regions is as important as the nature and loci of the regions (Buzsáki, 2006). For example, the presence or lack of interregional synchrony leads to different cognitive and behavioral outcomes (Hummel & Gerloff, 2005; see review of neuronal communication through "coherence" in Fries, 2005).

In 1929, E. G. Boring, the historian of psychology, claimed that the application of the experimental method to the problem of mind is *the* outstanding event in the history of the study of the mind, an event without comparison. Such enthusiasm can today be held for the study of human action, which is finally investigated at all levels of analysis and by diverse fields, with each camp yielding fruits that benefit the other. It is clear that, for this scientific challenge, these are the most exciting times in intellectual history. Still, it appears ironic that the most difficult thing to understand in the universe is our own very nature and how it enables us to act on the world.

Notes

1. It should be noted that, in the early 20th century, behaviorism may have served as a healthy reaction to the prevalent mentalism of structuralist, prebehaviorist psychology, which attempted to explain all operations in terms of reportable conscious processes and suffered from lacking rigorous experimental methods, the kind that were later introduced by the behaviorists (Hilgard, 1987). Behaviorism engendered a vast array of sophisticated experimental paradigms that continue to benefit mainstream psychology and behavioral neuroscience today. One of countless examples of such fruits can be found in experiments designed to assess the perceptual and cognitive capabilities of animals (e.g., color perception in the octopus).

2. Through reverse engineering, scientists intend to unravel what specific neural structures or complex nervous events (e.g., consciousness) are *for,* but seldom is it considered that, though today there is no controversy regarding what the heart is for, such was not the case until the late 17th century, when the English medical doctor William Harvey experimentally falsified the prevalent theory that "venous" blood originates in the liver. If reverse engineering the heart was difficult, it is no surprise that it is difficult to reverse engineer the nature of human action.

3. In a similar vein, Sperry (1952) proposed that the phenomenal percept (e.g., the shape of a banana) is more isomorphic with its related action plans (grabbing or drawing the banana) than with its sensory input (the proximal stimulus on the retina). With great influence, Gibson (1979) too proposed an "ecological theory" of perception in which perception is intimately related to action, but this approach is strictly nonrepresentational in that all the information necessary for action was provided and contained by the environment. For a treatment regarding the difference between ecological and representational ("cognitive") theories of action, see Hommel et al. (2001). See Sheerer (1984) for a review of the shortcomings of approaches in which the nature of percepts is based primarily on motor processing, as in "peripheralist," "motor," "efferent," and "reafferent" theories of thought (e.g., Festinger, Ono, Burnham, & Bamber, 1967; Hebb, 1968; Held & Rekosh, 1963; McGuigan, 1966; Münsterberg, 1891; Washburn, 1928; Watson, 1924). For contemporary treatments regarding how action influences the nature of conscious percepts, see Gray (1995), Hochberg (1998), and O'Regan and Noë (2001).

4. These approaches are similar in nature to what have been referred to as *analogical* or *situated* models of representation (see review in Wilson, 2002), which include *simulation* theory (Decety, 1996a, 1996b; Jeannerod, 2003). For example, the shape O can serve as an analogical representation of the concept CIRCLE because it possesses some "circularness," but the word "circle" or the formula $x^2 + y^2 = r^2$ cannot, for they are associated to CIRCLE only arbitrarily and by convention.

5. For some semantic knowledge, this information includes functional knowledge that is obtained via bodily interactions. For evidence regarding the role of functional knowledge in object identification, see Bub, Masson, and Bukach (2003).

6. The English empirical philosophers of the 18th century (e.g., John Locke, David Hume, James Hartley, James Mill, and George Berkeley) and the structuralist school of psychology led by E. B. Titchener (Titchener, 1896) in psychology are a few examples of the many intellectual movements that had "image-like" theories of mental representation (Hilgard, 1987; Schultz & Schultz, 1996).

7. Regarding memory research, embodied approaches are consonant with the notions of encoding specificity and state-dependent learning/retrieval and with the idea that, unlike computer memory, human memory is content-addressable memory rather than address-addressable memory (cf. Nyberg, Habib, McIntosh, & Tulving, 2000).

8. Early on, Hebb (1968) proposed the related hypothesis that the movements coincidental with mental events are not adventitious but necessary for the mental events to occur. Forty years earlier, Washburn (1928) proposed a similar hypothesis: "The motor innervations underlying the consciousness of effort are not mere accompaniments of directed thought, but an essential cause of directed thought" (p. 105).

9. See Georgopoulos (2002) regarding the shortcomings of the mirror-neuron hypothesis.

10. Interestingly, in virtue of such parietal signals and cellular recording technology, monkeys can control a cursor on a computer screen without any expressed movements (Andersen et al., 1987).

11. More specifically, by working in concert with the basal ganglia, the supplementary motor area contributes to actions that are "internally generated" and self-guided. By working in concert with the cerebellum and parietal cortex, the lateral premotor cortex contributes to actions that depend on external stimuli (Gazzaniga et al., 2002).

12. Unlike serial models, cascade models can also predict speech errors known as *mixed errors* (e.g., saying "sparcity" when attempting to say either "scarcity" or "sparse"). In these errors, the uttered word is semantically and phonologically related to the intended word (e.g., saying "rat" instead of "cat"). Cascade theories explain mixed errors as a product of the phonological activation of unselected word representations, which is a natural consequence of the cascade architecture (Dell, 1986; N. Martin, Gagnon, Schwartz, Dell, & Saffran, 1996). Specifically, mixed errors result from the phonological activation of word representations that are semantically related to the target word. For instance, when intending to say "cat," the semantically related word representations for RAT and PIG also send activation to the phonological processes. Because RAT happens to be phonologically related to CAT, its phonological features will also receive activation from the "cat." A lower activation level is reached by the phonological features of "pig" since they are activated only by the word representation PIG. If the probability of producing an erroneous word is in part proportional to the activation level reached by the word's phonological features, one is more likely to say "rat" instead of "cat" than "pig" instead of "cat."

13. According to the Chinese philosophy of feng shui, incidental action-related clutter (e.g., tools, pencils, and computer keyboards) influence behavior by causing "mental clutter," "distraction," and "mental disharmony." From a scientific standpoint, such disharmony could be interpreted as arising from stimulus-elicited, unconscious plans that interfere with cognitive processes and intended action.

14. The traditional view of intrabrain conflict is that the phylogenetically younger cortical areas of the brain are in conflict with the primitive impulses of the phylogenetically older brain regions (Bazett & Penfield, 1922; Luria, 1932). See Morsella (2005) and Chapter 30 for a reinterpretation of this view.

References

Aarts, H., & Dijksterhuis, A. (2003). The silence of the library: Environment, situational norm, and social behavior. *Journal of Personality and Social Psychology, 84,* 18–28.

Aflalo, T. N., & Graziano, M. S. A. (2006). Possible origins of the complex topographic organization of motor cortex: Reduction of a multidimensional space onto a two-dimensional array. *Journal of Neuroscience, 26,* 6288–6297.

Allman, J. M. (2000). *Evolving brains.* New York: Scientific American Library.

Andersen, R. A., Essick, G. K., & Siegel, R. M. (1987). Neurons of area 7 activated by both visual stimuli and oculomotor behavior. *Experimental Brain Research, 67,* 316–322.

Andersen, R., Meeker, D., Pesaran, B., Breznen, B., Buneo, C., & Scherberger, H. (2004). Sensorimotor transformations in the posterior parietal cortex. In M. S. Gazzaniga (Ed.), *The cognitive neurosciences III* (pp. 463–474). Cambridge, MA: MIT Press.

Arbib, M. A. (1981). Perceptual structures and distributed motor control. In V. Brooks (Ed.), *Handbook of physiology—The nervous system II: Motor control* (pp. 1449–1480). Bethesda, MD: American Physiological Society.

Arkin, R. C. (1998). *Behavior-based robotics.* Cambridge, MA: MIT Press.

Ashe, J., Taira, M., Smyrnis, N., Pellizer, G., Gerorakopoulos, T., Lurito, J. T., & Georgopoulos, A. P. (1993). Motor cortical activity preceding a memorized movement trajectory with an orthogonal bend. *Experimental Brain Research, 95,* 118–130.

Austin, J. L. (1962). *How to do things with words.* New York: Oxford University Press.

Baddeley, A. D. (1986). *Working memory.* Oxford: Oxford University Press.

Bagrat, A., & Georgopoulos, A. P. (1999). Cortical populations and behavior: Hebb's thread. *Canadian Journal of Experimental Psychology, 53,* 21–34.

Baker, T. B., Japuntich, S. J., Hogle, J. M., McCarthy, D. E., & Curtin, J. J. (2006). Pharmacological and behavioral withdrawal from addictive drugs. *Current Directions in Psychological Science, 5,* 232–236.

Baker, T. B., Piper, M. E., McCarthy, D. E., Majeskie, M. R., & Fiore, M. C. (2004). Addiction motivation reformulated: An affective processing model of negative reinforcement. *Psychological Review, 111,* 33–51.

Bargh, J. A. (1997). The automaticity of everyday life. In R. S. Wyer Jr. (Ed.), *The automaticity of everyday life: Advances in social cognition, 10*

(pp. 1–61). Mahwah, NJ: Lawrence Erlbaum Associates.

Bargh, J. A., & Chartrand, T. L. (2000). A practical guide to priming and automaticity research. In H. Reis & C. Judd (Eds.), *Handbook of research methods in social psychology* (pp. 253–285). New York: Cambridge University Press.

Bargh, J. A., Chen, M., & Burrows, L. (1996). Automaticity of social behavior: Direct effects of trait construct and stereotype activation on action. *Journal of Personality and Social Psychology, 71,* 230–244.

Bargh, J. A., Raymond, P., Pryor, J. B., & Strack, F. (1995). Attractiveness of the underling: An automatic power-sex association and its consequences for sexual harassment and aggression. *Journal of Personality and Social Psychology, 68,* 768–781 .

Barsalou, L. W. (1999). Perceptual symbol systems. *Behavioral and Brain Sciences, 22,* 577–560.

Barsalou, L. W. (2003). Situated simulation in the human conceptual system. *Language and Cognitive Processes, 18,* 513–562.

Bazett, H. C., & Penfield, W. G. (1922). A study of the Sherrington decerebrate animal in the chronic as well as the acute condition. *Brain, 45,* 185–265.

Beilock, S. L., & Holt, L. E. (2007). Embodied preference judgments: Can likeability be driven by the motor system? *Psychological Science, 18,* 51–57.

Berridge, K. C., & Robinson, T. E. (1995). The mind of an addicted brain: Neural sensitization of wanting versus liking. *Current Directions in Psychological Science, 4,* 71–76.

Berthoz, A. (2002). *The brain's sense of movement.* Cambridge, MA: Harvard University Press.

Berti, A., & Pia, L. (2006). Understanding motor awareness through normal and pathological behavior. *Current Directions in Psychological Science, 15,* 237–240.

Bindra, D. (1976). *A theory of intelligent behavior.* New York: Wiley-Interscience.

Bizzi, E., & Mussa-Ivaldi, F. A. (2004). Toward a neurobiology of coordinate transformations. In M. S. Gazzaniga (Ed.), *The cognitive neurosciences III* (pp. 413–425). Cambridge, MA: MIT Press.

Bizzi, E., Mussa-Ivaldi, F., & Giszter, S. (1991). Computations underlying the execution of movement: A biological perspective. *Science, 253,* 287–291.

Boroditsky, L., & Ramscar, M. (2002). The roles of body and mind in abstract thought. *Psychological Science, 13,* 185–188.

Botvinick, M. M., Braver, T. S., Carter, C. S., Barch, D. M., & Cohen, J. D. (2001). Conflict monitoring and cognitive control. *Psychological Review, 108,* 624–652.

Botvinick, M. M., & Bylsma, L. M. (2005). Distraction and action slips in an everyday task: Evidence for a dynamic representation of task context. *Psychonomic Bulletin and Review, 12,* 1011–1017.

Brass, M., Derffuss, J., Mattes-von Cramon, G., & von Cramon, D. Y. (2004). Imitative response tendencies in patients with frontal brain lesions. *Neuropsychology, 17,* 265–271.

Breiter, H. C., & Gasic, G. P. (2004). A general circuitry processing reward/aversion information and its implications for neuropsychiatric illness. In M. S. Gazzaniga (Ed.), *The cognitive neurosciences III* (pp. 1043–1065). Cambridge, MA: MIT Press.

Brown, J. W., & Braver, T. S. (2005). Learned predictions of error likelihood in the anterior cingulate cortex. *Science, 307,* 1118–1121.

Brown, S., & Martinez, M. J. (2007). Activation of premotor vocal areas during musical discrimination. *Brain and Cognition, 63,* 59–69.

Bryon, S., & Jedynak, C. P. (1972). Troubles du transfert interhemispherique: A propos de trois observations de tumeurs du corps calleux. Le signe de la main etrangère. *Revue Neurologique, 126,* 257–266.

Bub, D. N., Masson, M. E. J., & Bukach, C. M. (2003). Gesturing and naming: The use of functional knowledge in object identification. *Psychological Science, 14,* 467–472.

Burgess, C., & Lund, K. (1997). Modelling parsing constraints with high-dimensional context space. *Language and Cognitive Processes, 12,* 177–210.

Butterworth, B. (1992). Disorders of phonological encoding. *Cognition, 42,* 261–286.

Buzsáki, G. (2006). *Rhythms of the brain.* New York: Oxford University Press.

Cacioppo, J. T., Priester, J. R., & Berntson, G. G. (1993). Rudimentary determinants of attitudes: II. Arm flexion and extension have differential effects on attitudes. *Journal of Personality and Social Psychology, 65,* 5–17.

Campbell, D. T. (1974). Evolutionary epistemology. In P. A. Schilpp (Ed.), *The philosophy of Karl Popper* (pp. 413–463). La Salle, IL: Open Court.

Caramazza, A. (1997). How many levels of processing are there in lexical access? *Cognitive Neuropsychology, 14,* 177–208.

Carlson, N. R. (1994). *Physiology of behavior.* Needham Heights, MA: Allyn and Bacon.

Carpenter, W. B. (1874). *Principles of mental physiology.* New York: Appleton.

Carver, C. S., Ganellen, R. J., Froming, W. J., & Chambers, W. (1983). Modeling: An analysis in terms of category accessibility. *Journal of Experimental Social Psychology, 19,* 403–421.

Carver, C. S., & Scheier, M. F. (1990). Origins and functions of positive and negative affect: A control-process view. *Psychological Review, 97,* 19–35.

Chan, J.-L., & Ross, E. D. (1997). Alien hand syndrome: Influence of neglect on the clinical presentation of frontal and callosal variants. *Cortex, 33,* 287–299.

Chartrand, T. L., & Bargh, J. A. (1999). The chameleon effect: The perception-behavior link and social interaction. *Journal of Personality and Social Psychology, 76,* 893–910.

Chartrand, T. L., Maddux, W., & Lakin, J. (2005). Beyond the perception-behavior link: The ubiquitous utility and motivational moderators of unconscious mimicry. In R. Hassin, J. Uleman, & J. A. Bargh (Eds.), *The new unconscious* (pp. 334–361). New York: Oxford University Press.

Chen, M., & Bargh, J. A. (1999). Consequences of automatic evaluation: Immediate behavioral predispositions to approach or avoid the stimulus. *Personality and Social Psychology Bulletin, 25,* 215–224.

Chomsky, N. (1959). Review of "Verbal Behavior" by Skinner, B. F. *Language, 35,* 26–58.

Christensen, M. S., Lundbye-Jensen, J., Geertsen, S. S., Petersen, T. H., Paulson, O. B., & Nielsen, J. B. (2007). Premotor cortex modulates somatosensory cortex during voluntary movements without proprioceptive feedback. *Nature Neuroscience, 10,* 417–419.

Cisek, P., & Kalaska, J. F. (2005). Neural correlates of reaching decisions in dorsal premotor cortex: Specification of multiple direction choices and final selection of action. *Neuron, 45,* 801–814.

Damasio, A. R., Tranel, D., & Damasio, H. C. (1991). Somatic markers and the guidance of behavior: Theory and preliminary testing. In H. S. Levin et al. (Eds.), *Frontal lobe function and dysfunction* (pp. 217–229). London: Oxford University Press.

Damasio, H., Tranel, D., Grabowski, T., Adolphs, R., & Damasio, A. (2004). Neural systems behind word and concept retrieval. *Cognition, 92,* 179–229.

Daprati, E., & Sirigu, A. (2006). How we interact with objects: Learning from brain lesions. *Trends in Cognitive Sciences, 10,* 265–270.

Dawkins, R. (1976). *The selfish gene.* New York: Oxford University Press.

Decety, J. (1996a). Do executed and imagined movements share the same central structures? *Cognitive Brain Research, 3,* 87–93.

Decety, J. (1996b). Neural representations for action. *Reviews in the Neurosciences, 7,* 285–297.

Dell, G. S. (1986). A spreading activation theory of retrieval in sentence production. *Psychological Review, 93,* 283–321.

Dell, G. S., Burger, L. K., & Svec, W. R. (1997). Language production and serial order: A functional analysis and a model. *Psychological Review, 104,* 123–147.

DeLong, M. R. (2000). The basal ganglia. In E. R. Kandel, J. H. Schwartz, & T. M. Jessell (Eds.), *Principles of neural science* (4th ed., pp. 854–867). New York: McGraw-Hill.

Dempsey, E. W. (1951). Homeostasis. In S. S. Stevens (Ed.), *Handbook of experimental psychology* (pp. 209–235). New York: Wiley.

Dennett, D. C. (1991). *Consciousness explained.* Boston: Little, Brown.

DeSoto, M. C., Fabiani, M., Geary, D. C., & Gratton, G. (2001). When in doubt, do it both ways: Brain evidence of the simultaneous activation of conflicting responses in a spatial Stroop task. *Journal of Cognitive Neuroscience, 13,* 523–536.

de Waal, F. B. M. (2002). Evolutionary psychology: The wheat and the chaff. *Current Directions in Psychological Science, 11,* 187–191.

Dijkstra, K., Kaschak, M. P., & Zwaan, R. A. (2007). Body posture facilitates retrieval of autobiographical memories. *Cognition, 102,* 139–149.

Eichenbaum, H., & Cohen, N. J. (2001). *From conditioning to conscious recollection: Memory systems of the brain.* New York: Oxford University Press.

Eimer, M., Hommel, B., & Prinz, W. (1995). S-R compatibility and response selection. *Acta Psychologica, 90,* 301–323.

Eriksen, B. A., & Eriksen, C. W. (1974). Effects of noise letters upon the identification of a target letter in a nonsearch task. *Perception and Psychophysics, 16,* 143–149.

Eriksen, C. W., & Schultz, D. W. (1979). Information processing in visual search: A continuous flow conception and experimental results. *Perception and Psychophysics, 25,* 249–263.

Fazio, R. H., Sanbonmatsu, D. M., Powell, M. C., & Kardes, F. R. (1986). On the automatic activation of attitudes. *Journal of Personality and Social Psychology, 50,* 229–238.

Festinger, L., Ono, H., Burnham, C. A., & Bamber, D. (1967). Efference and the conscious experience of perception. *Journal of Experimental Psychology Monograph 74,* 1–36.

Flack, W. F., Jr. (2006). Peripheral feedback effects if facial expressions, bodily postures, and vocal expressions on emotional feelings. *Cognition and Emotion, 20,* 177–195.

Fries, P. (2005). A mechanism for cognitive dynamics: Neuronal communication through neuronal coherence. *Trends in Cognitive Sciences, 9,* 474–480.

Frith, C., & Wolpert, D. (Eds.). (2003). *The neuroscience of social interaction.* New York: Oxford University Press.

Gainotti, G., Silveri, M. C., Daniele, A., & Giustolisi, L. (1995). Neuroanatomical correlates of category-specific semantic disorders: A critical survey. *Memory, 3,* 247–264.

Galantucci, B., Fowler, C. A., & Turvey, M. T. (2006). The motor theory of speech perception reviewed. *Psychonomic Bulletin and Review, 13,* 361–377.

Gallistel, C. R. (1980). *The organization of action: A new synthesis.* Hillsdale, NJ: Lawrence Erlbaum Associates.

Gallistel, C. R., & Gibbon, J. (2001). Computational versus associative models of simple conditioning. *Current Directions in Psychological Science, 10,* 146–150.

Ganz, L. (1975). Temporal factors in visual perception. In E. C. Carterette & M. P. Friedman (Eds.), *Handbook of perception* (Vol. 5, pp. 169–231). New York: Academic Press.

Gazzaniga, M. S., Ivry, R. B., & Mangun, G. R. (2002). *Cognitive neuroscience, second edition.* New York: Norton.

Georgopoulos, A. P. (2002). Cognitive motor control: Spatial and temporal aspects. *Current Opinion in Biology, 12,* 678–683.

Georgopoulos, A. P., Caminiti, R., Kalaska, J. F., & Massey J. T. (1983). Spatial coding of movement: A hypothesis concerning the coding of movement direction by motor cortical populations. *Experimental Brain Research: Supplement, 7,* 327–336.

Ghez, C., & Thach, W. T. (2000). The cerebellum. In E. R. Kandel, J. H. Schwartz, & T. M. Jessell (Eds.), *Principles of neural science* (4th ed., pp. 832–852). New York: McGraw-Hill.

Gibson, J. J. (1979). *The ecological approach to visual perception.* Boston: Houghton Mifflin.

Giles, H., Coupland, J., & Coupland, N. (1991). *Contexts of accommodation: Developments in applied sociolinguistics.* New York: Cambridge University Press.

Glenberg, A. M. (1997). What memory is for. *Behavioral and Brain Sciences, 20,* 1–55.

Goldman-Rakic, P. S. (1992). Working memory and the mind. *Scientific American, 267,* 111–117.

Goldrick, M. (2006). Limited interaction in speech production: Chronometric, speech error, and neuropsychological evidence. *Language and Cognitive Processes, 21,* 817–855.

Goldrick, M., & Blumstein, S. E. (2006). Cascading activation from phonological planning to articulatory processes: Evidence from tongue twisters. *Language and Cognitive Processes, 21,* 649–683.

González, J., Barros-Loscertales, A., Pulvermüller, F., Meseguer, V., Sanjuán, A., Belloch, V., et al. (2006). Reading *cinnamon* activates olfactory brain regions. *NeuroImage, 32,* 906–912.

Goodale, M., & Milner, D. (2004). *Sight unseen: An exploration of conscious and unconscious vision.* New York: Oxford University Press.

Gould, J. L. (1982). *Ethology: The mechanisms and evolution of behavior.* New York: Norton.

Gould, S. J. (1977). *Ever since Darwin: Reflections in natural history.* New York: Norton.

Grafton, S. T., Fadiga, L., Arbib, M. A., & Rizzolatti, G. (1997). Premotor cortex activation during observation and naming of familiar tools. *NeuroImage, 6,* 231–236.

Grafton, S. T., & Ivry, R. B. (2004). The representation of action. In M. S. Gazzaniga (Ed.), *The cognitive neurosciences III* (pp. 441–451). Cambridge, MA: MIT Press.

Gray, J. A. (1995). The contents of consciousness: A neuropsychological conjecture. *Behavioral and Brain Sciences, 18,* 659–676.

Greenwald, A. G. (1970). Sensory feedback mechanisms in performance control: With special reference to the ideomotor mechanism. *Psychological Review, 77,* 73–99.

Grézes, J., & Decety, J. (2002). Does visual perception of object afford action? Evidence from a neuroimaging study. *Neuropsycholgia, 40,* 212–222.

Grill-Spector, K., Sayres, R., & Ress, D. (2006). High-resolution imaging reveals highly selective nonface clusters in the fusiform face area. *Nature Neuroscience, 9,* 1177–1185.

Grodzinsky, Y., & Amunts, K. (2006). *Broca's region.* New York: Oxford University Press.

Grossberg, S. (1999). The link between brain learning, attention, and consciousness. *Consciousness and Cognition, 8,* 1–44.

Halsband, U., & Freund, H. J. (1990). Premotor cortex and conditional motor learning in man. *Brain, 113,* 207–222.

Harleß, E. (1861). Der Apparat des Willens. *Zeitshrift für Philosophie und philosophische Kritik, 38,* 499–507.

Harnad, S. (1990). The symbol grounding problem. *Physica D, 42,* 335–346.

Hauk, O., Davis, M. H., Kherif, F., & Pulvermuller, F. (2008). Imagery or meaning? Evidence for a semantic origin of category-specific brain activity in metabolic imaging. *European Journal of Neuroscience, 27,* 1856–1866.

Hebb, D. O. (1968). Concerning imagery. *Psychological Review, 75,* 466–477.

Heckhausen, H., & Beckmann, J. (1990). Intentional action and action slips. *Psychological Review, 97,* 36–48.

Heilman, K. M., Rothi, L. J., & Valenstein, E. (1982). Two forms of ideomotor apraxia. *Neurology, 32,* 342–346.

Held, R., & Rekosh, J. (1963). Motor-sensory feedback and the geometry of visual space. *Science, 141,* 722–723.

Hilgard, E. R. (1987). *Psychology in America: A historical survey.* Orlando, FL: Harcourt Brace Jovanovich.

Hobson, J. A. (1999). *Consciousness.* New York: Scientific American Library.

Hochberg, J. (1998). Gestalt theory and its legacy: Organization in eye and brain, in attention and mental representation. In J. Hochberg (Ed.), *Perception and cognition at century's end: Handbook of perception and cognition* (2nd ed., pp. 253–306). San Diego, CA: Academic Press.

Hommel, B., Müsseler, J., Aschersleben, G., & Prinz, W. (2001). The theory of event coding: A framework for perception and action planning. *Behavioral and Brain Sciences, 24,* 849–937.

Hubel, D. H., & Wiesel, T. N. (1968) Receptive fields and functional architecture of monkey striate cortex. *Journal of Physiology (London), 195,* 215–243.

Hummel, F., & Gerloff, C. (2005). Larger interregional synchrony is associated with greater behavioral success in a complex sensory integration task in humans. *Cerebral Cortex, 15,* 670–678.

Iacoboni, M., & Dapretto, M. (2006). The mirror neuron system and the consequences of its dysfunction. *Nature Reviews Neuroscience, 7,* 942–951.

James, W. (1950). *Principles of psychology* (Vol. 2). New York: Dover. (Original work published 1890)

Jeannerod, M. (2003). Simulation of action as a unifying concept for motor cognition. In S. H.

Johnson-Frey (Ed.), *Taking action: Cognitive neuroscience perspectives on intentional acts* (pp. 139–163). Cambridge, MA: MIT Press.

Jenkins, A. C., Macrae, C. N., & Mitchell, J. P. (2008). Repetition suppression of ventromedial prefrontal activity during judgments of self and others. *Proceedings of the National Academy of Sciences, 105,* 4507–4512.

Kakei, S., Hoffman, D. S., & Strick, P. L. (1999). Muscle and movement representations in the primary motor cortex. *Science, 285,* 2136–2139.

Kan, I. P., Barsalou, L. W., Solomon, K. O., Minor, J. K., & Thompson-Schill, S. L. (2003). Role of mental imagery in a property verification task: fMRI evidence for perceptual representations of conceptual knowledge. *Cognitive Neuropsychology, 20,* 525–540.

Kandel, E. R., & Hawkins, R. D. (1992). The biological basis of learning and individuality. *Scientific American, 241,* 66–76.

Karni, A., Meyer, G., Rey-Hipolito, C., Jezzard, P., Adams, M., Turner, R., et al. (1998). The acquisition of skilled motor performance: Fast and slow experience-driven changes in primary motor cortex. *Proceedings of the National Academy of Sciences of the United States of America, 95,* 861–868.

Keele, S. W., & Ivry, R. (1991). Does the cerebellum provide a common computation for diverse tasks? A timing hypothesis. *Annals of the New York Academy of Sciences, 608,* 197–211.

Kellenbach, M. L., Wijers, A. A., & Mulder, G. (2000). Visual semantic features are activated during the processing of concrete words: Event-related potential evidence for perceptual semantic priming. *Cognitive Brain Research, 10,* 67–75.

Knight, R. T., Staines, W. R., Swick, D., & Chao, L. L. (1999). Prefrontal cortex regulates inhibition and excitation in distributed neural networks. *Acta Psychologica, 101,* 159–178.

Kolb, B., & Wishaw, I. Q. (2006). *An introduction to brain and behavior* (2nd ed.). New York: Worth.

Kosslyn, S. M., Ganis, G., & Thompson, W. L. (2003). Mental imagery: Against the nihilistic hypothesis. *Trends in Cognitive Science, 7,* 109–111.

LaBerge, D., & Samuels, S. J. (1974). Toward a theory of automatic information processing in reading. *Cognitive Psychology, 6,* 293–323.

Lakoff, G., & Johnson, M. (1999). *Philosophy in the flesh*. New York: Basic Books.

Landauer, T. K., & Dumais, S. T. (1997). A solution to Plato's problem: The latent semantic analysis theory of acquisition, induction, and representation of knowledge. *Psychological Review, 104,* 211–240.

Lang, P. J. (1994). The varieties of emotional experience: A meditation on James-Lange theory. *Psychological Review, 101,* 211–221.

Lashley, K. S. (1942). The problem of cerebral organization in vision. In H. Kluver (Ed.), *Visual mechanisms. Biological symposia, 7* (pp. 301–322). Lancaster, PA: Cattell Press.

Lashley, K. S. (1951). The problem of serial order in behavior. In L. A. Jeffress (Ed.), *Cerebral mechanisms in behavior. The Hixon symposium* (pp. 112–146). New York: Wiley.

Laurey, S. (2005). The neural correlate of (un)awareness: Lessons from the vegetative state. *Trends in Cognitive Sciences, 12,* 556–559.

Lavond, D. G., Kim, J. J., & Thompson, R. F. (1993). Mammalian brain substrates of aversive classical conditioning. *Annual Review of Psychology, 44,* 317–342.

LeDoux, J. E. (1996). *The emotional brain: The mysterious underpinnings of emotional life*. New York: Simon & Schuster.

LeDoux, J. E. (2000). Emotion circuits in the brain. *Annual Review of Neuroscience, 23,* 155–184.

Leslie, A. M. (1994). ToMM, To By, and agency: Core architecture and domain specificity. In L. Hirschfield & S. Gelman (Eds.), *Mapping the mind: Domain specificity in cognition and culture* (119–148). New York: Cambridge University Press.

Levelt, W. J. M. (1989). *Speaking: From intention to articulation*. Cambridge, MA: MIT Press.

Levelt, W. J. M., Roelofs, A., & Meyer, A. S. (1999). A theory of lexical access in speech production. *Brain and Behavioral Sciences, 22,* 313–335.

Lewin, K. (1935). *A dynamic theory of personality*. New York: McGraw-Hill.

Lhermitte, F. (1983). "Utilization behaviour" and its relation to lesions of the frontal lobe. *Brain, 106,* 137–255.

Liberman, A. M., & Mattingly, I. G. (1985). The motor theory of speech perception revised. *Cognition, 21,* 1–36.

Libet, B. (1999). Do we have free will? In B. Libet, A. Freeman, & J. K. B. Sutherland (Eds.), *The volitional brain: Towards a neuroscience of free will* (pp. 47–58). New York: Imprint Academic.

Libet, B. (2004). *Mind time: The temporal factor in consciousness*. Cambridge, MA: Harvard University Press.

Livnat, A., & Pippenger, N. (2006). An optimal brain can be composed of conflicting agents. *Proceeding of the National Academy of Sciences of the United States of America, 103,* 3198–3202.

Longcamp, M., Anton, J. L., Roth, M., & Velay, J. L. (2005). Premotor activations in response to visually presented single letters depend on the hand used to write: A study on left-handers. *Neuropsychologia, 43,* 1801–1809.

Lorenz, K. (1963). *On aggression.* New York: Harcourt Brace & World.

Lotze, R. H. (1852). *Medizinische Psychologie oder Physiologie der Seele.* Leipzig: Weidmann'sche Buchhandlung.

Luria, A. R. (1932). *The nature of human conflicts, or emotion, conflict and will: An objective study of the disorganisation and control of human behavior.* New York: Liverlight.

MacDonald, A. W., III, Cohen, J. D., Stenger, V. A., & Carter, C. S. (2000). Dissociating the role of the dorsolateral prefrontal and anterior cingulate cortex in cognitive control. *Science, 288,* 1835–1838.

Macrae, C. N., Heatherton, T. F., & Kelley, W. M. (2004). A self less ordinary: Medial prefrontal cortex and you. In M. S. Gazzaniga (Ed.), *The cognitive neurosciences III* (pp. 1067–1075). Cambridge, MA: MIT Press.

Mahon, B. Z., & Caramazza, A. (2008). A critical look at the embodied cognition hypothesis and a new proposal for grounding conceptual content. *Journal of Physiology–Paris, 102,* 59–70.

Marchetti, C., & Della Sala, S. (1998). Disentangling the alien and anarchic hand. *Cognitive Neuropsychiatry, 3,* 191–207.

Marcus, G. (2008). *Kluge: The haphazard construction of the mind.* Boston: Houghton Mifflin Company.

Markman, A. B., & Dietrich, E. (2000). Extending the classical view of representation. *Trends in Cognitive Sciences, 4,* 470–475.

Marr, D. (1982). *Vision.* New York: Freeman.

Martin, A. (2001). Functional neuroimaging of semantic memory. In R. Cabeza & A. Kingstone (Eds.), *Handbook of functional neuroimaging of cognition* (pp. 153–186). Cambridge, MA: MIT Press.

Martin, A., & Caramazza, A. (2003). Neuropsychological and neuroimaging perspectives on conceptual knowledge: An introduction. *Cognitive Neuropsychology, 20,* 195–212.

Martin, N., Gagnon, D. A., Schwartz, M. F., Dell, G. S., & Saffran, E. M. (1996). Phonological facilitation of semantic errors in normal and aphasic speakers. *Language and Cognitive Processes, 11,* 257–282.

Maynard Smith, J. (1982). *Evolution and the theory of games.* New York: Cambridge University Press.

McClelland, J. L. (1979). On the time-relations of mental processes: An examination of systems of processes in cascade. *Psychological Review, 86,* 287–330.

McGuigan, F. J. (1966). *Thinking: Studies of covert language processes.* New York: Appleton-Century-Crofts.

Meltzoff, A. N. (2002). Elements of a developmental theory of imitation. In A. N. Meltzoff & W. Prinz (Eds.), *The imitative mind: Development, evolution, and brain bases* (pp. 19–41). New York: Cambridge University Press.

Meltzoff, A. N., & Prinz, W. (2002). *The imitative mind: Development, evolution, and brain bases.* New York: Cambridge University Press.

Metcalfe, J., & Mischel, W. (1999). A hot/cool-system analysis of delay of gratification: Dynamics of willpower. *Psychological Review, 106,* 3–19.

Meyer, D. E., & Schvaneveldt, R. W. (1971). Facilitation in recognizing pairs of words: Evidence of a dependence between retrieval operations. *Journal of Experimental Psychology, 90,* 227–234.

Miller, E. K., & Cohen, J. D. (2001). An integrative theory of prefrontal cortex function. *Annual Review of Neuroscience, 24,* 167–202.

Miller, G. A., Galanter, E., & Pribram, K. H. (1960). *Plans and the structure of behavior.* New York: Holt.

Milner, A. D., & Goodale, M. (1995). *The visual brain in action.* New York: Oxford University Press.

Minsky, M. (1985). *The society of mind.* New York: Simon & Schuster.

Minsky, M. L. (1975). A framework for representing knowledge. In P. H. Winston (Ed.), *The psychology of computer vision* (pp. 211–277). New York: McGraw Hill.

Morsella, E. (2005). The function of phenomenal states: Supramodular interaction theory. *Psychological Review, 112,* 1000–1021.

Morsella, E., & Krauss, R. M. (2004). The role of gestures in spatial working memory and speech. *American Journal of Psychology, 117,* 411–424.

Münsterberg, H. (1891). Über Aufgaben und Methoden der Psychologie. *Schriften der Gesellschaft für psychologische Forschung, 1,* 93–272.

Muzur, A., Pace-Schott, E. F., & Hobson, J. A. (2002). The prefrontal cortex in sleep. *Trends in Cognitive Sciences, 6,* 475–481.

Nattkemper, D., & Ziessler, M. (2004): Editorial: Cognitive control of action: The role of action effects. *Psychological Research, 68,* 71–73.

Navarrete, E., & Costa, A. (2004). How much linguistic information is extracted from ignored pictures? Further evidence for a cascade model of speech production. *Journal of Memory and Language, 53,* 359–377.

Neisser, U. (1967). *Cognitive psychology.* New York: Appleton-Century-Crofts.

Neumann, R., Förster, J., & Strack, F. (2003). Motor compatibility: The bidirectional link between behavior and evaluation. In J. Musch & K. C. Klauer (Eds.), *The psychology of evaluation: Affective processes in cognition and emotion* (pp. 371–391). Mahwah, NJ: Lawrence Erlbaum Associates.

Neumann, R., & Strack, F. (2000). Approach and avoidance: The influence of proprioceptive and exteroceptive cues on encoding of affective information. *Journal of Personality and Social Psychology, 79,* 39–48.

Norman, D. A., & Shallice, T. (1980). *Attention to action: Willed and automatic control of behavior* (Technical Report 8006). San Diego: Center for Human Information Processing, University of California, San Diego.

Novick, J. M., Trueswell, J. C., & Thompson-Schill, S. L. (2005). Cognitive control and parsing: Re-examining the role of Broca's area in sentence comprehension. *Cognitive, Affective, and Behavioral Neuroscience, 5,* 263–281.

Nyberg, L., Eriksson, J., Larsson, A., & Marklund, P. (2006). Learning by doing versus learning by thinking: An fMRI study of motor and mental training. *Neuropsychologia, 44,* 711–717.

Nyberg, L., Habib, R., McIntosh, A. R., & Tulving, E. (2000). Reactivation of encoding-related brain activity during memory retrieval. *Proceedings of the National Academy of Sciences of the United States of America, 97,* 11120–11124.

Öhman, A., Carlsson, K., Lundqvist, D., & Ingvar, M. (2007). On the unconscious subcortical origin of human fear. *Physiology & Behavior, 92,* 180–185.

Öhman, A., & Mineka, S. (2001). Fears, phobias, and preparedness: Toward an evolved module of fear and fear learning. *Psychological Review, 108,* 483–522.

Oliveri, M., Finocchiaro, C., Shapiro, K., Gangitano, M., Caramazza, A., & Pascual-Leone, A. (2004). All talk and no action: A transcranial magnetic stimulation study of motor cortex activation during action word production. *Journal of Cognitive Neuroscience, 16,* 374–381.

Olsson, A., & Phelps, E. A. (2004). Learned fear of "unseen" faces after Pavlovian, observational, and instructed fear. *Psychological Science, 15,* 822–828.

O'Regan, J. K., & Noë, A. (2001). A sensorimotor account of vision and visual consciousness. *Behavioral and Brain Sciences, 24,* 939–973.

Padoa-Schioppa, C., & Bizzi, E. (2003). Neuronal plasticity in the motor cortex of monkeys acquiring a new internal model. In S. H. Johnson-Frey (Ed.), *Taking action: Cognitive neuroscience perspectives on intentional acts* (pp. 341–360). Cambridge, MA: MIT Press.

Paivio, A. (1979). *Imagery and verbal processes.* Hillsdale, NJ: Lawrence Erlbaum Associates.

Parsons, L. M., Fox, P. T., Downs, J. H., Glass, T., Hirsch, T. B., Martin, C. C., et al. (1995). Use of implicit motor imagery for visual shape discrimination as revealed by PET. *Nature, 375,* 54–58.

Pavlov, I. P. (1927). *Conditioned reflexes.* Oxford: Oxford University Press.

Pellionisz, A., & Llinas, R. (1980). Tensorial approach to the geometry of brain function: Cerebellar coordination via a metric tensor. *Neuroscience, 5,* 1125–1136.

Penfield, W., & Rasmussen, T. (1950). *The cerebral cortex of man.* New York: Macmillan.

Piaget, J. (1971). *Biology and knowledge: An essay on the relations between organic regulations and cognitive processes.* Chicago: University of Chicago Press.

Pickering, M. J., & Garrod, S. (2006). Do people use language production to make predictions during comprehension? *Trends in Cognitive Sciences, 11,* 105–110.

Pinker, S. (1997). *How the mind works.* New York: Norton.

Postle, B., Idzikowski, C., Della Sala, S., Logie, R., & Baddeley, A. (2006). The selective disruption of spatial working memory by eye movements. *Quarterly Journal of Experimental Psychology, 59,* 100–120.

Prescott, T. J., & Humphries, M. D. (2007). Who dominates who in the dark basements of the brain. *Behavioral and Brain Sciences, 30,* 104–105.

Prinz, W. (2003). How do we know about our own actions? In S. Maasen, W. Prinz, & Roth (Eds.), *Voluntary action: Brains, minds, and sociality* (pp. 21–33). London: Oxford University Press.

Pulvermuller, F. (2005). Brain mechanisms linking language and action. *Nature Reviews Neuroscience, 6,* 576–582.

Puttemans, V., Wenderoth, N., & Swinnen, S. P. (2005). Changes in brain activation during the acquisition of a multifrequency bimanual coordination task: From the cognitive stage to advanced levels of automaticity. *Journal of Neuroscience, 25,* 4270–4278.

Pylyshyn, Z. W. (2002). Mental imagery: In search of a theory. *Behavioral and Brain Sciences, 25,* 156–238.

Rapp, B., & Goldrick, M. (2000). Discreteness and interactivity in spoken word production. *Psychological Review, 107,* 460–499.

Rizzolatti, G., Fogassi, L., & Gallese, V. (2004). Cortical mechanisms subserving object grasping, action understanding, and imitation. In M. S. Gazzaniga (Ed.), *The cognitive neurosciences III* (pp. 427–440). Cambridge, MA: MIT Press.

Rizzolatti, G., Gentilucci, M., Camarda, R. M., Gallese, V., Luppino, G., Matelli M., et al. (1990). Neurons related to reaching-grasping arm movements in the rostral part of area 6 (area 6a beta). *Experimental Brain Research, 82,* 337–350.

Rizzolatti, G., Sinigaglia, C., & Anderson, F. (2008). *Mirrors in the brain: How our minds share actions, emotions, and experience.* New York: Oxford University Press.

Roe, A., & Simpson, G. G. (1958). *Behavior and evolution.* New Haven, CT: Yale University Press.

Rolls, E. T. (2007). *Emotions explained.* New York: Oxford University Press.

Rolls, E. T., & Treves, A. (1998). *Neural networks and brain function.* New York: Oxford University Press.

Rosenbaum, D. A. (2002). Motor control. In H. Pashler (Series Ed.) & S. Yantis (Vol. Ed.), *Stevens' handbook of experimental psychology: Vol. 1. Sensation and perception* (3rd ed., pp. 315–339). New York: Wiley.

Rosenbaum, D. A. (2005). The Cinderella of psychology: The neglect of motor control in the science of mental life and behavior. *American Psychologist, 60,* 308–317.

Rosenbaum, D. A., Slotta, J. D., Vaughan, J., & Plamondon, R. J. (1991). Optimal movement selection. *Psychological Science, 2,* 86–91.

Rossetti, Y., & Pisella, L. (2003). Mediate responses as direct evidence for intention: Neuropsychology of not-to, not-now, and not-there tasks. In S. H. Johnson-Frey (Ed.), *Taking action: Cognitive neuroscience perspectives on intentional acts* (pp. 67–105). Cambridge, MA: MIT Press.

Rumelhart, D. E., McClelland, J. L., & the PDP Research Group (1986). *Parallel distributed processing: Explorations in the microstructure of cognition* (Vols. 1 & 2). Cambridge, MA: MIT Press.

Schacter, D. L., & Addis, D. R. (2007). The cognitive neuroscience of constructive memory: Remembering the past and imagining the future. *Philosophical Transactions of the Royal Society of London, Series B: Biological Sciences, 362,* 773–786.

Schank, R. C., & Abelson, R. P. (1977). *Scripts, plans, goals, and understanding: An inquiry into human knowledge structures.* Hillsdale, NJ: Lawrence Erlbaum Associates.

Schmahmann, J. D. (1998). Dysmetria of thought: Clinical consequences of cerebellar dysfunction on cognition and affect. *Trends in Cognitive Sciences, 2,* 362–371.

Schultz, D. P., & Schultz, S. E. (1996). *A history of modern psychology* (6th ed.). Fort Worth, TX: Harcourt Brace College Publishers.

Schwoebel, J., Boronat, C. B., & Coslett, H. B. (2002). The man who executed "imagined" movements: Evidence for dissociable components of the body schema. *Brain and Cognition, 50,* 1–16.

Sechenov, I. M. (1863). *Reflexes of the brain.* Cambridge, MA: MIT Press.

Seligman, M. E. P., & Hager, J. L. (1972). *Biological boundaries of learning.* New York: Appleton-Century-Crofts.

Shallice, T. (1972). Dual functions of consciousness. *Psychological Review, 79,* 383–393.

Sheerer, E. (1984). Motor theories of cognitive structure: A historical review. In W. Prinz & A. F. Sanders (Eds.), *Cognition and motor processes* (pp. 77–98). Berlin: Springer-Verlag.

Shepherd, G. M. (1994). *Neurobiology* (3rd ed.). New York: Oxford University Press.

Sherrington, C. S. (1906). *The integrative action of the nervous system.* New Haven, CT: Yale University Press.

Simpson, G. G. (1949). *The meaning of evolution.* New Haven, CT: Yale University Press.

Skinner, B. F. (1953). *Science and human behavior.* New York: Macmillan.

Smith, E. R., & Semin, G. R. (2004). Socially situated cognition: Cognition in its social context. *Advances in Experimental Social Psychology, 36,* 53–117.

Solarz, A. (1960). Latency of instrumental responses as a function of compatibility with the meaning of eliciting verbal signs. *Journal of Experimental Psychology, 59,* 239–245.

Soon, C. S., Brass, M., Heinze, H.-J., & Haynes, J.-D. (2008). Unconscious determinants of free decisions in the human brain. *Nature Neuroscience, 11,* 543–545.

Sperry, R. W. (1952). Neurology and the mind-brain problem. *American Scientist, 40,* 291–312.

Starreveld, P. A., Theeuwes, J., & Mortier, K. (2004). Response selection in visual search: The influence of response compatibility of nontargets. *Journal* of *Experimental Psychology: Human Perception and Performance, 30,* 56–78.

Strick, P. L. (2004). Basal ganglia and cerebellar circuits with the cerebral cortex. In M. S. Gazzaniga (Ed.), *The cognitive neurosciences III* (pp. 453–461). Cambridge, MA: MIT Press.

Tan, S. K. H., Temel, Y., Blokland, A., Steinbusch, H. W. M., & Visser-Vandewalle, V. (2006). The subthalamic nucleus: From response selection to execution. *Journal of Clinical Neuroanatomy, 31,* 155–161.

Tetlock, P. E. (2002). Social functionalist frameworks for judgment and choice: Intuitive politicians, theologians, and prosecutors. *Psychological Review, 109,* 451–471.

Tettamanti, M., Buccino, G., Saccuman, M. C., Gallese, V., Danna, M., Scifo, P., et al. (2005). Listening to action-related sentences activates fronto-parietal motor circuits. *Journal of Cognitive Neuroscience, 17,* 273–281.

Thompson-Schill, S. L., Aguirre, G. K., D'Esposito, M., & Farah, M. J. (1999). A neural basis for category and modality specificity of semantic knowledge. *Neuropsychologia, 37,* 671–676.

Thorpe, W. H. (1964). *Learning and instinct in animals.* Cambridge, MA: Harvard University Press.

Tinbergen, N. (1952). "Derived" activities: Their causation, biological significance, origin and emancipation during evolution. *Quarterly Review of Biology, 27,* 1–32.

Titchener, E. B. (1896). *An outline of psychology.* New York: Macmillan.

Tolman, E. C. (1948). Cognitive maps in rats and men. *Psychological Review, 55,* 189–208.

Tolman, E. C., & Honzik, C. H. (1930). Introduction and removal of reward, and maze performance in rats. *University of California Publications in Psychology, 4,* 257–275.

Tops, M., & de Jong, R. (2006). Posing for success: Clenching a fist facilitates approach. *Psychonomic Bulletin and Review, 13,* 229–234.

Tranel, D., & Damasio, A. R. (1985). Knowledge without awareness: An autonomic index of facial recognition by prosopagnosics. *Science, 228,* 1453–1454.

Tranel, D., Damasio, H., & Damasio, A. R. (1997). A neural basis for the retrieval of conceptual knowledge. *Neuropsychologia, 35,* 1319–1327.

Tucker, M., & Ellis, R. (2001). The potentiation of grasp types during visual object categorization. *Visual Cognition, 8,* 769–800.

Tucker, M., & Ellis, R. (2004). Action priming by briefly presented objects. *Acta Psychologica, 116,* 185–203.

Ungerleider, L. G., & Mishkin, M. (1982). Two cortical visual systems. In D. J. Ingle, M. A. Goodale, & R. J. W. Mansfield (Eds.), *Analysis of visual behavior* (pp. 549–586). Cambridge, MA: MIT Press.

Utter, A. A., & Basso, M. A. (2008). The basal ganglia: An overview of circuits and function. *Neuroscience and Biobehavioral Reviews, 32,* 333–342.

van Turennout, M., Hagoort, P., & Brown, C. M. (1998). Brain activity during speaking: From syntax to phonology in 40 milliseconds. *Science, 280,* 572–574.

van Veen, V., & Carter, C. S. (2006). Conflict and cognitive control in the brain. *Current Directions in Psychological Science, 5,* 237–240.

van Veen, V., Cohen, J. D., Botvinick, M. M., Stenger, V. A., & Carter, C. C. (2001). Anterior cingulate cortex, conflict monitoring, and levels of processing. *NeuroImage, 14,* 1302–1308.

von Neumann, J. (1958). *The computer and the brain.* New Haven, CT: Yale University Press.

Vygotsky, L. S. (1962). *Thought and language.* Cambridge, MA: MIT Press.

Warrington, E. K. (1975). The selective impairment of semantic memory. *Quarterly Journal of Experimental Psychology, 27,* 635–657.

Washburn, M. F. (1928). Emotion and thought: A motor theory of their relation. In C. Murchison (Ed.), *Feelings and emotions: The Wittenberg Symposium* (pp. 99—145). Worcester, MA: Clark University Press.

Watson, J. B. (1919). *Psychology from the standpoint of a behaviorist.* Philadelphia: Lippincott.

Watson, J. B. (1924). *Behaviorism.* New York: Norton.

Wegner, D. M. (2002). *The illusion of conscious will.* Cambridge, MA: MIT Press.

Weiskrantz, L. (1992). Unconscious vision: The strange phenomenon of blindsight. *The Sciences, 35,* 23–28.

Wexler, M., Kosslyn, S. M., & Berthoz, A. (1998). Motor processes in mental rotation. *Cognition, 68,* 77–94.

Wickens, D. D. (1938). The transference of conditioned excitation and conditioned inhibition from one muscle group to the antagonistic muscle group. *Journal of Experimental Psychology, 22,* 101–123.

Wild, B., Rodden, F. A., Rapp, A., Erb, M., Grodd, W. R., & Ruch, W. (2006). Humor and smiling: Cortical regions selective for cognitive, affective, and volitional components. *Neurology, 66,* 887–893.

Wilson, M. (2002). Six views of embodied cognition. *Psychonomic Bulletin and Review, 9,* 625–636.

Wundt, W. (1900). *Die sprache.* Leipzig: Engelmann.

Yamadori, A. (1997). Body awareness and its disorders. In M. Ito, Y. Miyashita, & E. T. Rolls (Eds.), *Cognition, computation, and consciousness* (pp. 169–176). Washington, DC: American Psychological Association.

Zwaan, R. A., Stanfield, R. A., & Yaxley, R. H. (2002). Language comprehenders mentally represent the shapes of objects. *Psychological Science, 13,* 168–171.

PART 1

Basic Principles, Systems, and Phenomena

2 Cognition and Action

Wolfgang Prinz, Gisa Aschersleben, *and* Iring Koch

Abstract

This chapter addresses theoretical and experimental approaches to the cognitive underpinnings of action. It begins with a brief discussion of what the study of cognitive mechanisms can contribute to the study of action. It then focuses on the two levels by which cognitive mechanics of action can be studied: within and between task sets. The first kind of study addresses issues of action control. The representational resources and functional mechanisms involved in the cognitive mechanics of goal-directed action are considered. The second kind of study addresses issues of task control. The task-switching methodology is introduced to lay the ground for describing the currently pertinent theoretical frameworks of task-set control. Relevant empirical findings are presented to illustrate how action is modulated by task set.

Keywords: cognitive approaches, actions, action control, task control, task sets

In this chapter we address theoretical and experimental approaches to the cognitive underpinnings of action. We focus on two major issues. Before we get there, we briefly discuss what the study of cognitive mechanisms can contribute to the study of action.

Cognitive Approaches to Action

As has often been pointed out, action is hard to study. Human action is ambiguous in several respects. First, there is no obvious and unambiguous way of parsing the continuous stream of peoples' doings and of individuating well-defined tokens of action within that stream (Stränger & Hommel, 1995). That stream can be segmented at various brain levels and on various time scales, ranging from short and simple gestures like raising one's eyebrows to long-lasting and complex undertakings like enrolling in a graduate program. Second, since people tend to accompany their doings by accounts of what they think they are doing, these accounts may act back on what they actually do—and there is no easy and obvious way to disentangle the two (Wegner & Vallacher, 1986). Third, actions always arise from an intricate interplay between external factors pertaining to the current situation and internal factors pertaining to current motivational, volitional, and cognitive states (Lewin, 1926). Since these internal factors cannot be readily accessed and assessed, the study of action is not an easy game to play. No wonder that action is a neglected field of study in the cognitive sciences and that mainstream research has always focused on the study of "stimulus information and its vicissitudes" (Neisser, 1967)—that is, of stimulus-dependent cognitive functions like sensation, perception, imagery, pretention, and recall, where ambiguities are less severe.

The cognitive approaches that we discuss in this chapter are not meant to address the full picture of human action and its ambiguities. In fact, they avoid some of these ambiguities by concentrating on the study of well-individuated and well-defined actions in well-controlled experimental settings. Accordingly, the scope of what they can contribute to the understanding of the complexities of full-fledged action in everyday life has its natural limitations. Importantly, the approaches we discuss do not address the motivational and volitional precursors of action. They focus on the *cognitive mechanics* of action planning and execution, leaving *volitional dynamics* to participants' willingness to follow the experimenter's instruction.

Cognitive Mechanics: Action Knowledge

What does it mean to study the cognitive mechanics of action, and what do we need to embark on for such studies? For the prototypical case of voluntary action on which we focus here, two basic conditions must be met. One is that individuals need to entertain certain goals. The other is that they need to plan and eventually perform certain actions to attain them. The key issue of cognitive mechanics then refers to the interaction between goals and actions and their respective representations: How can goals select appropriate actions—appropriate in the sense of being suited to realize them? In other words, what kinds of representational mechanisms do we need to understand how goal-directed action becomes possible?

For this we need to study how both goals and actions are represented and how their representations interact. Goals and actions are not enough, however. There is always a third partner in the game: the current situation. The current situation may interact with goals and actions in two different ways. One is that it may constrain and specify the goals to be pursued. The other is that it may constrain and specify the actions required to attain given goals. Thus, in order to provide a full picture of the cognitive mechanics of action, we need to explain how goals and knowledge about the current situation give rise to the selection and production of appropriate action. In this chapter we address these three basic components and their mutual relationships under the notion of *action knowledge*.

The study of action knowledge addresses the functional architecture of the representational resources for action planning and execution. One set of pertinent questions addresses structural issues. How are goals, actions, and the current situation represented, and how are these representations related to each other? Another set of questions addresses functional issues, pertaining to backward and forward computation (Frith, Blakemore, & Wolpert, 2000; Jordan, 1996; Kawato, 1997; Wolpert, 1997). Backward computation determines appropriate actions and/or situations for the realization of given goals. It starts from desired and intended states of affairs in the future, acting back to states required to precede them (e.g., action selection and selection of action opportunities). Conversely, forward computation determines expected consequences of given actions and/or situations. It starts from given states of affairs, acting forward to states expected to follow them in the future (e.g., deliberations about actions and action monitoring).

In this chapter we discuss voluntary action in performance, learning, and development. Performance studies focus on mechanisms of backward computation, acting back from goals to actions. However, as we will see in studies on learning and development, action knowledge is initially built up through forward learning, acting forward from movements to movement outcomes.

Volitional Dynamics: Task Instructions

The study of cognitive mechanics of action takes goals and goal pursuit for granted, leaving out of consideration both the motivational issue of where the goals come from and the volitional issue of what energizes their pursuit and shelters it from competing attractions and seductions (Gollwitzer, 1999). However, the fact that these dynamical sources of action are not explicitly considered does not mean that they are altogether ignored. Rather, they are implicitly taken into account by task instructions.

In experimental settings, participants are instructed to perform certain actions under certain conditions. For instance, they may be required to press the left key of two keys in response to a red light and the right key in response to a green light, delivering responses as fast as they can after light onset. A task like this can be conceived in two different ways. In one conceptualization—the traditional one—the task requires assigning responses to stimuli according to prespecified rules (S-R mapping). In the other conceptualization—the one that we adopt here—it requires selecting voluntary actions under given internal and external circumstances (action selection). As concerns cognitive mechanics, action selection relies on backward computation of appropriate actions based on representations of goals and current stimulus conditions. As concerns volitional dynamics, it relies on task instructions and participants' willingness to follow them. Thus, obedience to well-controlled experimental instructions replaces the imponderables of motivational and volitional dynamics in real life.

Task Sets: Within and Between

In typical experimental paradigms, the task environment will, beyond providing volitional dynamics, also provide specific sets of rules that apply to the task. Such rules may either be communicated through instructions (e.g., as prescriptive rules for mapping actions to stimuli) or be gradually acquired while performing the task (e.g., as descriptive rules that apply to relations between stimuli, actions, and outcomes). Task environments provide, in other words, specific contexts for action and action production. In the literature it is generally assumed that task contexts to which individuals are exposed are represented in terms of *task sets* (Meiran, 1996; Rogers & Monsell, 1995). Task sets are context-specific configurations of action knowledge, providing the knowledge base for a given task. This knowledge base may comprise both prescriptive rules and descriptive regularities inherent in the task.

The cognitive mechanics of action can be studied at two levels: within and between task sets. The first kind of study addresses issues of *action control,* to which we turn in section 2. The second kind of study addresses issues of *task control,* to which we turn in section 3.

Action Control

In this section we consider representational resources and functional mechanisms involved in the cognitive mechanics of goal-directed action. We start with ideomotor theory. This theory provides a simple but powerful conceptual framework for explaining goal-directed action in terms of performance, learning, and development. Then we move on discussing pertinent evidence from two domains of study. One concerns the modulation of ongoing action through perception. The other concerns the emergence of goal-directed action in early infancy.

Ideomotor Theory

Ideomotor theory offers an answer to the question of how goal-directed action is possible at all. Historically, the ideomotor approach to action is much younger than the sensorimotor approach. The sensorimotor framework regards actions as reactions—that is, as responses that are selected and triggered by stimuli. Strict versions of the approach (like hard-core S-R theories) claim that the stimulus is both a necessary and a sufficient condition for the action to occur. Ideomotor theory, in contrast, stresses the role of internal, volitional causes of action. This framework views actions as creations of the will—that is, as events that come into being by virtue of the fact that people pursue goals and entertain intentions to realize them.

The basic ideas underlying ideomotor theory were first spelled out by Lotze (1852) and James (1890). According to Lotze, in order to carry out a voluntary action, two conditions must be fulfilled. First, there must be an idea or mental image of what is being willed (*Vorstellung des Gewollten*). Second, all conflicting ideas or images must be absent or removed (*Hinwegräumung aller Hemmungen*). When these two conditions are met, the mental image acquires the power to guide the movements required to realize the intention, thus converting ideas in the mind into facts in the world.

Thirty years later, James summarized these ideas in what he called the ideomotor principle of voluntary action:

> Every representation of a movement awakens in some degree the actual movement which is its object; and awakens it in a maximum degree whenever it is not kept from doing so by an antagonistic representation present simultaneously in the mind. (James, 1890, vol. II, p. 526)

At first glance this sounds like magic (Prinz, 1987; Thorndike, 1913). How should it be possible for representations of movements to awaken the actual movements to which they refer? Both Lotze and James argue that these links arise from learning. Whenever a movement is performed, it goes along with perceivable consequences, or action effects. Some are directly linked to carrying out the movement itself, such as the kinesthetic sensations that accompany each movement. Others are linked to the movement in a more indirect way since they occur in the agent's environment at a certain spatial and/or temporal distance from the actual movement. For example, when one's fingers operate a light switch, the light does not appear at the location of the switch but comes on at a distance. Likewise, when one throws a basketball, it will travel some time before it lands in the basket—at quite a distance from the throwing movement.

Ideomotor theory posits that the regularities between actual movements and their resident and remote perceivable consequences are captured in associations. In other words, representations coding the perceivable bodily and environmental consequences of movements will become associated with representations coding the movements themselves. Such associations can then become functional in two ways. First, they allow individuals to expect certain outcomes, given certain movements or motor commands—that is, to predict perceivable consequences of given movements (forward computation). Second, they allow them to select certain movements or motor commands, given certain intentions to achieve desired states of affairs in the environment—that is, to select movements required to achieve predefined goals (backward computation).

According to ideomotor theory, action knowledge is built on such bidirectional associations, and voluntary action relies on backward computations performed on that knowledge base. Accordingly, the representation of any event that has been learned to go along with or follow from a particular action will hereafter exhibit the power to call that action forth. Importantly, this applies not only to representations of body-related action effects (e.g., thinking of one's finger operating a light switch) but also to representations of more remote action effects in the environment (e.g., thinking of the light going on).

Ideomotor theory was initially meant to explain how actions are prompted and guided through internally generated thoughts and intentions. Yet, if it is true that *thinking of an action* and/or its remote consequences can prompt and instigate that action, this should be even more true of *perceiving that action* and/or its outcome. An extension of the ideomotor principle along these lines was in fact suggested by Greenwald (1970, 1972). Greenwald showed that perceiving a particular event (say, a red light) that has first been learned to follow from a particular action (i.e., as a red feedback flash following pressing a particular response key) will hereafter prompt and/or facilitate the execution of that action. With this extension, ideomotor theory claims that the perception of an event that shares features with an event that has been learned to accompany or follow from one's own action will tend to prompt that action. In other words, the perception of events will prompt the production of similar events.

This theoretical claim has three important implications pertaining to the functional organization of action knowledge: ideomotor mapping, common coding, and distal reference.

The notion of *ideomotor mapping* refers to the learning requirements implied by the theory. In order for the ideomotor principle to work, two requirements must be met. One is that the system is capable of learning regular associations between actions and their ensuing (resident and remote) effects. The other is that these associations, once established, can also be used in the

reverse direction, that is, from representations of action effects to actions effectuating them (Elsner, 2000; Elsner & Hommel, 2001, 2004; Koch, Keller, & Prinz, 2004; Kunde, 2001, 2003; Kunde, Koch, & Hoffmann, 2004; Stock & Hoffmann, 2002).

The notion of *common coding* refers to the functional architecture of action knowledge. Ideomotor theory requires a common representational domain for perception and action, with shared resources for perceiving events and planning actions (Hommel, Müsseler, Aschersleben, & Prinz, 2001; MacKay, 1987; Prinz, 1984, 1990, 1997). In this domain, actions are represented through their perceivable effects. As a consequence, perception and action are entirely commensurate—and this is why similarity can work between them.

The notion of *distal reference* refers to the representational content of entries in the common representational domain for perception and action. Distal reference is fairly obvious on the perceptual side. What we see and hear are patterns of neither sensory stimulation nor brain activation. Instead, we perceive objects and events in the environments—distal events rather than proximal stimuli or even central activations (Brunswick, 1944, 1952, 1955). No less obvious is distal reference on the action side. For instance, when we plan to hammer a nail into the wall, action planning does not refer to muscle contractions in the arm or to activations in the motor cortex. Instead, it refers to the planned action and its intended outcome in the environment (James, 1890; Prinz, 1992). Distal reference guarantees that perception and action planning draw on commensurate representations—representations that refer to events in the distal world—and not to activation patterns in the proximal body or the central brain, where afferent and efferent codes are incommensurate since one refers to activations in sense organs and the other to activations in muscles.

Action Modulation Through Perception

Ideomotor theory opens new avenues to the study of the cognitive mechanics of action planning and action control. The similarity principle inherent in the notion of common coding implies that perception and action will modulate each other reciprocally whenever they are similar. Perception will modulate production, and likewise production will modulate perception, depending on representational overlap.

Here we focus on one of these two routes, that is, from perception to production. For this route, ideomotor theory has a straightforward prediction to offer. Since it claims that action perception draws on representational resources that are also involved in action production, it predicts that planning and control of ongoing action is modulated through concurrent perception of actions and action effects. This modulation is content specific: It depends on the representational overlap between the events that are being perceived and the actions that are being planned.

Performance

How does action modulation through perception work? Pertinent evidence is provided by various kinds of experimental paradigms, such as S-R compatibility, action interference, action induction, and action coordination.

S-R Compatibility

A rich body of evidence concerning the workings of similarity in the interplay between perception and action comes from studies on S-R compatibility (Fitts, 1964; Fitts & Seeger, 1953; Kornblum, Hasbroucq, & Osman, 1990; Proctor & Vu, 2002). Although most of these studies are grounded in the logic of the sensorimotor framework, their results often pose a severe challenge to that logic.

S-R compatibility effects can be observed in choice reaction time tasks when one manipulates the mapping rules, that is, the rules for assigning responses to stimuli. When a given set of responses (Rs) is mapped onto a given set of stimuli (Ss) under different mapping rules, or S-R assignments, it is often the case that faster reactions and lower error rates are obtained for one assignment as compared to the other. A simple example is provided by a choice reaction task with two stimuli and two responses. Suppose that on each trial a stimulus light is flashed either to the left or to the right of a fixation mark and that the task requires pressing one of two response keys, either the left one or the right one. A setup like this allows for two assignments of responses to stimuli. With the compatible assignment, stimuli and responses share a common feature (both left or both right) in contrast to the incompatible assignment, where they always exhibit different features (right-left or left-right). As has been shown in numerous studies, response performance for compatible assignments is clearly superior to incompatible assignments (cf., e.g., Fitts & Seeger, 1953).

Although most classical studies address spatial compatibility between stimuli and responses, S-R compatibility effects are not limited to the spatial domain. For instance, when the stimulus set comprises visually presented letters like A, B, and C and the response set is made up of the spoken names of these letters, one may arrange for one "natural" assignment and a number of less natural, arbitrary assignments between stimuli and responses. Here, too, response times are shorter and error rates lower for the compatible than the incompatible assignments (Morin & Forrin, 1962; Van Duren & Sanders, 1988).

Unlike spatial S-R compatibility, which relies on physical similarity between stimulus and response locations, symbolic S-R compatibility seems to rely on acquired symbolic equivalence. However, in both cases the two assignments differ in terms of representational overlap between stimulus and response features. When that overlap is sufficiently large (as in compatible assignments), automatically activated stimulus features will prespecify, or prime, responses exhibiting the same features. Accordingly, S-R compatibility effects rely on similarity-based priming of action through perception (Greenwald, 1970; Kornblum et al., 1990).

S-R compatibility effects are also obtained when response features overlap with stimulus features that are irrelevant for response selection. An example from the spatial domain is provided by the Simon paradigm (Simon, 1990; Simon & Rudell, 1967). In a typical Simon task, two response keys (left/right) are assigned to two stimuli that differ on a nonspatial dimension like color (say, red/green). On each trial the stimulus is presented on either the right-hand or the left-hand side of the display. Stimulus color is thus relevant and stimulus position irrelevant for response selection. Still a substantial spatial compatibility effect is regularly observed: Responses are faster and error rates lower for trials in which the stimulus is presented on the side on which the response is produced.

A powerful demonstration of the same effect in the symbolic domain is provided by the Stroop task (Stroop, 1935): In this task, color words (e.g., red, green, and blue) are shown in different colors, and the task requires to name the colors in which the words are printed, ignoring their names altogether. Still, there is no way to suppress those names—to the effect that word reading heavily interferes with color naming.

In sum, these effects suggest that perception may prime action, based on similarity between mandatory features of perceived events ("stimuli") and mandatory features of to-be-produced events ("responses").

These effects pose a challenge to the sensorimotor framework since it provides no obvious rule for the workings of similarity between stimuli and responses. In contrast, ideomotor theory provides a natural framework to account for these effects.

Perception/Action Interference

Ideomotor theory claims that the perception of a particular action performed by someone else draws on representational resources that are also involved in the perceiver's planning and control of same or similar own actions. Pertinent evidence comes from studies in which action perception interferes with concurrent action production. For instance, it has been shown that the production of particular hand gestures is modulated through concurrent perception of related gestures (Brass, Bekkering, & Prinz, 2001). In these studies, participants had to initiate, as fast as possible, a particular finger gesture on command while watching either the same or a different gesture performed by a hand on a computer screen. The task required initiating the predetermined gesture as soon as the hand on the screen started moving. Results indicated that participants could initiate the required gesture much faster when the same gesture was shown on the screen as compared to a different one.

A similar interference effect applies to the selection of gestures: The time to select a particular gesture on command is shorter when the imperative stimulus that specifies which gesture to select is superimposed on a hand performing the same gesture as compared to conditions in which the gesture to be produced is different from the gesture being perceived (Brass, Bekkering, Wohlschläger, & Prinz, 2000). Remarkably, the same interference effect is obtained when dynamic gestures are replaced by static postures. Interference is particularly pronounced for what may be called "target postures," that is, postures reflecting anticipated end states or goals of the gestures to be produced (Stürmer, Aschersleben, & Prinz, 2000).

Action Imitation

A strong role for action goals is also supported from studies on action imitation (see Chapter 22; Bekkering & Prinz, 2002; Bekkering & Wohlschläger, 2002; Gattis, Bekkering, & Wohlschläger, 2002; Gleissner, Meltzoff, & Bekkering, 2000). In these experiments, 3- to 5-year-olds took part in an imitation game requiring them to imitate one out of four possible gestures, namely, reaching for their left or right ear with their left or right arm. In two cases (left ear/right arm and right ear/left arm), the reaching arm had to cross the body midline, whereas no such crossing was involved in the other two cases. Kids made virtually no errors in uncrossed tasks, but a substantial number of errors was observed in crossed tasks. In crossed tasks, two kinds of error can be made: effector errors (correct ear/wrong arm) and goal errors (wrong ear/correct arm). Virtually all errors that occurred were effector errors: In their own actions, infants reached for the same ear at which the model's action was directed but chose a simpler movement to attain that goal. In a further study it was shown that this error pattern is obtained only when the gestures are really goal directed: In a control condition without goal attainment (in which the same gestures were shown without eventually reaching for the ear), both types of errors were equally frequent (Gleissner et al., 2000).

There are two lessons to be learned here. First, as far as imitation succeeds, it demonstrates the operation of shared representational resources for action perception and production. Second, as far as imitation fails, it elucidates the nature of these resources, suggesting that they contain more information than just the kinematics of movement patterns. They contain information about full-fledged goal-directed actions, with goals (ends) taking the lead over movements (means) in the control of action imitation. These observations support the central claim of ideomotor theory that actions are represented in terms of what they lead to.

Action Induction

Further support for a key role of goals for both action perception and production comes from studies on induced, or ideomotor, movements. This term refers to actions that become spontaneously induced when people watch other people's actions and their outcomes (Prinz, 1987). For instance, while watching, in a slapstick movement, an actor who walks along the edge of a plunging precipice, observers are often unable to sit still and watch quietly. They will move their legs and their arms or displace their body weight to one side or another.

How is the pattern of induced movements related to the pattern of perceived events that call them forth? Two answers to this question have been proposed: perceptual and intentional induction (Prinz, De Maeght, & Knuf, 2004). Perceptual induction posits that spontaneous movements mirror what observers *see* happening in the scene. This answer regards induced action as a special kind of imitative action—nonvoluntary imitation, as it were. Intentional induction posits that spontaneous movements realize what observers *want to see* happening in the scene. This answer regards induced action as a special kind of goal-directed action—futile instrumental action, as it were.

Experimental studies have shown that both principles may be effective at the same time, depending on task conditions. For instance, in studies in which individuals watched the outcome of self-performed actions, the pattern of induced movements was different for instrumental and noninstrumental effectors. When they watched a rolling ball whose course they had before determined through their own hand movements, the instrumental effector (hand) exhibited strong intentional induction but no perceptual induction at all, whereas noninstrumental effectors (like the head) showed both intentional and perceptual induction (Knuf, Aschersleben, & Prinz, 2001).

A different picture emerged when individuals watched the outcome of goal-directed actions performed by somebody else. In this situation, both perceptual and intentional induction were observed. Importantly, intentional induction was always guided by the observer's intentions and not by the observee's intentions. This was shown in experimental settings in which the two competed with each other; that is, their respective intentions and goals opposed each other. In this situation, intentional induction always followed the observer's intentions, disregarding the observee's goals altogether (De Maeght & Prinz, 2004).

These studies support both perceptual and intentional induction. Perceptual induction is stimulus triggered and works bottom up, whereas intentional induction is goal directed and works top down. In any case, action induction is not just a matter of imitation. Perceptual induction is imitative, but intentional induction is not. It makes people act as if they could change what they see happening into what they want to see happening. Goals and goal-related intentions thus play a key role in the representational resources shared between action perception and production.

Bimanual Coordination

The basic claim that actions are represented in terms of their (anticipated or intended) outcomes can also be applied to situations in which individuals need to coordinate two different actions, as, for instance, in bimanual coordination. A key assumption in classical theories of action coordination has been that the coordination of the two actions is achieved mainly by the coupling of efferent motor signals (Kelso, 1984). Ideomotor theory suggests a different view. The scope of the claim that actions are controlled through representations of their perceptual outcomes is not limited to the planning of single actions. It applies to the coordination and coupling of concurrent actions as well.

There is now substantial evidence in support of this claim. In one of their experiments, Mechsner, Kerzel, Knoblich, and Prinz (2001) first replicated a classical paradigm. They instructed participants to perform bimanual index-finger oscillations either in symmetry or in parallel. Participants started at slow pace and then went faster and faster. The typical finding in this paradigm is a symmetry bias: as people move faster, parallel oscillations become increasingly harder to maintain and, at some point, switch into symmetrical ones. The converse is never observed: Never will symmetrical oscillations switch into parallel ones. According to the received view, the symmetry bias supports motor coupling, that is, coupling at the level of efferent commands. This is because symmetrical oscillations rely on concurrent activation of homologous muscles in the two hands, whereas parallel oscillations recruit nonhomologous muscles.

This view seems to be unwarranted, however. In a further condition, participants were required to carry out the same finger oscillations, with one hand held palm up and the other palm down. In this case, concurrent activation of homologous muscles applies to parallel, not to symmetrical, oscillations. Therefore, parallel oscillations should now be more stable than symmetrical ones. Results showed the opposite: Under this condition, too, symmetrical oscillations were stable, whereas parallel oscillations were harder to maintain and tended to switch into symmetrical ones at high speeds. This suggests that the symmetry pertains to perceivable action outcomes, not to motor signals and muscle activations.

The same conclusion is supported from the result of a bimanual circling task (Mechsner et al., 2001). In this task, participants had to carry out circular movements with both hands simultaneously. The usual finding here is that only a small number of coordination patterns is stable at high velocities. For untrained individuals it is almost impossible to produce circling patterns that are characterized by nonharmonic frequency ratios for the two hands. For instance, when asked to complete four circles with one hand and three circles with the other during a certain interval, participants will fail to produce the required pattern and switch to patterns with harmonic frequency ratios (like 4:4 or 4:2 instead of 4:3, as required).

The standard interpretation of this finding, too, is that efferent muscle commands can be coupled only with harmonic frequency ratios. However, if one posits that bimanual coupling relies on action outcomes, one must predict that couplings with nonharmonic frequency ratios should become possible when one arranges the task in such a way that the perceptual outcomes of the two movements exhibit a harmonic frequency ratio. This was in fact shown in an experimental setting in which participants had to perform movements exhibiting a nonharmonic frequency ratio (hand movements at a ratio of 4:3) in order to achieve perceivable movement outcomes exhibiting a harmonic ratio (movements of visible action effects at a ratio of 4:4). Under these conditions, participants could easily produce stable movement outcomes, even at

high velocities, by moving their hands in a seemingly impossible manner. Once more we may conclude that actions are guided by representations of their outcomes.

Learning

How is action knowledge acquired? How do individuals create a knowledge base that allows for both forward and backward computation? In other words, how do individuals learn to link actions to action outcomes in the first place, and how do they then come to use these linkages in the reverse order, leading them from anticipated or intended outcomes to actions? This issue has been explored in a variety of learning paradigms.

Action–Effect–Learning

Ideomotor theory claims that events that follow from given actions will hereafter gain the power to trigger those actions. Ideomotor learning thus converts former action effects into potential goals for future action. For instance, when an individual learns that pressing a particular key will always trigger a red light flash (action effect), that knowledge can also be used to trigger that particular key press when the individual, for whatever reason, wants to produce a red light flash (action goal). Theory requires two steps here: acquisition of associations between actions and their ensuing effects and inverting these associations for goal-directed action (learning through forward computation and action selection through backward computation, respectively).

These two steps have been explored in a number of studies (Elsner & Hommel 2001, 2004; Hommel, 1996). In these studies, participants first went through an acquisition phase in which they were exposed to contingencies between actions and action effects (say, left versus right key presses followed by low- versus high-pitched tones). On each trial they chose one of the actions, and that action was then followed by its assigned effect. Importantly, these action effects were entirely irrelevant during acquisition. In the test phase the order of events was reversed: Previous action effects (tones) now preceded the actions to be performed in forced- and free-choice tasks. Results indicated that both response frequencies in free-choice tasks and reaction times in forced-choice tasks depended on the associations learned during acquisition. In free-choice designs the tones would bias action selection and, hence, affect response frequencies. In forced-choice designs the tones would shorten or lengthen reaction times depending on whether they had before been learned to follow from the required action.

These findings match precisely the basic claims of ideomotor theory. As concerns acquisition, they provide evidence for automatic integration between actions and action outcomes through associations (forward computation). As concerns performance at test, they provide evidence for automatic action priming through learned action effects (backward computation). The logic of the paradigm implies that the perceptual priming effect serves as a probe for demonstrating what the learning of action effects leads to: the automatic integration of action effects into the representational resources subserving action planning and action control.

Stimulus–Effect Compatibility

Reaction time tasks require one to select and perform certain actions in response to certain stimulus events. A trial is completed when the action has been performed. In these tasks the outcome of the action always resides in the action itself. Therefore, if one wants to study the impact of action outcomes independent from actions proper, one needs to arrange for a task that separates the two and allows one to dissociate their respective effects. A task like this should help one to tell stimulus–response compatibility (S-R: based on similarity between stimuli and actions proper) from stimulus–effect compatibility (S-E: based on similarity between stimuli and action effects).

This issue was explored in a study by Hommel (1993). The study was based on an auditory Simon task in which participants responded to high- versus low-pitched tones by pressing right-hand versus left-hand response keys, respectively (say, right-hand responses for high tones and left-hand responses for low tones). Tones were randomly presented in one of two loudspeakers, one on the left-hand and the other on the right-hand side. This setting was designed to yield a regular Simon effect: Responses should be fast when the stimuli triggering them are presented in the loudspeaker on the same side as the responses, but they should be slow when stimulus presentation is on the opposite side. Hommel extended the paradigm by introducing visual action effects. These effects were perfectly contingent on the two responses, but they were always located on the opposite side. When participants pressed a right-hand key (in response to a high-pitched tone), a light would turn on on the left-hand side, and when they pressed the left-hand key (in response to a low-pitched tone), a light would turn on on the right-hand side. The task was administered under two instructions. In the control group, participants were instructed to ignore the lights altogether and just press keys in response to tones according to instructions. In the experimental group, participants were instructed to turn on lights in response to tones according to instructions, ignoring response keys altogether. The idea was to implement two different task sets: one featuring the actions themselves (key presses) and one featuring their remote effects (light onsets).

Results for the control group showed a regular Simon effect, as expected. In the experimental group the Simon effect was reversed, however. Under this instruction, performance was determined by the compatibility relationship between stimulus locations and effect location (S-E compatibility): Responses were fast when the stimulus and the light shared the same location (despite the fact that the location of the response itself was always on the opposite side). Conversely, responses were slow when the stimulus and the light appeared in different locations (despite the fact that the location of the action itself was in this case always on the same side as the stimulus). S-E compatibility may thus overrule S-R compatibility when one creates a situation in which actions and effects can be dissociated (see also Hommel, 2004; Chapter 18).

Response–Effect Compatibility

If it is true that goal-directed action relies on exploiting action–effect associations in the reverse direction, one should expect that the efficiency of action control depends, among other things, on representational overlap, or similarity between actions and their ensuing effects. The greater this overlap, the easier it should be to establish those associations and the stronger they should be. Therefore, when a given action needs to be selected in response to some arbitrary imperative stimulus, response times should, other things being equal, depend on response–effect compatibility.

This has in fact been demonstrated in a number of studies. For example, Kunde (2001) required participants to respond to each of two color stimuli by pressing a key either forcefully or softly. In the compatible condition a forceful key press triggered a loud tone, whereas a soft key press triggered a quiet tone. In the incompatible condition these response–effect contingencies were reversed. Results indicated that key presses

could be initiated faster in the compatible than in the incompatible condition. This finding has been confirmed in subsequent studies (e.g., Keller & Koch, 2006; Koch & Kunde, 2002; Kunde, 2003; Kunde et al., 2004). In recent studies R-E compatibility has also been shown to apply to music-like sequential skills, that is, to compatibility relationships between sequences of finger movements and sequences of tones following from them (Keller & Koch, 2008; Koch, Keller, & Prinz, 2004).

Conclusion

Effect-related compatibility effects provide perhaps the most direct and most elegant proof for the basic claim of ideomotor theory that voluntary actions are guided by anticipations of intended action effects. Although action–effect learning supports this claim, too, it does not unambiguously show that action selection really relies on internally generated anticipations of action effects. Here it may not be necessary to invoke internally generated anticipations since action effects are in this paradigm also provided as external stimuli. This is not the case for stimulus–effect and response–effect compatibility, however. Here the action is always selected before the action effect comes up. Therefore, effect-related compatibility effects point to the secret workings of anticipatory representations of action effects in the representational machinery for action control.

Goal-Directed Action in Early Infancy

While there is a long-lasting history on the role of the anticipation of action effects in adult action control (see, e.g., Aschersleben, 2002; Hommel et al., 2001; Prinz, 1997), only recently has research focused on the question of the emergence of goal-directed action in early infancy. As outlined previously, it is important to have a clear definition of what constitutes an action—as opposed to a movement, actions differ from movements in their intentional character; that is, actions are directed toward goals. As a consequence, it is important for both theoretical considerations and practical experimental planning to distinguish the two constituents of an action: the movement and the goal. This distinction corresponds to the well-established distinction between means and ends. One important consequence for infant research is that infants have to be able to differentiate means from ends, and they need this discrimination not only to perform their own goal-directed actions but also to interpret the goal-directed actions expressed by others.

How are these two aspects of goal-directed actions interrelated in development? As we will see in the next paragraphs, understanding our own actions and other peoples' actions are two capacities that are intimately linked. However, there is disagreement in the literature regarding the direction of influence, that is, whether understanding oneself as an agent precedes the understanding of others as agents or vice versa (see, e.g., Hauf & Prinz, 2005). The notion of a common representational domain for perception and action as proposed by the common coding approach (Hommel et al., 2001; Prinz, 1990, 1997) leads to two main assumptions. First, even young infants have an abstract representation of actions (see Chapter 18). This representation is used by both the perceptual system to perceive and interpret actions of other persons as goal directed and by the motor system to perform goal-directed actions. Second, the format of this representation is a distal one; that is, actions are represented in terms of their anticipated effects in the environment. As a consequence, action effects should play an important role in infant action perception as well as in infant action production (Aschersleben, 2006).

The idea of common representations can also be found in Meltzoff's (1993, 2002) active intermodal mapping (AIM) approach, which has been suggested to account for neonatal imitation. It is assumed that humans have the inborn ability to actively match visible movements of others with nonvisible but felt movements of one's self. This account assumes a supramodal, abstract representational system that matches the perceptual information of the seen act with the proprioceptive information of the produced act.

Common representations for perception and action mean that infants have a commensurate action representation system; they can, by matching own and other people's actions, get to know about the subjective side of the other person by drawing inferences on the basis of their own experiences or vice versa. By underlining equivalence, both directions of influence are feasible in a common coding approach.

However, most theories propose an influence of action production on action perception. Infants first have to acquire a specific level of reasoning about their own actions in order to be able to understand other people's actions (e.g., Tomasello, 1995, 1999). To achieve an understanding of intentions in other people, infants must first come to act in an intentional fashion themselves, which in turn requires infants to be able to differentiate between means and ends. Infants pass the means–end task typically at the age of 8 months (Willatts, 1999). In this task, infants are shown an interesting toy, which is placed on a table out of their reach. However, beneath the toy is a cloth with its front edge being in infants' reach. At the age of 8 months but not earlier, the infant will pull the cloth in order to get the toy. To come closer to an answer to the question of how action interpretation and action production are interrelated in development and how action knowledge develops in general, we give a brief review of the evidence on each aspect of action control separately in the following paragraphs.

Action Production

From very early on, infants consider the outcomes of a movement in movement control. Infants learn to act on their environment in order to bring about desired consequences. By exploring the contingencies between self-performed movements and environmental events, infants learn to predict the effects of their actions. This is important for the development of goal-directed action, in which an action must be chosen that is suitable to bring about a desired effect. For example, 2- to 5-month-old infants learn the relations between leg kicks and the contingent movements of a mobile (e.g., Rovee & Rovee, 1969; Rovee-Collier & Shyi, 1993). In these studies, infants lie in a crib with a ribbon running between their ankle and an overhead mobile. Within a few minutes, infants recognize the contingency between their foot kicks and the movement of the mobile—their rate of kicking increases dramatically. In further studies, very young infants learned the relations between leg kicks and the sounds of a rattle (Rochat & Morgan, 1998) or to turn their heads in anticipation of a bottle (Papousek, 1967). Even newborns learn to suck in a certain frequency in order to hear their mother's voice (De Casper, & Fifer, 1980). The main characteristic of this instrumental learning is that the production of the movement is influenced by an interesting event that follows it. Learning about actions and their effects helps the infant produce a desired effect by performing a given movement. Thus, action–effect learning can be seen as a prerequisite for goal-directed action.

However, following ideomotor theory (see the section "Ideomotor Theory"), the acquisition of action–effect associations is only the first step. What needs to follow in individual learning as well as in early development is to invert these associations for goal-directed actions. Thus, we need to show that infants use the anticipation of action effects to control their actions. Moreover, infants' learning about the consequences of self-produced actions is constrained by motor development. Especially in the first year of life, the range of possible self-performed actions is quite narrow; therefore, it seems rather unlikely that infants acquire all their knowledge about actions and their effects by instrumental learning. As a consequence, imitation becomes the prominent way of learning actions during infancy. In order to imitate, infants must watch other persons' actions, use the visual input as a basis for an action plan, and execute the motor output. As infants have ample opportunity to observe other people, their actions, and the consequences of these actions in the environment, imitative learning is an efficient way to acquire knowledge about actions. Various authors have shown that at 6 months of age, infants start to understand other people's actions as goal directed (e.g., Hofer, Hohenberger, Hauf, & Aschersleben, 2008; Jovanovic et al., 2007; Kamewari, Kato, Kanda, Ishiguro, & Hiraki, 2005; Woodward, 1998, 1999). However, imitative learning requires not only action–effect knowledge as provided by observational learning but, furthermore, the transfer of the observed action–effect relations to own actions.

Research on infant imitation indicates that imitative learning develops not before the age of 6 to 9 months (Barr, Dowden, & Hayne, 1996; Elsner, Hauf, & Aschersleben, 2007; Heimann & Nilheim, 2004; Meltzoff, 1988). In a typical study, infants watch a model performing various new actions on one or several objects. After a delay, which amounts to 1 day up to several months, infants come back to the lab and are handed over the objects. It is then coded whether the infants perform the action(s) they had seen in the modeling phase some time ago. Thus, most of the imitation studies focus on memory aspects, that is, on whether and how long infants can remember actions presented by a human model. Only recently has research started to focus on the role of action effects in infant action control. Carpenter, Nagell, and Tomasello (1998) delayed the effect of the infant's action (i.e., colored lights or a colorful spinning wheel) and checked whether infants would look expectantly to the end result following their action. Ten- and 12-month-olds copied the target actions, but only the latter checked whether their actions would bring about an effect. Thus, 12-month-olds have encoded that the model's actions had produced an effect, and they expected their own actions to be effective, too. Elsner and Aschersleben (2003) tested whether infants expected the effects to be the same as they had seen in the model's presentation. Infants observed a model performing two target actions on an object, producing an interesting effect with each action. Results showed that 9-month-olds did not yet learn the relations between the movements and the effects by observation. In contrast, 12-month-olds benefited from observing the model but did not yet understand the specific relations between the movements and effects. By 15 months, infants detected whether their own actions were followed by the same effects as the model's actions, which requires that they had encoded which specific movement led to which effect.

Supporting evidence for the fact that 12-month-olds consider the observed action–effect relations comes from a study by Hauf, Elsner, and Aschersleben (2004). They showed that 12- and 18-month-olds produced a target action that elicited an interesting action effect more often and with shorter latency than other actions that were not combined with such an interesting action effect. Thus, the observation of

an action–effect relation led to selective production of different action steps. Most important, this study provides clear evidence for effect anticipation in infancy: The action step, for which the infant expected to elicit an interesting effect, was produced as the first action in most cases, indicating that the infants anticipated this effect when producing the action step for the first time (see also Klein, Hauf, & Aschersleben, 2006). Follow-up studies using a more simple paradigm suggest that infants start to benefit from watching other persons' action–effect contingencies at even younger ages (Hauf & Aschersleben, 2008).

The findings about the role of action effects in infant action control can be taken as evidence of a goal representation that is defined in terms of action effects. At the age of 9–12 months, infants seem to have goal representations in terms of action effects in their minds. Moreover, it seems that at this age, they already treat other persons as having goals in mind (Aschersleben, 2007). One conclusion that can be drawn concerns the direction of influence between the two aspects of action control. It seems that infants first are able to perceptually detect relations between other persons' actions and their effects in the middle of their first year of life, whereas the transfer of observed action–effect relations to own behavior seems to emerge not before the first birthday. Before discussing this problem in more detail, we give a brief review of the evidence on action perception.

Action Perception

Interpreting the actions of other persons as goal directed has been viewed as a precursor of intentional understanding. Understanding that other persons have intentions that drive their actions is probably the first mental state that infants subscribe to persons. Thus, it is an important step toward a full-fledged "theory of mind" that does not develop before the age of 4 years (Aschersleben, Hofer, & Jovanovic, in press; Wellmann, Phillips, Dunphy-Lelii, & Lalonde, 2004).

Various studies were able to show that already in their second year of life, infants develop a sophisticated understanding of other persons' actions and their corresponding mental states. In his seminal study, Meltzoff (1995) showed that 18-month-old infants who observed a model trying but failing to achieve the end result of a target action (e.g., to pull apart a dumbbell) produced about as many target actions as infants who observed a successful demonstration. Instead of just copying the surface features of the failed attempts, infants completed the observed actions, indicating that at the age of 18 months, infants are already able to infer the goals of actions performed by other persons (see also Bellagamba & Tomasello, 1999).

At the age of 14 months, infants are able to evaluate whether an action was made on purpose. Carpenter, Akhtar, and Tomasello (1998) showed infants different actions and marked them vocally as accidental ("Whoops!") or intentional ("There!"). Infants took into account whether the modeled action was done on purpose or by accident and imitated more actions that were marked as intentional. Gergely, Bekkering, and Király (2002) demonstrated that 14-month-olds also encode situational constraints that may force the model to choose a certain action. The infants imitated seemingly irrational actions (like touching a box with the head to produce a light; Meltzoff, 1988) only when the model's hands were free during demonstration. When the model's hands were occupied, most infants used their hands to touch the box and make the light appear, indicating that they considered this action to be the more rational alternative.

By the second year of life, children achieve a quite sophisticated level of knowledge about other persons' actions. They understand intentional actions, distinguish between intentional and nonintentional actions, and infer action goals from other people's actions. At the beginning of the second year of life, infants seem to pass a transition phase between the understanding of goals as end states of actions in a nonmentalistic manner and the interpretation of action goals in a mentalistic way (Aschersleben, 2006, 2007). The understanding of actions as goal directed is an important milestone on the way to the mentalistic understanding of intentions and can already be observed in the first year of life. However, it is important to note that although the goal of an action can be interpreted in the sense of an intention preceding that action, in the first year of life reasoning about goals is usually meant in a nonmentalistic way, that is, in terms of perceivable outcomes of actions or end states.

Most studies on action interpretation reveal that goal directedness of a seen action is not interpreted by infants before the age of 9 to 12 months (e.g., Csibra, Gergely, Biro, Koos, & Brockbank, 1999; Gergely, Nadasdy, Csibra, & Biro, 1995; Hofer, Hauf, & Aschersleben, 2005; Johnson, Slaughter, & Carey, 1998; Kuhlmeier, Wynn, & Bloom, 2003; Philipps & Wellman, 2005; Premack & Premack, 1997; Sodian, Schoeppner, & Metz, 2004). For example, Gergely and colleagues (Csibra et al., 1999; Gergely et al., 1995) could show that 9- and 12-month-olds but not 6-month-olds interpret the goal directedness of a computer-animated ball by distinguishing between rational and irrational movement patterns. Twelve-month-old infants can also recognize the underlying positive or negative "valence" of an action; the helping actions of one computer-animated actor toward another are seen as similar to caressing actions, whereas a hindering act is seen as similar to a hitting act (Premack & Premack, 1997). Finally, Kuhlmeier et al. (2003) report evidence suggesting that

12-month-old infants not only recognize goal-related actions but also interpret future actions of an actor on the basis of previously witnessed behavior in another context.

This body of evidence seems to support the notion that infants must first come to act in a goal-directed fashion themselves to achieve an understanding of goal directedness in other people. However, there are arguments against this interpretation both from the theoretical side and from an empirical point of view. First, it has to be noted that most of the previously cited studies used nonhuman agents. There is an ongoing discussion in the literature about the question at what age (and if at all) infants understand the goal directedness of nonhuman actors. Theorists holding a constructivist view assume that infants acquire an understanding of actions as goal directed through gradual experience with particular actions of exclusively *human* agents (Meltzoff, 1995; Poulin-Dubois, Lepage, & Ferland, 1996; Tomasello, 1999; Woodward, 1998). On the contrary, the nativist view assumes that goal attribution is rooted in a specialized system of reasoning that is activated whenever infants encounter entities with appropriate features (e.g., self-propulsion), thus predicting that infants attribute goals to human and inanimate agents from early on (Csibra et al., 1999; Gergely et al., 1995; Johnson, 2000; Leslie, 1995; Premack & Premack, 1997). The available evidence at least leads to the interpretation that infants are not able to interpret actions as goal directed when performed by a nonhuman agent before the age of 9 to 12 months (for a single exception, see Luo & Baillargeon, 2005).

Second, on the empirical side, it has recently been shown that already at the age of 5 to 6 months, infants are able to interpret human actions as goal directed. In her seminal habituation studies, Woodward (1998, 1999) could show that 5- to 6-month-old infants already perceive and interpret human reaching and grasping movements as goal directed. She habituated infants to an event in which a human actor grasped a toy. On subsequent test trials, she recorded the infants' novelty responses (as revealed by looking times) for two different kinds of events. Results indicated that infants demonstrated a stronger novelty response to events in which the actor's goal had changed while preserving the physical properties of the reach as compared to events in which the physical properties of the reach had changed while preserving the same goal (new toy at old location versus old toy at new location). Similarly, Kamewari et al. (2005) demonstrated goal attribution in 6.5-month-olds to human action (as well as to humanoid-robot motion but not to a moving box) by using the paradigm developed by Gergely et al. (1995). Finally, in a recent study, Daum and colleagues (Daum, Prinz, & Aschersleben, 2008) could show that 6-month-old infants even encode the goal of an object-directed uncompleted reaching action.

Infants in Woodward's studies did not show this pattern when the grasping human hand was replaced by an unfamiliar action of a human agent, consisting of dropping the back of the hand on the object or when the grasping human hand was replaced by inanimate agents (e.g., mechanical claws, rods, or occluders). Woodward suggested that infants' understanding of actions as goal directed is restricted to familiarity and experience with human actions; thus, she assumed that infants do not extend this understanding to similar motions of inanimate agents. Recent studies applying a modified Woodward paradigm were able to extend Woodward's argumentation about familiarity by showing that already 6- to 10-month-olds are able to interpret even unfamiliar human actions as goal directed if and only if the action leads to a salient action effect (i.e., a salient change in the object's state; Hofer, Hauf, & Aschersleben, 2007; Hofer et al., 2008; Jovanovic et al., 2007; Király, Jovanovic, Prinz, Aschersleben, & Gergely, 2003). These studies can be interpreted as showing that infants need a clear action effect to identify the goal of an unfamiliar action and, as a consequence, to interpret even new actions as goal directed.

Another important role of action effects is that they help to parse action sequences and to infer intentions of other persons. Action analysis is central to inferring intentions. At natural breakpoints, the links between action and intention are especially strong (Baldwin & Baird, 1999). For example, it has been shown that 10-month-old infants parse observed sequences of continuous everyday actions along intention boundaries (Baldwin, Baird, Saylor, & Clark, 2001). This supports the notion that infants are sensitive to the occurrence of action effects that mark the completion of intentions. Moreover, these studies demonstrate the important role of action effects for infants' perception and interpretation of human actions.

Taken together, there is strong evidence suggesting that infants as young as 6 months of age treat human agents as having goals in mind. This questions the traditional account assuming that infants first have to acquire a specific level of reasoning about their own actions in order to be able to understand other people's actions. However, one has to be very careful in drawing this conclusion, as evidence about infants' ability to perform goal-directed actions relies mostly on imitation studies. In these studies, infants first have to understand and encode the model's action before they can imitate what they have seen. Thus, it might be just for methodological reasons that action understanding seems to come first in development.

From Forward Learning to Backward Computation

Starting with instrumental learning, infants learn the contingencies between self-performed movements and the effects they produce during their first few months of life. According to ideomotor theory, this first phase of acquisition of associations between actions and their ensuing effects results in abstract goal representations in terms of action effects. These abstract representations, which form the basis for infant action knowledge, can then be used both to understand goal-directed actions performed by other persons and to produce own goal-directed actions. Whereas infants are able to interpret other persons' actions as goal directed at the age of 6 months, the production of means–end behavior seems to emerge not before the age of 9 to 12 months.

Does this mean that infants first learn to perceive and understand other persons' actions and only then transfer this knowledge to their own self-performed actions? This seems reasonable not only from the state of the art regarding literature on infant action perception and action production but also from the fact that action production—at least as measured by imitative learning—requires not only action–effect knowledge as provided by observational learning but, furthermore, the transfer of the observed action–effect relations to own actions. Thus, an additional step is required that might take some time in development.

However, there are various caveats in this argumentation. First, there are two recent studies suggesting the opposite, that is, that action experience facilitates action perception. Hauf, Aschersleben, and Prinz (2007) found that 9- and 11-month-old infants (but not 7-month-olds) who had first played with a toy later on preferred to watch a video presenting an adult acting on the same object instead of a different one. Sommerville, Woodward, and Needham

(2005) tested 3-month-old infants who first got some experience in object manipulation (wearing "sticky" mittens). These infants focused on the relation between the actor and her goal during a subsequent habituation task, whereas infants without this experience failed. Converging evidence is reported by Sommerville and Woodward (2005) using a means–end task (pulling a cloth to retrieve a toy). Some of the 10-month-olds understood that the initial step of the cloth-pulling sequence was directed toward the ultimate goal of attaining the toy but only if they were able to solve a similar sequence in their own action production. These findings indicate a developmental link between infants' goal-directed action production and their ability to detect such goals in the actions of others.

Second, as already mentioned, evidence about infants' ability to perform goal-directed actions relies mostly on imitation studies with the problem that infants first have to understand and encode the model's action before they can imitate what they have seen. Moreover, action production is constrained by motor development. Especially in the first year of life, the range of possible self-performed actions is quite narrow. Thus, it might well be that just for methodological reasons (application of demanding motor tasks or use of imitation tasks), action understanding seems to come first in development. As a consequence, to decide the question about the direction of influence between the two aspects of action control, new paradigms are required in which these two aspects are studied within the same infants using rather simple actions, that can be applied in both action perception and action production tasks (similarly to what Sommerville and Woodward, 2005, did but probably at younger ages). From the point of view of theories assuming a common representational level for own and other people's actions, all kinds of influences are feasible, even that both aspects of action control develop independently as soon as the abstract representations of actions are established.

Task Control

In a previous section, we described research on the question as to how the mechanisms underlying action control unfold during early development in infancy. In particular, we discussed findings suggesting that the acquisition of action knowledge (i.e., learning of action–effect contingencies) can become dependent on the situational context (e.g., Elsner & Aschersleben, 2003). The notion of context refers to features of the situation that serve as a cue to trigger goal-directed action. Importantly, the developmental perspective on action control can be viewed as a reconstruction of the issue of action control as a basic learning problem, relating actions to situational contexts.

In cognitive accounts of action control, the term "context" is often used to refer to the behavioral task in which a given action is to be performed. The mental representation of task context has also been termed "task set." The notion of task set has a long tradition in psychology (Ach, 1910), but only recently has there been a renewed interest in task set as a major determinant of action in variable and changing situations (Monsell, 2003). In view of the preceding sections, a task set can be defined as context-specific configuration of action knowledge; that is, it determines the currently relevant subset of action–effect contingencies that are part of the available general action knowledge.

In the psychological laboratory, task sets are typically adopted on the basis of some form of explicit task instructions (e.g., "please read these words"). Evidently, the existence of a task set is the precondition to observe the phenomena of action induction and interference as described previously.

However, in single-task situations, it is not possible to study the influence of task set directly because the task set supposedly remains constant. The present section aims to describe recent research on task set.

The exploration of task set requires experimental situations in which subjects need to select a task set in the face of potentially competing task sets. To this end, multitask paradigms are a viable avenue to explore the processes and representations underlying task set. One of these paradigms is the dual-task paradigm (e.g., Pashler, 2000), in which processing of two tasks overlaps in time. However, despite some recent developments in this paradigm suggesting that it can be useful to study processes related to task set (e.g., Koch & Rumiati, 2006; Luria & Meiran, 2003; Schuch & Koch, 2004), here we focus on models and findings based on research using task switching, which is currently the most frequently used paradigm to investigate the mechanisms underlying task-set control (Monsell, 2003).

First, we briefly introduce the task-switching methodology to lay the ground for describing the currently pertinent theoretical frameworks of task-set control. Then, we discuss relevant empirical findings to illustrate how action is modulated by task set.

Task-Set Switching

In task-switching studies, the individual tasks are usually simple. Unlike tasks such as coffee making, which requires a sequence of actions to accomplish the task goal, cognitive psychology typically uses tasks in which the goal is accomplished by performing a single action. For example, such a task may be to name the color of a visually presented stimulus. If this stimulus happens to be a word, an alternate task may be to read the word aloud. Word reading with such ambiguous, "bivalent" stimuli is typically more dominant than color naming (Stroop, 1935). Therefore, performing color naming instead of word reading with ambiguous stimuli requires a strong task set. The rationale underlying task-switching studies is to explore the processing dynamics of rapid sequential selections of task sets.

Early studies (e.g., Jersild, 1927) compared performance in single-task blocks (e.g., AAAA) with that in mixed blocks, in which two tasks alternate (e.g., ABAB), and found "alternation costs." More recent studies used mixed blocks containing also task repetitions. Regardless of the specific experimental procedure, task switches typically result in worse performance than task repetitions, indicating "switch costs" (for reviews, see Allport & Wylie, 1999; Monsell, 2003).

Costs when switching tasks are a ubiquitous phenomenon. Most studies had subjects switch between tasks that differ in stimulus categories, and a wide range of different tasks have been used so far. However, similar switch costs can be observed when the "input side" of the tasks remain unchanged and processing requirements differ in terms of output modality only (e.g., manual versus pedal responses; Philipp & Koch, 2005). Thus, switch costs arise whenever subjects had to switch a processing component (no matter whether "early" or "late" in the cascade of cognitive processes) that needs to be specified in the task set. Thus, the selection and implementation of a task set is clearly essential for endowing behavior with the flexibility to act successfully in a dynamic and variable environment.

Theoretical Frameworks for Task-Set Control

A variety of theoretical accounts of task-set control have been proposed. A major difference between these accounts refers to the issue of whether switching tasks requires an "executive" control mechanism that operates exclusively in case of a task switch.

There is a class of accounts that propose the existence of such an executive mechanism, such as "task-set reconfiguration" (Goschke, 2000; Meiran, 1996; Rogers & Monsell, 1995) or "goal shifting" (Rubinstein, Meyer, & Evans, 2001). Viewed in this theoretical framework, one obvious and attractive possibility is that switch costs provide a "direct" measure of the duration of the hypothesized task-set reconfiguration process (for a discussion, cf. Rogers & Monsell, 1995).

Evidence for reconfiguration accounts comes from studies manipulating the time available for preparation of task switches. For example, Rogers and Monsell (1995) used a predictable sequence of tasks (*alternating-runs procedure,* e.g., AABB) and manipulated the response–stimulus interval (RSI). Because the task sequence was predictable, the RSI can arguably be used for task preparation (for a discussion, cf. Koch, 2003). Rogers and Monsell found significantly reduced switch costs with prolonged RSI. Converging evidence comes from studies conducted by Meiran and colleagues. Meiran (1996; Meiran, Chorev, & Sapir, 2000), however, argued that manipulations of RSI allow not only for active preparation of task set but also for "passive" decay of the preceding set, which would also result in reduced switch costs. To disentangle these two hypothesized processes, Meiran used unpredictable task sequences but provided explicit task cues in each individual trial (see also Sudevan & Taylor, 1987). This so-called *explicit cuing procedure* allows one to manipulate the cue–target interval (CTI) independently from the response–cue interval (RCI). Such studies showed that switch costs are reduced with long RCIs, suggesting that task sets indeed decay over time to some degree (Altmann, 2005; Gade & Koch, 2005; Koch, 2001; Koch & Allport, 2006; Meiran et al., 2000; Sohn & Anderson, 2001). However, these studies also found

that switch costs are reduced with long CTIs (see, e.g., Meiran et al., 2000), nicely confirming Rogers and Monsell's (1995) proposal that task sets can be selected and prepared in advance.

Importantly, however, preparation was not complete in almost all the studies, and there remained substantial "residual" switch costs (Allport, Styles, & Hsieh, 1994; De Jong, 2000; Hübner, Futterer, & Steinhauser, 2001; Nieuwenhuis & Monsell, 2002). The finding of residual switch costs and other findings described further later in this chapter are taken as supporting the other, alternative class of theoretical framework. This framework proposes that there is no specific "reconfiguration" mechanism but only a general set-selection or goal-setting process that operates both in switch and in repetition trials, albeit at varying degrees of effectiveness that are determined by differential amounts of interference in switch and repetition trials (Koch, 2005). Accordingly, switch costs are attributed to a prolongation of the duration of task-specific processes such as response selection (Allport & Wylie, 1999). For example, Allport et al. (1994) suggested that switch costs simply reflect proactive interference on the level of task sets—a slowing of response selection produced by persisting activation of the previously implemented set or persisting inhibition of the intended new set (see also Gilbert & Shallice, 2002).

Current theorizing suggests that "switch cost" is not a unitary construct and that several processes contribute to it (Monsell, 2003). Most current researchers endorse some or other variant of a whole family of theories postulating two functionally different levels of task control. One initial set-selection level can be termed goal setting, or configuration, and serves to "tune" the system to process stimuli according to a new task goal ("biased competition"; cf. Duncan, Humphreys, & Ward, 1997;

Miller, 2000; Miller & Cohen, 2001; see also Koch & Allport, 2006). The other level can be broadly subsumed under the label of "task implementation," which refers to a variety of processes that subserve current task performance but that are also responsible for producing proactive interference in a subsequent task switch. We now describe relevant empirical findings.

Empirical Findings Related to Task-Set Switching

We have already described findings related to task-set preparation. In this section, we describe a set of further findings. Most of these findings relate to phenomena that appear to be more readily explained by accounts assuming that switch costs represent interference effects rather than effects of "executive" control.

Exogenous, Stimulus-Based Priming of Task Set

One level on which task-set interference occurs is related to stimulus processing. For example, Rogers and Monsell (1995) had subjects switch between a numerical parity judgment task (odd versus even) and a letter judgment task (consonant versus vowel) using bivalent stimuli such as "G4." The stimulus categories in both tasks were assigned (by instruction) to response keys in such a way that both stimulus attributes were mapped onto the same response ("congruent") or to different responses ("incongruent"). When comparing performance with congruent stimuli with that of "neutral" stimuli (e.g., G#), for which the task-irrelevant attribute was not mapped to a response, Rogers and Monsell observed higher RTs for congruent than for neutral stimuli. Because there should be redundant response activation for congruent stimuli, increased RT for such stimuli relative to neutral stimuli suggests a process of stimulus-based reactivation of the competing

task set, giving rise to interference on the level of task sets. Allport and Wylie (2000) confirmed this observation. They had subjects switch between color naming and word reading, using compound color-word Stroop stimuli that were always "incongruent" (such as the word GREEN presented in the color blue). In Allport and Wylie's (2000) experiment 5, some color words were uniquely associated with the word-reading task, whereas the remaining color words occurred in both tasks. Allport and Wylie found that switch costs in the word-reading task were significantly greater with color words primed by their occurrence in the competing, color-naming task than with color words that had not appeared in the context of the color-naming task. This finding has been replicated by Waszak, Hommel, and Allport (2003) using picture-word Stroop stimuli.

Note, however, that the stimulus-specific priming effect reported by Allport and Wylie (2000) could have been due to S-R priming because incongruent stimuli are associated not only with the competing task but also with the competing response. To disentangle the role of task versus response priming, Koch and Allport (2006) had subjects practice the tasks with stimuli that were uniquely mapped to only one of the two tasks. Then this stimulus-task mapping was reversed. If practicing the tasks resulted in establishing associations between stimulus codes and task sets, then reversing the mapping should create strong interference because the stimuli would associatively activate the incorrect, now competing task set. In fact, RT in general and switch costs in particular were significantly increased after the mapping reversal. Importantly, this was observed even for congruent stimuli, for which response priming could have played no role because the S-R relation remained unchanged by the mapping reversal (see also Waszak et al., 2003).

A further test of this "exogenous" priming component in task switching was provided by Rubin and Koch (2006). They used bivalent stimuli and included a task-irrelevant color as a third stimulus feature. This irrelevant stimulus feature was correlated with the correct task but was not mapped to any response. After practice, this correlation was reversed, which indeed resulted in transiently increased switch costs. This result strongly suggests that extraneous features of the stimulus situation that thus form part of the situational, "episodic" context of task processing can come to be associated with task sets and can trigger them in a completely involuntary way (see also Koch, Prinz, & Allport, 2005).

It has been speculated that this kind of stimulus-based priming of tasks is largely responsible for residual switch costs (Allport & Wylie, 2000; Rogers & Monsell, 1995; Waszak et al., 2003). However, recent studies found that this priming effect is markedly reduced or even eliminated with long preparation intervals (Koch & Allport, 2006; Rubin & Koch, 2006), suggesting that this process is not responsible for residual switch costs. What, then, might be the basis of residual switch costs?

To explain residual switch costs, Meiran (2000a, 2000b) suggested that there are two separable components of task set, which he termed "stimulus set" and "response set." According to this distinction, preparation effects influence mainly stimulus set. Stimulus set refers to the type of input processing, including perceptual "filter settings" (or "biases") and the task-relevant stimulus categories. Given that preparation interacts with stimulus priming of tasks, it appears likely that this kind of priming is actually related to stimulus set (cf. Koch & Allport, 2006). In contrast, the likely source of residual switch costs is related to the second component of task set, response set, which is described next.

Response-Related Components of Switch Costs

The notion of "response set" refers to the task-specific stimulus and response categories that are assigned to the physical responses (e.g., manual key presses). For example, in a color discrimination task, a right key press could code a color attribute (e.g., blue), whereas the same key press could code a shape attribute (e.g., curved) in the context of a shape task. That is, one and the same response can be associated with two different "response meanings" (Schuch & Koch, 2003). According to Meiran (2000b), the process of response recoding, that is, the internal reweighting of the sets of response meanings, is not amenable to preparation and is thus the main source of residual switch costs. Thus, response codes remain biased (or weighted) for one task even if the subject prepares a different task, giving rise to a kind of "inertia" (Allport et al., 1994) on the level of response set.

According to an account proposed by Schuch and Koch (2003; Koch & Philipp, 2005), the response set persists and interferes when switching the task in subsequent trials because then the response set needs to be readjusted during the process of response selection. Evidence for this kind of response-related carryover in task switching came from studies using a go/no-go methodology. For example, using explicitly cued task switching, Koch and Philipp (2005) introduced an auditory go/no-go signal (high versus low tone) simultaneous with onset of the imperative task stimulus. The authors found cue-based task preparation effects in go trials. This finding clearly indicated that subjects prepared the task also in no-go trials because the sequence of go versus no-go trials was entirely unpredictable. However, switch costs were strongly reduced after no-go trials. This reduction suggests that preparation alone is not sufficient to result in switch costs (but see

Kleinsorge, Gajewski, & Heuer, 2005). Rather, the reweighting (or recoding) of response codes during the response process appears to be responsible for the carryover that produces residual switch costs (Schuch & Koch, 2003). This response-based account of residual switch costs was recently supported by studies using a variant of the go/no-go paradigm (i.e., the stop-signal paradigm) that also found no switch costs when no response was executed in the preceding trial (Philipp, Jolicoeur, Falkenstein, & Koch, 2007; Verbruggen, Liefooghe, Szmalec, & Vandierendonck, 2005; Verbruggen, Liefooghe, & Vandierendonck, 2006).

Carryover, Switch Cost Asymmetries, and Inhibitory Processes

A likely mechanism to explain the response-related carryover responsible for residual switch costs is persisting inhibition of the upcoming task. This explanation is based mainly on the observation of switch-cost asymmetries (for a review, see Monsell, Yeung, & Azuma, 2000). For example, using a digit-naming task, Meuter and Allport (1999) had subjects switch between their first and second language (L1 and L2, respectively). Switch costs were significantly larger when switching from L2 to L1 than vice versa. This asymmetry in switch costs could be explained by assuming that the "stronger" (or more dominant) L1 interferes more strongly with performing the naming task in the nondominant L2, requiring strong inhibition of L1. This inhibition persists and slows down performance when subjects switch back to L1 (cf. Costa & Santesteban, 2004; Green, 1998; Philipp, Gade, & Koch, 2007). Likewise, in Stroop tasks, switch costs are typically larger for the dominant word-reading task as compared to color naming, suggesting an explanation in terms of persisting inhibition (Allport et al., 1994; Masson, Bub,

Woodward, & Chan, 2003), similar to that of the findings in language switching.

However, it is possible to account for these findings by assuming strong persisting activation of the preceding task rather than persisting inhibition of the currently required task and that this carryover of activation interferes with selecting and establishing a new task set. To demonstrate unambiguously the role of inhibitory processes in task-set control, Mayr and Keele (2000) developed a new measure of inhibition. They had subjects switch among three tasks and compared performance in n-2 task repetition trials (e.g., ABA) with that of n-2 nonrepetition trials (CBA). Persisting activation would lead to facilitation effects in n-2 repetitions. However, the results indicate n-2 repetition costs, suggesting persisting inhibition of previously abandoned tasks. Using n-2 repetition costs as a measure of relative task inhibition and applying it to language switching, Philipp et al. (2007) were recently able to demonstrate inhibition of competing languages, with the most dominant language (L1) suffering most from inhibition.

To examine the likely functional locus of this inhibitory effect in task control, Schuch and Koch (2003) tested whether n-2 repetition costs occur also following no-go trials, in which no task-specific response is selected and executed. In fact, they found substantial n-2 repetition costs after go trials but only a very small and nonsignificant effect following no-go trials. This finding clearly suggests that response set is an important contributor to n-2 repetition costs (cf. Gade & Koch, 2007; Koch, Gade, & Philipp, 2004). Furthermore, n-2 repetition costs suggest not only the existence of persisting inhibition in task switching but also their likely contribution to residual switch costs (Mayr & Keele, 2000; Schuch & Koch, 2003).

Taken together, the previously mentioned findings provided a substantial database related to the mechanisms involved in task-set control. Yet, so far, the data do not seem to provide the crucial constraints for deciding among competing theoretical accounts. In particular, they do not provide decisive evidence for or against "reconfiguration" views based on the notion of "executive" control. By comparison, the involvement of interference mechanisms in task-set control does not seem to be under dispute.

Current and Future Directions of Research on Task-Set Control

The recent literature offers several mathematically specified models of task-set control that seem to fit well to a subset of the empirical data (e.g., Altmann, 2002; Gilbert & Shallice, 2002; Meiran, 2000; Schneider & Logan, 2005; Yeung & Monsell, 2003a, 2003b). However, currently there is not yet a consensus as to the range of phenomena that can be used for benchmark testing to decide among these competing models. Therefore, to provide crucial empirical constraints for further development of these models, it is important to delineate relevant future research issues. Here we briefly discuss four research issues for which the connection to computationally explicit models still needs to be specified.

First, there is a growing number of studies relating to the neuronal substrate of task control. Generally, these studies point to a crucial role of the prefrontal cortex (PFC) in task control (e.g., Miller & Cohen, 2001). Specifically, a recent meta-analysis suggested that a lateral PFC area close to the junction of the precentral sulcus and the inferior frontal sulcus is implicated in task preparation processes (Derrfuss, Brass, Neumann, & von Cramon, 2005). With regard to task implementation processes, recent research suggests that the right inferior frontal cortex is crucially involved in inhibitory processes in task control (Aron,

Robbins, & Poldrack, 2004). However, current neuroscience studies of task control are still not sufficiently linked to cognitive models and mechanisms so that there remains an important theoretical challenge to bridge this gap in future joint research efforts.

Second, there is a recent line of research exploring processes of online response monitoring. This research employs a different class of experimental paradigm to investigate interference, namely, the so-called flanker paradigm (Eriksen & Eriksen, 1974), to examine processes of "conflict monitoring" (cf. Botvinick, Braver, Barch, Carter, & Cohen, 2001). Monitoring processes have been hardly investigated in task switching so that it is important to relate these two research areas. One potential point of contact is the finding of reduced (or even eliminated) switch costs following no-go trials (e.g., Koch & Philipp, 2005; Philipp et al., 2007). No-go trials do not require response selection, but they prevent processes related to response execution, too. It is thus possible that online monitoring processes during or even after response execution play a crucial but yet largely unexplored role in task switching (see Steinhauser & Hübner, 2006). Moreover, it might well be that these hypothesized monitoring processes are very closely related to those currently examined in the context of research on conflict monitoring. However, this conceptual link still needs to be established empirically.

A third line of research is concerned with monitoring processes on a different level. In particular, there is a long tradition assuming that action is monitored and controlled on the basis of verbal self-instructions (Luria, 1961; Wygotski, 1934/1969; see also Goschke, 2000). However, verbal mediation of task-set control has been explored in only a few studies so far. For example, Miyake, Emerson, Padilla, and Ahn (2004) used explicitly cued task switching and, in addition, had subjects perform secondary tasks. These authors found that articulatory suppression, which can be assumed to interfere with verbal (and subvocal) self-instruction, strongly increases switch costs, whereas equally demanding secondary tasks do not affect switch costs if these tasks do not require active vocal production (see also Emerson & Miyake, 2003; Goschke, 2000). This line of research suggests that there is a level of monitoring and control that is not yet adequately captured in any of the previously mentioned models of task-set control.

The final issue to be discussed here is "inversely" related to the previous issue of verbal mediation, which is a quite "high" level of control. This final issue is concerned with the question as to whether successful action in task-switching situations can be explained more adequately entirely on the basis of elementary learning mechanisms (see Chapter 19). Two-process models of performance in explicitly cued task switching were recently questioned by Logan and Bundesen (2003), who examined the effect of the change of the task cue independently from the effect of a task switch. This independent examination is usually not possible in the explicitly cued task-switching paradigm because a task switch is strictly associated with a cue switch. To dissociate task switching from cue switching, these authors used a 2:1 mapping of cue to task so that a cue change could still result in a task repetition. Using this method, it was found that there are indeed substantial costs of cue switching even if the associated task remains unchanged and that there are circumstances in which no "true" task-switch costs at all are detectable. This finding suggests that traditionally measured switch costs (i.e., the performance difference between task switches and task repetitions) have a large component that is attributable to processes associated with cue switching.

The processes associated with cue switching are beginning to receive more attention in the task-switching literature (Forstmann, Brass, & Koch, 2007; Mayr & Kliegl, 2003; Schneider & Logan, 2005). Currently, the debate centers around the issue of whether cue processing is just one more out of several already known component processes that contribute to switch costs or whether the issue of cue processing really suggests an account of task-switching performance based on low-level elementary learning mechanisms. Given that task-set control ultimately needs to be explained without referring to an all-knowing omnipotent control "homunculus," it appears advisable to study the learning mechanisms underlying flexible and adaptive behavior very thoroughly before this provocative alternative is prematurely dismissed. In fact, this issue might be a good candidate to bridge the gap to other research traditions, such as to social cognition.

Task Sharing

Typical experiments on action and task control rely on the study of isolated individuals. In this section we take a brief look at a paradigm in which two (or potentially more) individuals share a given task in a division-of-labor mode of operation, each of them taking care of a different aspect of the task. This kind of paradigm allows one to study whether the task set on which each individual's performance relies is limited to the action knowledge required for his or her own share of the task or whether it takes the other individual's share into account as well. This issue has recently been addressed for both spatial and symbolic tasks (Atmaca, Sebanz, Prinz, & Knoblich, in press; Sebanz, Knoblich, & Prinz, 2003).

Consider, for instance, two individuals sharing a spatial Simon task (Sebanz et al., 2003). In this task a color cue (red versus green) served as the imperative stimulus.

The color cue specified which response key to press (i.e., left versus right). The color cue was superimposed on an irrelevant spatial cue pointing left or right. That cue could be provided, such as by a hand or an arrow pointing in one of the two directions or by a pair of eyes looking to the left or to the right. As a result, there were two types of trials: compatible and incompatible. On compatible trials the irrelevant spatial cue corresponded to the response required by the color cue (left/left or right/right), whereas cues and responses did not correspond on incompatible trials (left/right or right/left).

The task was administered in three settings: standard, partial, and shared. The standard setting required participants to perform the full task. As expected, a marked interference effect was obtained in this setting: Responses were faster and errors less frequent on compatible than on incompatible trials. Results from a third condition with a neutral spatial cue indicated that this difference reflected both facilitation in the compatible and inhibition in the incompatible case. In the partial setting, a go/no-go task was administered. Participants were required to respond to stimuli with one of the two colors (go) and to withhold responses to the other color (no-go). They were seated either left or right in front of the computer screen so that the spatial cue could be pointing either toward them or away from them. Accordingly, one can still distinguish between compatible and incompatible trials on both go and no-go trials. As expected, the interference effect was gone in this setting. This finding indicates that when only a single response is available, that response is not represented in terms of spatial features like relative position.

In the shared setting the full task was divided up among two participants sitting next to each other in front of the screen, one in charge of the red stimuli and the other in charge of the green stimuli. Note that this setting implies, for each participant, exactly the same go/no-go task as before. Still, the shared setting differs from the partial setting in terms of social context. In the shared setting each of the two participants acts as a contributor to a common task to which the other is contributing as well. There are two options here. One is that each individual acts on his or her own, like in the partial task. The other is that each of them forms a kind of a joint task set for the common task in which the other's actions are equivalent to one's own actions. If that were the case, the interference effect that was gone in the partial setting should be back in the shared setting. In that setting the left/right dimension should be reestablished on the response side since one's own position in front of the screen is now either left or right to one's partner's position.

This is exactly what the results showed, indicating that in the shared task setting, two individuals may coordinate their activities such that they act like the two hands of one. Individuals thus treat the other's actions like their own. Of course, they do not do what the other is doing. Rather, they do what their own share of the task requires, but they take the other's share into account as well. Importantly, as has been shown in further experiments, the interference effect is not obtained in the shared setting when one participant is performing the task, whereas the other sitting next to him or her is doing nothing at all. This suggests that the mere presence of another individual is not sufficient to establish interference. Interference between the two requires that one knows or believes that the other is sharing the task.

An even stronger interference effect was obtained when one participant responded selectively to one of the two colors (as before), whereas the other responded to the spatial cue, that is, direction (Sebanz,

Knoblich, & Prinz, 2005). This lends strong support to the notion of shared task sets. When the participant in charge of color knows that the spatial dimension is relevant for the other participant, this acts to increase the spatial interference effect for her own task. This, then, is what task sharing affords: Performance on one's own share is affected by knowing the other's share.

Concluding Remark: Context for Action

This chapter has focused on the cognitive underpinnings of action control and task control in human agents. In our concluding remark we would like to point out how the study of the cognitive machinery for task performance and action control can become part of a more comprehensive framework that combines the cognitive mechanics with the motivational dynamics of action and task control. A framework like this would have to consider human voluntary action as a special kind of reward-driven animal behavior.

One way of broadening the theoretical framework along this line is suggested by the way the term "context" is used in cognitive research and in research on animal learning. It seems that this term is used with two different meanings. First, in the cognitive tradition, the term "context" has been defined as "task" and the corresponding mental representation as "task set." Broadly speaking, a task set determines the currently relevant subset of the action knowledge; that is, it specifies the type of actions that are required in response to certain stimulus situations in order to accomplish a desired behavioral goal.

In contrast, "context" in animal learning usually refers to the whole bundle of background stimuli that constitute the experimental setting in which learning (i.e., conditioning) takes place. Thus, "context" can refer to any stimulus or set of stimuli

associated with successful action in response to a specific trigger stimulus. In his descriptive analysis of behavior, Skinner (1938) termed this trigger stimulus "discriminative stimulus," and he asserted that stimuli can set the "occasion" for successful behavior. However, more recent models of "occasion setting" in the conditioning literature have elaborated the way contextual stimuli are processed (see, e.g., Pearce & Bouton, 2001; Rescorla, 1988; Schmajuk, Lamoureux, & Holland, 1998), suggesting that representations of context can modulate stimulus-specific behavior (for a review, see, e.g., Swartzentruber, 1995).

Some conditioning theories treat context as something that can compete for associative strength with other, more specific stimuli in order to predict some other events, such as biologically important other stimuli, or response outcomes. In that sense, the imperative stimulus would combine with contextual stimuli to form a "compound cue." Other theories posit that contextual stimuli can serve as "occasion setters" to signal the predictive value of certain other stimuli (for a review, see Pearce & Bouton, 2001). That is, conditioning can be associatively linked to context representations, and the function of context is to signal current reward contingencies. If we draw the analogy that such context-based reward contingencies are just the motivational counterparts of more cognitive, or volitional, entities, such as task set–based action–effect contingencies (or action codes), then it should become possible to delineate further points of conceptual contact between animal learning and control of human action and task set, explaining human voluntary action in terms of both cognitive mechanics and motivational dynamics.

In fact, it appears that such contact is already beginning to emerge. Consider, as an example for studying the role of context, an experimental setting in which a predictive stimulus is accompanied by a second stimulus that modulates the predictive value of the other one. One theoretical approach to a setting like this would be that subjects learn "stimulus compounds," that is, that they learn to treat the combination of both stimuli as a new, compound stimulus that requires an adaptive response. This line of reasoning appears to be closely related to Logan and Bundesen's (2003; Schneider & Logan, 2005) approach to explain behavior in explicitly cued task switching. They suggest that subjects learn to respond to the compound of the cue and the imperative task stimulus and that no actual set switching needs to be assumed to explain successful action in task switching. This view competes with more conventional theoretical views that treat explicit task cues as occasion setters so that context representations indicate response–outcome contingencies. This is analogous to the idea that task set is a temporally enduring representation that serves to "bias" the cognitive system to interpret stimuli in a way that allows for successful action in that given situation. This biasing role for context representations in human performance is assumed in many neuroscience models (e.g., Braver & Cohen, 2000; Miller & Cohen, 2001; Ruge et al., 2005; see also Koch & Allport, 2006).

It appears that social cognition research attributes a similar role to social context. Research in social cognition usually refers to the modulating influence of social aspects of a situation on cognitive and behavioral processes (e.g., Wyer & Srull, 1989). Here, the use of the term "context" seems to be located somewhere in between the rather narrow notion of "task" and the broad notion of episodic representations of the entire stimulus situation and behavioral requirements. In fact, Wyer and Gruenfeld (1995) have complained that early social

cognition research has taken the notion of context too narrowly and thus failed to fully recognize the important modulating role of representations of social context on cognition and behavior. More recently, it appears to have become a well-received view that social context can serve to prime the way other people's behavior is interpreted and explained, and this priming can persist and produce "inertia" phenomena akin to those examined in task-switching research (for a review, see Bargh & Ferguson, 2000; Chapters 5 and 9).

Likewise, the cognitive approach to action has begun to include social elements in its empirical investigation of action control, so there is already some evidence for a confluence of theoretical ideas about the contextual causation of cognitive and behavioral processes. Moreover, social-cognitive research on imitative behavior (for a review, see, e.g., Dijksterhuis & Bargh, 2001) has recently strongly benefited from animal research. Animal research has discovered cortical neurons that are responsive to the action intentions of other animals ("mirror neurons"; for a recent review, see Rizzolatti & Craighero, 2004) and are potentially involved both in producing actions and in perceiving actions in others. Thus, we are optimistic that cognitive research, animal learning, and social cognition research have a strong potential for cross-fertilization.

However, despite potential analogies concerning the role of context, the three research areas of animal learning—human action, task set, and social cognition—have not yet been sufficiently connected so far. It would be clearly worthwhile to elaborate in more detail how the use of context representations in cognitive, social-cognitive, and animal learning models relates conceptually to each other. We believe that this elaboration would help deepen our understanding of how human action is controlled in variable social situations and complex task environments.

References

Ach, N. (1910). *Über den Willensakt und das Temperament.* Leipzig: Quelle und Meyer.

Allport, A., Styles, E. A., & Hsieh, S. (1994). Shifting intentional set: Exploring the dynamic control of tasks. In C. Umiltà & M. Moscovitch (Eds.), *Attention and performance XV: Conscious and nonconscious information processing* (pp. 421–452). Cambridge, MA: MIT Press.

Allport, A., & Wylie, G. (1999). Task-switching: Positive and negative priming of task-set. In G. W. Humphreys, J. Duncan, & A.M. Treisman (Eds.), *Attention, space and action: Studies in cognitive neuroscience* (pp. 273–296). Oxford: Oxford University Press.

Allport, A., & Wylie, G. (2000). Selection-for-action in competing (Stroop) tasks: "Task-switching," stimulus-response bindings, and negative priming. In S. Monsell & J. S. Driver (Eds.), *Attention and performance XVIII: Control of cognitive processes* (pp. 35–70). Cambridge, MA: MIT Press.

Altmann, E. M. (2005). Repetition priming in task switching: Do the benefits dissipate? *Psychonomic Bulletin and Review, 12,* 535–540.

Aron, A. R., Robbins, T. W., & Poldrack, R. A. (2004). Inhibition and the right inferior frontal cortex. *Trends in Cognitive Sciences, 8,* 170–177.

Aschersleben, G. (2002). Temporal control of movements in sensorimotor synchronization. *Brain and Cognition, 48,* 66–79.

Aschersleben, G. (2006). Early development of action control. *Psychology Science, 48,* 405–418.

Aschersleben, G. (2007). Handlungswahrnehmung in der frühen Kindheit [Action perception in early infancy]. In L. Kaufmann, H.-C. Nuerk, K. Konrad, & K. Willmes (Eds.), *Kognitive Entwicklungsneuropsychologie* [Developmental cognitive neuroscience] (pp. 287–299). Göttingen: Hogrefe.

Aschersleben, G., Hofer, T., & Jovanovic, B. (in press). The link between infant attention to goal-directed action and later theory of mind abilities. *Developmental Science.*

Atmaca, S., Sebanz, N., Prinz, W., & Knoblich, G. (in press). Action co-representation: The joint SNARC effect. *Social Neuroscience.*

Baldwin, D. A., & Baird, J. A. (1999). Action analysis: A gateway to intentional inference. In P. Rochat (Ed.), *Early social cognition: Understanding others in the first months of life* (pp. 215–240). Mahwah, NJ: Lawrence Erlbaum Associates.

Baldwin, D., Baird, J., Saylor, M. M., & Clark, M. A. (2001). Infants parse dynamic action. *Child Development, 72,* 708–717.

Bargh, J. A., & Ferguson, M. L. (2000). Beyond behaviorism: On the automaticity of higher mental processes. *Psychological Bulletin, 126,* 925–945.

Barr, R., Dowden, A., & Hayne, H. (1996). Developmental changes in deferred imitation by 6- to 24-month-old infants. *Infant Behavior and Development, 19,* 159–170.

Bekkering, H., & Prinz, W. (2002). Goal representations in imitative actions. In K. Dautenhahn & C. L. Nehaniv (Eds.), *Imitation in animals and artifacts* (pp. 555–572). Cambridge, MA: MIT Press.

Bekkering, H., & Wohlschläger, A. (2002). Action perception and imitation: A tutorial. In W. Prinz & B. Hommel (Eds.), *Attention and performance XIX. Common mechanisms in perception and action* (pp. 294–314). Oxford: Oxford University Press.

Bellagamba, F., & Tomasello, M. (1999). Re-enacting intended acts: Comparing 12- and 18-month-olds. *Infant Behavior and Development, 22,* 277–282.

Botvinick, M. M., Braver, T. S., Barch, D. M., Carter, C. S., & Cohen, J. D. (2001). Conflict monitoring and cognitive control. *Psychological Review, 108,* 624–652.

Brass, M., Bekkering, H., & Prinz, W. (2001). Movement observation affects movement execution in a simple response task. *Acta Psychologica, 106,* 3–22.

Brass, M., Bekkering, H., Wohlschläger, A., & Prinz, W. (2000). Compatibility between observed and executed finger movements: Comparing symbolic, spatial, and imitative cues. *Brain and Cognition, 44,* 124–143.

Braver, T. S., & Cohen, J. D. (2000). On the control of control: The role of dopamine in regulating prefrontal function and working memory. In S. Monsell & J. Driver (Eds.), *Attention and performance XVIII: Control of cognitive processes* (pp. 713–737). Cambridge, MA: MIT Press.

Brunswik, E. (1944). Distal focussing of perception: Size constancy in a representative sample of situations. *Psychological Monographs, 56,* 1–49.

Brunswik, E. (1952). Conceptual framework of psychology. In U. Neurath, R. Karnap, & C. Morris (Eds.), *International encyclopedia of united science* (Vol. 1[10]). Chicago: University of Chicago Press.

Brunswik, E. (1955). Representative design and probabilistic theory in a functional psychology. *Psychological Review, 62,* 193–217.

Carpenter, M., Akhtar, N., & Tomasello, M. (1998). Fourteen- through 18-month-old infants differentially imitate intentional and accidental actions. *Infant Behavior and Development, 21,* 315–330.

Carpenter, M., Nagell, K., & Tomasello, M. (1998). Social cognition, joint attention, and communicative competence from 9 to 15 months of age. *Monographs of the Society for Research in Child Development, 63*(4).

Costa, A., & Santesteban, M. (2004). Lexical access in bilingual speech production: Evidence from language switching in highly proficient bilinguals and L2 learners. *Journal of Memory and Language, 50,* 491–511.

Csibra, G., Gergely, G., Biro, S., Koos, O., & Brockbank, M. (1999). Goal attribution without agency cues: The perception of "pure reason" in infancy. *Cognition, 72,* 237–267.

Daum, M. M., Prinz, W., & Aschersleben, G. (2008). Encoding the goal of an object-directed but uncompleted reaching action in 6- and 9-month-old infants. *Developmental Science, 11,* 607–619.

De Casper, A. J., & Fifer, W. P. (1980). Of human bonding: Newborns prefer their mothers' voices. *Science, 208,* 1174–1176.

De Jong, R. (2000). An intention-activation account of residual switch costs. In S. Monsell & J. Driver (Eds.), *Attention and performance XVIII: Control of cognitive processes* (pp. 357–376). Cambridge, MA: MIT Press.

De Maeght, S., & Prinz, W. (2004). Action induction through action observation. *Psychological Research, 68,* 97–114.

Derrfuss, J., Brass, M., Neumann, J., & von Cramon, D. Y. (2005). Involvement of the inferior frontal junction in cognitive control: Meta-analyses of switching and Stroop studies. *Human Brain Mapping, 25,* 22–34.

Dijksterhuis, A., & Bargh, J. A. (2001). The perception-behavior expressway: Automatic effects of social perception on social behavior. In M. P. Zanna (Ed.), *Advances in experimental social psychology* (Vol. 33, pp. 1–40). San Diego, CA: Academic Press.

Duncan, J., Humphreys, G., & Ward, R. (1997). Competitive brain activity in visual attention. *Current Opinion in Neurobiology, 7,* 255–261.

Elsner, B. (2000). *Der Erwerb kognitiver Handlungsrepräsentationen* [The acquisition of cognitive representations of action]. Berlin: Wissenschaftlicher Verlag.

Elsner, B., & Aschersleben, G. (2003). Do I get what you get? Learning about effects of self-performed and observed actions in infants. *Consciousness and Cognition, 12,* 732–751.

Elsner, B., Hauf, P., & Aschersleben, G. (2007). Imitating step by step: A detailed analysis of 9- to 15-month old's reproduction of a three-step action sequence. *Infant Behavior and Development, 30,* 325–335.

Elsner, B., & Hommel, B. (2001). Effect anticipation and action control. *Journal of Experimental Psychology: Human Perception and Performance, 27,* 229–240.

Elsner, B., & Hommel, B. (2004). Contiguity and contingency in action-effect learning. *Psychological Research, 68,* 138–154.

Emerson, M. J., & Miyake, A. (2003). The role of inner speech in task switching: A dual-task investigation. *Journal of Memory and Language, 48,* 148–168.

Eriksen, B. A., & Eriksen, C. W. (1974). Effects of noise letters upon the identification of a target letter in a nonsearch task. *Perception and Psychophysics, 16,* 143–149.

Fitts, P. M. (1964). Perceptual-motor skill learning. In A. W. Melton (Ed.), *Categories of human learning* (pp. 243–285). New York: Academic Press.

Fitts, P. M., & Seeger, C. M. (1953). S-R compatibility: Spatial characteristics of stimulus and response codes. *Journal of Experimental Psychology, 46,* 199–210.

Forstmann, B., Brass, M., & Koch, I. (2007). Methodological and empirical issues when dissociating cue-related from task-related processes in the explicit task-cuing procedure. *Psychological Research, 71,* 393–400.

Frith, C. D., Blakemore, S.-J., & Wolpert, D. M., (2000). Abnormalities in the awareness and control of action. *Philosophical Transactions of the Royal Society London B*(355), 1771–1788.

Gade, M., & Koch, I. (2005). Linking inhibition to activation in the control of task sequences. *Psychonomic Bulletin and Review, 12,* 530–534.

Gade, M., & Koch, I. (2007). The influence of overlapping response sets on task inhibition. *Memory & Cognition, 35,* 603–609.

Gattis, M., Bekkering, H., & Wohlschläger, A. (2002). Goal-directed imitation. In A. W. Meltzoff & W. Prinz (Eds.), *The imitative mind: Development, evolution, and brain bases* (pp. 183–205). Cambridge: Cambridge University Press.

Gergely, G., Bekkering, H., & Király, I. (2002). Rational imitation in preverbal infants. *Nature, 415,* 755.

Gergely, G., Nadasdy, Z., Csibra, G., & Biro, S. (1995). Taking the intentional stance at 12 months of age. *Cognition, 56,* 165–193.

Gilbert, S., & Shallice, T. (2002). Task switching: A PDP model. *Cognitive Psychology, 44,* 297–337.

Gleissner, B., Meltzoff, A. W., & Bekkering, H. (2000). Children's coding of human action: Cognitive factors influencing imitation in 3-year-olds. *Developmental Science, 3,* 405–414.

Gollwitzer, P. M. (1999). Implementation intentions and effective goal pursuit: Strong effects of simple plans. *American Psychologist, 54,* 493–503.

Goschke, T. (2000). Intentional reconfiguration and involuntary persistence in task-set switching. In S. Monsell & J. Driver (Eds.), *Attention and performance XVIII: Control of cognitive processes* (pp. 333–355). Cambridge, MA: MIT Press.

Green, D. W. (1998). Mental control of the bilingual lexico-semantic system. *Bilingualism: Language and Cognition, 1,* 67–81.

Greenwald, A. G. (1970). Sensory feedback mechanisms in performance control: With spatial reference to the ideo-motor mechanism. *Psychological Review, 77,* 73–99.

Greenwald, A. G. (1972). On doing two things at once: Time sharing as a function of ideomotor compatibility. *Journal of Experimental Psychology, 94,* 52–57.

Hauf, P., & Aschersleben, G. (2008). Action-effect anticipation in infant action control. *Psychological Research, 72,* 203–210.

Hauf, P., Aschersleben, G., & Prinz, W. (2007). Baby do, baby see! How action production influences action perception in infants. *Cognitive Development, 22,* 16–32.

Hauf, P., Elsner, B., & Aschersleben, G. (2004). The role of action effects in infant's action control. *Psychological Research, 68,* 115–125.

Hauf, P., & Prinz, W. (2005). The understanding of own and others' actions during infancy. *Interaction Studies, 6,* 429–445.

Heimann, M., & Nilheim, K. (2004). 6-months olds and delayed actions: An early sign of an emerging explicit memory? *Cognitie Creier Comportament, 8,* 249–254.

Hofer, T., Hauf, P., & Aschersleben, G. (2005). Infant's perception of goal-directed actions performed by a mechanical device. *Infant Behavior and Development, 28,* 466–480.

Hofer, T., Hauf, P., & Aschersleben, G. (2007). Infant's perception of goal-directed actions on television. *British Journal of Developmental Psychology, 25,* 485–498.

Hofer, T., Hohenberger, A., Hauf, P., & Aschersleben, G. (2008). The link between maternal interaction style and infant action understanding. *Infant Behavior and Development, 31,* 115–126.

Hommel, B. (1993). Inverting the Simon effect by intention: Determinants of direction and extent of effects of irrelevant spatial information. *Psychological Research, 55,* 270–279.

Hommel, B. (1996). The cognitive representation of action: Automatic integration of perceived action effects. *Psychological Research, 59,* 176–186.

Hommel, B. (2004). Coloring an action: Intending to produce color events eliminates the Stroop effect. *Psychological Research, 68,* 74–90.

Hommel, B., Müsseler, J., Aschersleben, G., & Prinz, W. (2001). The theory of event coding (TEC): A framework for perception and action planning. *Behavioral and Brain Sciences, 24,* 849–878.

Hübner, R., Futterer, T., & Steinhauser, M. (2001). On attentional control as source of residual shift costs: Evidence from two-component task shifts. *Journal of Experimental Psychology: Learning, Memory, and Cognition, 27,* 640–653.

James, W. (1890). *The principles of psychology.* New York: Holt.

Jersild, A. T. (1927). Mental set and shift. *Archives of Psychology* (Whole No. 89).

Johnson, S. (2000). The recognition of mentalistic agents in infancy. *Trends in Cognitive Sciences, 4,* 22–28.

Johnson, S., Slaughter, V., & Carey, S. (1998). Whose gaze will infants follow? The elicitation of gaze-following in 12-month-olds. *Developmental Science, 1,* 233–238.

Jordan, M. I. (1996). Computational aspects of motor control and motor learning. In E. H. Heuer & E. S. Keele (Eds.), *Handbook of perception and action* (pp. 71–118). New York: Academic Press.

Jovanovic, B., Király, I., Elsner, B., Gergely, G., Prinz, W., & Aschersleben, G. (2007). The role of effects for infants' perception of action goals. *Psychologia, 50,* 273–290.

Kamewari, K., Kato, M., Kanda, T., Ishiguro, H., & Hiraki, K. (2005). Six-and-a-half-month-old children positively attribute goals to human action and to humanoid-robot motion. *Cognitive Development, 20,* 303–320.

Kawato, M. (1997). Bidirectional theory approach to consciousness. In I. Masao, Y. Miyashita, & E. T. Rolls (Eds.), *Cognition, computation, and consciousness* (pp. 233–248). New York: Oxford University Press.

Keller, P., & Koch, I. (2006). Exogenous and endogenous response priming in voluntary action. *Advances in Cognitive Psychology, 2,* 269–276.

Keller, P., & Koch, I. (2008). Action planning in sequential skills: Relations to music performance. *Quarterly Journal of Experimental Psychology, 61,* 275–291.

Kelso, J. A. S. (1984). Phase transitions and critical behavior in human bimanual coordination. *American Journal of Physiology, 15,* R1000–R1004.

Király, I., Jovanovic, B., Prinz, W., Aschersleben, G., & Gergely, G. (2003). The early origins of goal attribution in infancy. *Consciousness and Cognition, 12,* 752–769.

Klein, A., Hauf, P., & Aschersleben, G. (2006). The role of action effects in 12-month-olds' action control: A comparison of televised model and live model. *Infant Behavior and Development, 29,* 535–544.

Kleinsorge, T., Gajewski, P., & Heuer, H. (2005). Task sets under reconstruction: Effects of partially incorrect precues. *Quarterly Journal of Experimental Psychology, 58A,* 521–546.

Knuf, L., Aschersleben, G., & Prinz, W. (2001). An analysis of ideomotor action. *Journal of Experimental Psychology: General, 130,* 779–798.

Koch, I. (2001). Automatic and intentional activation of task sets. *Journal of Experimental Psychology: Learning, Memory, and Cognition, 27,* 1474–1486.

Koch, I. (2003). The role of external cues for endogenous advance reconfiguration in task switching. *Psychonomic Bulletin and Review, 10,* 488–492.

Koch, I. (2005). Sequential task predictability in task switching. *Psychonomic Bulletin and Review, 12,* 107–112.

Koch, I., & Allport, A. (2006). Cue-based preparation and stimulus-based priming of tasks in task switching. *Memory and Cognition, 34,* 433–444.

Koch, I., Gade, M., & Philipp, A. (2004). Inhibition of response mode in task switching. *Experimental Psychology, 51,* 52–58.

Koch, I., Keller, P., & Prinz, W. (2004). The ideomotor approach to action control: Implications for skilled performance. *International Journal of Sport and Exercise Psychology, 2,* 362–375.

Koch, I., & Kunde, W. (2002). Verbal response-effect compatibility. *Memory and Cognition, 30,* 1297–1303.

Koch I., & Philipp, A. M. (2005). Effects of response selection on the task repetition benefit in task switching. *Memory and Cognition, 33,* 624–634.

Koch, I., Prinz, W., & Allport, A. (2005). Involuntary retrieval in alphabet-arithmetic tasks: Task-mixing and task-switching costs. *Psychological Research, 69,* 252–261.

Koch, I., & Rumiati, R. I. (2006). Task-set inertia and memory-consolidation bottleneck in dual tasks. *Psychological Research, 70,* 448–458.

Kornblum, S., Hasbroucq, T., & Osman, A. (1990). Dimensional overlap: Cognitive basis for stimulus-response compatibility: A model and taxonomy. *Psychological Review, 97,* 253–270.

Kuhlmeier, V., Wynn, K., & Bloom, P. (2003). Attribution of dispositional states by 12-month-olds. *Psychological Science, 14,* 402–408.

Kunde, W. (2001). Response-effect compatibility in manual choice-reaction tasks. *Journal of Experimental Performance: Human Perception and Performance, 27,* 387–394.

Kunde, W. (2003). Temporal response-effect compatibility. *Psychological Research, 67,* 153–159.

Kunde, W., Koch, I., & Hoffmann, J. (2004). Anticipated action effects affect the selection, initiation, and execution of actions. *Quarterly Journal of Experimental Psychology, 57A,* 87–106.

Leslie, A. M. (1995). A theory of agency. In D. Sperber & D. Premack (Eds.), *Causal cognition: A multidisciplinary debate. Symposia of the Fyssen Foundation* (pp. 121–149). New York: Clarendon Press/Oxford University Press.

Lewin, K. (1926). Untersuchungen zur Handlungs- und Affekt-Psychologie. II. Vorsatz, Wille und Bedürfnis [Intention, will and need]. *Psychologische Forschung, 7,* 330–385.

Logan, G. D., & Bundesen, C. (2003). Clever homunculus: Is there an endogenous act of control in the explicit task cuing procedure? *Journal of Experimental Psychology: Human Perception and Performance, 29,* 575–599.

Lotze, R. H. (1852). *Medicinische Psychologie oder Physiologie der Seele.* Leipzig: Weidmann'sche Buchhandlung.

Luo, Y., & Baillargeon, R. (2005). Can a self-propelled box have a goal? Psychological reasoning in 5-month-old infants. *Psychological Science, 16,* 601–608.

Luria, A. R. (1961). *The role of speech in the regulation of normal and abnormal behavior.* New York: Liveright.

Luria, A. R., & Meiran, N. (2003). Online order control in the psychological refractory period paradigm. *Journal of Experimental Psychology: Human Perception and Performance, 29,* 556–574.

MacKay, D. (1987). *The organisation of perception and action: A theory of language and other cognitive skills*. Berlin: Springer.

Masson, M. E., Bub, D. N., Woodward, T. S., & Chan, J. C. (2003). Modulation of word-reading processes in task switching. *Journal of Experimental Psychology: General, 132*, 400–418.

Mayr, U., & Keele, S. W. (2000). Changing internal constraints on action: The role of backward inhibition. *Journal of Experimental Psychology: General, 129*, 4–26.

Mayr, U., & Kliegl, R. (2003). Differential effects of cue changes and task changes on task-set selection costs. *Journal of Experimental Psychology: Learning, Memory, and Cognition, 29*, 362–372.

Mechsner, F., Kerzel, D., Knoblich, G., & Prinz, W. (2001). Perceptual basis of bimanual coordination. *Nature, 414*, 69–73.

Meiran, N. (1996). Reconfiguration of processing mode prior to task performance. *Journal of Experimental Psychology: Learning, Memory, and Cognition, 22*, 1423–1442.

Meiran, N. (2000a). Modeling cognitive control in task-switching. *Psychological Research, 63*, 234–249.

Meiran, N. (2000b). The reconfiguration of the stimulus task-set and the response task-set during task switching. In S. Monsell & J. Driver (Eds.), *Attention and performance XVIII: Control of cognitive processes* (pp. 377–400). Cambridge, MA: MIT Press.

Meiran, N., Chorev, Z., & Sapir, A. (2000). Component processes in task switching. *Cognitive Psychology, 41*, 211–253.

Meltzoff, A. N. (1988). Infant imitation after a 1-week delay: Long-term memory for novel acts and multiple stimuli. *Developmental Psychology, 24*, 470–476.

Meltzoff, A. N. (1993). The centrality of motor coordination and proprioception in social and cognitive development: From shared actions to shared mind. In G. J. P. Savelsbergh (Ed.), *The development of coordination in infancy* (pp. 463–496). Amsterdam: Free University Press.

Meltzoff, A. N. (1995). Understanding the intentions of others: Re-enactment of intended acts by 18-month-old children. *Developmental Psychology, 31*, 838–850.

Meltzoff, A. N. (2002). Elements of a developmental theory of imitation. In A. Meltzoff & W. Prinz (Eds.), *The imitative mind: Development, evolution and brain bases* (pp. 19–41). New York: Cambridge University Press.

Meuter, R. F. I., & Allport, A. (1999). Bilingual language switching in naming: Asymmetrical costs of language selection. *Journal of Memory and Language, 40*, 25–40.

Miller, E. K. (2000). The prefrontal cortex and cognitive control. *Nature Reviews Neuroscience, 1*, 59–65.

Miller, E. K., & Cohen, J. D. (2001). An integrative theory of prefrontal cortex function. *Annual Review of Neuroscience, 24*, 167–202.

Miyake, A., Emerson, M. J., Padilla, F., & Ahn, J. (2004). Inner speech as a retrieval aid for task goals: The effects of cue type and articulatory suppression in the random task cuing paradigm. *Acta Psychologica, 115*, 123–142.

Monsell, S. (2003). Task switching. *Trends in Cognitive Sciences, 7*, 134–140.

Monsell, S., Yeung, N., & Azuma, R. (2000). Reconfiguration of task-set: Is it easier to switch to the weaker task? *Psychological Research, 63*, 250–264.

Morin, R. E., & Forrin, B. (1962). Mixing of two types of S-R associations in a choice reaction time task. *Journal of Experimental Psychology, 64*, 137–141.

Neisser, U. (1967). *Cognitive psychology*. New York: Appleton-Century-Crofts.

Nieuwenhuis, S., & Monsell, S. (2002). Residual costs in task-switching: Testing the failure-to-engage account. *Psychonomic Bulletin and Review, 9*, 86–92.

Papousek, H. (1967). Experimental studies of appetitional behavior in human newborns and infants. In H. W. Stevenson, E. H. Hess, & H. L. Rheingold (Eds.), *Early behavior: Comparative and developmental approaches* (pp. 249–277). New York: Wiley.

Pashler, H. (2000). Task switching and multitask performance. In S. Monsell & J. Driver (Eds.), *Attention and performance XVIII: Control of cognitive processes* (pp. 277–307). Cambridge, MA: MIT Press.

Pearce, J. P., & Bouton, M. E. (2001). Theories of associative learning in animals. *Annual Reviews of Psychology, 52*, 111–139.

Philipp, A. M., Gade, M., & Koch, I. (2007). Inhibitory processes in language switching: Evidence from switching language-defined response sets. *European Journal of Cognitive Psychology, 19*, 395–416.

Philipp, A. M., & Koch, I. (2005). Switching of response modalities. *Quarterly Journal of Experimental Psychology, 58A*, 1325–1338.

Philipp, A. M., Jolicoeur, P., Falkenstein, M., & Koch, I. (2007). Response selection and response execution in task switching: Evidence from a go-signal paradigm. *Journal of Experimental Psychology: Learning, Memory, & Cognition, 33,* 1062–1075.

Phillips, A., & Wellman, H. M. (2005). Infants' understanding of object-directed action. *Cognition, 98,* 137–155.

Poulin-Dubois, D., Lepage, A., & Ferland, D. (1996). Infants' concept of animacy. *Cognitive Development, 11,* 19–36.

Premack, D., & Premack, A. J. (1997). Infants attribute value +- to the goal-directed actions of self-propelled objects. *Journal of Cognitive Neuroscience, 9,* 848–856.

Prinz, W. (1984). Modes of linkage between perception and action. In W. Prinz & A.-F. Sanders (Eds.), *Cognition and motor processes* (pp. 185–193). Berlin: Springer.

Prinz, W. (1987). Ideomotor action. In H. Heuer & A.-F. Sanders (Eds.), *Perspectives on perception and action* (pp. 47–76). Hillsdale, NJ: Lawrence Erlbaum Associates.

Prinz, W. (1990). A common coding approach to perception and action. In O. Neumann & W. Prinz (Eds.), *Relationships between perception and action: Current approaches* (pp. 167–201). Berlin: Springer.

Prinz, W. (1992). Why don't we perceive our brain states? *European Journal of Cognitive Psychology, 4,* 1–20.

Prinz, W. (1997). Perception and action planning. *European Journal of Cognitive Psychology, 9,* 129–154.

Prinz, W., De Maeght, S., & Knuf, L. (2004). Intention in action. In G. W. Humphreys & M. J. Riddoch (Eds.), *Attention in action: Advances from cognitive neuroscience* (pp. 93–107). Hove: Psychology Press.

Proctor, R., & Vu, K.-P. L. (2002). Eliminating, magnifying, and reversing spatial compatibility effects with mixed location-relevant and irrelevant trials. In W. Prinz & B. Hommel (Eds.), *Common mechanisms in perception and action* (Attention and Performance, Vol. XIX) (pp. 443–474). Oxford: Oxford University Press.

Rescorla, R. A. (1988). Pavlovian conditioning: It's not what you think it is. *American Psychologist, 43,* 151–160.

Rizzolatti, G., & Craighero, L. (2004). The mirror-neuron system. *Annual Review of Neuroscience, 27,* 169–192.

Rochat, P., & Morgan, R. (1998). Two functional orientations of self-exploration in infancy. *British Journal of Developmental Psychology, 16,* 139–154.

Rogers, R. D., & Monsell, S. (1995). Costs of a predictable switch between simple cognitive tasks. *Journal of Experimental Psychology: General, 124,* 207–231.

Rovee, C. K., & Rovee, D. T. (1969). Conjugate reinforcement of infants' exploratory behavior. *Journal of Experimental Child Psychology, 8,* 33–39.

Rovee-Collier, C. & Shyi, G. (1993). A functional and cognitive analysis of infant long-term retention. In M. L. Howe, C. J. Brainerd, & V. F. Reyna (Eds.), *Development of long-term retention.* New York: Springer, 3–55.

Rubin, O., & Koch, I. (2006). Exogenous influences on task-set activation in task switching. *Quarterly Journal of Experimental Psychology, 59A,* 1033–1046.

Rubinstein, J., Meyer, D. E., & Evans, J. E. (2001). Executive control of cognitive processes in task switching. *Journal of Experimental Psychology: Human Perception and Performance, 27,* 763–797.

Ruge, H., Brass, M., Koch, I., Rubin, O., Meiran, N. & von Cramon, D. Y. (2005). Advance preparation and stimulus-induced interference in cued task switching: Further insights from BOLD fMRI. *Neuropsychologia, 43,* 340–355.

Schmajuk, N. A., Lamoureux, J. A., & Holland, P. C. (1998). Occasion setting: A neural network framework. *Psychological Review, 105,* 3–32.

Schneider, D., & Logan, G. D. (2005). Modelling task switching without switching tasks: A short-term priming account of explicitly cued performance. *Journal of Experimental Psychology: General, 134,* 343–367.

Schuch, S., & Koch, I. (2003). The role of response selection for inhibition of task sets in task shifting. *Journal of Experimental Psychology: Human Perception and Performance, 29,* 92–105.

Schuch, S., & Koch, I. (2004). The costs of changing the representation of action: Response repetition and response-response compatibility in dual tasks. *Journal of Experimental Psychology: Human Perception and Performance, 30,* 566–582.

Sebanz, N., Knoblich, G., & Prinz, W. (2003). Representing others' actions: Just like one's own? *Cognition, 88,* B11–B21.

Sebanz, N., Knoblich, G., & Prinz, W. (2005). How to share a task: Co-representing stimulus-response mappings. *Journal for Experimental Psychology: Human Perception and Performance, 31,* 1234–1246.

Simon, J. R. (1990). The effects of an irrelevant directional cue on human information processing. In R. W. Proctor, & T. G. Reeve (Eds.), *Stimulus-*

response compatibility: An integrated perspective (pp. 31–86). Amsterdam: North-Holland.

Simon, J. R., & Rudell, A. P. (1967). Auditory S-R compatibility: The effect of an irrelevant cue on information processing. *Journal of Applied Psychology, 51,* 300–304.

Skinner, B. F. (1938). *The behavior of organisms.* New York: Appleton-Century-Crofts.

Sodian, B., Schoeppner, B., & Metz, U. (2004). Do infants apply the principle of rational action to human agents? *Infant Behavior and Development, 27,* 31–41.

Sohn, M.-H., & Anderson, J. R. (2001). Task preparation and task repetition: Two-component model of task switching. *Journal of Experimental Psychology: General, 130,* 764–778.

Sommerville, J. A., & Woodward, A. L. (2005). Pulling out the intentional structure of action: The relation between action processing and action production in infancy. *Cognition, 95,* 1–30.

Sommerville, J. A., Woodward, A. L., & Needham, A. (2005). Action experience alters 3-month-old infants' perception of others' actions. *Cognition, 96,* B1–B11.

Steinhauser, M., & Hübner, R. (2006). Response-based strengthening in task-shifting: Evidence from shift effects produced by errors. *Journal of Experimental Psychology: Human Perception and Performance, 32,* 517–534.

Stock, A., & Hoffmann, J. (2002). Intentional fixation of behavioral learning, or how R-O learning blocks S-R learning. *European Journal of Cognitive Psychology, 14,* 127–153.

Stränger, J., & Hommel, B. (1995). The perception of action and movement. In W. Prinz & B. Bridgeman (Eds.), *Handbook of perception and action: Vol. I. Perception* (pp. 397–451). London: Academic Press.

Stroop, J. R. (1935). Studies of interference in serial verbal reactions. *Journal of Experimental Psychology, 28,* 643–662.

Stürmer, B., Aschersleben, G., & Prinz, W. (2000). Correspondence effects with manual gestures and postures: A study of imitation. *Journal of Experimental Psychology: Human Perception and Performance, 26,* 1746–1759.

Sudevan, P., & Taylor, D. A. (1987). The cueing and priming of cognitive operations. *Journal of Experimental Psychology: Human Perception and Performance, 13,* 89–103.

Swartzentruber, D. (1995). Modulatory mechanisms in Pavlovian conditioning. *Animal Learning and Behavior, 23,* 123–143.

Thorndike, E. L. (1913). Ideo-motor action. *Psychological Review, 20,* 91–106.

Tomasello, M. (1995). Joint attention as social cognition. In C. Moore & P. J. Dunham (Eds.), *Joint attention: Its origins and role in development* (pp. 103–130). Hillsdale, NJ: Lawrence Erlbaum Associates.

Tomasello, M. (1999). Having intentions, understanding intentions, and understanding communicative intentions. In P. D. Zelazo, J. W. Astington, & D. R. Olson (Eds.), *Developing theories of intention: Social understanding and self-control* (pp. 63–75). Mahwah, NJ: Lawrence Erlbaum Associates.

Van Duren, L., & Sanders, A. F. (1988). On the robustness of the additive factors stage structure in blocked and mixed choice reaction designs. *Acta Psychologica, 69,* 83–94.

Verbruggen, F., Liefooghe, B., Szmalec, A., & Vandierendonck, A. (2005). Inhibiting responses when switching: Does it matter? *Experimental Psychology, 52,* 125–130.

Verbruggen, F., Liefooghe, B., & Vandierendonck, A. (2006). Selective stopping in task switching: The role of response selection and response execution. *Experimental Psychology, 53,* 48–57.

Waszak, F., Hommel, B., & Allport, A. (2003). Task-switching and long-term priming: Role of episodic S-R bindings in task-shift costs. *Cognitive Psychology, 46,* 361–413.

Wegner, D. M., & Vallacher, R. R. (1986). Action identification. In R. M. Sorrentino (Ed.), *Handbook of motivation and cognition: Foundations of social behavior* (pp. 550–582). New York: Guilford Press.

Wellmann, H. M., Phillips, A., Dunphy-Lelii, S., & Lalonde, N. (2004). Infant social attention predicts pre-school social cognition. *Developmental Science, 7,* 283–288.

Willatts, P. (1999). Development of means-end behavior in young infants: Pulling a support to retrieve a distant object. *Developmental Psychology, 35,* 651–667.

Wolpert, D. M. (1997). Computational approaches to motor control. *Trends in Cognitive Sciences, 1,* 209–216.

Woodward, A. L. (1998). Infants selectively encode the goal object of an actor's reach. *Cognition, 69,* 1–34.

Woodward, A. L. (1999). Infant's ability to distinguish between purposeful and non-purposeful behaviors. *Infant Behavior and Development, 22,* 145–160.

Wyer, R. S., & Gruenfeld, D. H. (1995). Information processing in social contexts: Implications for social memory and judgment. In M. P. Zanna (Ed.), *Advances in experimental social psychology* (Vol. 27, pp. 49–91). San Diego, CA: Academic Press.

Wyer, R. S., & Srull, T. K. (1989). *Memory and cognition in its social context.* Hillsdale, NJ: Lawrence Erlbaum Associates.

Wygotski, L. S. (1969). *Denken und Sprechen* [Thought and language]. Stuttgart: S. Fischer Verlag. (Original work published 1934)

Yeung, N., & Monsell, S. (2003a). The effects of recent practice on task switching. *Journal of Experimental Psychology: Human Perception and Performance, 29,* 919–936.

Yeung, N., & Monsell, S. (2003b). Switching between tasks of unequal familiarity: The role of stimulus-attribute and response-set selection. *Journal of Experimental Psychology: Human Perception and Performance, 29,* 455–469.

The Inhibition of Unwanted Actions

Clayton E. Curtis *and* Mark D'Esposito

Abstract

This chapter discusses key studies of inhibitory control, focusing on cognitive neuroscience studies. It provides insights into the potential neural mechanisms that may underlie our ability to inhibit unwanted action. Based on these findings, it is argued that inhibitory control is best modeled as the process by which we select the best response among the competing responses, including not responding at all. One implication of this model is that no single area of the brain is specialized for inhibiting all unwanted actions.

Kewords: inhibitory control, cognitive neuroscience, response, goal-directed behavior

Inhibitory control is one of many high-level cognitive processes that fall under the rubric of "executive" or "cognitive" control. Successfully withholding an overlearned, prepotent, or planned motor response is a critical demonstration of inhibitory control. Here we briefly review key studies of inhibitory control with a special emphasis on cognitive neuroscience studies. We aim to provide some insights into the potential neural mechanisms that may underlie our ability to inhibit unwanted action. Leveraged with these findings, we argue that inhibitory control, like voluntary control more generally, is best modeled as the process by which we select the best response among the competing responses, including not responding at all. One implication of this model is that no single area of the brain is specialized for inhibiting all unwanted actions.

All animals are endowed with the capability of motor behavior. With that endowment they are faced with the continuous responsibility of selecting certain courses of action over others in order to ascertain their goals. A distinguishing feature of the higher animal species, like primates, is their exceptional ability to voluntarily control their actions. Voluntary control is necessary when an optimal motor response is uncertain or when a competing motor response must be overcome. A special case of voluntary control, or the more general term "executive" or "cognitive" control, is the ability to inhibit an unwanted action. Successfully withholding an overlearned, prepotent, or planned motor response is a critical demonstration of inhibitory control. Indeed, the ecological validity of such a construct is high, and we can all think of a multitude of instances when we have had to inhibit our behavior. In social situations, our gaze at any given instant communicates to others information about our internal thoughts. For example, you might find it prudent to inhibit your glances toward an attractive person sitting at an adjacent table especially if you are dining with your partner. Here we briefly review key cognitive neuroscience studies that have investigated the neural responses of monkeys and humans performing tasks that are laboratory analogs of everyday response inhibition. We aim to provide some insights into the potential neural mechanisms that may underlie our ability to inhibit unwanted action.

Laboratory Tests of Inhibition

A variety of tasks are used to study inhibitory control in some form or another pitting an overlearned, stereotyped, prepotent, or naturally compatible response against a response contingent upon a novel or unnatural mapping. For example, the Stroop task (Stroop, 1935) requires subjects to say aloud the font color of a word instead of reading the word itself (e.g., say "blue" if presented with the word "RED" printed in a blue font). Vocal response times and errors increase when subjects have to say the font color compared to when they have to read the word. The Eriksen flanker task (Eriksen & Eriksen, 1974) requires subjects to press a left or right button if a centrally presented arrow stimulus is pointed to the left or right, respectively. If the central target arrow stimulus is flanked by arrows that are incongruent in direction with the target (e.g., "<<<<><<<<" indicates respond right), response times and errors increase. The Simon task (Simon, 1969) requires subjects to press a left or right button depending on the color of a stimulus cue. Response times and errors increase when the stimulus is presented to the side that is opposite to the button with which the

stimulus is associated (e.g., if ● = left button and ○ = right button, response times will be slower when ● compared to ○ is presented on the right side of the display). The Stroop task requires inhibition of the overlearned behavior of reading text. The Eriksen flanker task requires inhibiting the incompatible and competing response indicated by the flanking distracters. The Simon task requires inhibiting the button press that is congruent with the spatial position of the stimulus cue.

Although these classic tasks have a long prominent history in cognitive psychology studies of inhibitory control, for a variety of reasons and with a few notable exceptions they have not been used as regularly in cognitive neuroscience studies. Here we focus on three tasks that have strong response inhibition demands and that have been widely and successfully used to study the neural correlates of response inhibition: antisaccade tasks, go/no-go tasks, and stop-signal tasks (Figure 3.1).

We first describe each task, including the similarities and differences, and then we delve into the basic research into the neural mechanisms supporting inhibition in each of these tasks and finally draw some conclusions across the studies using the various tasks.

Antisaccade Task

In an antisaccade task (Hallett, 1978), subjects make a saccade (i.e., shift their gaze with a rapid ballistic eye movement) to the opposite hemifield, away from a visually cued location (Figure 3.1a). Correct performance requires that the subject, first, inhibit the "reflex-like" prepotent tendency to shift their gaze to the visual cue and, second, generate a saccade to the mirror imaged location of the cue. Prosaccade trials, where gaze is simply shifted to the visual cue, are commonly performed in separate blocks or randomly intermixed with antisaccade trials. Compared to prosaccades,

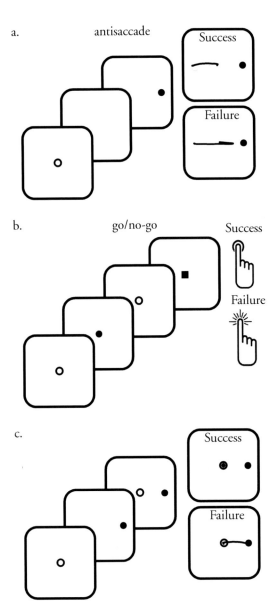

Fig. 3.1 Tasks that require inhibitory control.

a. Antisaccade task. The subject maintains central fixation until a visual target appears. On prosaccade trials, the subject makes a saccade to the target. On antisaccade trials, the reflex-like prosaccade must be inhibited so that an antisaccade can be generated to the target's mirror-image location. Inhibitory failures take on the prototypical form of small prosaccades followed rapidly by corrective antisaccades.

b. Go/no-go task. The subject makes a speeded button press whenever a GO stimulus is presented, in this example, a black circle. On rare occasions, a NO-GO stimulus, a black square in this example, is presented, and the subject must inhibit responding.

c. Stop-signal task. On frequent GO trials, the subject maintains central fixation and makes speeded saccades to the appearance of a peripheral target to the left or right of fixation. On rare STOP trials, a visual cue, in this case the reappearance of the fixation point, is emitted after a period of time known as the stop-signal delay. This signals to the subject to cancel or inhibit the planned movement. Sometimes the subject is successful at withholding the saccade but sometimes fails canceling the planned saccade.

Go/No-Go Task

In a go/no-go task, subjects make a speeded manual response, typically a button press, as soon as a go cue, typically a visual stimulus, is detected (Figure 3.1b). On rare trials, the go cue is replaced with a stimulus that instructs the subject to withhold the response, the no-go cue. Responding gains potency because speeded responses are generated so frequently and are often erroneously generated following the no-go cue. The power of the go/no-go task stems from the fact that the difficulty of suppressing the response increases as the response is habitualized through the relative infrequency of no-go trials.

Stop-Signal Task

Stop-signal, or countermanding, tasks (Logan, 1994), as they are called, require the voluntary control over the production of movements because an imperative stop signal is infrequently presented instructing the subject that the planned movements should be withheld. In a stop-signal task,

antisaccades are slower because of the extra time required to inhibit the automatic saccade plus the time to program the antisaccade. Errors on antisaccade trials are characterized by small-amplitude saccades generated toward the visual cue and are thought to reflect inhibitory failures. The power of the antisaccade task stems from the fact that one must suppress a response with high stimulus–response spatial compatibility (i.e., shift gaze to a location that matches the location of the visual cue).

subjects make a speeded response, typically a manual button press or an eye movement, on the presentation of a visual go cue (Figure 3.1c). On rare trials, just after the presentation of the go cue, an imperative stop signal is presented instructing the subject to withhold the planned movement. Intuitively, as the stop signal is delayed, the motor plan has more time to evolve toward execution, and the probability that the subject will be able to inhibit the response decreases. Similar to the go/no-go task, the power of the stop-signal task relies on the difficulty of suppressing the speeded habitualized response.

Although each task similarly requires withholding a prepotent response, they differ in terms of when in the perception–action cycle inhibition is thought to begin. During a stop-signal task, inhibition begins late, after the go cue has been presented and therefore during the planning of the motor response. During a go/no-go task, inhibition begins earlier, simultaneous with the no-go cue. During an antisaccade task, before a block or before a trial the subject must be instructed whether the trial is an antisaccade or prosaccade trial. Therefore, inhibition can begin even earlier, as soon as the subject is cued that the trial is an antisaccade trial.

Neural Mechanisms of Inhibition

Here we describe human and nonhuman primate research that has provided insights into the potential neural mechanisms of response inhibition. Although the construct of inhibition can be operationalized at many levels, from the molecular to psychological level, we limit our scope of analysis to the systems level (i.e., populations or networks of neurons).

Eye movements are used as the response modality most often in studies of monkeys chiefly because we know more about the oculomotor system than any other motor system (Figure 3.2) (Carpenter, 2000; Glim-cher, 2003). The use of eye movements as a dependent variable has several advantages specifically for investigations into inhibition. Since the cost of making unwanted reaches, for example, is often greater than the cost of making unwanted glances (i.e., touching someone or something may be more costly than just looking), the neural mechanisms for the executive control over eye movements may be simpler. In addition, since eye movements can be generated with very fast response latencies (e.g., typically less than 200 milliseconds in humans and 150 milliseconds in monkeys), control processes such as inhibition must act quickly, or errors are likely to be made. Increased frequency of errors can be advantageous for experimentation because if we want to really understand inhibition, we need to investigate the causes of failures of inhibition. Finally, another advantage of using the oculomotor system is that the position of gaze is experimentally controlled at all times. This is important because much of the work on inhibition deals explicitly or implicitly with the spatial compatibility of visual cues and motor responses, and the position of a visual stimulus on the retina changes with regard to the position of gaze.

Electrophysiological studies of the monkey frontal eye field (FEF) have yielded promising clues to the neural mechanisms of response inhibition. FEF neurons are traditionally thought to play a critical role in transforming visual information into saccade commands (Bruce, Friedman, Kraus, & Stanton, 2004). Indeed, several types of neurons exist in the FEF. Visual FEF neurons respond when a visual stimulus falls within the neuron's response field (i.e., a spatially localized portion of the visual field). Motor FEF neurons respond just prior to the execution of a saccade into the neuron's response field. Visuomotor FEF neurons are hybridizations; they show both visually evoked and saccade-evoked activity.

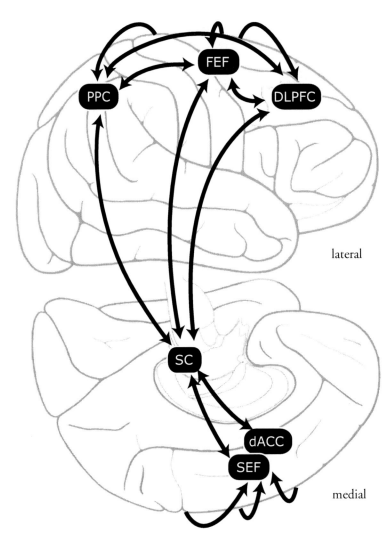

lateral

medial

Fig. 3.2 Key connections between nodes of the oculomotor network in the human brain. This network, with the superior colliculus (SC) serving as the final common pathway, is thought to govern the generation of saccades. Together, these areas are also thought to play important roles in visuospatial and visuomotor behavior, such as that required for the production and inhibition of saccades.

Abbreviations: PPC = posterior parietal cortex; FEF = frontal eye fields; DLPFC = dorsal lateral prefrontal cortex; SEF = supplementary eye fields; dACC = dorsal anterior cingulate cortex.

Saccades (i.e., fast ballistic eye movements) with specific vectors can be elicited by electrical microstimulation of FEF motor neurons. These motor neurons possess all the characteristics of a cell that controls the production of movement (Schall, 2002). For example, the stochastic variability in the time it takes to initiate a saccade to a flashed visual target is directly related to the time it takes for the firing rate of motor FEF neurons to reach a fixed threshold (Thompson, Bichot, & Schall, 1997). Figure 3.3 illustrates this relationship by showing the rate of growth in firing rate in the same neuron during numerous trials in which the response time tended to be fast, medium, or slow. Note that the variability in response

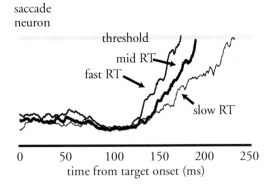

Fig. 3.3 The stochastic variability in the time it takes to initiate a saccade to a flashed visual target is directly related to the time it takes for the firing rate of motor FEF neurons to reach a fixed threshold. The rate of growth in firing rate in the same FEF neuron during numerous trials in which the response time tended to be fast, medium, or slow. Note that the variability in response time is a function of the time needed to reach the threshold. Based on Thompson et al. (1997).

time is a function of the time needed to reach the threshold. Therefore, FEF motor neurons control the production of saccades. In direct opposition to these saccade neurons are another class of neurons in the FEF that are active when the monkey is actively fixating gaze on a stationary position. If fixation neurons are microstimulated during the course of smooth pursuit or saccadic eye movements, oculomotion is immediately halted (Burman & Bruce, 1997). Overall, saccades are produced when activity in FEF motor neurons that drive the eyes to a stimulus increases and activity in FEF fixation neurons that lock gaze in place decreases (Everling & Munoz, 2000; Hanes & Schall, 1996).

With these two different types of FEF neurons in mind, now let us consider the behavior of FEF saccade and fixation neurons during prosaccade compared to antisaccade trials. Saccade neurons in the monkey FEF exhibit a greater firing rate during prosaccade compared to antisaccade trials (Figure 3.4a) (Everling & Munoz, 2000). Moreover, the difference in firing rate can be seen as early as the fixation interval, well before the target even appears. Fixation neurons in the FEF exhibit a greater firing rate just prior to antisaccades compared to prosaccades (Figure 3.4b), again hundreds of milliseconds before the appearance of the target. Therefore, on antisaccade trials when the animal anticipates that he will need to inhibit the prepotent reflex-like saccade, the firing rate of FEF saccade neurons decreases, while the firing rate of fixation neurons increases. These changes are thought to bias the oculomotor system toward a less motile state where the onset of the target and its associated capture of attention is less likely to result in an unwanted saccade (Munoz & Everling, 2004). If activity in saccade neurons can be kept below a critical threshold (e.g., Figure 3.3) just long enough for the voluntary an-

tisaccade to be programmed and initiated, then the decision to make a correct antisaccade is likely to be achieved. Indeed, activity in FEF saccade neurons is greater on trials in which the animal failed to inhibit the saccade toward the target (Figure 3.4c) (Everling & Munoz, 2000).

Therefore, with these observations we can posit a simple neuronal mechanism that determines the ability to inhibit an unwanted saccade. At the time when the peripheral visual target stimulus appears, competition between FEF gaze-holding and gaze-shifting mechanisms determines whether a reflexive saccade is triggered. Moreover, the difference in firing rate between prosaccade and antisaccade trials and the difference in firing rate between successful and failed antisaccades trials can be seen several hundred milliseconds before the visually guided saccade must be inhibited. These competitive interactions may give rise to a psychological preparatory set that primes the oculomotor system toward a gaze-holding or a gaze-shifting state. Stochastic fluctuations in the firing rates of FEF neurons may destabilize the preparatory state, leading to failures in the ability to inhibit the unwanted prosaccade.

The voluntary control of behavior, of which withholding an action is a critical demonstration, can be exerted at any point along the series of processes that evolve over time from sensation to action. In the context of a stop-signal task, inhibition takes place far downstream in this evolution, after the movement has been planned. Inhibiting or canceling a planned movement following an imperative stop signal can be modeled as a race between independent GO and STOP mechanisms (Hanes & Carpenter, 1999; Logan, Cowan, & Davis, 1984) (Figure 3.5). Which process first reaches a critical threshold, or finish line, determines whether the planned response is generated. By adjusting the time between the presentation of the stimulus

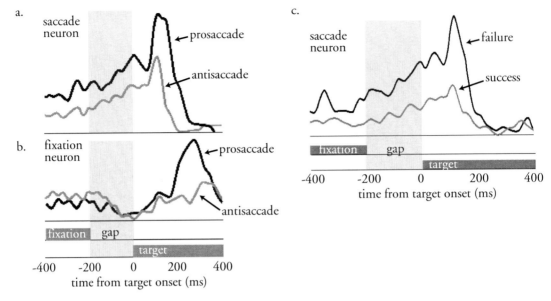

Fig. 3.4 FEF neuronal firing during prosaccade and antisaccade trials.
a. The firing rate of saccade neurons is greater prior to prosaccade than antisaccades.
b. The firing rate of fixation neurons is greater prior to antisaccade than prosaccades.
c. The firing rate of saccade neurons is greater on antisaccade trials where the animal failed to inhibit the prosaccade compared to when the animal was successful. Based on Everling and Munoz (2000).

that initiates the GO response processes and the presentation of the stop stimulus, an interval known as the stop-signal delay, the probability that either one of the two possible responses will win the race can be adjusted (Logan, 1994). Canceling is easier when the stop-signal delay is short because one has more time to cancel the movement. Importantly, using the saccadic response time distribution for GO trials and the probability of successful saccade cancellation at different stop-signal delays, one can estimate the time needed to cancel a planned saccade once the stop signal had been given; this time is referred to as the *stop-signal reaction time* (SSRT).

The presaccadic growth of activity in FEF saccade neurons is correlated with saccade production, while the growth of activity in FEF fixation neurons is correlated with saccade withholding during the performance of stop-signal tasks (Schall, 2001). FEF saccade neurons show a phasic burst of activity

within 100 milliseconds following the appearance of the visual target, while FEF fixation neurons activity declines rapidly (Hanes, Patterson, & Schall, 1998). These early changes in neuronal firing reflect the planning and preparation of the visually guided saccade. When no stop-signal is emitted (i.e., GO trials), the firing rate of saccade neurons continues to build until the critical threshold is breached and a saccade is finally generated (Figures 3.6a and 3.6b). When a stop-signal is emitted (i.e., STOP trials) and the animal is successful at inhibiting the planned saccade, fixation neurons exhibit a burst of firing that coincides with a sharp decrease in the firing rate of saccade neurons (Figures 3.6a and 3.6b). However, if these changes in firing invoked by the stop signal do not occur quickly enough or, to be more precise, do not occur within the SSRT, then the animal is not able to withhold the movement, and a failure of inhibition occurs (Figure 3.6c). Overall, the

a.

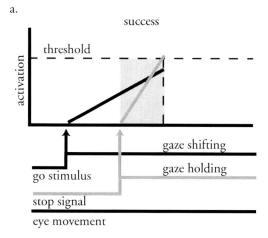

b.

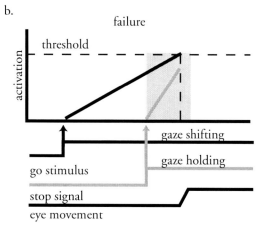

Fig. 3.5 Race model of stop-signal task. Performance on the stop-signal task has been conceptualized to be a race between GO and STOP processes. The activation of neural GO processes related to shifting gaze (black line) race against the activation of neural STOP processes related to holding gaze (gray line) toward a winner-take-all threshold (dashed horizontal line) that determines whether a saccade is triggered. The gray bar represents the time needed to cancel a saccade after a stop signal has been emitted, a time known as the stop-signal reaction time (SSRT).

a. If the processes leading to holding gaze reach a critical threshold before the processes that lead to shifting gaze, then successful saccade cancellation will occur.

b. However, if the gaze shifting processes reach threshold first, then a saccade will be triggered. Notice that in b, the stop-signal delay was longer, which resulted in less time for the processes leading to holding gaze to grow to threshold. Manipulating this delay can reliably affect successful saccade countermanding.

activity pattern of FEF saccade and fixation neurons corresponds very well with the hypothetical GO and STOP processes of the race model where the outcome of a race

between saccade and fixation neurons determines whether a saccade is generated.

Functional magnetic resonance imaging (fMRI) studies have provided critical support in humans for the findings from monkey electrophysiology. For example, the generation of antisaccades compared to prosaccades causes greater activation in the human FEF (Connolly, Goodale, Menon, & Munoz, 2002; Curtis & D'Esposito, 2003). The increase is presumably due to the coactivation of saccade and fixation neurons in the FEF during antisaccade trials. Similarly, during a stop-signal task, the successful cancellation of a planned saccade (i.e., STOP trial) causes greater human FEF activation than the generation of a saccade on no-stop signal, or GO, trials (Curtis, Cole, Rao, & D'Esposito, 2005). Again, the increased activation likely reflects the coactivation of saccade and fixation neurons on STOP trials.

An important implication of these data is that the inhibition of an unwanted action emerges or is the consequence of the competition between different potential responses. Therefore, inhibitory control, like voluntary control more generally, may be best modeled as the process by which we select the best response among all competing responses, including not responding at all. At least at the level of premotor structures, a mechanism specialized for inhibiting actions, per se, does not seem necessary for the behavioral expression of inhibiting an unwanted action.

Functional MRI studies consistently activate the inferior frontal gyrus (IFG) in ventral premotor cortex during tasks that require inhibiting a manual button press (Aron, Fletcher, Bullmore, Sahakian, & Robbins, 2003). For instance, during go/no-go task performance, IFG activity time locked to NO-GO trials is higher than activity time locked to GO trials in both humans (Garavan, Ross, & Stein, 1999; Konishi, Nakajima, Uchida, Sekihara, & Miyashita, 1998; Konishi et al., 1999;

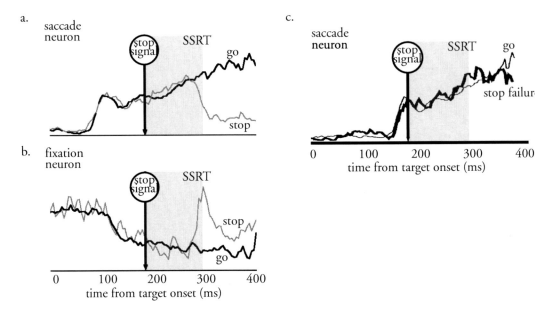

Fig. 3.6 FEF neuronal firing during a stop-signal task.

a. The firing rate of a saccade neuron during a GO and a STOP trial. Following the initial visually evoked response, the firing rate increases, presumably toward a threshold that when breached results in a saccade. On STOP trials the firing rate declines rapidly following the presentation of the stop signal. Importantly, this decline occurs within the SSRT.

b. The firing rate of a fixation neuron on GO and STOP trials.

c. The firing rate of a saccade neuron on trials in which the no stop signal was given (GO) and when a stop signal was given but the animal did not cancel the saccade in time. Based on Hanes et al. (1998).

Liddle, Kiehl, & Smith, 2001) and monkeys (Morita, Nakahara, & Hayashi, 2004) (Figures 3.7a and 3.7c). This activation is thought to reflect some process related to inhibiting the unwanted motor response. In addition, activity in right IFG is greater on STOP trials compared to GO trials during a manual version of the stop-signal task (Figure 3.7b) (Aron & Poldrack, 2006). This difference is greater in individuals with faster SSRTs, perhaps suggesting that the larger activation difference reflects more efficient inhibitory control. Moreover, damage to the right IFG in humans impairs one's ability to inhibit responding and lengthens the SSRT (i.e., the time needed to inhibit a planned action) (Aron et al., 2003). In summary, it appears that the IFG is critically involved in the inhibition of unwanted manual motor responses just as the FEF is involved in suppressing eye movements.

However, the precise mechanisms reflected by IFG activity to support inhibitory control over manual motor responses needs several lines of clarification. First, most of the human studies find that IFG activity is right lateralized. Given that ventral premotor cortex, as well as all other motor systems, has a strong contraversive organization (i.e., neurons in one hemisphere largely code for movements toward the opposite side of space or movements made with limbs on the opposite side of the body), one would predict that activation should be greater in the hemisphere contralateral to the hand that is used for the response. With this assumption, one would predict that the left IFG should be more active when canceling movements with the right hand, which is the hand that most of the studies have used for responding. Therefore, the right lateralization of the IFG activation does not concur with what we know about the functional organization of

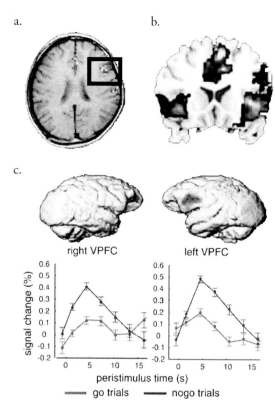

Fig. 3.7 Functional magnetic resonance imaging of GO/NO-GO task performance.

a. Subtracting activation during NO-GO performance from GO performance yields activation in right inferior frontal gyrus (Konishi et al., 1998).

b. Subtracting activation during STOP from GO trials on a stop-signal task yields activation that is greater in right compared to left inferior frontal gyrus (Aron & Poldrack, 2006).

c. A homologous frontal cortical area in the monkey has recently been identified with fMRI (Morita et al., 2004). Although a bilateral response is found, it is larger in the left hemisphere, contralateral to the hand used for responding.

the motor system. To date, there is not a clear explanation for why the activations are right lateralized other than the speculation that inhibitory control may be right lateralized just as language is left lateralized. Another intriguing possibility is that the right lateralization may be related to the lateralized bias of attention. For instance, the clinical syndrome of unilateral spatial neglect and numerous human functional imaging studies of spatial attention (Corbetta & Shulman, 2002) have found that the right

hemisphere is dominant for selective attentional processes. For example, in the neglect syndrome, after right hemisphere lesions, patients fail to attend, look at, and respond to stimuli located on the left side of space. Possibly more pertinent for the current discussion, it has been proposed that some neglect patients have a premotor "intentional" deficit (Coslett, Bowers, Fitzpatrick, Haws, & Heilman, 1990; Heilman & Valenstein, 1998). In other words, impairment exists within an intentional system, which serves to select among many locations in which to act. These patients have a disinclination to initiate movements or move toward or into contralateral hemispace. Thus, it is possible that the right IFG that is engaged during response inhibition tasks is part of this intentional motor system, and in this way, inhibition of a motor response may be a special form of disengaging attention or, in this case, disengaging *intention*.

Second, it has been proposed that the right IFG is a cortical region that is involved in inhibiting actions regardless of the response effector (e.g., hand, eye, voice), a general "cognitive brake" of sorts (Aron, Robbins, & Poldrack, 2004). It has even been suggested that the right IFG may be involved in inhibiting nonmotor responses, such as emotional responses (Lieberman, Hariri, Jarcho, Eisenberger, & Bookheimer, 2005). However, not all inhibition tasks evoke activity in the right (or left) IFG. Inhibiting eye movements, as compared to manual movements, does not typically evoke activity in the right IFG (Ford, Goltz, Brown, & Everling, 2005). Additionally, it remains unclear, in terms of neural circuitry, how neurons in the right IFG would exert their influence in the control of all types of movements. There is a paucity of electrophysiological recordings of neurons in ventral premotor cortex during motor inhibition tasks, which leaves open the possibility that the activations reported in IFG may not be directly related to inhibition. They could be related to the emotional sequelae of inhibiting a prepotent response or the conscious awareness of the conflicting responses. For example, one might experience an emotional reaction when attempting to inhibit an unwanted response when the chances of task failure are high. Similarly, the simple conscious awareness of conflicting motor plans, even without an emotional reaction, could also invoke neural activity in the IFG (Nieuwenhuis, Ridderinkhof, Blom, Band, & Kok, 2001). In any case, whether or not the hypothesis that the right IFG is an area specialized for general inhibitory control is correct, more research is needed in this area. Specifically, the response effector and types of inhibition tasks should be systematically manipulated.

Two other important components of tasks that require inhibitory control are the need to detect conflicting motor responses and the ability to monitor performance so that strategic adjustments can be implemented to optimize behavior. There is clear evidence that animals adjust their behavior following errors and even after successfully avoiding an error, say, on an antisaccade trial (Fecteau & Munoz, 2003; Gratton, 1992; Rabbitt, 1966). In the oculomotor system, motor regions along the medial frontal wall have been associated with both error detection and conflict monitoring (Botvinick, Cohen, & Carter, 2004; Schall, Stuphorn, & Brown, 2002). Thus, neurons in the supplementary eye field (SEF) have an increased rate of firing prior antisaccades compared to prosaccades (Figure 3.8a) (Schlag-Rey, Amador, Sanchez, & Schlag, 1997).

This difference can be seen several hundreds of milliseconds before the saccade is generated, essentially as soon as the instructional cue is given as the animal prepares for the appearance of the stimulus and contingent response. We have demonstrated an identical pattern in humans, where voxels near the SEF begin to ramp up during the preparation interval when the subjects know only that the trial is an antisaccade trial (Figures 3.8b and 3.8c) (Curtis & D'Esposito, 2003). Moreover, the amount of activity in the preparation interval predicts how successful the subject will be in subsequently inhibiting the reflexive saccade to the visual target. In both monkeys and humans, activity in the SEF was much lower on trials in which the subject failed to inhibit the unwanted glance. In fact, the preparatory activity is on par with the amount of activity during trials in which inhibition is not required (Curtis & D'Esposito, 2003; Schlag-Rey et al., 1997). Therefore, neurons in the SEF may somehow anticipate that conflict between the reflexive response to the visual target's location and the controlled need to maintain fixation until the antisaccade can be computed and generated. An output signal from the SEF may bias other nodes in the oculomotor network, making it less likely that the system is reactive to external visual inputs. For example, SEF projections to the FEF may increase the firing rate of fixation neurons or decrease the firing rate of saccade neurons, making it less likely that an error will be produced when the target appears.

Additionally, there must be a mechanism or set of mechanisms that allow animals to monitor their performance such that strategic changes can be implemented. Detecting the production of errors is necessary for one to make adaptive changes in future behavior. Neurons in the SEF show a pattern of activity during stop-signal tasks that suggest that they may play an important role in monitoring performance. Some SEF neurons show a burst of activity following errors on STOP trials (Figure 3.8d), and some show a burst of activity following successfully cancelled STOP trials (Figure 3.8e) (Stuphorn, Taylor, & Schall, 2000). Note that the onset of the activity is after the SSRT, so these signals are too late to be critically involved

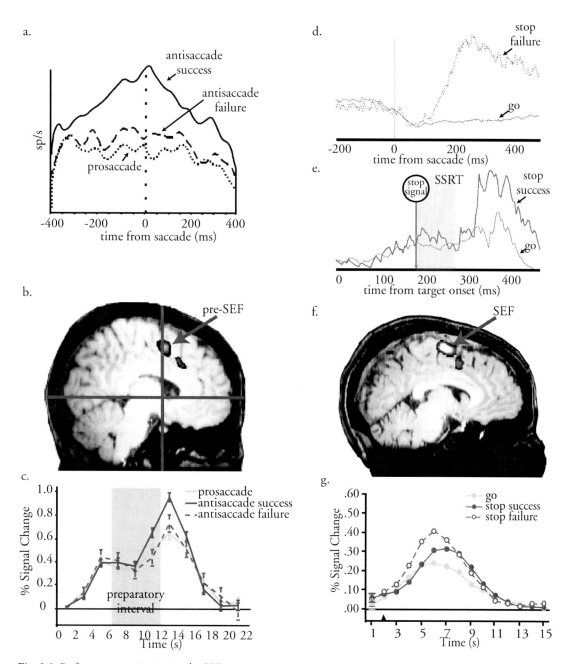

Fig. 3.8 Performance monitoring in the SEF.

a. The firing rate of SEF neurons is greater prior to antisaccades than prosaccades and antisaccade failures (Schlag-Rey et al., 1997). b. and c. Activity in an area just anterior to the human SEF shows greater activity just prior to antisaccades compared to prosaccades and antisaccade failures (Curtis & D'Esposito, 2003). d. Some monkey SEF neurons show a burst of activity following errors on STOP trials of a stop-signal task and e. some show a burst of activity following successfully cancelled STOP trials (Stuphorn et al., 2000). f. and g. Similarly in humans, the SEF shows increased activation related to success and failures of inhibition (Curtis et al., 2005).

in the act of inhibition. Instead, they signal how successful or not the animal is performing the required task. Moreover, activity in the human SEF is greater for both successful and unsuccessful STOP trials compared to

GO trials (Figures 3.8f and 3.8g) (Curtis et al., 2005), suggesting that the human SEF contains the requisite signals for monitoring performance that could be used in feedback learning. Presumably, these signals cause changes in the oculomotor system by biasing the activity of saccade and fixation neurons on the upcoming trials. In sum, during oculomotor tasks that require inhibiting unwanted saccades, neurons in frontal areas along the medial wall, like the SEF, may contain signals that can be used to optimize performance. These include increased activity when one anticipates and prepares for conflicting oculomotor responses and activity that signals both successes and failures inhibiting the unwanted responses.

Conclusions

Goal-directed behavior involves the engagement of a wide array of cognitive processes that allow us to bridge the gap between the processing of incoming sensory input and the execution of actions adaptively suited to the current environment. Achieving our goals requires higher-level influences over sensory input, internal states, and motor output. By exerting influence over these domains, humans have evolved increasingly more sophisticated control over interactions with both the natural world and each other. This control permits the goal-directed override of primitive and inflexible reactions to environmental stimuli as occurs in other animals, what Mesulam (2002) refers to as the "default mode." In this chapter, we have reviewed the potential neural mechanisms mediating the voluntary control of an action, which is necessary when an optimal motor response is uncertain or when a competing motor response must be overcome. Determining the mechanisms of such control may lead to greater insight regarding more general control mechanisms. The empirical findings we reviewed in this chapter support the notion that the inhibition of actions is best modeled as the process by which we select the best response among the competing responses, including not responding at all.

The empirical evidence we have reviewed derives from both human and nonhuman primate research, using electrophysiological and functional neuroimaging methods. It is important to note the tremendous value of using both approaches for gaining an understanding of brain–behavior relationships. Since both types of research have particular strengths as well as limitations, neither approach is ideal in isolation. Rather, the data derived from each are complimentary and convergent, and the sum is greater than its parts. For example, single-unit recording in awake behaving monkeys has the temporal and spatial resolution that cannot be achieved by functional neuroimaging methods in humans. However, human imaging methods provides whole-brain recording, allowing for investigations of an entire neural circuit and its interactions.

In this chapter, we emphasized studies of the oculomotor system, which serves as an excellent model for studying the neural mechanisms underlying our ability to inhibit unwanted actions. When we intend to move our eyes, there is competition between FEF gaze-holding and gaze-shifting mechanisms that will determine whether an eye movement occurs. Withholding of an action, such as an eye movement, can obviously be exerted at any point along the series of processes that evolve over time from sensation to action. Overall, the activity pattern of FEF saccade and fixation neurons corresponds very well with the hypothetical GO and STOP processes of the race model derived from behavioral studies. In this model, the outcome of the race between saccade and fixation neurons determines whether a saccade is generated. In addition, this mechanism seems to be initiated before the actual action, which likely serves as a preparatory set that primes the oculomotor system toward a gaze-holding or a gaze-shifting state. Another node of the oculomotor circuit, the SEF, appears critically involved in detecting conflicting motor responses and monitoring performance so that strategic adjustments can be implemented to optimize behavior.

There are two important implications of these empirical data. First, inhibition of an unwanted action emerges or is the consequence of the competition between different potential responses and is not due to an "inhibitory" signal per se. This idea is similar to that put forth by other investigators studying other domains of cognition, such as language (Thompson-Schill, D'Esposito, Aguirre, & Farah, 1997; Thompson-Schill et al., 1998). For example, in a verb-generation task, the need to overcome a prepotent response may occur when choosing one associated verb for a given noun from among competing alternatives. That is, some nouns (e.g., "cat") have many weakly associated verbs, whereas others (e.g., "scissors") have only a few strongly associated verbs ("cut"). In a human fMRI study, Thompson-Schill and colleagues found that generating verbs to nouns with many possible responses (as in the case of "cat") was associated with increased left ventral PFC activity. Interestingly, this region is homologous to that activated in the right hemisphere during the response inhibition tasks discussed in this chapter. Furthermore, patients with damage to this region were impaired at retrieving verbs only under conditions of increased competition. These findings were interpreted in the context of the demands for the selection of information among competing alternatives. Kimberg and Farah (1993) have put forth a similar idea, implemented as a computation model, demonstrating that tasks such as the Stroop tasks can be successfully performed without an "inhibitory" module in their model. Rather, correct responses are achieved by a module (presumably in the PFC) that mediates the selection of an action by the weighting of information active in working memory. Thus, at least at the level of premotor structures such as the FEF and SEF and possibly at the level of the PFC, a mechanism specialized for inhibiting actions, per se, does not seem necessary for the behavioral expression of inhibiting an unwanted action.

A second implication that arises from our review is that it is unlikely that there is a single area of the brain that is specialized for the computations necessary for *withholding all unwanted actions* (see Chapter 30). As we have discussed regarding the oculomotor system, selecting an appropriate eye movement for the task at hand requires the interplay between different premotor structures, such as the FEF and SEF, and is also likely under the control of higher level regions, such as the PFC. Moreover, it is likely that different neural circuitry is required for withholding other types of output modalities, such as speech and manual responses.

References

Aron, A. R., Fletcher, P. C., Bullmore, E. T., Sahakian, B. J., & Robbins, T. W. (2003). Stop-signal inhibition disrupted by damage to right inferior frontal gyrus in humans. *Nature Neuroscience, 6,* 115–116.

Aron, A. R., & Poldrack, R. A. (2006). Cortical and subcortical contributions to stop signal response inhibition: Role of the subthalamic nucleus. *Journal of Neuroscience, 26,* 2424–2433.

Aron, A. R., Robbins, T. W., & Poldrack, R. A. (2004). Inhibition and the right inferior frontal cortex. *Trends in Cognitive Science, 8,* 170–177.

Botvinick, M. M., Cohen, J. D., & Carter, C. S. (2004). Conflict monitoring and anterior cingulate cortex: An update. *Trends in Cognitive Science, 8,* 539–546.

Bruce, C. J., Friedman, H. R., Kraus, M. S., & Stanton, G. B. (2004). The primate frontal eye field. In L. M. Chalupa & J. S. Werner (Eds.), *The visual neurosciences* (Vol. 1, pp. 1428–1448). Cambridge, MA: MIT Press.

Burman, D. D., & Bruce, C. J. (1997). Suppression of task-related saccades by electrical stimulation in the primate's frontal eye field. *Journal of Neurophysiology, 77,* 2252–2267.

Carpenter, R. H. (2000). The neural control of looking. *Current Biology, 10,* R291–R293.

Connolly, J. D., Goodale, M. A., Menon, R. S., & Munoz, D. P. (2002). Human fMRI evidence for the neural correlates of preparatory set. *Nature Neuroscience, 5,* 1345–1352.

Corbetta, M., & Shulman, G. L. (2002). Control of goal-directed and stimulus-driven attention in the brain. *Nature Reviews. Neuroscience, 3,* 201–215.

Coslett, H. B., Bowers, D., Fitzpatrick, E., Haws, B., & Heilman, K. M. (1990). Directional hypokinesia and hemispatial inattention in neglect. *Brain, 113*(Pt. 2), 475–486.

Curtis, C. E., Cole, M. W., Rao, V. Y., & D'Esposito, M. (2005). Canceling planned action: An fMRI study of countermanding saccades. *Cerebral Cortex, 15,* 1281–1289.

Curtis, C. E., & D'Esposito, M. (2003). Success and failure suppressing reflexive behavior. *Journal of Cognitive Neuroscience, 15,* 409–418.

Eriksen, B. A., & Eriksen, C. W. (1974). Effects of noise letters upon the identification of a target letter in a nonsearch task. *Perception and Psychophysics, 16,* 143–149.

Everling, S., & Munoz, D. P. (2000). Neuronal correlates for preparatory set associated with pro-saccades and anti-saccades in the primate frontal eye field. *Journal of Neuroscience, 20,* 387–400.

Fecteau, J. H., & Munoz, D. P. (2003). Exploring the consequences of the previous trial. *Nature Reviews. Neuroscience, 4,* 435–443.

Ford, K. A., Goltz, H. C., Brown, M. R., & Everling, S. (2005). Neural processes associated with antisaccade task performance investigated with event-related fMRI. *Journal of Neurophysiology, 94,* 429–440.

Garavan, H., Ross, T. J., & Stein, E. A. (1999). Right hemispheric dominance of inhibitory control: An event-related functional MRI study. *Proceedings of the National Academy of Sciences of the United States of America, 96,* 8301–8306.

Glimcher, P. W. (2003). The neurobiology of visual-saccadic decision making. *Annual Review of Neuroscience, 26,* 133–179.

Gratton, G. (1992). Optimizing the use of information: The strategic control of the activation of responses. *Dissertation Abstracts International, 52*(7-B), 3940.

Hallett, P. (1978). Primary and secondary saccades to goals defined by instructions. *Vision Research, 18,* 1279–1296.

Hanes, D. P., & Carpenter, R. H. (1999). Countermanding saccades in humans. *Vision Research, 39,* 2777–2791.

Hanes, D. P., Patterson, W. F., II, & Schall, J. D. (1998). Role of frontal eye fields in countermanding saccades: Visual, movement, and fixation activity. *Journal of Neurophysiology, 79,* 817–834.

Hanes, D. P., & Schall, J. D. (1996). Neural control of voluntary movement initiation. *Science, 274,* 427–430.

Heilman, K. M., & Valenstein, E. Frontal lobe neglect in man. *Neurology.* 22(6):660–64.

Kimberg, D. Y., & Farah, M. J. (1993). A unified account of cognitive impairments following frontal lobe damage: The role of working memory in complex, organized behavior. *Journal of Experimental Psychology: General, 122,* 411–428.

Konishi, S., Nakajima, K., Uchida, I., Kikyo, H., Kameyama, M., & Miyashita, Y. (1999). Common inhibitory mechanism in human inferior prefrontal cortex revealed by event-related functional MRI. *Brain, 122*(Pt. 5), 981–991.

Konishi, S., Nakajima, K., Uchida, I., Sekihara, K., & Miyashita, Y. (1998). No-go dominant brain activity in human inferior prefrontal cortex revealed by functional magnetic resonance imaging. *European Journal of Neuroscience, 10,* 1209–1213.

Liddle, P. F., Kiehl, K. A., & Smith, A.M. (2001). Event-related fMRI study of response inhibition. *Human Brain Mapping, 12,* 100–109.

Lieberman, M. D., Hariri, A., Jarcho, J. M., Eisenberger, N. I., & Bookheimer, S. Y. (2005). An fMRI investigation of race-related amygdala activity in African-American and Caucasian-American individuals. *Nature Neuroscience, 8,* 720–722.

Logan, G. D. (1994). On the ability to inhibit thought and action: A user's guide to the stop signal paradigm. In D. Dagenbach & T. H. Carr (Eds.), *Inhibitory processes in attention, memory, and language* (pp. 189–239). San Diego, CA: Academic Press.

Logan, G. D., Cowan, W. B., & Davis, K. A. (1984). On the ability to inhibit simple and choice reaction time responses: A model and a method. *Journal of Experimental Psychology: Human Perception and Performance, 10,* 276–291.

Mesulam, M.-Marsel (2002). The human frontal lobes: Transcending the default mode through contingent encoding. In D. T. Stuss & R. T. Knight (Eds.), *Principles of frontal lobe function* (pp. 8–30). New York: Oxford University Press.

Morita, M., Nakahara, K., & Hayashi, T. (2004). A rapid presentation event-related functional magnetic resonance imaging study of response inhibition in macaque monkeys. *Neuroscience Letters, 356,* 203–206.

Munoz, D. P., & Everling, S. (2004). Look away: The anti-saccade task and the voluntary control of eye movement. *Nature Reviews. Neuroscience, 5*, 218–228.

Nieuwenhuis, S., Ridderinkhof, K. R., Blom, J., Band, G. P., & Kok, A. (2001). Error-related brain potentials are differentially related to awareness of response errors: Evidence from an antisaccade task. *Psychophysiology, 38*, 752–760.

Rabbitt, P. M. (1966). Errors and error correction in choice-response tasks. *Journal of Experimental Psychology, 71*, 264–272.

Schall, J. D. (2001). Neural basis of deciding, choosing and acting. *Nature Reviews. Neuroscience, 2*, 33–42.

Schall, J. D. (2002). The neural selection and control of saccades by the frontal eye field. *Philosophical Transactions of the Royal Society of London. Series B, Biological Sciences, 357*, 1073–1082.

Schall, J. D., Stuphorn, V., & Brown, J. W. (2002). Monitoring and control of action by the frontal lobes. *Neuron, 36*, 309–322.

Schlag-Rey, M., Amador, N., Sanchez, H., & Schlag, J. (1997). Antisaccade performance predicted by neuronal activity in the supplementary eye field. *Nature, 390*, 398–401.

Simon, J. R. (1969). Reactions toward the source of stimulation. *Journal of Experimental Psychology, 81*, 174–176.

Stroop, J. R. (1935). Studies of interference in serial verbal reactions. *Journal of Experimental Psychology, 18*, 643–662.

Stuphorn, V., Taylor, T. L., & Schall, J. D. (2000). Performance monitoring by the supplementary eye field. *Nature, 408*, 857–860.

Thompson, K. G., Bichot, N. P., & Schall, J. D. (1997). Dissociation of visual discrimination from saccade programming in macaque frontal eye field. *Journal of Neurophysiology, 77*, 1046–1050.

Thompson-Schill, S. L., D'Esposito, M., Aguirre, G. K., & Farah, M. J. (1997). Role of left inferior prefrontal cortex in retrieval of semantic knowledge: A reevaluation. *Proceedings of the National Academy of Sciences of the United States of America, 94*, 14792–14797.

Thompson-Schill, S. L., Swick, D., Farah, M. J., D'Esposito, M., Kan, I. P., & Knight, R. T. (1998). Verb generation in patients with focal frontal lesions: A neuropsychological test of neuroimaging findings. *Proceedings of the National Academy of Sciences of the United States of America, 95*, 15855–15860.

The Visual Control of Object Manipulation

David A. Westwood

Abstract

This chapter discusses the visual control of object manipulation, focusing on the question of whether conscious perception is necessary for the control of manipulation. Research supporting the two-streams hypothesis of action and perception is reviewed. It is argued that apart from the task of programming and controlling the intended action, the selection of an appropriate response depends on perceptual processing that takes place in the ventral stream because deciding how to interact with an object first requires that object to be identified.

Keywords: conscious perception, object perception, action, perceptual processing

Objects figure prominently in most facets of everyday human behavior. Whether eating, playing, or working, there is usually an object involved out of either necessity or perhaps convenience. Humans are remarkably adept at reaching out, picking up, and using objects (i.e., object manipulation), except in cases where the physical or neurological plant has been compromised. Although objects can be manipulated with the hands, feet, or the mouth, attention here is restricted to manual object manipulation, also referred to as manual prehension. The control of object manipulation has been the focus of a considerable amount of research in a number of fields, ranging from kinesiology, neuroscience, physiology, and psychology to philosophy, engineering, computer science, and rehabilitation. There have been tremendous advances made in understanding the sensory, cognitive, and motor mechanisms that lie behind the planning and control of manipulatory actions, and a thorough review would scarcely fit in a single book let alone a single chapter in a book. This chapter focuses on the visual control of object manipulation, addressing the rather specific question of whether conscious perception is necessary for the control of manipulation.

The control of object manipulation can be conceived as a sequence of somewhat distinct tasks that can be illustrated with a familiar scenario. Imagine arriving home at the end of the day to hear the phone ringing. Because you just bought this particular cordless phone, you cannot remember exactly where you left it. Moreover, the ringer for the phone is located on the home base, not on the handset itself; the ringing sound is thus useless for locating the most important piece of apparatus. In this scenario, one must first consider the question of intention: Do you wish to answer the phone or ignore it? If you decide to answer the phone, then it must be located; because the ringing noise is coming from the base rather than the handset, auditory information is not helpful in this regard. A visual search must be initiated with the phone as the target of interest. While searching for the phone, it may be necessary to move other objects that are blocking a direct line of sight; object recognition mechanisms would be required to determine which objects are movable and which are not. When (and if) the phone is located, a decision about how to pick it up may be required (i.e., response selection). In this case, the possible responses could include an overhand grasp with the left hand or perhaps an inverted grasp with the right hand. Because the phone is not moving, a decision about precisely when to initiate the grasping action is not critical. In situations requiring interception of a moving object, such as catching a ball, deciding when to start the movement is of paramount importance. To begin the grasping action, appropriate motor commands must be generated and sent to the muscles of the upper limb (i.e., response programming). Those motor commands must specify a grasping trajectory that takes into consideration the size, location, and orientation of the handset, or else the action will surely fail. Once the action has begun, the unfolding movement must be monitored and adjusted to fix execution errors or to respond to changes in the environment such as if the phone suddenly slips from its precarious perch (i.e., response execution). Assuming that each of the tasks outlined here is completed, a stable grasp on the phone can be effected, and appropriate lifting dynamics (i.e., forces) can be used to bring the phone to the ear to hear the discordant tones of the telemarketer's sales pitch.

Object Perception and Object Manipulation

The study of object perception and recognition has a rich history in psychology and neuroscience. Contemporary views of object perception and recognition adopt a representational perspective (e.g., Marr, 1982) according to which the task of the perceptual system is to generate an internal representation of a distal stimulus. That representation serves as a starting point for generating conscious perceptual experience—perhaps through reciprocal connections to the earliest regions of the visual cortex (Llinas, Ribary, Contreras, & Pedroarena, 1998)—and it forms an interface with the cognitive system, making contact with semantic memory. Although considerable research has focused on perception in the auditory, olfactory, and somatosensory modalities, discussion here is restricted to the visual modality.

Visual object recognition consists of several stages (Grill-Spector, 2003). After the object's retinal image has been transduced into neural impulses and carried into the visual cortex, abstract features such as location, edges, orientations, color, and disparity are extracted and encoded. In the middle stages of visual processing, feature codes are combined to represent contours and surfaces; at this stage, an object can be conceived of as a distributed representation of visual features. In the later stages of visual processing, distributed object representations make contact with semantic memory, which consists of object names, functions, and characteristics.

Some of the stages of object perception—particularly those related to the analysis and representation of object shape—would appear to overlap with those necessary for guiding interactions with objects. Whereas Woodworth (1899) was the first to demonstrate empirically that vision is critical for the accurate programming and execution of simple reaching movements, it was Jeannerod

(1986) who showed that intrinsic object features such as size and shape influence the posture of the grasping hand (i.e., the "grasping" component of prehension) while it is moving toward the target. Larger objects (versus smaller objects) lead to greater opening of the finger–thumb aperture, and the shape of the object affects the locations where the grasping digits make contact with the object: The opposition axis between the finger and thumb passes through or close to the object's center of mass (Paulignan, Frak, Toni, & Jeannerod, 1997).

Because both recognition and grasping require information about object form, one might predict that a single representation of the object would drive both processes. However, as is reviewed next, considerable evidence has amassed indicating that this is not the case. Distinct computations of object form lie behind object perception and object manipulation, and these computations are implemented by anatomically segregated brain regions.

Separate Visual Pathways for Perception and Action

Goodale, Milner, Jakobson, and Carey (1991) studied the perceptual and motor abilities of D. F., a patient with a disorder known as visual form agnosia. Patients with this disorder cannot perceive the shape of visual objects and consequently have profound difficulty recognizing black-and-white line drawings of objects, among other things. Consistent with her perceptual disorder, D. F. could not report the orientation of a tilted slot by rotating a handheld manipulandum, and neither could she verbally discriminate between matched versus unmatched pairs of tilted slots. Surprisingly, despite her profound perceptual deficit, she was remarkably adept at orienting her hand to the angle of a tilted slot when "posting" a letter into it. Appropriately oriented hand postures were

seen very early in D. F.'s reaching movements, well before tactile feedback from the target slot could be used to modify the response. Thus, the control of her hand orientation was clearly guided by visual information about the orientation of the slot—information that did not reach her conscious perceptual awareness.

Earlier reports had already demonstrated that the visual control of action does not require conscious perception of the target object. Weiskrantz, Warrington, Sanders, and Marshall (1974) showed that a patient with cortical blindness (also known as "blindsight") could point toward visual targets with greater-than-chance accuracy despite performing at chance when asked to verbally report the locations of those targets. Moreover, Goodale, Pelisson, and Prablanc (1986) showed that reaching movements ended up at the proper location of a target whose position was deliberately changed during an accompanying eye movement. This would not be particularly noteworthy except that participants demonstrated no awareness that the target had changed position at all. Unlike Goodale et al.'s (1991) study of D. F.'s manipulatory abilities, the two experiments just described focused on object location, not object form. Because object location is not fundamental to the perception of object identity, a dissociation between motor and perceptual sensitivity to location is easier to explain—and somewhat less surprising—than the dissociation between motor and perceptual sensitivity to object form seen in D. F.'s case; after all, analysis of object form is critical to both recognition and manipulation.

Low-resolution magnetic resonance imaging (MRI) scans of D. F.'s brain taken in 1991 suggested a lesion in the ventral visual stream (Milner et al., 1991), a pathway carrying visual information from the primary visual area in the occipital lobe through to the cortex in the inferior temporal lobe.

The location of D. F.'s lesion was recently confirmed using high-resolution MRI images, indicating a loss of neural tissue in the lateral occipital cortex (LOC), a region at the junction of the occipital and temporal lobes in the ventral stream (James, Culham, Humphrey, Milner, & Goodale, 2003).

Based on the neurological and behavioral evidence from D. F., in concert with extensive data from neuroanatomical and neurophysiological studies of monkey visual cortex, Goodale and Milner (1992) proposed a reinterpretation of the functions of the dorsal and ventral visual streams as first described by Ungerleider and Mishkin (1982). Goodale and Milner proposed that the ventral stream—consisting of occipital and temporal cortex—is responsible for perceptual aspects of vision, such as conscious experience and object recognition, whereas the dorsal stream—consisting of brain regions in the occipital and posterior parietal cortex—is responsible for the visuomotor transformations required for the control of actions such as manual prehension. According to this view, D. F.'s ventral stream lesion disrupted her visual perception of object form, but her intact dorsal stream enabled her to nevertheless manipulate objects using visual information about object form.

Strong support for this dorsal/ventral division of labor was provided by a study of grasping and object perception in two patients with complementary lesions to dorsal and ventral visual cortex (Goodale, Meenan, et al., 1994). Patient D. F., the visual form agnosic described earlier, had damage to the ventral stream, whereas patient R. V., a patient with optic ataxia, had bilateral damage to the posterior parietal cortex. In the study, the two patients grasped or made perceptual judgments about a variety of irregularly shaped objects. In the grasping task, D. F.'s opposition axis tended to pass through the object's center of mass, whereas R. V.'s did not. In the perceptual task, pairs of randomly rotated objects were presented that either matched in form or did not. In stark contrast to the results from the grasping task, D. F. performed at chance in this perceptual discrimination task, whereas R.V. performed quite well. This clear double dissociation between perceptual and motor performance is consistent with the idea that damage to the ventral stream disrupts perceptual aspects of vision—explaining D. F.'s inability to discriminate between objects with different shapes—whereas damage to the dorsal stream disrupts sensorimotor aspects of vision—explaining R.V.'s inability to properly align the grasping axis on the surface of irregularly shaped objects.

Further Support for the Two-Streams Hypothesis of Action and Perception

In an extensive exposition of their two-streams hypothesis, Milner and Goodale (1995) pulled together evidence from diverse fields ranging from human neuropsychology, monkey neurophysiology, and neuroanatomy to psychophysics and cognitive psychology. Since the publication of *The Visual Brain in Action* (Milner & Goodale, 1995), a tremendous amount of research has been inspired by the idea that perception and action are mediated by distinct brain systems. Although much of this research has been supportive of the two-streams hypothesis, some findings have required clarification—and in some cases modification—of the original proposal. Some of those key studies are reviewed here, with emphasis given to experiments in which object form—rather than position or motion—is the primary manipulated variable.

Functional Neuroimaging

In the years since Milner and Goodale's (1995) seminal work, there has been an explosion of research using functional MRI (fMRI) to explore the functional organization of the human brain. Whereas conventional MRI is used primarily to image static neural structures, physiological aspects of brain function can be imaged using modified MRI parameters. Local changes in blood oxygenation (i.e., BOLD imaging) can be measured with reasonable spatial ($1 \times 1 \times 3$-mm voxel sizes are typical) and temporal (one image of the entire cerebrum can be collected in about 1–3 seconds) resolution while participants carry out various cognitive and motor tasks. Logothetis, Pauls, Augath, Trinath, and Oeltermann (2001) have recently demonstrated that BOLD signals are tightly linked to changes in local neural activity, giving validity to this technique as a method for imaging neural processing.

Selective activation in circumscribed regions of the ventral stream has been reported for complex objects like faces (fusiform face area: Haxby et al., 1994; Kanwisher, McDermott, & Chun, 1997), places (parahippocampal place area: Epstein & Kanwisher, 1998), and bodies (superior temporal gyrus: Grossman et al., 2000) and distinct object features such as color (V4: McKeefry & Zeki, 1997), motion (V5 or middle temporal area: Watson et al., 1993), and form (LOC: Malach et al., 1995). Such visual specificity is consistent with a role for the ventral stream in building the internal representations necessary for visual perception and object recognition. Although there is debate in this field about whether ventral stream processing is truly modular (e.g., Ishai, Ungerleider, Martin, Schouten, & Haxby, 1999) and even more disagreement about what these selectively activated brain regions are actually processing (e.g., Gauthier, Tarr, Anderson, Skudlarski, & Gore, 1999), the findings here are generally consistent with a role for the ventral stream in visual perception.

The neural substrates of object manipulation have been difficult to explore using fMRI because overt movements create artifacts in the measured signals. Nevertheless,

using careful event-related designs that temporally segregate movement artifacts and the somewhat sluggish vascular response to these movements, a number of groups have been able to study the neural correlates of object manipulation using fMRI. Binkofski and colleagues (1998) identified an area in the anterior intraparietal sulcus (AIP) of the dorsal stream that showed selective activation when participants made grasping movements. In a parallel behavioral study of patients with parietal lesions, those authors also report grasping deficits in patients whose lesions included AIP. Selective activation of area AIP during grasping has also been found by Culham and colleagues (2003), who used a sophisticated methodology in which objects of varying sizes and orientations could be displayed—and grasped—on individual trials. A number of other studies have since provided further support for the role of intraparietal regions in control of grasping (e.g., Creem-Regehr & Lee, 2005; Ehrsson, Fagergren, Johansson, & Forssberg, 2003; Frey, Vinton, Norlund, & Grafton, 2005). A recent fMRI study of the visual form agnosic patient D. F. (James et al., 2003) showed normal activation in area AIP during grasping performance but little to no activation in area LOC of the ventral stream when she attempted (unsuccessfully) to identify line drawings of familiar objects. These findings are consistent with earlier behavioral studies demonstrating D. F.'s intact visuomotor abilities but impaired visual perception.

Neurophysiological Studies of Nonhuman Primates

At the time Milner and Goodale (1995) published *The Visual Brain in Action*, it was already established that neurons in the posterior parietal cortex of the macaque monkey were selectively activated during visually guided tasks such as saccades (Lynch, Mountcastle, Talbot, & Yin, 1977;

Yin & Mountcastle, 1977), reaching movements (Mountcastle, Lynch, Georgopoulos, Sakata, & Acuna, 1975), and grasping (Taira, Mine, Georgopoulos, Murata, & Sakata, 1990). Since that time, considerably more evidence has accumulated that not only replicates the earlier findings but also begins to shed light on the nature of the information and sensorimotor transformations that take place in the posterior parietal cortex. The available evidence—derived from studies using a variety of methodologies including single-unit recording, reversible inactivation, neural ablation, and neural connectivity analysis—suggests that grasping is mediated by an extensively interconnected circuit of occipital (V3A: Nakamura et al., 2001; V6A: Battaglini et al., 2002; Caminiti et al., 1999), parietal (areas 5 and 7: Debowy, Ghosh, Ro, & Gardner, 2001; AIP: Gallese, Murata, Kaseda, Niki, & Sakata, 1994; Murata, Gallese, Luppino, Kaseda, & Sakata, 2000), and frontal (ventral premotor cortex [F5]: Fogassi et al., 2001) brain regions, in which progressive transformations of visual object features into motor commands takes place (for a recent and comprehensive review, see Castiello, 2005; Cohen & Andersen, 2002).

Transcranial Magnetic Stimulation

In transcranial magnetic stimulation (TMS), neural activity is disrupted in a localized region by applying a brief, powerful magnetic field at the surface of the head. Unlike observational techniques like fMRI and single-unit recording, TMS can be used to determine the causal role of a particular brain region in a targeted behavior. Although a number of studies have used TMS to explore the neural substrates of visually guided action, only two studies were found that used the technique to explore manual prehension. Tunik, Frey, and Grafton (2005) applied TMS over three brain regions (V6A, AIP, and primary motor cortex) thought to be important for the control of grasping movements while participants reached to objects whose size or orientation was changed during the response. Only when the TMS was applied over AIP were appropriate hand adjustments disrupted: TMS pulses delivered over the primary motor cortex and over V6A in the occipital cortex did not disrupt online grip adjustments. This study provides strong evidence for a causal link between the neural processing carried out in AIP and the online control of grasping. Consistent with this finding, Glover, Miall, and Rushworth (2005) showed that repetitive TMS applied over the left intraparietal sulcus during grasping disrupted the initiation but not the execution of online grip modifications when the target object changed size midflight.

Psychophysics

Although the evidence presented thus far provides strong support for the idea that distinct neural systems are involved in perceptual and sensorimotor aspects of vision, that evidence does not address what is arguably the most important and most controversial postulate of the two-streams hypothesis—that conscious perception of object form is not necessary for the control of object manipulation. The fMRI and neurophysiological evidence presented previously argues neither for nor against the idea that the visual transformations of object form necessary for perceptual and sensorimotor tasks are fundamentally different, simply that different regions of the cortex are implicated in the two tasks. Compelling, albeit controversial, evidence for the functional independence of object perception and object manipulation has been found in a number of psychophysical experiments that show striking differences between perceptual and sensorimotor sensitivities to visual illusions.

Visual illusions have long been used as a tool for studying the underlying mechanisms of perception, providing important insight into the visual cues and computations that lie behind conscious experience (Gregory, 1997). More recently, visual illusions have been used to explore the relationship between conscious perceptual experience and sensorimotor behavior (for a review, see Carey, 2001). Wong and Mack (1981) showed that saccadic eye movements to a target presented in an induced-motion display were quite accurate despite the fact that participants incorrectly judged the target to be oscillating back and forth. In a similar vein, Bridgeman, Peery, and Anand (1997) found that participants could point accurately to a target whose location was judged inaccurately because of a large visual frame centered slightly to the left or right of the body midline; a recent extension and reinterpretation of these results was carried out by Dassonville, Bridgeman, Kaur Bala, Thiem, and Sampanes (2004).

In what appears to be the first study to look at the effect of a perceptual illusion of object form on manipulatory action, Aglioti, DeSouza, and Goodale (1995) found that an Ebbinghaus size-contrast illusion (in which a target disk surrounded by larger flanking circles appears smaller than the very same disk surrounded by smaller flanking circles) affected participants' judgments of the relative sizes of two target disks but not the peak grip aperture measured when participants actually grasped the individual disks. In other words, somehow the grasping hand "knew" the true sizes of the disks despite the fact that participants were not consciously aware of this information. Haffenden and Goodale (1998) replicated and extended Aglioti et al.'s results using improved methods: Parametric measurements of size perception were used, and visual information was removed at the onset of the grasping movements, thereby preventing the use of updated visual information to adjust the action as the hand homed in on the target object.

The seminal studies described previously spawned a large research effort into the effects of visual illusions on perceptual and sensorimotor responses. By and large, with some notable exceptions (for a discussion, see Franz, 2001), most experiments report that the peak aperture of visually guided grasping is not affected by pictorial illusions such as the Ponzo "railroad tracks" illusion or the Titchener circles (Ebbinghaus) size-contrast illusion despite the clear and robust effects of these visual displays on conscious perception of object size. Indeed, Westwood, King, and Christensen (revised manuscript submitted January, 2008) have recently demonstrated that there is no correlation between the perceptual effects of a size-contrast illusion and the effects of the illusion on grip aperture at any point in time during visually guided grasping movements.

Although it may seem surprising that the grasping hand can behave in a manner that disagrees with the individual's own conscious perceptual experience, this finding provides important clues about the nature of the visual computations that lie behind perception and action. One possible explanation for the observed difference between perception and action is that the two tasks require different types of information about the object's form (Goodale & Humphrey, 1998). In order to execute an accurate grasp—so that the object is not bumped, knocked over, or perhaps dropped—the motor system requires information about the size, orientation, and location of the target object that is specified in absolute metrics. It is not sufficient to know that the target object is bigger or smaller than a breadbox, for example; rather, one needs to know that it is 12 centimeters in width. Because of its requirement for metrical precision, the sensorimotor system must rely on visual computations that use accurate cues to the object's size and location, such as binocular depth cues like stereopsis and vergence angle and retinal image size. Unreliable cues like the geometric scene elements used in pictorial illusions to invoke inappropriate size-constancy mechanisms will not suffice and are thus ignored.

With regard to perceptual experience, the requirements for metrical precision are quite different. Because the ultimate goal of visual perception is to make sense of the world by linking currently available visual inputs with stored semantic memory, it is imperative that the perceptual system is not wedded to the absolute metrics of the visual array. Imagine how difficult life would be if you could not somehow realize that a cup of coffee is a cup of coffee no matter how large or small the particular cup is and no matter where it is located relative to your current position. For that matter, if perceptual experience were yoked to the absolute metrics of the visual array, it would not be possible to identify people or objects on television or on a movie screen. In other words, it is the relative rather than absolute metrics of the visual world that are fundamental to the successful operation of perceptual mechanisms. Perception is an inherently relative process whereby objects are judged in relation to other objects and landmarks in the visual scene and indeed relative to other objects and information represented in semantic memory. This is why perception is so susceptible to pictorial illusions; these illusions work only when the target object is compared in an obligatory way with the other visual elements in the scene.

Action Is Not Always Separate From Perception

By and large, discussion to this point has centered on important differences between the visual mechanisms that deliver object form information to the sensorimotor versus perceptual system. The mechanisms for the former utilize absolute metrics and reside in the dorsal stream, and the mechanisms

for the latter utilize relative metrics and are located in the ventral stream. However, from an evolutionary point of view, any visual pathway in the brain would have evolved only if it served some useful purpose in the control of behavior. That is, in one way or another, the perceptual mechanisms proposed to exist within the ventral stream of visual cortex must be able to influence movement. This point was made quite clearly in Milner and Goodale's (1995) exposition of their two-visual streams hypothesis and is emphasized in the epilogue that accompanies the release of the second edition of that book.

The key difference between the dorsal "action" and ventral "perception" systems is not that the former can influence motor control whereas the latter cannot but that the dorsal pathway has an immediate or proximal influence on motor responses whereas the ventral pathway has an indirect or distal influence on motor responses. To make this distinction clear, one need only consider the commonplace scenario of making a bowl of cereal for breakfast. In order to accomplish this task, one must identify which of the objects in the kitchen is a bowl and which is a box of cereal. Once this task has been completed, appropriate patterns of muscle activity can then be generated that will allow the bowl and cereal to be brought together in a manner conducive to the final goal of a wholesome meal. In this scenario, the task of identifying the appropriate target object (i.e., discriminating between a bowl versus a plate) would require the services of the perceptual mechanisms in the ventral stream. However, the end point for this perceptual task is not simply to distinguish between pieces of flatware but to flag an object as the target for an action. In other words, the goal of this "perceptual" activity is linked in a very fundamental way to "action." The task of reaching toward the target object and effecting a stable grasp would surely be mediated by the dorsal stream since the computations carried out in this pathway are intended to deliver absolute object metrics to the motor system for the purpose of controlling movement. Thus, this task is also clearly linked to "action" but in a more immediate and direct way than the object discrimination task carried out previously.

Given this reasoning, then, one might wonder which aspects of object manipulation are handled by the dorsal stream and which are handled by the ventral stream. There are four lines of research that speak to the relationship between ventral and dorsal stream processing in control of manipulatory actions.

Memory

With some notable exceptions, such as in drama, communication, or teaching, people do not try to grasp objects that are not physically present in the surrounding environs. By and large, the to-be-grasped object is not only physically present but also visible when the action is required (an obvious exception is when one must fumble to find the switch on a bedside lamp on waking up in a dark room). Thus, it would seem reasonable that the dorsal stream mechanisms charged with programming and controlling grasping movements would capitalize on the wealth of current visual information about the target object that is available when the action is about to be initiated. By using the most current visual information, the dorsal stream can avoid continuously updating the movement plan every time the actor or target object moves before response initiation. As is discussed next, considerable evidence suggests that this is exactly how the dorsal stream operates; the system is engaged for response programming just before the action is initiated, and it appears to depend on the visibility of the target object at that time. A quite different mode of action control is

engaged when the target is not visible—a mode of control that draws on a perceptual representation of the object laid down by the ventral visual stream.

Goodale, Jakobson, and Keillor (1994) showed that D. F., the visual form agnosic patient, scaled her grip aperture to the size of target objects when grasping with current vision of the environment but not when the target object was removed from view 2 seconds prior to initiating the action (i.e., a "pantomimed" grasp). Jakobson et al. proposed that the dorsal stream does not have a memory of its own: The ventral stream stores object features in memory and delivers this information to the motor system when an action to a remembered object is required. On the flip side of the neuropsychological coin, Milner and colleagues (2001) demonstrated a paradoxical improvement in grasping performance for the optic ataxic patient I. G.—who had bilateral damage to the posterior parietal cortex—when that patient grasped an object 2 seconds after it had been removed from view. When the object was visible and the action was initiated immediately on seeing the object, I. G. showed a poor correlation between peak grip aperture and object size. That deficit in visually guided action is consistent with I. G.'s lesion in the posterior parietal cortex. The correlation between object size and I. G.'s grip aperture was much clearer in the delayed grasping task, suggesting that the control of memory-guided action was driven by I. G.'s intact ventral stream. Interestingly, there was some evidence that I. G. learned to make use of stored object features to control actions even when the object in fact remained visible, hinting at a possible rehabilitation strategy for patients with dorsal stream lesions.

In a series of experiments using visual illusions in neurologically healthy individuals, Westwood and colleagues have shown that conscious form perception is important for the control of memory-guided grasping but not visually guided grasping (Westwood, Chapman, & Roy, 2000; Westwood, Heath, & Roy, 2000; Westwood & Goodale, 2003). Westwood and Goodale (2003) had participants grasp and estimate the sizes of rectangular objects that were presented beside larger, same-sized, or smaller flanking rectangles. Participants were highly sensitive to the perceptual effects of this size-contrast display, judging the object to be smaller when it was presented beside a larger (as compared to smaller) flanker. In a set of open-loop grasping trials, the objects remained visible until the onset of the action, at which point liquid-crystal occlusion goggles blocked any further visual input. In a randomly intermixed set of no-vision trials, the objects were blocked from view at the same instant an auditory tone cued the grasping response; on average, participants initiated their grasping movement about 300 milliseconds after this. Grip aperture was measured using a 3-D optoelectronic recording system. The results showed no significant effect of flanker size on peak grip aperture in the open-loop trials but a robust effect of the flankers on peak grip aperture in the no-vision trials. Because the only difference between the open-loop and no-vision trials was the visibility of the target display during the 300 milliseconds between response cuing and response initiation, Westwood and Goodale reasoned that this immediate premovement period must be critical for the programming of the subsequent action. To the extent that the target object is visible during this period of time, it would appear that this is when the dorsal stream visuomotor mechanisms are engaged—leading to grasping actions that are insensitive to the pictorial illusion. If the object is not visible during this period, the programming of the action is instead driven by a perceptual representation of the target object generated and likely maintained

within the ventral stream. In other words, the dorsal stream does not generate an action program until the moment the action is actually required. Hence, the visual control of action by the dorsal stream operates in real time, based on currently visual input from the environment.

Monocular Viewing

Binocular visual cues are important for the control of grasping and reaching movements (Jackson, Newport, & Shaw, 2002; Mon-Williams & Dijkerman, 1999; Servos, Goodale, & Jakobson, 1992). When binocular cues are manipulated or removed, predictable decreases in grasping accuracy and consistency are observed. Not only are monocular actions less accurate than their binocular counterparts, but it appears that the two types of actions might be controlled by quite different brain systems. Dijkerman, Milner, and Carey (1996) showed that D. F.'s grasping movements were dramatically impaired when binocular cues were removed, suggesting that the dorsal stream cannot work properly without such inputs. Marotta, DeSouza, Haffenden, and Goodale (1998) showed in neurologically healthy participants that monocular (versus binocular) grasps were much more sensitive to a size-contrast illusion, but only when the object's height—a monocular cue to object distance—was varied unpredictably (versus predictably) on a trial-by-trial basis. Marotta et al.'s findings suggest that the perceptual stream is engaged for response programming and control when binocular cues are unavailable. Otto-de Haart, Carey, and Milne (1999) failed to replicate Marotta et al.'s finding, but the former study used a different type of illusion and did not vary object height in a random fashion.

Lifting Dynamics

The programming and control of grasping requires information about object size and shape, which can in principle be derived unambiguously from the binocular projection of the object's image on the two retinas. The control of lifting dynamics—the forces and torques used to hold and lift the object—however, requires information about object mass and the distribution of that mass (Westling & Johansson, 1984). This information cannot be derived exclusively from currently available binocular inputs: Some stored knowledge about the density of the object or the familiar mass of the object is necessary (Goodale, 2000). Because access to stored knowledge is thought to be the domain of the perceptual (rather than visuomotor) system, one would predict that the control of lifting dynamics—unlike the control of the grasping aperture—might require a perceptual analysis of the object.

Consistent with this prediction, at least two studies (Brenner & Smeets, 1996; Jackson & Shaw, 2000) have shown that participants use greater lifting forces when picking up objects erroneously perceived to be larger because of a surrounding pictorial illusion—despite the fact that the maximum grip aperture used during the approach phase of the action was not similarly influenced by the size illusion. These findings suggest that a perceptual analysis of object form is utilized to access stored knowledge about mass or density for the purpose of controlling lifting dynamics, whereas this is not true for the control of grip aperture. Although Westwood, Dubrowski, Carnahan, and Roy (2000) found that a Ponzo pictorial illusion did not affect lifting dynamics, those results cannot be directly compared with the studies just described because, unlike those studies, the objects in Westwood et al.'s study were intentionally designed to violate expected correlations between size and mass.

The story has recently become complicated, however, by findings reported first by Flanagan and Beltzner (2000) and then

recently extended by Grandy and Westwood (2006). Both studies investigated the effect of the size-weight illusion on perception and action, but for the sake of clarity only the latter study is discussed here. In the size-weight illusion, the larger of two objects is perceived to weigh less than the smaller despite the identical or at least very similar masses of the two objects. In Grandy and Westwood's study, the smaller object weighed only slightly less than the larger object despite its dramatically smaller size; nevertheless, participants erroneously reported that the smaller object felt heavier than the larger object throughout all 20 lifting trials in the study. Analysis of lifting dynamics told a completely different story, however. Participants correctly used larger forces (and force rates) to lift the larger object (versus the smaller object) in direct opposition to the participants' own reports that the larger object felt lighter than the smaller. The dramatic difference between perceptual and sensorimotor responses to the size-weight illusion challenges the idea proposed earlier that control of lifting dynamics is driven by a perceptual analysis of the object. Perhaps the key difference between the size-weight illusion studies and the pictorial size illusion studies is that, in the former, perceptually unambiguous visual input is used to access distinct sensorimotor and perceptual representations of object mass, whereas, in the latter, perceptually ambiguous visual input is used to drive both perceptual and sensorimotor computations of object heaviness. Further research is required to clarify the mechanisms underlying the perception of object heaviness and the control of lifting dynamics.

Response Selection

The hand posture most suitable for picking up an object depends on how the object will be used once it has been grasped (Rosenbaum, Vaughan, Barnes, & Jorgensen,

1992). This is particularly important when interacting with tools. Consider a hammer resting on a table with its handle pointed away from rather than toward the body. Although it would be most comfortable to pick the hammer up using a simple overhand grasp, the hammer would then be upside down once lifted. It would make more sense to sacrifice some initial discomfort by grasping the hammer with an inverted grasp so that the tool will be in the upright position once lifted. In order to select the most efficient way to grasp an object, one must appreciate its functional semantics, that is, the ways in which the object can be used. Because this would require an appreciation of the object's identity, it is conceivable that response selection—unlike response programming and execution—would be driven by a perceptual analysis of the target object.

In a clever experiment, Creem and Proffitt (2001) presented handled tools at various orientations and asked participants to pick the tool up and pantomime its use. For some tool orientations (i.e., handles pointing away from the actor), efficient pantomimes required the adoption of an initially awkward hand posture. In some sets of trials, participants were given a sequence of numbers or spatial locations to retain in memory while performing the grasp-pantomime task (i.e., dual-task trials) whereas in other trials this secondary memory task was not required (i.e., single-task trials). In the dual-task trials (versus single-task trials), participants were less likely to use awkward hand postures in the critical orientation conditions. In other words, the requirement to remember irrelevant information interfered with the participants' ability to select a grasping posture appropriate to the ultimate goal of pantomiming the use of the tool. Regardless of whether or not the secondary memory task was required, however, participants used metrically appropriate grip apertures and

hand orientations to enclose the handle of the tool. Thus, the working memory load did not interfere with the programming and execution of the chosen action, only the selection of the action in the first place. This study strongly suggests that response selection is driven by the perceptual mechanisms of the ventral stream—mechanisms intimately connected to cognitive and memory systems that have capacity limitations and that are thus subject to overload from secondary task performance. Response programming and execution, by way of contrast, do not appear to require the perceptual mechanisms of the ventral stream unless, as outlined earlier, binocular vision of the target object is not available during the immediate premovement period.

Conclusion

Over the past 20 or so years, considerable evidence has accumulated that is consistent with the idea that conscious perception of object form is not necessary for the control of object manipulation. The control of grasping can be driven by computations that take place in the dorsal stream of occipital and parietal cortex—computations that utilize currently available binocular inputs to deliver the absolute metrics of the object to the motor system. Conscious perception of object form is mediated by computations that take place in the ventral stream of occipital and temporal cortex—computations that lead to the creation of an internal representation of the object that can be used to access stored semantic information. Whereas the dorsal stream computes the exact metrics of the object—which are fundamental to precise motor control—the ventral stream computes its relative metrics—which are fundamental to perceptual constancy. Although functionally and anatomically distinct, both of the two visual streams contribute to the control of object manipulation but in quite different ways. The dorsal stream appears to be restricted to the programming and control of grasping when binocular inputs from the target object are available at the moment the action is required. The ventral stream appears to deliver object information to the motor system for response programming and control when binocular vision of the object is unavailable. Quite apart from the task of programming and controlling the intended action, the selection of an appropriate response depends on perceptual processing that takes place in the ventral stream because deciding how to interact with an object first requires that object to be identified.

Acknowledgments

Thank you to Camilla M. Holmvall for providing helpful comments on an earlier version of this chapter. Thank you to Mel Goodale for the many insightful discussions we have shared on the topics discussed in this chapter. Preparation of this chapter was made possible in part by funding from the Natural Sciences and Engineering Research Council of Canada to David A. Westwood.

References

Aglioti, S., DeSouza, J. F., & Goodale, M. A. (1995). Size-contrast illusions deceive the eye but not the hand. *Current Biology, 5,* 679–685.

Battaglini, P. P., Muzur, A., Galletti, C., Skrap, M., Brovelli, A., & Fattori, P. (2002). Effects of lesions to area V6A in monkeys. *Experimental Brain Research, 144,* 419–422.

Binkofski, F., Dohle, C., Posse, S., Stephan, K. M., Hefter, H., Seitz, R. J., et al. (1998). Human anterior intraparietal area subserves prehension: A combined lesion and functional MRI activation study. *Neurology, 50,* 1253–1259.

Brenner, E., & Smeets, J. B. (1996). Size illusion influences how we lift but not how we grasp an object. *Experimental Brain Research, 111,* 473–476.

Bridgeman, B., Peery, S., & Anand, S. (1997). Interaction of cognitive and sensorimotor maps of visual space. *Perception and Psychophysics, 59,* 456–469.

Caminiti, R., Genovesio, A., Marconi, B., Mayer, A. B., Onorati, P., Ferraina, S., et al. (1999). Early coding of reaching: Frontal and parietal association connections of parieto-occipital cortex. *European Journal of Neuroscience, 11,* 3339–3345.

Carey, D. P. (2001). Do action systems resist visual illusions? *Trends in Cognitive Sciences, 5,* 109–113.

Castiello, U. (2005). The neuroscience of grasping. *Nature Reviews Neuroscience, 6,* 726–736.

Cohen, Y. E., & Andersen, R. A. (2002). A common reference frame for movement plans in the posterior parietal cortex. *Nature Reviews Neuroscience, 3,* 553–562.

Creem, S. H., & Proffitt, D. R. (2001). Grasping objects by their handles: A necessary interaction between cognition and action. *Journal of Experimental Psychology: Human Perception and Performance, 27,* 218–228.

Creem-Regehr, S. H., & Lee, J. N. (2005). Neural representations of graspable objects: Are tools special? *Cognitive Brain Research, 22,* 457–469.

Culham, J. C., Danckert, S. L., DeSouza, J. F., Gati, J. S., Menon, R. S., & Goodale, M. A. (2003). Visually guided grasping produces fMRI activation in dorsal but not ventral stream brain areas. *Experimental Brain Research, 153,* 180–189.

Dassonville, P., Bridgeman, B., Kaur Bala, J., Thiem, P., & Sampanes, A. (2004). The induced Roelofs effect: Two visual systems or the shift of a single reference frame? *Vision Research, 44,* 603–611.

Debowy, D. J., Ghosh, S., Ro, J. Y., & Gardner, E. P. (2001). Comparison of neuronal firing rates in somatosensory and posterior parietal cortex during prehension. *Experimental Brain Research, 137,* 269–291.

Dijkerman, H. C., Milner, A. D., & Carey, D. P. (1996). The perception and prehension of objects oriented in the depth plane. I. Effects of visual form agnosia. *Experimental Brain Research, 112,* 442–451.

Ehrsson, H. H., Fagergren, A., Johansson, R. S., & Forssberg, H. (2003). Evidence for the involvement of the posterior parietal cortex in coordination of fingertip forces for grasp stability in manipulation. *Journal of Neurophysiology, 90,* 2978–2986.

Epstein, R., & Kanwisher, N. (1998). A cortical representation of the local visual environment. *Nature, 392,* 598–601.

Flanagan, J. R., & Beltzner, M. A. (2000). Independence of perceptual and sensorimotor predictions in the size-weight illusion. *Nature Neuroscience, 3,* 737–741.

Fogassi, L., Gallese, V., Buccino, G., Craighero, L., Fadiga, L., & Rizzolatti, G. (2001). Cortical mechanism for the visual guidance of hand grasping movements in the monkey: A reversible inactivation study. *Brain, 124,* 571–586.

Franz, V. H. (2001). Action does not resist visual illusions. *Trends in Cognitive Sciences, 5,* 457–459.

Frey, S. H., Vinton, D., Norlund, R., & Grafton, S. T. (2005). Cortical topography of human anterior intraparietal cortex active during visually guided grasping. *Cognitive Brain Research, 23,* 397–405.

Gallese, V., Murata, A., Kaseda, M., Niki, N., & Sakata, H. (1994). Deficit of hand preshaping after muscimol injection in monkey parietal cortex. *Neuroreport, 5,* 1525–1529.

Gauthier, I., Tarr, M. J., Anderson, A. W., Skudlarski, P., & Gore, J. C. (1999). Activation of the middle fusiform "face area" increases with expertise in recognizing novel objects. *Nature Neuroscience, 2,* 568–573.

Glover, S., Miall, R. C., & Rushworth, M. F. (2005). Parietal rTMS disrupts the initiation but not the execution of on-line adjustments to a perturbation of object size. *Journal of Cognitive Neuroscience, 17,* 124–136.

Goodale, M. A. (2000). A visible difference. *Current Biology, 10,* R46–R47.

Goodale, M. A., & Humphrey, G. K. (1998). The objects of action and perception. *Cognition, 67,* 181–207.

Goodale, M. A., Jakobson, L. S., & Keillor, J. M. (1994). Differences in the visual control of pantomimed and natural grasping movements. *Neuropsychologia, 32,* 1159–1178.

Goodale, M. A., Meenan, J. P., Bulthoff, H. H., Nicolle, D. A., Murphy, K. J., & Racicot, C. I. (1994). Separate neural pathways for the visual analysis of object shape in perception and prehension. *Current Biology, 4,* 604–610.

Goodale, M. A., & Milner, A. D. (1992). Separate visual pathways for perception and action. *Trends in Neuroscience, 15,* 20–25.

Goodale, M. A., Milner, A. D., Jakobson, L. S., & Carey, D. P. (1991). A neurological dissociation between perceiving objects and grasping them. *Nature, 349,* 154–156.

Goodale, M. A., Pelisson, D., & Prablanc, C. (1986). Large adjustments in visually guided reaching do not depend on vision of the hand or perception of target displacement. *Nature, 320,* 748–750.

Grandy, M. S., & Westwood, D. A. (2006). Opposite effects of a size-weight illusion on perception and action. *Journal of Neurophysiology, 95,* 3887–3892.

Gregory, R. L. (1997). Knowledge in perception and illusion. *Philosophical Transactions of the Royal Society of London. Series B, Biological Sciences, 352,* 1121–1127.

Grill-Spector, K. (2003). The neural basis of object perception. *Current Opinion in Neurobiology, 13,* 159–166.

Grossman, E., Donnelly, M., Price, R., Pickens, D., Morgan, V., Neighbor, G., et al. (2000). Brain areas involved in perception of biological motion. *Journal of Cognitive Neuroscience, 12,* 711–720.

Haffenden, A. M., & Goodale, M. A. (1998). The effect of pictorial illusion on prehension and perception. *Journal of Cognitive Neuroscience, 10,* 122–136.

Haxby, J. V., Horwitz, B., Ungerleider, L. G., Maisog, J. M., Pietrini, P., & Grady, C. L. (1994). The functional organization of human extrastriate cortex: A PET-rCBF study of selective attention to faces and locations. *Journal of Neuroscience, 14,* 6336–6353.

Ishai, A., Ungerleider, L. G., Martin, A., Schouten, J. L., & Haxby, J. V. (1999). Distributed representation of objects in the human ventral visual pathway. *Proceedings of the National Academy of Sciences of the United States of America, 96,* 9379–9384.

Jackson, S. R., Newport, R., & Shaw, A. (2002). Monocular vision leads to a dissociation between grip force and grip aperture scaling during reach-to-grasp movements. *Current Biology, 12,* 237–240.

Jackson, S. R., & Shaw, A. (2000). The Ponzo illusion affects grip-force but not grip-aperture scaling during prehension movements. *Journal of Experimental Psychology: Human Perception and Performance, 26,* 418–423.

James, T. W., Culham, J., Humphrey, G. K., Milner, A. D., & Goodale, M. A. (2003). Ventral occipital lesions impair object recognition but not object-directed grasping: An fMRI study. *Brain, 126,* 2463–2475.

Jeannerod, M. (1986). The formation of finger grip during prehension: A cortically mediated visuomotor pattern. *Behavioural Brain Research, 19,* 99–116.

Kanwisher, N., McDermott, J., & Chun, M. M. (1997). The fusiform face area: A module in human extrastriate cortex specialized for face perception. *Journal of Neuroscience, 17,* 4302–4311.

Llinas, R., Ribary, U., Contreras, D., & Pedroarena, C. (1998). The neuronal basis for consciousness. *Philosophical Transactions of the Royal Society of London. Series B, Biological Sciences, 353,* 1841–1849.

Logothetis, N. K., Pauls, J., Augath, M., Trinath, T., & Oeltermann, A. (2001). Neurophysiological investigation of the basis of the fMRI signal. *Nature, 412,* 150–157.

Lynch, J. C., Mountcastle, V. B., Talbot, W. H., & Yin, T. C. (1977). Parietal lobe mechanisms for directed visual attention. *Journal of Neurophysiology, 40,* 362–389.

Malach, R., Reppas, J. B., Benson, R. R., Kwong, K. K., Jiang, H., Kennedy, W. A., et al. (1995). Object-related activity revealed by functional magnetic resonance imaging in human occipital cortex. *Proceedings of the National Academy of Sciences USA, 92,* 8135–8139.

Marotta, J. J., DeSouza, J. F., Haffenden, A. M., & Goodale, M. A. (1998). Does a monocularly presented size-contrast illusion influence grip aperture? *Neuropsychologia, 36,* 491–497.

Marr, D. (1982). *Vision.* San Francisco: Freeman.

McKeefry, D. J., & Zeki, S. (1997). The position and topography of the human colour centre as revealed by functional magnetic resonance imaging. *Brain, 120,* 2229–2242.

Milner, A. D., Dijkerman, H. C., Pisella, L., McIntosh, R. D., Tilikete, C., Vighetto, A., et al. (2001). Grasping the past: Delay can improve visuomotor performance. *Current Biology, 11,* 1896–1901.

Milner, A. D., & Goodale, M. A. (1995). *The visual brain in action.* New York: Oxford University Press.

Milner, A. D., Perrett, D. I., Johnston, R. S., Benson, P. J., Jordan, T. R., Heeley, D. W., et al. (1991). Perception and action in "visual form agnosia." *Brain, 114,* 405–428.

Mon-Williams, M., & Dijkerman, H. C. (1999). The use of vergence information in the programming of prehension. *Experimental Brain Research, 128,* 578–582.

Mountcastle, V. B., Lynch, J. C., Georgopoulos, A., Sakata, H., & Acuna, C. (1975). Posterior parietal association cortex of the monkey: Command functions for operations within extrapersonal space. *Journal of Neurophysiology, 38,* 871–908.

Murata, A., Gallese, V., Luppino, G., Kaseda, M., & Sakata, H. (2000). Selectivity for the shape, size, and orientation of objects for grasping in neurons of monkey parietal area AIP. *Journal of Neurophysiology, 83,* 2580–2601.

Nakamura, H., Kuroda, T., Wakita, M., Kusunoki, M., Kato, A., Mikami, A., et al. (2001). From three-dimensional space vision to prehensile hand movements: The lateral intraparietal area links the area V3A and the anterior intraparietal area in macaques. *Journal of Neuroscience, 21,* 8174–8187.

Otto-de Haart, E. G., Carey, D. P., & Milne, A. B. (1999). More thoughts on perceiving and grasping the Muller-Lyer illusion. *Neuropsychologia, 37,* 1437–1444.

Paulignan, Y., Frak, V. G., Toni, I., & Jeannerod, M. (1997). Influence of object position and size on human prehension movements. *Experimental Brain Research, 114,* 226–234.

Rosenbaum, D. A., Vaughan, J., Barnes, H. J., & Jorgensen, M. J. (1992). Time course of movement planning: Selection of handgrips for object manipulation. *Journal of Experimental Psychology: Learning, Memory, and Cognition, 18,* 1058–1073.

Servos, P., Goodale, M. A., & Jakobson, L. S. (1992). The role of binocular vision in prehension: A kinematic analysis. *Vision Research, 32,* 1513–1521.

Taira, M., Mine, S., Georgopoulos, A. P., Murata, A., & Sakata, H. (1990). Parietal cortex neurons of the monkey related to the visual guidance of hand movement. *Experimental Brain Research, 83,* 29–36.

Tunik, E., Frey, S. H., & Grafton, S. T. (2005). Virtual lesions of the anterior intraparietal area disrupt goal-dependent on-line adjustments of grasp. *Nature Neuroscience, 8,* 505–511.

Ungerleider, L. G., & Mishkin, M. (1982). Two cortical visual systems. In D. J. Ingle, M. A. Goodale, & R. J. W. Mansfield (Eds.), *Analysis of visual behaviour* (pp. 549–586). Cambridge, MA: MIT Press.

Watson, J. D., Myers, R., Frackowiak, R. S., Hajnal, J. V., Woods, R. P., Mazziotta, J. C., et al. (1993). Area V5 of the human brain: Evidence from a combined study using positron emission tomography and magnetic resonance imaging. *Cerebral Cortex, 3,* 79–94.

Weiskrantz, L., Warrington, E. K., Sanders, M. D., & Marshall, J. (1974). Visual capacity in the hemianopic field following a restricted occipital ablation. *Brain, 97,* 709–728.

Westling, G., & Johansson, R. S. (1984). Factors influencing the force control during precision grip. *Experimental Brain Research, 53,* 277–284.

Westwood, D. A., Chapman, C. D., & Roy, E. A. (2000). Pantomimed actions may be controlled by the ventral visual stream. *Experimental Brain Research, 130,* 545–548.

Westwood, D. A., Dubrowski, A., Carnahan, H., & Roy, E. A. (2000). The effect of illusory size on force production when grasping objects. *Experimental Brain Research, 135,* 535–543.

Westwood, D. A., & Goodale, M. A. (2003). Perceptual illusion and the real-time control of action. *Spatial Vision, 16,* 243–254.

Westwood, D. A., Heath, M., & Roy, E. A. (2000). The effect of a pictorial illusion on closed-loop and open-loop prehension. *Experimental Brain Research, 134,* 456–463.

Westwood, D. A., King, J. P., & Christensen, B. (revised manuscript submitted January, 2008). *A dissociation between perception and action but not planning and control.* Manuscript submitted for publication.

Wong, E., & Mack, A. (1981). Saccadic programming and perceived location. *Acta Psychologica, 48,* 123–131.

Woodworth, R. S. (1899). The accuracy of voluntary movement. *Psychological Review, 3*(Suppl. 13), 1–119.

Yin, T. C., & Mountcastle, V. B. (1977). Visual input to the visuomotor mechanisms of the monkey's parietal lobe. *Science, 197,* 1381–1383.

The Two Horses of Behavior: Reflection and Impulse

Fritz Strack, Roland Deutsch, *and* Regina Krieglmeyer

Abstract

This chapter examines the most important psychological concepts that have been used to explain human behavior. It begins by describing how psychological theories have moved from explanations at the situational level to explanations at the level of mental processes. It then discusses the most central theoretical constructs that have been proposed as determinants of behavior: attitudes, behavioral decisions, goal pursuit, habits, needs, and motivational orientations. Although each of these concepts has shortcomings, each still possesses great and distinct explanatory power to the extent that they can be included in a coherent theoretical model. The dual-system model integrates a number of psychological processes and specifies how they interact and determine social behavior.

Keywords: attitudes, behavioral decisions, goal pursuit, habits, needs, motivation, orientations, dual-system model, social behavior

In the tripartite definition of psychology, behavior has always played a dominant role. It has been a central phenomenon of interest not only during the period of *behaviorism,* where studying anything other than observable behavior was considered unscientific (e.g., Skinner, 1953), but even for psychologists today who are primarily concerned with thinking or feeling.

On one hand, research often aims at understanding how cognition and affect interact with behavior as behavioral precursors or consequences (e.g., Kuhl, 1985). On the other hand, behavior necessarily serves an important pragmatic role in psychological research. In many paradigms, it is interpreted as the observable manifestation of an unobservable mental process and

thereby lends itself as a convenient measure to inspect and assess aspects of thinking and feeling (e.g., Lachman, Lachman, & Butterfield, 1979). Both perspectives, the theoretical and the methodological, are concerned with the link among affect, cognition, and behavior. Therefore, these perspectives either are based on or aim at extending theories of human behavior.

In this chapter, we begin by describing how psychological theories have moved from explanations at the situational level to explanations at the level of mental processes. We then turn to what we believe to be the most central theoretical constructs that have been proposed as determinants of behavior. From this overview, we conclude that although each of these concepts has shortcomings, each still possesses great and distinct explanatory power to the extent that it can be included in a coherent theoretical model. Such a model is described. It is a dual-system model that integrates a number of psychological processes and specifies how they interact and determine social behavior.

Theories of Behavior

Psychology has offered numerous accounts that attempt to explain why and how people behave in a particular way. Theories of behavior differ in many ways, but one important difference is the degree to which they invoke the existence of elaborate cognitive or affective processes that mediate how resulting behavior emerges from situational inputs. Such mediation was almost absent in the models of early learning psychology and behaviorism. Radical behaviorists totally refrained from speculating about inner processes (Skinner, 1938; Watson, 1913), and many other theories were limited to postulating the existence of stimulus–response (S-R) associations in memory that are energized by an unspecific drive (e.g., Hull, 1943). In addition to *habit, needs,* and *drive,* such theories featured learning rules, describing how practice and reward shape habits (e.g., Thorndike, 1898).

As research in the behaviorist tradition progressed, it became clear that habits and drives were not even capable of explaining the behavior of lower mammals (e.g., rats). Based on the observation that changes in the quality or amount of rewards could produce sudden, dramatic changes in behavior (e.g., Crespi, 1942), researchers came to conclude that the *anticipated outcomes* of behaviors exerted strong effects. Consequently, researchers started to incorporate *incentive* as an explanatory concept into learning theories (Hull, 1952).

With the demise of behaviorism and the advent of the cognitive revolution (Neisser, 1967), mental processes took the leading role in explaining behavior (Bargh & Ferguson, 2000). While behaviorism has long been the dominant paradigm of psychology, social psychology has assumed a special role in that it has never adopted the behaviorist perspective to the degree it was taken on in other fields. Partly because it has its roots in gestalt psychology (Danziger, 2000), social psychology did not exclude the mental level of analysis from scientific analysis. As a consequence, for social psychology, it was the mental representation of the environment that became the basis for behavioral predictions. For instance, Lewin's idea of a *life space* represents the self in relation to its goals in a dynamic account in which behavior is the result of operating forces (Lewin, 1939).

Opening psychology to theorizing about inner mechanisms has created a wealth of mental constructs aimed at explaining human behavior, such as goals, intentions, decision making, needs, or attitudes. Just as modern versions of behaviorist concepts such as habit and drive continue to inspire research (e.g., Lambert et al., 2003; Ouellette & Wood, 1998; see Chapter 21), many mental constructs proved to be useful tools for understanding aspects of human behavior. In what follows, we give a short overview of what we believe to be the most central explanatory constructs.

Determinants of Behavior
Attitudes

Historically, social psychologists strongly relied on the concept of *attitudes* to explain behavior. Attitudes, defined as predispositions to evaluate persons, objects, or issues, were assumed to manifest themselves in specific behaviors. From the outset, attitudes were assessed to predict behavior (Thurstone, 1928), and popular definitions (e.g., Allport, 1935; Rosenberg & Hovland, 1960) identify behavior as a component of an attitude. After some doubts were expressed about this relationship (LaPiere, 1934; Wicker, 1969), theories emerged to explain how and under which circumstances behavior could be predicted by attitudes (e.g., Fazio, 1990; Fishbein & Ajzen, 1975).

The attitude–behavior relationship is moderated by a number of factors (Fazio & Olson, 2003). First, attitudes and behaviors can be manifest at very different levels of abstraction (e.g., liking and protecting bumblebees versus liking and protecting the environment), and only if the levels *correspond* can one expect attitudes to reliably predict behavior (Ajzen & Fishbein, 1977). Second, beliefs about how other people would appreciate the behavior and one's belief that one could perform the behavior must be taken into account when predicting what people will do in a given situation (Ajzen, 1991; Fishbein & Ajzen, 1975).

A second set of moderators relates to a fundamental distinction between different processes that bring about evaluations: On the one hand, evaluations may be stored and therefore be immediately accessible from memory (Fazio, Sanbonmatsu, Powell, & Kardes, 1986). On the other hand, processes of reasoning may construe evaluations or modify those retrieved from memory (Fazio, 1990; Wilson, Lindsey, & Schooler, 2000). There is now converging evidence that automatically retrieved evaluations may predict different behaviors than construed evaluations (e.g., Poehlman, Uhlmann, Greenwald, & Banaji, 2006; Wilson et al., 2000). There is also evidence that the two types of evaluations predict different behaviors, especially in the case where people are motivated and able to adjust what they retrieve from memory, as when the retrieved attitude is socially undesirable (Fazio & Towles-Schwen, 1999). Moreover, evidence indicates that the more accessible attitudes are in memory, the greater their influence on behavior (e.g., Fazio &

Williams, 1986). Thus, the predictive power of attitudes depends on moderating variables, which allows attitudes to be integrated into models that include these underlying cognitive processes.

Behavioral Decisions

One of the most successful concepts used to explain behavior is *behavioral decision*. By this term, we refer to cognitive processes that precede forming intentions and that concern, broadly speaking, the potential costs and benefits of performing a particular behavior (e.g., Feather, 1990). Theories focusing on behavioral decisions come in many variants and are widely used not only in social psychology (e.g., Bandura, 1977; Fishbein & Ajzen, 1975) but also in health psychology (Schwarzer, 1999), organizational behavior (e.g., Vroom, 1964), and economic theory (e.g., Becker, 1993). As different as these individual approaches are, they share the assumption that intentions are determined by thoughts about the likelihood and desirability of behavioral outcomes, and that intentions have a privileged access to those psychomotor processes that determine overt behavior. From this perspective, behavior is presumed to be a function of its anticipated outcomes. If we know exactly what people anticipate, we can predict what they intend. And when we know what they intend to achieve, we can predict how they will behave. Fishbein and Ajzen's model of social behavior has been aptly named by the authors both *theory of reasoned action* (e.g., Fishbein & Ajzen, 1975) and *theory of planned behavior* (e.g., Ajzen, 1988).

Compared to the concepts of habit and drive, the concept of behavioral decision significantly improves the understanding of many facets of human behavior (e.g., Fishbein & Mittelstadt, 1989). It helps explain behavior that is driven by very delayed consequences and by complex, spontaneously assembled plans. Moreover, it allows for a type of learning that is not based on the repetitive coupling of situations and behaviors. Instead, learning can occur through observation or communication (e.g., Bandura, 1977), whereby knowledge is conveyed by language or other symbolic means.

As successful as these models were in predicting intentions and ultimately behavior (Fishbein & Ajzen, 1975), they contribute little to our understanding of how goals and intentions actually translate into behavior. In addition, the concept of behavioral decision has a hard time explaining entirely thoughtless behaviors (Langer, Blank, & Chanowitz, 1978) or behaviors that people pursue despite their explicit belief that the overall outcomes will be negative, as is sometimes the case of addictive behaviors (e.g., Robinson & Berridge, 2003; see Chapter 24). These examples suggest that a considerable number of behaviors cannot be predicted by knowing the expected value of outcomes, partly because the resulting intentions may fail to translate into behavior and partly because people sometimes do not engage in such evaluations. Other concepts, such as habits, need states, or goal pursuit, are better suited to fill these explanatory gaps.

Goal Pursuit

Theories of goal pursuit specifically seek to explain how goals—once they are set—translate into overt behavior. Research has established numerous features of goal pursuit (see Förster, Liberman, & Friedman, 2007; see Chapter 9), distinguishing it from other determinants of behavior. Most important, goal pursuit can be best understood as a regulative process that monitors the distance between the actual and desired state, and selects appropriate means to minimize the distance to the goal (e.g., Carver & Scheier, 1998; Miller, Galanter, & Pribram, 1960; see Chapter 15). In many situations, multiple means exist to reach a given goal (Kruglanski et al., 2002; see Chapter 17). As part of its regulative nature, goal pursuit selects new means if obstacles block a planned path to the goal.

Apart from regulative feedback loops, goal pursuit was demonstrated to go hand in hand with numerous cognitive processes that support goal attainment, such as a reduced attention toward conflicting goals (Kruglanski et al., 2002) or more positive evaluations of goal-relevant stimuli (e.g., Ferguson & Bargh, 2004). Once they are formed, *implementation intentions* increase the accessibility of intention-relevant representations in memory (Webb & Sheeran, 2007). This way, the appropriate behavior may be more easily activated by situational cues (Gollwitzer, 1999; see Chapter 29). Once the goal has been reached, the maintaining motivational processes stop, and the accessibility of corresponding representations decreases (Förster, Liberman, & Higgins, 2005; Chapter 9).

Habits

In the behaviorist tradition, habits were defined as learned associations between stimuli and behaviors, which may determine behavior directly through situational stimulation (e.g., Hull 1943; Skinner, 1938; Watson, 1913). Whereas this traditional and narrow view of habits has not proven successful in explaining voluntary human behavior (Bargh & Ferguson, 2000), modern variants of the concepts seem indispensable (Aarts & Dijksterhuis, 2000; Dijksterhuis & Bargh, 2001; Ouelette & Wood, 1998). Extending James's (1890) *ideomotor principle* (see Chapters 2 and 18), a large body of research suggests that some perceptual and motorical representations are strongly interconnected. This, for example, might occur if a social stereotype that includes behavioral information is activated in memory (Dijksterhuis & Bargh,

2001). For example, Bargh, Chen, and Burrows (1996) have demonstrated that being exposed to the elderly stereotype caused participants to walk more slowly. Likewise, activating general concepts or perceptions that are by experience linked to behaviors or goals were demonstrated to have a directing effect on ongoing behavior, even outside of people's awareness (e.g., Holland, Hendriks, & Aarts, 2005).

It is important to note that the behaviors were emitted not immediately after they had been primed but only later when the situation required engaging in a certain action, like walking. It can thus be assumed that, as in studies on priming effects on various cognitive tasks (e.g., Meyer & Schvaneveldt, 1971), spreading activation may operate for behaviors as well. That is, a behavior will be elicited if the activation reaches a certain threshold, while the different sources may contribute in an additive manner. Similarly, the priming itself may occur in a subthreshold manner that is not accompanied by a subjective experience (Draine & Greenwald, 1998). In addition, habits can be well understood in terms of memorized "action plans," which may receive activation not from situations but from goals (Aarts & Dijksterhuis, 2000).

Needs and Motivational Orientations

In recent years, there has been a surge in research on the impact of motivational states on affect and cognition, both of which ultimately influence behavior (e.g., Sorrentino & Higgins, 1986). For instance, it has become apparent that need states have various effects. Many studies illuminate the operation of basic motivational orientations. Specifically, perceiving positive or negative stimuli automatically facilitates approach or avoidance behaviors (Chen & Bargh, 1999; Förster & Strack, 1996). Evidence also suggests that the link between valence and behavior is bidirectional: Performing approach or avoidance behavior also facilitates the processing of compatible information (Förster & Strack, 1997; Neumann & Strack, 2000).

While motivational orientations influence behavior very broadly, recent evidence suggests that need states may have a more specific impact. Particularly, there is growing evidence that being deprived of basic needs, such as nutrition or hydration, establishes a *behavioral preparedness* and a *perceptual readiness* for relevant information in the environment. For instance, hunger and thirst were demonstrated to lower perceptual thresholds for need-relevant stimuli (Aarts, Dijksterhuis, & De Vries, 2001). In addition, some evidence suggests that the valence of objects or behaviors varies depending on deprivation (Cabanac, 1971). Particularly, objects that can serve the function of reducing deprivation acquire a more positive meaning in a deprived than in a satiated state (Ferguson & Bargh, 2004; Sherman, Rose, Koch, Presson, & Chassin, 2003). At the same time, they are more likely to facilitate approach behaviors (Seibt, Häfner, & Deutsch, 2007).

Interim Summary

This review suggests that the determinants of human behavior are manifold and multifaceted. For at least two reasons, we deem it important to integrate these explanatory concepts into a coherent model. First, we suggest that despite some overlap, each of the reviewed concepts—attitudes, decisions, goals, habits, needs, and motivational orientations—makes a unique and indispensable contribution to the understanding of human behavior. For example, goals allow behavior to be influenced by delayed consequences, choices create links to rationality, attitudes allow quick evaluations, habits capitalize on regularity and allow for automatization, needs connect behavior to biological necessities, and motivational orientations allow quick and global behavioral orientations.

We suggest that focusing on only one or two concepts may result in a satisfactory explanation for a limited range of behaviors but at the same time may result in explanatory gaps regarding other phenomena. For instance, models of choice are excellent in predicting economic behavior when the motivation and capacity for thorough decision making are high. At the same time, they have a hard time explaining truly irrational behaviors such as addictions, which are presumably best understood in terms of habits or need activation (Deutsch & Strack, 2006; Robinson & Berridge, 2003; Tiffany, 1990). An integrative model can close such explanatory gaps by using a minimum number of principles necessary to explain a maximum number of behavioral phenomena.

Second, we suggest that the previously mentioned concepts are best understood in terms of their interaction with each other rather than in terms of each operating independently. That is, a model should explain how and under what circumstances relevant mechanisms influence one another. As explained in this chapter, the standard sequence of information processing may provide an appropriate temporal structure.

Dual-Process Models of Social Behavior

Such an integration was aspired by dual-process models in social (and cognitive) psychology. Typically, these models postulate two types of information processing that are more or less elaborate regarding their mechanisms. For example, the more elaborate processes have been assumed to be "rule based" and the less elaborate ones to be "associative" (Sloman, 1996). Other models have made a distinction between a "systematic" and a "heuristic" type of processing (e.g., Chaiken, Liberman, & Eagly,

1989) or between a "central" and a "peripheral route" on which attitudinal decisions can be reached (Petty & Cacioppo, 1986). However, most models focus on people's attitudes as the final outcome of the process. That is, attitudes are assumed to be generated by different mental mechanisms. Very few approaches (e.g., Metcalfe & Mischel, 1999) propose a direct link to behavior. A second issue concerns the parallel versus sequential operation of the two processes. Some models assume that the processes are driven by either one or the other type of mechanism (see Smith & DeCoster, 2000). Others propose two parallel systems that jointly generate outcomes.

In the remainder of this chapter, we focus on a model that concentrates on behavior as an outcome of two distinct systems that process information in an interactive manner.

The Reflective Impulsive Model
Basic Components of the Model

The Reflective Impulsive Model (RIM; Strack & Deutsch, 2004) explains behavior as the joint product of two mental systems that have different operating principles but interact in the course of processing. One system is called "impulsive," the other "reflective." Although their operations are described at a mental level of analysis, it is worth noting that neuroscientists have subsequently proposed a similar distinction at a biological level of analysis (e.g., Bechara, 2005). The two systems are assumed to run in parallel and to interact at different stages of processing. Specifically, the impulsive system is permanently active, while the operation of the reflective system depends on the amount of cognitive capacity that is available.

The Impulsive System

In its most basic version, the impulsive system is identical with James's (1890) ideomotor principle (see also Lotze, 1852). That is, a perceived or imagined content may elicit a behavior without an intention or a goal. More recently, evidence from the neurosciences suggests that the ideomotor principle can be extended to concepts that include a motor component (Gallese, Fadiga, Fogassi, & Rizzolatti, 1996; see Chapters 11 and 13).

However, perceptual or conceptual inputs and behavior may also be linked in a less immediate fashion. That is, behavioral implications of a concept may be activated by a concept (or an image) that is only indirectly associated to a behavioral schema. For example, Bargh et al. (1996) found that being exposed to a stereotype about elderly persons may cause people to walk more slowly (see also Cesario, Plaks, & Higgins, 2006). If such behaviors are not elicited by a decision or a goal, a more complex structure of the impulsive system must exist. In fact, the RIM assumes that in the impulsive system, the link between perceptual input and behavioral output is created by an associative network that is shaped by past operations. Thus, this network serves as an associative memory connecting the past to the present. As in other associative-network models (e.g., Anderson & Bower, 1973), links between elements are created and strengthened by their joint activation as a function of frequency and recency. A particular element may be activated either by one element with which it is strongly associated (like "black" and "white") or by several other elements that are activated at the same time. For example, in the Bargh et al. (1996) study, activating the elderly stereotype was not sufficient to induce the slow walking; additionally, participants' walking behavior had to be elicited by other means. Thus, it seems likely that the behavioral effect was the result of a joint activation.

It is important to note that operations of the impulsive system require little effort. If the link is sufficiently preactivated, the

mere exposure to the appropriate stimulus may suffice to elicit a behavior. Because these principles also apply to more complex sequences, the execution of behavior is greatly facilitated. It has become habitualized and can be performed with little attention. Unfortunately, the advantage of effortless execution comes with a serious disadvantage. That is, the creation of stable links occurs slowly (Devine, Plant, & Buswell, 2000), and once they are created, they are rigid and resistant to change.

THE ROLE OF AFFECT AND VALENCE

Other than through a strong link to a behavioral schema, behavior can be influenced by the valence that is engendered in the course of its execution. That is, a behavior that is associated with feeling better will be more likely to be elicited than a behavior that is associated with feeling worse. This hedonic mechanism obeys the same associative principles mentioned previously. As a result, a stimulus that is associated with a particular behavior may elicit the associated feeling and thereby facilitate or inhibit ongoing behavior. For example, a spider may trigger fear, which facilitates behavioral withdrawal.

In general, the impulsive system is oriented toward approach or avoidance, and this "motivational orientation" (Cacioppo, Priester, & Berntson, 1993) can be triggered by the (a) experience of positive or negative affect, (b) processing of positive or negative stimuli, (c) perception of approach or avoidance, or (d) execution of approaching or avoiding behaviors. In the RIM, one's preparedness to change the distance between oneself and an aspect of the environment defines the dominant motivational orientations. That is, a decrease stands for approach and an increase for avoidance. The latter can be achieved by either moving away from a target (flight) or causing the target to be removed (fight). These changes may occur in physical locomotions, symbolic operations (see Markman & Brendl, 2005), or imagination. Within both motivational orientations, contextual influences may determine the specific type of response.

The mechanism of motivational orientation is further defined by the principles of compatibility and bidirectionality. The compatibility principle implies that facilitation occurs for the processing of information, the experience of affect, and the execution of behavior if they are compatible with the prevailing motivational orientation, that is, if approach goes with positive and avoidance with negative valence. The bidirectionality principle states that this influence may operate in both directions. Thus, affect and evaluation may influence behavior and vice versa.

For certain, self-perception theory (Bem, 1967) has long posited that behavior may exert a causal influence on attitudes. However, the underlying mechanisms of the two approaches are quite different from each other. Specifically, self-perception theory assumes that people's behavior provides a basis to draw inferences about underlying attitudes. In contrast, the impulsive mechanisms of the RIM do not require that inferences be drawn. Moreover, the effects are predicted to occur even when the meaning of a behavior remains obscured (e.g., Strack, Martin, & Stepper, 1988). Therefore, the motivational orientation can be seen as a global predisposition of the impulsive system that serves to facilitate the processing of information and the execution of behavior in a specific manner.

In addition, an adaptive processing system also needs to be guided by the specific requirements for the survival of the organism. For example, the impulsive system of one's approaching responses toward stimuli that are food related should be facilitated if one is starving. In fact, evidence (Seibt et al., 2007) suggests that people who are hungry react faster to food-related words

if the required response involves moving a lever toward the stimulus and react slower if the lever has to be moved in the opposite direction.

Taken together, the impulsive system is specialized to afford fast and automatic adjustments of the organism to the environment.

The Reflective System

However, the advantages of the impulsive system are accompanied by serious shortcomings. Specifically, its fast and effortless processing goes along with a substantial rigidity and an outright failure with respect to performing certain tasks. Particularly, the principle of *frequency* impairs the impact of pieces of information that are processed only once and diminishes the impact of remote consequences. Similarly, the *recency* principle creates a disadvantage for information whose impact occurred in the distant past. Moreover, adaptation would be quicker and better if learning-related changes did not require individuals to be exposed firsthand to particular stimuli and situations but allowed them to learn vicariously from the experiences of others. Specifically, being able to learn from others' mistakes without suffering the negative consequences of their errors is a great benefit.

Hence, to achieve these gains, there exists a second, reflective system with different operating principles. As a whole, the reflective system is concerned with *the generation and transformation of knowledge.* Specifically, the reflective system assigns and transforms truth values using syllogistic operations. For example, perceiving a particular person may activate the characteristic "old" in the impulsive systems. In addition, the reflective system would create a noetic relationship between the perceptual input and the characteristic and assign it the value "true." Such a propositional categorization allows further transformations. In the simplest case, the operation of a negation may be applied to reverse the truth value. Alternatively, categorical information may be used to draw inferences about features of a target that are not open to immediate perception.

In this epistemic process, the reflective system performs a series of operations. It starts with a deictic procedure ("pointing and referring") that assigns a perceptual or imaginal input to a category. The resulting "propositional categorization" may then become the basis of a "noetic decision" that may be factual and/or evaluative in nature. An evaluative decision may provide the basis for a subsequent "behavioral decision" that focuses on the reduction of a discrepancy between a current state of the self and a positively evaluated possibility. A process of "intending" (e.g., Gollwitzer, 1999) links a behavioral decision to the actual execution of behavior. This process is terminated once the behavior is executed or the preceding behavioral decision has been fulfilled by other means.

Reflective-Impulsive Interactions

Thus far, we have described each of the two systems with respect to their major elements and operating principles. Now we describe the general characteristics of how the two systems interact and how these interactions are manifest at various stages of processing. Above all, reflective operations need an informational basis on which to generate various decisions. Because this information is rarely contained in perceptual input, it must come from a preexistent store. The reflective-impulsive model assumes that different types of memory processes are featured in the two systems. Specifically, the reflective system possesses a working memory with a very limited capacity but has the capability of directly addressing its contents (Baddeley, 1986). In contrast, the impulsive system has associative structures that are gradually formed into a long-term store of

unlimited capacity (e.g., Johnson & Hirst, 1991). For the effective functioning of the reflective system, this associative store plays an important role by providing the contents that are used for its computational, syllogistic operations. At the most basic level, a propositional categorization can be performed only if the category is already available in memory. Similarly, inferences from general knowledge can be drawn only if an appropriate schema is found.

Retrieval may be prompted by the input. If the input is strongly associated with a given category, it will most likely be activated in both the impulsive and the reflective system, and the informational input will undergo further processing. If there exists no strong link between the input and a category, the spreading activation across the associative links may be weak and "trickle away." However, because operations in the reflective system require that the input be categorized, categorical information from the associative store must be retrieved. Thus, ensuing processing of the input depends not only on the nature of the search cue but also on the accessibility of the stored information. As a function of the frequency and recency of prior activation, each piece of information is assumed to have a specific activation potential (Higgins, 1996) that reflects the probability with which it enters into reflective operations. Therefore, reflective operations may be strongly influenced by processes in the impulsive system. For example, a person may be categorized as "adventurous" simply because people had previously been exposed to this category (e.g., in a different context; Higgins, Rholes, & Jones, 1977).

However, the activation potential of a piece of information is determined not only by the frequency and recency with which the impulsive system is exposed to a stimulus but also by its prior use in the reflective system. In other words, thinking about a content will increase the probability that the same (or related) information will be retrieved at a later time. This may have severe consequences on judgment and decision making. For example, if a preceding judgment implies a selective search for a particular type of information, a subsequent judgment will be biased by the selectively increased accessibility. This mechanism of selective accessibility was found to underlie the so-called anchoring heuristic (Mussweiler & Strack, 1999; Strack & Mussweiler, 1997).

These mechanisms describe the nature of two types of interaction between the impulsive and reflective systems. While levels of accessibility in the associative store determine how likely it is that a given piece of information is used for reflective purposes, reflective processes influence the activation potential for subsequent operations.

Synergisms and Antagonisms in the Determination of Behavior

In the described model, the two systems converge in the final pathway to behavior. In the reflective system, behavior is based on a noetic decision about the desirability and feasibility of a particular action (cf. Ajzen, 1991; Bandura, 1977). As argued before, those decisions may have been indirectly influenced by the impulsive system, which may have had its effect through the accessibility of the activated information. A behavioral decision, however, may not immediately result in behavior: The impulsive system may interfere by activating behavioral schemata that are incompatible with the behavioral decision. As another possibility, the behavioral decision may reflect delaying a response and behaving at a later point in time.

The previous discussion implies that overt behavior depends on the magnitude of the compatibility of the outputs from both systems. If both systems contribute to the activation of the same schema, the execution of the behavior will be facilitated. It may be smoothened even further if the contribution of the impulsive system eases the execution by creating a feeling of fluency and positive affect (Csikszentmihalyi, 1988; Winkielman & Cacioppo, 2001).

However, if they activate incompatible schemata or if the execution of impulsive behaviors is inhibited by the reflective system, the two systems may stand in competition. Such antagonistic activation may trigger feelings of conflict and temptation (see Chapter 30). To prevail, the reflective system may apply metacognitive knowledge about the functioning of the impulsive mechanisms and divert attention away from the tempting stimulus. Finally, although both systems may contribute to the execution of a behavior, the impulsive system can assume primary control if the operating conditions for the reflective system are not satisfied (Hofmann, Rauch, & Gawronski, 2007). As a result, behaviors will be less likely to be determined by assessments of feasibility and future consequences than by immediate associations and hedonic quality. Sometimes, this may be adaptive; other times, impulsive determination may also be disruptive and even damaging (Deutsch & Strack, 2005).

A second issue is the delay that may be necessary for a behavioral decision to be executed. For example, a person watches an advertisement for a candy bar on television and decides to buy the advertised product the next day. In such a case, the temporal gap between the behavioral decision and behavioral execution must be bridged. To keep the behavioral schemata from being permanently activated, we suggest that the gap is bridged by a process of *intending* (e.g., Gollwitzer, 1999) that causes only an appropriate situation to be capable of reactivating the behavioral decision. In turn, such a situation triggers a behavioral schema that is conducive in that particular context. That is, the sight of a candy bar (or a picture thereof) may reactivate the behavioral decision to buy the product. We also assume the intending process to be self-terminating in that it will be turned off once the goal of the behavioral decision has been reached.

Conclusions

It was the purpose of this chapter to identify the most important psychological concepts that have been used to explain human behavior. In doing this, it became obvious that although some concepts seem incompatible, each has its unique significance under certain circumstances. For example, a behavior that is the result of habit may stand in contrast to a behavior that is driven by the anticipation of delayed consequences. However, both kinds of determinant play a crucial role. Therefore, we suggested that these elements can be integrated into a coherent model that allows one to predict their mutual influence under given conditions. For such a model to have explanatory power, several conditions had to be fulfilled. First, it had to be defined by underlying systems that are compatible with knowledge from the neurosciences. Second, it had to describe the interaction between the two systems at various stages of processing and to specify the relative contribution of each system under different conditions. Third, it had to be able to integrate motivational and emotional processes. Finally, it had to be focused on emergent behavior. The RIM (Strack & Deutsch, 2004) was portrayed as a model that may fulfill these requirements. Of course, many implications of the model have not yet been thoroughly tested. Therefore, future research must provide additional insights regarding the underlying mechanisms featured in the model and their relation to existing phenomena and processes that have been investigated at different levels of analysis.

References

Aarts, H., & Dijksterhuis, H. (2000). Habits as knowledge structures: Automaticity in goal-directed behavior. *Journal of Personality and Social Psychology, 78,* 53–63.

Aarts, H., Dijksterhuis, A., & De Vries, P. (2001). The psychology of drinking: Being thirsty and Perceptually Ready. *British Journal of Psychology, 92,* 631–642.

Ajzen, I. (1988). *Attitudes, personality, and behavior.* Chicago: Dorsey Press.

Ajzen, I. (1991). The theory of planned behavior. *Organizational Behavior and Human Decision Processes, 50,* 179–211.

Ajzen, I., & Fishbein, M. (1977). Attitude-behavior relations: A theoretical analysis and review of empirical research. *Psychological Bulletin, 84,* 888–918.

Allport, G. W. (1935). Attitudes. In C. Murchison (Ed.), *A handbook of social psychology* (pp. 798–844). Worcester, MA: Clark University Press.

Anderson, J. R., & Bower, G. H. (1973). *Human associative memory.* Washington, DC: Winston.

Baddeley, A. (1986). *Working memory.* Oxford: Clarendon Press.

Bandura, A. (1977). Self-efficacy: Toward a unifying theory of behavioral change. *Psychological Review, 84,* 191–215.

Bargh, J. A., Chen, M., & Burrows, L. (1996). Automaticity of social behavior: Direct effects of trait construct and stereotype activation on action. *Journal of Personality and Social Psychology, 71,* 230–244.

Bargh, J. A., & Ferguson, M. J. (2000). Beyond behaviorism: On automaticity of higher mental processes. *Psychological Bulletin, 126,* 925–945.

Bechara, A. (2005). Decision making, impulse control and loss of willpower to resist drugs: A neurocognitive perspective. *Nature Neuroscience, 8,* 1458–1463.

Becker, G. S. (1993). The economic way of looking at behavior. *Journal of Political Economy, 101,* 385–409.

Bem, J. W. (1967). Self perception—An alternative interpretation of cognitive dissonance phenomena. *Psychological Review, 74,* 183–200.

Cabanac, M. (1971). Physiological role of pleasure. *Science, 173,* 1103–1107.

Carver, C. S., & Scheier, M. F. (1998). *On the self-regulation of behavior.* Cambridge: Cambridge University Press.

Cacioppo, J. T., Priester, J. R., & Berntson, G. G. (1993). Rudimentary determinants of attitudes. II: Arm flexion and extension have differential effects on attitudes. *Journal of Personality and Social Psychology, 65,* 5–17.

Cesario, J., Plaks, J. E., & Higgins, E. T. (2006). Automatic social behavior as a motivated preparation to interact. *Journal of Personality and Social Psychology, 90,* 893–910.

Chaiken, S., Liberman, A., & Eagly, A. (1989). Heuristic and systematic information processing within and beyond the persuasion context. In J. Uleman & J. Bargh (Eds.), *Unintended thought* (pp. 212–252). New York: Guilford Press.

Chen, M., & Bargh, J. A. (1999). Consequences of automatic evaluation: Immediate behavioral predispositions to approach or avoid the stimulus. *Personality and Social Psychology Bulletin, 25,* 215–224.

Crespi, L. P. (1942). Quantitative variation of incentive and performance in the white rat. *American Journal of Psychology, 55,* 467–517.

Csikszentmihalyi, M. (1988). The flow experience and its significance for human psychology. In M. Csikszentmihalyi & I. S. Csikszentmihalyi (Eds.), *Optimal experience: Psychological studies of flow in consciousness* (pp. 15–35). Cambridge: Cambridge University Press.

Danziger, K. (2000). Making social psychology experimental: A conceptual history, 1920–1970. *Journal of the History of the Behavioral Sciences, 34,* 329–347.

Deutsch, R., & Strack, F. (2005). Impulsive and reflective determinants of addictive behavior. In R. W. Wiers & A. W. Stacy (Eds.), *Handbook of implicit cognition and addiction* (pp. 45–57). Thousand Oaks, CA: Sage.

Deutsch, R., & Strack, F. (2006). Duality-models in social psychology: From opposing processes to interacting systems. *Psychological Inquiry, 17,* 166–172.

Devine, P. G., Plant, E. A., & Buswell, B. N. (2000). Breaking the prejudice habit: Progress and obstacles. In S. Oskamp (Ed.), *Reducing prejudice and discrimination* (pp. 185–208). Thousand Oaks, CA: Sage.

Dijksterhuis, A., & Bargh, J. A. (2001). The perception-behavior expressway: Automatic effects of social perception on social behavior. In M. P. Zanna (Ed.), *Advances in experimental social psychology* (Vol. 33, pp. 1–40). San Diego, CA: Academic Press.

Draine, S. C., & Greenwald, A. G. (1998). Replicable unconscious semantic priming. *Journal of Experimental Psychology: General, 127,* 286–303.

Fazio, R. H. (1990). Multiple processes by which attitudes guide behavior: The mode model as an integrative framework. *Advances in Experimental Social Psychology, 23,* 75–109.

Fazio, R. H., & Olson, M. A. (2003). Implicit measures in social cognition research: Their meaning and use. *Annual Review of Psychology, 54,* 297–327.

Fazio, R. H., Sanbonmatsu, D. M., Powell, M. C., & Kardes, F. R. (1986). On the automatic evaluation of attitudes. *Journal of Personality and Social Psychology, 50,* 229–238.

Fazio, R. H., & Towles-Schwen, T. (1999). The MODE model of attitude-behavior processes. In S. Chaiken & Y. Trope (Eds.), *Dual process theories in social psychology* (pp. 97–116). New York: Guilford Press.

Fazio, R. H., & Williams, C. J. (1986). Attitude accessibility as a moderator of the attitude-perception and attitude-behavior relations: An investigation of the 1984 presidential election. *Journal of Personality and Social Psychology, 5,* 505–514.

Feather, N. T. (1990). Bridging the gap between values and actions. In E. T. Higgins & R. M. Sorrentino (Eds.), *Handbook of motivation and cognition: Foundations of social behavior* (Vol. 2, pp. 151–192). New York: Guilford Press.

Ferguson, M. J., & Bargh, J. A. (2004). Liking is for doing: The effects of goal pursuit on automatic evaluation. *Journal of Personality and Social Psychology, 87,* 557–572.

Fishbein, M., & Ajzen, I. (1975). *Belief, attitude, intention, and behavior: An introduction to theory and research.* Reading, MA: Addison-Wesley.

Fishbein. M, & Mittelstadt, S. E. (1989). Using the theory of reasoned action as a framework for understanding and changing AIDS-related behaviors. In V. M. Mays, G. W. Albee, & S. F. Schneider (Eds.), *Psychological approaches to the primary prevention of AIDS* (pp. 142–167). Beverly Hills, CA: Sage.

Förster, J., Liberman, N., & Higgins, E. T. (2005). Accessibility from active and fulfilled goals. *Journal of Experimental Social Psychology, 41,* 220–239.

Förster, J., Liberman, N., & Friedman, S. (2007). Seven principles of goal activation: A systematic approach to distinguishing goal priming from priming of non-goal constructs. *Personality and Social Psychology Review, 11,* 211–233.

Förster, J., & Strack, F. (1996). The influence of overt head movements on memory for valenced words: A case of conceptual-motor compatibility. *Journal of Personality and Social Psychology, 71,* 421–430.

Förster, J., & Strack, F. (1997). Motor actions in retrieval of valenced information: A motor congruence effect. *Perceptual and Motor Skills, 85,* 1419–1427.

Gallese, V., Fadiga, L., Fogassi, L., & Rizzolatti, G. (1996). Action recognition in the premotor cortex. *Brain, 119,* 593–609.

Gollwitzer, P. M. (1999). Implementation intentions: Strong effects of simple plans. *American Psychologist, 54,* 493–503.

Greenwald, A. G., Poehlman, A., Uhlmann, E., & Banaji, M. R. (in press). Understanding and interpreting the Implicit Association Test III: Meta-analysis of predictive validity. *Journal of Personality and Social Psychology.*

Higgins, E. T. (1996). Knowledge activation: Accessibility, applicability, and salience. In E. T. Higgins & A. W. Kruglanski (Eds.), *Social psychology: Handbook of basic principles* (pp. 133–168). New York: Guilford Press.

Higgins, E. T., Rholes, W. S., & Jones, C. R. (1977). Category accessibility and impression formation. *Journal of Experimental Social Psychology, 13,* 141–154.

Hofmann, W., Rauch, W., & Gawronski, B. (2007). And deplete us not into temptation: Automatic attitudes, dietary restraint, and self-regulatory resources as determinants of eating behavior. *Journal of Experimental Social Psychology, 43,* 497–504.

Holland, R. W., Hendriks, M., & Aarts, H. (2005). Smells like clean spirit: Nonconscious effects of scent on cognition and behavior. *Psychological Science, 16,* 689–693.

Hull, C. L. (1943). *Principles of behavior.* New York: Appleton-Century-Crofts.

Hull, C. L. (1952). *A behavior system: An introduction to behavior theory concerning the individual organism.* New Haven, CT: Yale University Press.

James, W. (1890). *The principles of psychology.* New York: Holt.

Johnson, M. K., & Hirst, W. (1991). Processing subsystems of memory. In R. G. Lister & H. J. Weingartner (Eds.), *Perspectives on cognitive neuroscience* (pp. 197–217). New York: Oxford University Press.

Kruglanski, A. W., Shah, J. Y., Fishbach, A., Friedman, M. R., Chun, W. Y., & Sleeth-Keppler, D. (2002). A theory of goal systems. *Advances in Experimental Social Psychology, 34,* 331–378.

Kuhl, J. (1985). Volitional mediators of cognition-behavior consistency: Self-regulatory processes and action versus state orientation. In J. Kuhl & J. Beckman (Eds.), *Action control: From cognition to behavior* (pp. 101–128). New York: Springer-Verlag.

Lachman, R., Lachman, J. L., & Butterfield, E. C. (1979). *Cognitive psychology and information processing.* Hillsdale, NJ: Lawrence Erlbaum Associates.

Lambert, A. J., Payne, B. K., Jacoby, L. L., Shaffer, L. M., Chasteen, A. L., & Khan, S. K. (2003). Stereotypes as dominant responses: On the "social facilitation" of prejudice in anticipated public contexts. *Journal of Personality and Social Psychology, 84,* 277–295.

Langer, E. J., Blank, A., & Chanowitz, B. (1978). The mindlessness of ostensibly thoughtful action: The role of "placebic" information in interpersonal interaction. *Journal of Personality and Social Psychology, 36,* 635–642.

LaPiere, R. T. (1934). Attitudes vs. actions. *Social Forces, 13,* 230–237.

Lewin, K. (1939). Field theory and experiment in social psychology: Conceptual methods. *American Journal of Sociology, 44,* 868–896.

Lotze, H. R. (1852). *Medicinische Psychologie oder Physiologie der Seele.* Leipzig: Weidmann.

Markman, A. B., & Brendl, C. M. (2005). Research report constraining theories of embodied cognition. *Psychological Science, 16,* 6–10.

Metcalfe, J., & Mischel, W. (1999). A hot/cool-system analysis of delay of gratification: Dynamics of willpower. *Psychological Review, 106,* 3–19.

Meyer, D. E., & Schvaneveldt, R. W. (1971). Facilitation in recognizing pairs of words: Evidence of a dependence between retrieval operations. *Journal of Experimental Psychology, 90,* 227–234.

Miller, G. A., Galanter E., & Pribram, K. H. (1960). *Plans and the structure of behavior.* New York: Holt, Rinehart and Winston.

Mussweiler, T., & Strack, F. (1999). Comparing is believing: A selective accessibility model of judgmental anchoring. In W. Stroebe & M. Hewstone (Eds.), *European review of social psychology* (Vol. 10, pp. 135–167). Chichester: Wiley.

Neisser, U. (1967). *Cognitive psychology.* New York: Appleton-Century-Crofts.

Neumann, R., & Strack, F. (2000). Approach and avoidance: The influence of proprioceptive and exteroceptive cues on encoding of affective information. *Journal of Personality and Social Psychology, 79,* 39–48.

Ouellette, J. A., & Wood, W. (1998). Habit and intention in everyday life: The multiple processes by which past behavior predicts future behavior. *Psychological Bulletin, 124,* 54–74.

Petty, R. E., & Cacioppo, J. T. (1986). *Communication and persuasion: Central and peripheral routes to attitude change.* New York: Springer-Verlag

Robinson, T. E., & Berridge, K. C. (2003). Addiction. *Annual Review of Psychology, 54,* 23–53.

Rosenberg, M. J., & Hovland, C. I. (1960). *Attitude organization and change: An analysis of consistency among attitude components.* New Haven, CT: Yale University Press.

Schwarzer, R. (1999). Self-regulatory processes in the adoption and maintenance of health behaviors: The role of optimism, goals, and threats. *Journal of Health Psychology, 4,* 115–127.

Seibt, B., Häfner, M., & Deutsch, R. (2007). Prepared to eat: How immediate affective and motivational responses to food cues are influenced by food deprivation. *European Journal of Social Psychology, 37,* 359–379.

Sherman, S. J., Rose, J. S., Koch, K., Presson, C. C., & Chassin, L. (2003). Implicit and explicit attitudes toward cigarette smoking: The effects of context and motivation. *Journal of Social and Clinical Psychology, 22,* 13–39.

Skinner, B. F. (1938). *The behavior of organisms.* New York: Appleton-Century-Crofts.

Skinner, B. F. (1953). *Science and human behavior.* New York: Macmillan.

Sloman, S. A. (1996). The empirical case for two systems of reasoning. *Psychological Bulletin, 119,* 3–22.

Smith, E. R., & DeCoster, J. (2000). Dual process models in social and cognitive psychology: Conceptual integration and links to underlying memory systems. *Personality and Social Psychology Review, 4,* 108–131.

Sorrentino, R. M., & Higgins, E. T. (1986). *Handbook of motivation and cognition.* New York: Wiley.

Strack, F., & Deutsch, R. (2004). Reflective and impulsive determinants of social behavior. *Personality and Social Psychology Review, 8,* 220–247.

Strack, F., Martin, L. L., & Stepper, S. (1988). Inhibiting and facilitating conditions of the human smile: A nonobtrusive test of the facial feedback hypothesis. *Journal of Personality and Social Psychology, 54,* 768–777.

Strack, F., & Mussweiler, T. (1997). Explaining the enigmatic anchoring effect: Mechanisms of selective accessibility. *Journal of Personality and Social Psychology, 73,* 437–446.

Thorndike, E. L. (1898). Animal intelligence: An experimental study of associative processes in animals. *Psychological Review Monographs Supplement, 5,* 551–553.

Thurstone, L. L. (1928). Attitudes can be measured. *American Journal of Sociology, 33,* 529–554.

Tiffany, S. T. (1990). A cognitive model on drug urges and drug-use behavior: Role of automatic and nonautomatic processes. *Psychological Review, 97,* 147–168.

Vroom, V. H. (1964). *Work and motivation.* New York: Wiley.

Watson, J. B. (1913). Psychology as the behaviorist views it. *Psychological Review, 20,* 158–177.

Webb, T. L., & Sheeran, P. (2007). How do implementation intentions promote goal attainment? A test of component processes. *Journal of Experimental Social Psychology, 43,* 295–302.

Wicker, A. W. (1969). Attitudes versus actions: The relationship of verbal and overt behavioral responses to attitude objects. *Journal of Social Issues, 25,* 41–78.

Wilson, T. D., Lindsey, S., & Schooler, T. Y. (2000). A model of dual attitudes. *Psychological Review, 107,* 101–126.

Winkielman, P., & Cacioppo, J. T. (2001). Mind at ease puts a smile on the face: Psychophysiological evidence that processing facilitation elicits positive affect. *Journal of Personality and Social Psychology, 81,* 989–1000.

PART 2

The Activation, Selection, and Expression of Action

Smart Moves: The Psychology of Everyday Perceptual-Motor Acts

David A. Rosenbaum, Jonathan Vaughan, Ruud G. J. Meulenbroek, Steven Jax, *and* Rajal G. Cohen

Abstract

This chapter presents a theory of motor planning. Topics discussed include a cognitive model of motion planning and control, posture-based motion planning, and evidence for knowledge of future body position.

Keywords: motor planning, motion planning, motion control, body position

In 1996, when IBM's Deep Blue computer beat the world's greatest chess player (Gary Kasparov), a person rather than Deep Blue was responsible for looking at the board and moving the pieces. IBM may have chosen to use a person rather than a computer for the perceptual-motor aspects of chess playing because those aspects may have seemed too uninteresting to simulate. Nevertheless, no computer in 1996—and none now—can begin to do what any normal 4-year-old can do—climb trees, pick strawberries, or set up a chess board and lift and move the chess pieces to and from desired locations. The problems to be solved in such tasks are not just physical; they are also psychological. Our understanding of the psychological bases of everyday perceptual-motor acts is miniscule compared to our

understanding of the psychological bases of more intellectual activities such as chess playing. However, progress is being made on the psychology of physical action. This chapter reviews some progress in this area of research as instantiated in the theory of motor planning developed by the authors and their colleagues.

As just indicated, there is a gulf between what normal 4-year-olds can do and what modern computers can do when it comes to the control of physical action. Computers are very good at planning chess moves, whereas most young children are not. (For a report about IBM's Deep Blue chess-playing abilities, see Hsu, 1999.) Meanwhile, computers, embodied in robots, cannot climb trees, pick strawberries, or set up a chess board and lift and move pieces to and from desired locations—all of which are easily achieved by many 4-year-old children. The reason that modern cognitive science has done so well with symbolic actions but has done so poorly with perceptual-motor actions is easy to surmise. The computational challenges of perceptual-motor actions are much greater than those of symbolic action. In the case of chess, for example, moves are easy to define. A given piece goes from one grid position to another. The number of possible moves at any point in a chess game can be large, and the number of possible move sequences afterward can be much larger still. Despite this complexity, one at least knows what primitives are being counted. In the case of perception and movement, the primitives are neither easily visible nor readily graspable. For movement—the focus of this chapter and our area of specialization—the number of ways that even simple acts can vary is infinite. One can move one's hand from one point to another such that the number of body positions at the end of the movement is infinite. For any given final body position, the number of paths that can lead to it from the starting postures is infinite. And for any of these paths, the number of timing patterns, reflecting where the body is at any given moment, is likewise infinite. A scientist facing this plethora of choices might be tempted to throw up his or her hands, but doing so would not be constructive, and contemplating how that physical act is generated would only lead to more frustration.

What is a psychologist of motor action to do, then? One alternative to throwing up one's hands is to follow the lead offered by B. F. Skinner (1969). Here we refer not to Skinner's rejection of mentalism but rather to his advocacy of instrumentalism. Skinner eschewed the analysis of body movements, a point not often appreciated. Following the pragmatic tradition in which he was raised (i.e., the pragmaticism of the American philosopher and educator John Dewey, 1929), Skinner spoke only of instrumental responses. He did not care whether a pigeon closed a key with its beak or its leg. All that mattered was that the key was closed, causing a pellet of food to be either delivered or not, depending on where in the reinforcement schedule the pigeon happened to be. Likewise, a rat in a Skinner box could depress a lever with its right paw, its left paw, or its head. How the lever was pressed was of no concern to Skinner.

This attitude allowed Skinner to collect data quickly and easily, but the data so amassed reflected the instrumental consequences of the movements Skinner's subjects made, not the movements themselves.

Surprisingly, Skinner's attitude toward movement was concordant with the view put forth by Edward Tolman (1948), one of the leading critics of the behaviorists during the era in which their views held so much sway. Tolman argued that it was not movements that rats in a maze remembered but rather the spatial configuration of the maze itself. This was why, if the rat was placed in a different place in the maze from the place it started before, it still found its way to the food. And this was also why, if the maze was suddenly flooded, the rat could swim to the reward though it had not swum there before. The specific movements made by rat were not what the rat learned. Instead, what the rat acquired was a set of places arranged in a coherent spatial representation, or *cognitive map*, as Tolman called it.

Putting Skinner and Tolman together in the same bed, so to speak, is an odd twist considering their radically different views of mental representation. Odd, too, is the fact that Tolman and Skinner actually spoke past each other when it came to motor control, for neither of them actually identified the "response" with "movement." Skinner did not do so, as mentioned previously, so when Tolman argued that his demonstrations deflated Skinner's claims, his argument rested on too "muscular" an interpretation of what Skinner meant by "response." This is not to belittle or challenge what Tolman argued, which we agree with wholeheartedly. More to the point is that neither of these two giants of American psychology really was concerned with movements per se. Neither of them actually grappled with the question of which movements emerge out of all the movements that are possible for a given instrumental outcome. This question, which became the focus of thinking for the Russian physiologist Nicolai Bernstein (1967), also comprises the focus of our own research, which is briefly summarized in the remainder of this chapter.

A Cognitive Approach to Motion Planning

We have developed a cognitive model of the planning and control of movements or, more specifically, movements that involve reaching and grasping of objects (Jax, Rosenbaum, Vaughan, & Meulenbroek, 2003; Rosenbaum, Loukopoulos, Meulenbroek, Vaughan, & Engelbrecht, 1995; Rosenbaum, Meulenbroek, Vaughan, & Jansen, 2001). In pursuing a cognitive model, we, like Tolman (1948), assume that memory representations play a central role in performance, both for evaluating the success of just-performed movements and for establishing goals of forthcoming movements. Understanding the content of such representations and the manner in which they are formed is a fundamental aim of cognitively oriented research on motor control.

Before delving into the particulars of the cognitive model we have developed, we wish to explain how our cognitive approach contrasts with other approaches to motor control. We want to do this to point to the special insights that may be gained by pursuing a cognitive (or "information processing") approach to this problem as opposed to or in addition to other approaches.

One complementary approach is *feedback control* theory, where the main idea is that performers use feedback to try to optimize performance (Jagacinski & Flach, 2003; Meyer, Abrams, Kornblum, Wright, & Smith, 1988; Stark, 1968). For feedback to be used effectively, the actor must have a goal, departures from which (errors) can be corrected. How goals are formed is not something that concerns most researchers

steeped in feedback control theory. By contrast, cognitive psychologists interested in motor control take as their primary focus the structure of goals and the processes by which goals are formed.

Another complementary approach to cognitively inspired research on motor control is *dynamical systems* theory. Here the main idea is that the state of the system evolves over time, often in some complex, typically nonlinear, way. Advocates of dynamical systems theory (e.g., Kelso, 1996; Turvey, 1990) use sophisticated quantitative techniques to describe how the state of the system being studied, as embodied in some measurable quantity such as the angle of a handheld pendulum at a given moment in time, depends on the prior states of the system. It is harder for such investigators to measure or model mental representations of *future* states. One could argue, however, that understanding how performance is modulated both by the past and by expectancies about the future is fundamentally important for a complete account of voluntary movement. Motor-control researchers who advocate dynamical systems theory have generally avoided appeals to mental representations, subscribing instead to the ecological approach to perception and action. Our view is that this confluence of adherence to dynamical systems analysis and adherence to the ecological approach is more of an incidental than a necessary feature of either approach. Neither approach strictly needs the other. By the same token, a cognitive approach that omits the rich quantitative models afforded by dynamical systems may be needlessly limited.

A third complementary approach to the cognitive approach is traditional *neuroscience*. Here one asks how neural structures are physically organized and interconnected (neuroanatomy) and what role is played by these neural structures (neurophysiology/cognitive neuroscience). Neurophysiological insights are limited by the tasks for which their involvement is assessed. For example, it is well accepted that the left hemisphere is more involved in motor planning than is the right hemisphere, judging from results of brain damage (Banich, 2004), brain imaging (Johnson-Frey, Newman-Norlund, & Grafton, 2005), and language lateralization (Banich, 2004). However, this conclusion has so far been based on relatively crude evaluations of motor planning in tasks that either have questionable relevance to everyday performance (e.g., pantomiming) or rely on informal clinical judgments of individuals' performance. Motor planning is a complex process, as demonstrated by the many years it takes children to learn motor skills (e.g., Meulenbroek & Van Galen, 1990) and as demonstrated by the very slow advent of autonomous motion planning of manipulation skills in robots, as mentioned at the outset of this chapter. A more sophisticated understanding is needed of both the contents and the real-time formation of motor plans. Such an understanding would allow the functions subserved by neural structures putatively involved in motor planning to be delineated in more detail than has been the case so far.

The proper context for the pursuit of this more detailed understanding is, we believe, cognitive psychology, where one tries to discern the functional processes leading to overt performance. Surprisingly, this approach has been pursued by remarkably few investigators. (For a discussion of the reasons for this state of affairs, see Rosenbaum, 2005, 2006.) One consequence of this situation is that the only cognitive model of motor planning that has been developed in sufficient detail to permit detailed simulations of a natural class of voluntary movements—reaching and grasping of objects—is the one developed in our laboratory (Rosenbaum, Vaughan, Jorgensen, Barnes, & Stewart, 1993; Rosenbaum

et al., 1995, 2001). This is not to say, however, that no one else has pondered the same questions, albeit from other vantage points. Motor planning models have been developed in the dynamical systems perspective (Bullock & Grossberg, 1988, 1989; Erlhagen & Schöner, 2002), in the feedback control perspective (Harris & Wolpert, 1998), and in the neuroscience perspective (Bizzi, Hogan, Mussa-Ivaldi, & Giszter, 1992; Bullock & Grossberg, 1989; Feldman, 1966). It is important to keep these other models in mind and draw on insights from them in pursuit of a cognitive model.

Posture-Based Motion Planning

One of the most influential ideas in neuroscience-based models of motor planning is the *equilibrium point hypothesis* (Bizzi et al., 1992; Feldman, 1966). According to this hypothesis, neuromuscular goal states are established prior to movement such that details of the movements to the goal states need not be specified in detail, nor must special corrective processes be employed to allow the effector to resist mechanical perturbations on the way to the goal. One version of the equilibrium point hypothesis says that muscle stiffnesses can be adjusted so a limb that was in equilibrium is no longer in equilibrium, and the only way to reach the new equilibrium point is to move to a new position (Bizzi et al., 1992). Another way of setting a new equilibrium point that does not entail adjusting muscle stiffnesses directly is changing the thresholds of muscle stretch reflexes, so a limb that was just in equilibrium now finds itself out of equilibrium given the new stretch–reflex thresholds; a movement must be made to correct the self-imposed error (Feldman, 1966).

Evidence for the equilibrium point hypothesis comes from neurophysiological and behavioral studies (for a review, see

Latash, 1993). The equilibrium hypothesis has been challenged (e.g., Gomi & Kawato, 1996), but answers to those challenges have been provided (Feldman & Latash, 2005; Feldman, Ostry, Levin, Gribble, & Mitinski, 1998; Gribble & Ostry, 2000). Striking evidence for the hypothesis that trajectories are defined by goal postures comes from Graziano, Taylor, and Moore (2002), who showed that sustained electrical stimulation to particular cells in the monkey motor cortex and premotor cortex caused unrestrained monkeys to adopt characteristic postures regardless of the monkeys' starting postures.

If one incorporates the main idea of the equilibrium-point hypothesis into a cognitive model, one has a model like the one developed in our lab. According to our *posture-based motion planning* model (Jax et al., 2003; Rosenbaum, Engelbrecht, Bushe, & Loukopoulos, 1993; Rosenbaum et al., 1995, 2001), goal postures are known before positioning movements begin.

The idea that intended goal postures have special representational status accords with the observations of Graziano et al. (2002) cited previously as well as the observations that initial movement directions anticipate final movement directions (Brown, Moore, & Rosenbaum, 2002) and also that initial hand speeds anticipate subsequent distances to be covered (Atkeson & Hollerbach, 1985; Gordon, Ghilardi, & Ghez, 1992; Hogan, 1984). With a few additional assumptions, the model accounts for a wide range of movement phenomena (for reviews, see Jax et al., 2003; Rosenbaum et al., 1995, 2001), including detailed features of hand and finger kinematics during prehension (Meulenbroek, Rosenbaum, Jansen, Vaughan, & Vogt, 2001; Rosenbaum et al., 2001), detailed features of manual obstacle-avoidance behavior (Vaughan, Rosenbaum, & Meulenbroek, 2001), and the capacity to compensate immediately for changes in joint mobility (Rosenbaum et al., 1995). It

is important to appreciate that the model applies to feedback correction as well as open-loop control because each time a correction is made, whether on the basis of visual feedback, kinesthetic feedback, or some other source of information, a multiplicity of possible solutions exists. The planning problem for which the posture-based motor planning model was developed must be solved for both initial and corrective movements.

The posture-based motion planning model assumes that during motor planning, goal postures are specified before movements are specified. This idea is motivated partly by the belief that for manual positioning movements, end positions have functional primacy over movements, an idea supported by the observation that position variance is minimized at end positions (Harris & Wolpert, 1998). The idea is also inspired by the fact that in models of another performance domain, language production, it is virtually universally accepted that there are higher and lower levels of representation (semantic, syntactic, morphological, phonological, phonetic, and execution). Hypothesizing that goal postures are specified before movements are specified—what we call the *goal-posture-first* hypothesis—introduces a distinct level of representation between location coding in external space (a high-level representation) and the movement execution level (a low-level representation). The addition of this intermediate level allows one to explain many findings in the motor control literature, including, in addition to those mentioned previously, that end positions of movements are remembered better than movements to end positions (Rosenbaum, Meulenbroek, & Vaughan, 1999; Smyth, 1984).

Evidence for Knowledge of Future Body Positions

As noted previously, there is evidence for the view that goal postures are known before movements are performed. A landmark study that established this point was conducted by Marteniuk, MacKenzie, Jeannerod, Athenes, and Dugas (1987), who showed that the shape of the function relating hand speed to pregrasp time differed for reaches to an object that was going to be tossed or carefully positioned.

Rosenbaum et al. (1990) obtained further evidence for intention effects in grasping. They did so by asking university students to reach out with the right hand to take hold of a horizontal cylinder that the students knew would be moved to different final positions. As shown in Figure 6.1, the cylinder lay on a pair of cradles. Two flat target disks lay on either side of the cylinder, one near the left end and one near the right end. Participants were asked to grasp the cylinder firmly with the right hand and bring the cylinder's left end or right end down onto the left or right target. As shown in Figure 6.1, the postures that participants adopted depended on what they planned to do with the cylinder. When the *right* end of the cylinder was going to be placed down on either target, participants grasped the cylinder with an overhand grip, but when the *left* end of the cylinder was going to be placed down on either target, participants grasped the cylinder with an *underhand* grip. Thus, participants anticipated the goal positions for movement 2 by the time they completed movement 1. Said another way, they knew how they would complete the second move before starting it, as demonstrated by the fact that they tolerated initial discomfort for the sake of later comfort or control. Ratings of comfort confirmed that underhand grasps were less comfortable than overhand grasps.

Subsequent studies explored the source and generality of this *end-state comfort* effect. When participants reached out to turn a handle to bring a pointer to a designated orientation (Rosenbaum et al., 1993), they

(A)

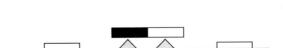

(B)

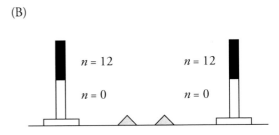

(C)

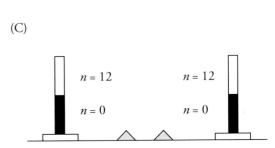

Fig. 6.1 (A) Cylinder lying flat before being picked up by the participant with the right hand. (B) Cylinder has been brought to the left or right target with the white side down. (C) Cylinder has been brought to the left or right target with the black side down. Numbers indicate how many participants took hold of the horizontal cylinder with the thumb toward the corresponding end. All subjects in B used an overhand grip, and all subjects in C used an underhand grip. Based on Rosenbaum, Marchak, Barnes, Vaughan, Slotta, and Jorgensen (1990).

likewise tolerated initial discomfort for later comfort or control. This outcome was obtained with the left hand as well as the right and was obtained even if the wheel containing the handle was placed on the floor so the arm hung down. Obtaining the end-state comfort effect in this situation ruled out an explanation of the effect based on exploitation of gravity.

End-state comfort was also observed for displacement tasks that entailed large vertical movements in which a cylinder was picked up at one location and then placed with a prescribed orientation at a target whose height ranged from near the feet to well above the head. The fact that the end-state comfort effect was obtained in this wide range of positions argues against exploitation of muscle or tendon elasticity as a source of the effect. The effect could also be eliminated if aiming accuracy was minimized (Rosenbaum, Heugten, & Caldwell, 1996), which indicated that end-state *control* was perhaps more important than end-state *comfort* per se.

A reaction-time study by Rosenbaum, Vaughan, Barnes, and Jorgensen (1992) shed light on the real-time processes behind the emergence of the end-state comfort effect (Figure 6.2). Subjects stood facing a wall-mounted panel with a removable handle that had magnetic "feet" protruding from its two ends. The feet rested

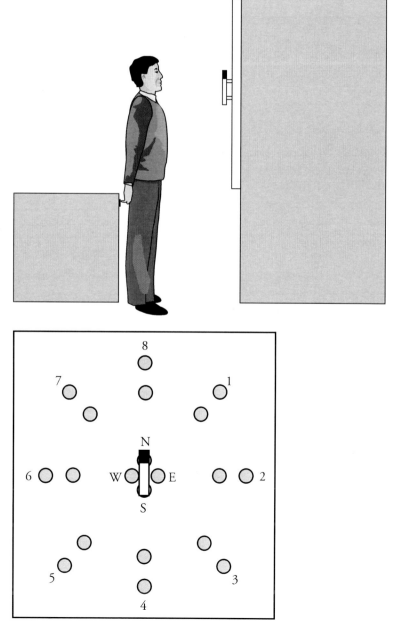

Fig. 6.2 Apparatus used in the RT-and-grasping study of Rosenbaum, Vaughan, Barnes, and Jorgensen (1992). Top panel: The subject's hand pressed gently against a switch. Bottom panel: Subject's view of the response panel. Here, the handle is attached via magnets beneath its feet to two iron disks, with the "pointer" end of the handle pointing up, or "North." The other three home positions had the handle pointing "East," "West," or "South." Around the home region were eight pairs of iron disks with small lights beside them (where the numbers appear here). When a target light turned on, the subject reached out to pull the handle from the home disks and placed it onto the signaled pair of target disks. The subject next returned his or her hand to the start switch and waited for one of the four home lights to turn on (where the letters N, E, W, and S appear here), indicating the home position to which the handle had to be brought. Based on Rosenbaum, Vaughan, Barnes, and Jorgensen (1992).

on two iron disks mounted on the panel. The orientation of the handle depended on which pair of iron disks the handle stood on at the start of each trial. When the subject was ready, as indicated by the fact that he or she pressed his or her right hand against a button located down by his or her side, a target light appeared beside another pair of iron disks located in one of eight radial positions around the home area. The task was to reach out and pull the handle from its home disks and place it as quickly as possible on the pair of disks designated by the target light. The dependent measures were (a) the delay between illumination of the target light and release of the start button, (b) the orientation of the hand when it grasped the handle (thumb toward the pointer or away from the pointer), (c) the time to move the handle from its home position to the target position, and (d) the handle's final orientation. Subjects were told to minimize the time between appearance of the target light and placement of the handle on the target. They were not told that the reaction time (RT) to release the hand from the start button would be recorded separately from the time to grasp the handle and carry it from the home to the target (the movement time).

As shown in Figure 6.3, subjects behaved in accordance with the end-state comfort effect: The way they took hold of the handle at its home position anticipated their final postures at the targets. Moreover, reaches culminating in thumb-toward grasps had shorter RTs than reaches culminating in thumb-away grasps even though the handle's start position and target position were the same. Thus, the spontaneous choice of thumb-toward versus thumb-away grasp had correspondingly shorter or longer RTs. The RT differences suggested that subjects decided even before starting their physical reaches how they would grasp the handle. Because the longer of the two reaction times was only about 0.3 seconds, participants made the decision within that amount of time.

The end-state comfort effect, as described previously, was reflected in a dichotomous measure of performance—overhand versus underhand grasps or, equivalently, thumb toward one end or the other of a grasped tube. A more recent study showed that end-state planning can also be demonstrated with a *continuous* measure. Cohen and Rosenbaum (2004) asked university students to stand in front of an empty bookshelf (Figure 6.4). A platform protruded from the bookshelf at stomach level, and a large plunger stood

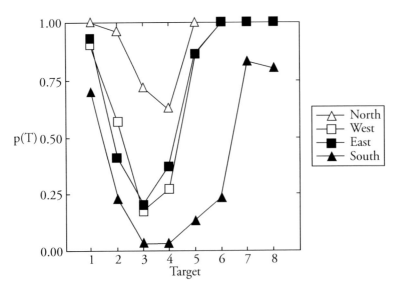

Fig. 6.3 Probability, p(T), of grasping the bar with the thumb toward the pointer when the pointer was toward the North, West, East, or South and the bar would be brought to targets 1 to 8. Based on Rosenbaum, Vaughan, Barnes, and Jorgensen (1992).

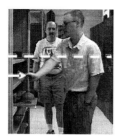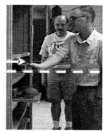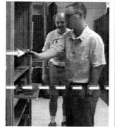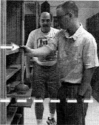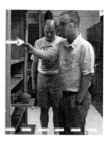

Fig. 6.4 Reaching for a plunger. A subject (who gave permission to have his photo shown here) grasps the plunger at the home platform with different grasp heights (white arrows) before moving the plunger to target platforms at different heights (white dashed lines). The first author, also shown here, was responsible for setting up the target platforms.

on this *home* platform. To the right of the home platform was another protruding *target* platform. The subject was asked to stand with his or her hands by his or her sides and, when ready, to take hold of the plunger with the right hand and move it to the target platform. After doing this, the subject was asked to return the hand to his or her side. The height of the home platform was constant, whereas the height of the target platform varied across trials. The dependent variable was the height along the length of the plunger where the subject took hold of it on the home platform—what Cohen and Rosenbaum (2004) called the *grasp height.* Figure 6.5 shows the result: The higher the

target platform, the lower the grasp height. Cohen and Rosenbaum (2004) interpreted this result, which was replicated with several different home and target shelf configurations, to mean that participants grasped the plunger in a way that allowed the hand to come close to the middle of the arm's range of motion at the end of the transport phase, consistent with the end-state comfort effect.

In these same studies, the end-state comfort effect was attenuated when, after moving the plunger to the target and lowering the arm, subjects returned the plunger to the home position. Had there been a complete end-state comfort effect for the

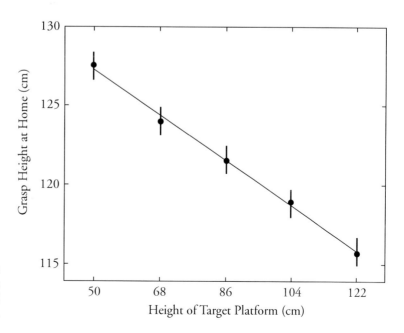

Fig. 6.5 Mean grasp heights (±1 SE) for home-to-target grasps. Based on Cohen and Rosenbaum (2004).

return moves, participants would have adopted grasp heights that afforded the same posture back at the home platform regardless of the target platform height. Instead, subjects adopted grasp heights at the target sites that were close to the grasp heights they had just adopted when they brought the plunger from the home to the target sites. A control experiment in which the height of the home platform was varied instead of the target platform showed that initial-state comfort could not explain all the grasp height variation in target-to-home movements. Cohen and Rosenbaum (2004) suggested that participants relied on a strategy in which they *generated* plans for object transports when new transports were required but *recalled* just-used grasp heights for return moves. Such a strategy was computationally convenient, for if the plunger could be grasped at some height for the move from the home platform to the target platform, it was reasonable to grasp the plunger at the same height for the return trip even if this compromised the end-state comfort effect to some extent. The idea that people can switch from generation to recall of motor plans is reminiscent of the well-known idea from cognitive psychology that the development of automaticity is accompanied by a switch from generation to recall of problem solutions (Logan, 1988, 2002).

Constraint Hierarchies

The foregoing discussion summarizes evidence for the view that goal postures are known before movements are initiated. But how are the goal postures chosen? There are generally many possible goal postures that allow a positioning task to be completed, so establishing that goal postures are represented in advance does not establish how they are selected.

The proposed solution to this problem in the posture-based motion planning model is that candidate goal postures are selected by eliminating possible goal postures, beginning with those candidates that fail to satisfy the most important constraints and ending with the one candidate that fails to satisfy only the lowest-level constraint.

Saying that there are levels of constraints implies a prioritized list of requirements in the actor's mind, or what we called a *constraint hierarchy* (Rosenbaum et al., 2001). In the posture-based motion planning model, a constraint hierarchy constitutes the actor's definition of the task to be performed. This concept is an important feature of the model because virtually all laboratory-based psychological research is about one task or another. The recent spate of interest in task switching (e.g., Monsell, 2003) indicates that there is interest in understanding how tasks are internally represented. The constraint hierarchy is one possible *structural* account of tasks that may complement the *process* accounts of tasks that have emerged in the task-switching literature.

In the posture-based motion planning theory, the constraint hierarchy for a reaching task is defined with respect to all the factors that potentially affect the experienced cost and benefit of the goal posture to be adopted and the movement made to it. (The movement to a goal posture is assumed in the theory to be the interpolated path from the starting posture to the goal posture.) Which constraints are deployed and with what priority depends on the task to be performed. Thus, as shown in Table 6.1, the constraint hierarchy for turning off a rotating electric saw is quite different from the constraint hierarchy for tackling one's opponent in American football. Within either of these tasks, goal postures and movements to those goal postures are chosen through elimination by aspects, a procedure that consists of eliminating candidates that fail to satisfy the most important constraint, then eliminating candidates that fail to satisfy the second most important constraint

Table 6.1 Two Constraint Hierarchies

Reach for the "Off" switch of a rotating electric saw
1. Don't collide with obstacles
2. Don't miss the target
3. Expend little energy

Tackle one's (American) football opponent
1. Do collide with opponents
2. Don't miss the target (his or her knees)
3. Expend lots of energy

and so on (Tversky, 1972). If more than one candidate is left at the end, the winner is chosen at random.

Several points are worth making in connection with this approach to planning. One is that elimination by aspects has proven to be a more workable solution than one we considered in an earlier version of our theory (Rosenbaum et al., 1995). There, we took a weighted average of candidate solutions where the weights were assigned to different features of each candidate solution, such as its movement cost, its proximity to an obstacle, and so on. The weights themselves reflected the relative importance of minimizing each feature. The problem with this approach was that the weighted average of different goal postures often turned out to be a goal posture that was worse than any of the plausible candidate goal postures. Elimination by aspects yields a single winner rather than an average of candidates and so avoids this problem.

A second point to be made about the constraint hierarchy approach is that this way of tackling the action planning problem contrasts with the prevailing method that has been pursued in robotics and neuroscience for generating controllers for specific tasks. That method relies on optimization (Harris & Wolpert, 1998; Hogan, 1984; Todorov, 2004) and focuses on the idea that the system minimizes or maximizes certain values. An attraction of the optimization approach is that it

draws on powerful mathematical tools. A drawback is that it is often unclear, using conventional mathematics, how to optimize many variables at once, although the nervous system apparently has little or no trouble doing so. This seeming paradox suggests either that the nervous system does not optimize or that, if it does, it does so through methods not yet contemplated by mathematicians.

By appealing to constraint hierarchies and elimination by aspects in the posture-based motion planning model, we reject optimization altogether. Instead, we embrace *satisficing,* a term introduced by Herbert Simon (1955) to refer to the fact that choices are often made to incur costs of any acceptable amount below some criterion and to adduce benefits of any acceptable amount above some criterion. Simon won the Nobel Prize in Economics for this idea as applied to business managers, who, by satisficing rather than optimizing, violated the axioms of rational choice theory, which exemplifies optimization par excellence. Simon observed that optimization is computationally very expensive and in some cases nearly impossible (Simon, 1989). Whether optimization is impossible in the motor system is impossible to prove, but it is obvious that actors do not always move optimally. Were this not the case (if we moved optimally), we might not need chiropractors, practitioners of the Alexander technique, and so on.

A third point to be made about the constraint hierarchy approach concerns the role of recall versus generation of candidate goal postures and movements. If candidate goal postures and movements are evaluated with respect to constraint hierarchies, where do the candidate goal postures and movements come from? In the posture-based motion planning theory, there are two sources. One is instance recall. The other is instance generation. Instance recall entails retrieval and evaluation of representations of recently adopted goal postures. The evaluation is made with respect to the constraint hierarchy defining the current task. From the set of recently adopted goal postures, one is selected as the most promising candidate goal posture (i.e., the one that satisfies the most constraints in the constraint hierarchy). If time permits, a potentially better candidate goal posture is sought in a second stage of processing by searching in posture space around the most promising candidate goal posture. The latter process entails *generation* of possible goal postures and may yield new, never-before-adopted goal postures, as can be important when new tasks arise.

A fourth and final point about the constraint hierarchy approach is that this approach has within it the kernel of a theory of skill development. As one gets more and more skilled at a task, one can perform the task more and more quickly, as is well known from the literature on the Power Law of learning (Crossman, 1959; Heathcote, Brown, & Mewhort, 2000; Newell & Rosenbloom, 1981). However, skill learning is not just manifested through faster performance. It is also manifested through more graceful flow in dance, more expressive phrasing in music, more finely shaded lines in painting, and so on. By appreciating these changing features of performance accompanying skill development, one can suggest, within the framework of the constraint hierarchy idea, that one way of understanding skill learning is to suppose that ever-deeper constraint hierarchies are formed for a task or, more properly, a task *class* (since the task itself changes when its constraint hierarchy does). This perspective predicts that variation in the way a task class is performed changes over the course of skill development such that variation with respect to broad features of the task are supplanted by variation with respect

to more microscopic features. A growing body of work on variability in performance accords with this view (Muller & Sternad, 2004; Newell, Liu, & Mayer-Kress, 2001).

Trial-and-error learning may also be understood in a new way from the perspective of the constraint hierarchy. As mentioned earlier, candidate solutions that satisfy lowest-level requirements are chosen at random. Therefore, one may understand trial-and-error learning as consisting of refinements in performance following the discovery that solutions of a particular kind prove more satisfactory than solutions of another kind, in which case the successful kind becomes a new constraint in the constraint hierarchy, albeit at a lower level than any constraint previously available for that task class. Such a process could give rise to the ever-finer discriminations that distinguish expert performers from less expert performers.

Conclusions

The foregoing discussion provides a thumbnail sketch of the theory of motor planning that we have been working on for the past several years. Many computational details have been omitted. These can be found in Rosenbaum et al. (2001). The theory, via its simulations, can account for many features of motor performance observed both in the laboratory and in everyday life. For example, with some simple extensions, the theory can be used to simulate reaching around obstacles (Rosenbaum et al., 2001; Vaughan et al., 2001), grasping (Meulenbroek et al., 2001; Rosenbaum et al., 2001), handwriting (Meulenbroek, Rosenbaum, Thomassen, & Loukopoulos, 1996), compensation for changes in joint mobility (Rosenbaum et al., 1995), and movement in three spatial dimensions (Klein Breteler & Meulenbroek, 2006; Vaughan, Rosenbaum, & Meulenbroek, 2006).

Many challenges remain for the theory. One of the most important is extending it from kinematics, the description of positions without regard to forces, to kinetics, the description of position with regard to forces. In principle, goal postures can be defined with respect to muscle tensions as well as joint angles. This is clearly needed insofar as a given joint angle can be maintained with different muscle tensions. When muscle tensions are specified, joint angles are determined, provided that external forces on the body are taken into account. However, the converse is not true: Knowing joint angles does not imply the corresponding forces (and torques). It will be important in future elaborations of the theory to have it specify muscle forces and torques as well as joint angles. Other remaining challenges are to have the model generate entire series of movements rather than single movements, to have it move more than one hand at a time, and, as intimated previously, to simulate learning in more detail than has been done before (for simulations of the effects of reaching for targets that were recently or not so recently reached, see Rosenbaum et al., 1995).

Recognizing the limited nature of the model developed so far highlights the importance of humility about our knowledge of motor control at this time. Would that there were some other, more advanced cognitive model of movement control than ours, but there is none, as far as we know. When we speak of smart moves, then, as in the title of this chapter, we do not mean moves performed only by elite athletes and brilliant virtuosi. When one looks closely at everyday motor acts and appreciates their computational complexity, one sees that virtually all moves are smart.

References

Atkeson, C. G., & Hollerbach, J. M. (1985). Kinematic features of unrestrained arm movements. *Journal of Neuroscience, 5,* 2318–2330.

Banich, M. T. (2004). *Cognitive neuroscience and neuropsychology* (2nd ed.). Boston: Houghton Mifflin.

Bernstein, N. (1967). *The coordination and regulation of movements.* London: Pergamon.

Bizzi, E., Hogan, N., Mussa-Ivaldi, F., & Giszter, S. (1992). Does the nervous system use equilibrium-point control to guide single and multiple joint movements? *Behavioral and Brain Sciences, 15,* 603–613.

Brown, L. E., Moore, C. M., & Rosenbaum, D. A. (2002). Feature-specific processing dissociates action from recognition. *Journal of Experimental Psychology: Human Perception and Performance, 28,* 1330–1344.

Bullock, D., & Grossberg, S. (1988). Neural dynamics of planned arm movements: Emergent invariants and speed-accuracy properties during trajectory formation. *Psychological Review, 95,* 49–90.

Bullock, D., & Grossberg, S. (1989). VITE and FLETE: Neural modules for trajectory formation and postural control. In W. A. Hershberger (Ed.), *Volitional action* (pp. 253–297). Amsterdam: North-Holland/Elsevier.

Cohen, R. G., & Rosenbaum, D. A. (2004). Where objects are grasped reveals how grasps are planned: Generation and recall of motor plans. *Experimental Brain Research, 157,* 486–495.

Crossman, E. R. F. W. (1959). A theory of the acquisition of speed skill. *Ergonomics, 2,* 153–166.

Dewey, J. (1929). *The quest for certainty.* New York: Minton, Balch.

Erlhagen, W., & Schöner, G. (2002). Dynamic field theory of movement preparation. *Psychological Review, 109,* 545–573.

Feldman, A. G. (1966). Functional tuning of the nervous system with control of movement or maintenance of a steady posture: II. Controllable parameters of the muscles. *Biophysics, 11,* 565–578.

Feldman, A. G., & Latash, M. L. (2005). Testing hypotheses and the advancement of science: Recent attempts to falsify the equilibrium point hypothesis. *Experimental Brain Research, 161,* 91–103.

Feldman, A. G., Ostry, D. J., Levin, M. F., Gribble, P. L., & Mitniski, A. B. (1998). Recent tests of the equilibrium-point hypothesis (lamda model). *Motor Control, 2,* 189–205.

Gomi, H., & Kawato, M. (1996). Equilibrium-point control hypothesis examined by measured arm stiffness during multijoint movement. *Science, 272,* 117–120.

Gordon, J., Ghilardi, M. F., & Ghez, C. (1992). In reaching, the task is to move the hand to a target. *Behavioral and Brain Sciences, 15,* 337–338.

Graziano, M. S., Taylor, C. S. R., & Moore, T. (2002). Complex movements evoked by microstimulation of precentral cortex. *Neuron, 34,* 841–851.

Gribble, P. L., & Ostry, D. J. (2000). Compensation for loads during arm movements using equilibrium-point control. *Experimental Brain Research, 135,* 474–482.

Harris, C. H., & Wolpert, D. (1998). Signal-dependent noise determines motion planning. *Nature, 394,* 780–784.

Heathcote, A., Brown, S., & Mewhort, D. J. K. (2000). The power law repealed: The case for an exponential law of practice. *Psychonomic Bulletin and Review, 7,* 185–207.

Hogan, N. (1984). An organizing principle for a class of voluntary movements. *Journal of Neuroscience, 4,* 2745–2754.

Hsu, F. H. (1999). IMB's Deep Blue chess grandmaster chips. *IEEE Computer Society, 19,* 70–81.

Jagacinski, R. J., & Flach, J. M. (2003). *Control theory for humans: Quantitative approaches to modeling performance.* Mahwah, NJ: Lawrence Erlbaum Associates.

Jax, S. A., Rosenbaum, D. A., Vaughan, J., & Meulenbroek, R. G. J. (2003). Computational motor control and human factors: Modeling movements in real and possible environments. *Human Factors, 45,* 5–27. (Special issue on "Quantitative Formal Models of Human Performance," M. Byrne & W. G. Gray, Eds.)

Johnson-Frey, S. H., Newman-Norlund, R., Grafton, S. T. (2005). A distributed network in the left cerebral hemisphere for planning everyday tool use actions. *Cerebral Cortex, 15,* 681–695.

Kelso, J. A. S. (1996). *Dynamic patterns.* Cambridge, MA: MIT Press.

Klein Breteler, M. D., & Meulenbroek, R. G. J. (2006). Modeling 3D object manipulation: synchronous single-axis joint rotations? *Experimental Brain Research, 168,* 395–408.

Latash, M. L. (1993). *Control of human movement.* Champaign, IL: Human Kinetics.

Logan, G. D. (1988). Toward an instance theory of automatization. *Psychological Review, 95,* 492–527.

Logan, G. D. (2002). An instance theory of attention and memory. *Psychological Review, 109,* 376–400.

Marteniuk, R. G., MacKenzie, C. L., Jeannerod, M., Athenes, S., & Dugas, C. (1987). Constraints on human arm movement trajectories. *Canadian Journal of Psychology, 4,* 365–378.

Meulenbroek, R. G. J., Rosenbaum, D. A., Jansen, C., Vaughan, J., & Vogt, S. (2001). Multijoint grasping movements: Simulated and observed effects of object location, object size, and initial aperture. *Experimental Brain Research, 138,* 219–234.

Meulenbroek, R. G. J., Rosenbaum D. A., Thomassen, A. J. W. M., Loukopoulos, L. D., & Vaughan, J. (1996). Adaptation of a reaching model to handwriting: How different effectors can produce the same written output, and other results. *Psychological Research, 59,* 64–74.

Meulenbroek, R. G. J., & Van Galen, G. P. (1990). Perceptual-motor complexity of printed and cursive letters. *Journal of Experimental Education, 58,* 95–110.

Meyer, D. E., Abrams, R. A., Kornblum, S., Wright, C. E., & Smith, J. E. K. (1988). Optimality in human motor performance: Ideal control of rapid aimed movements. *Psychological Review, 95,* 340–370.

Monsell, S. (2003). Task switching. *Trends in Cognitive Sciences, 7,* 134–140.

Muller, H., & Sternad, D. (2004). Decomposition of variability in the execution of goal-oriented tasks: Three components of skill improvement. *Journal of Experimental Psychology, 30,* 212–233.

Newell, K. M., Liu, Y-T., & Mayer-Kress, G. (2001). Time scales in motor learning and development. *Psychological Review, 108,* 57–82.

Newell, K. M., & Rosenbloom, P. S. (1981). Mechanisms of skill acquisition and the power law of learning. In J. R. Anderson (Ed.), *Cognitive skills and their acquisition* (pp. 1–55). New York: Lawrence Erlbaum Associates.

Rosenbaum, D. A. (2005). The Cinderella of psychology: The neglect of motor control in the science of mental life and behavior. *American Psychologist, 60,* 308–317.

Rosenbaum, D. A. (2006). Cinderella after the ball. *American Psychologist, 61,* 78–79.

Rosenbaum, D. A., Engelbrecht, S. E., Bushe, M. M., & Loukopoulos, L. D. (1993). A model for reaching control. *Acta Psychologica, 82,* 237–250.

Rosenbaum, D. A., Heugten, C., & Caldwell, G. C. (1996). From cognition to biomechanics and back: The end-state comfort effect and the middle-is-faster effect. *Acta Psychologica, 94,* 59–85.

Rosenbaum, D. A., Loukopoulos, L. D., Meulenbroek, R. G. M., Vaughan, J., & Engelbrecht, S. E. (1995). Planning reaches by evaluating stored postures. *Psychological Review, 102,* 28–67.

Rosenbaum, D. A., Marchak, F., Barnes, H. J., Vaughan, J., Slotta, J., & Jorgensen, M. (1990). Constraints for action selection: Overhand versus underhand grips. In M. Jeannerod (Ed.), *Attention and performance XIII* (pp. 321–342). Hillsdale, NJ: Lawrence Erlbaum Associates.

Rosenbaum, D. A., Meulenbroek, R. G., & Vaughan, J. (1999). Remembered positions: Stored locations or stored postures? *Experimental Brain Research, 124,* 503–512.

Rosenbaum, D. A., Meulenbroek, R. G., Vaughan, J., & Jansen, C. (2001). Posture-based motion planning: Applications to grasping. *Psychological Review, 108,* 709–734.

Rosenbaum, D. A., Vaughan, J., Barnes, H. J., & Jorgensen, M. J. (1992). Time course of movement planning: Selection of hand grips for object manipulation. *Journal of Experimental Psychology: Learning, Memory, and Cognition, 18,* 1058–1073.

Rosenbaum, D. A., Vaughan, J., Jorgensen, M. J., Barnes, H. J., & Stewart, E. (1993). Plans for object manipulation. In D. E. Meyer & S. Kornblum (Eds.), *Attention and performance XIV—A silver jubilee: Synergies in experimental psychology, artificial intelligence and cognitive neuroscience* (pp. 803–820). Cambridge, MA: MIT Press, Bradford Books.

Simon, H. (1955). A behavioral model of rational choice. *Quarterly Journal of Economics, 69,* 99–118.

Simon, H. (1989). *Models of thought.* New Haven, CT: Yale University Press.

Skinner, B. F. (1969). *Contingencies of reinforcement: A theoretical analysis.* New York: Appleton-Century-Crofts.

Smyth, M. M. (1984). Memory for movements. In M. M. Smyth & A. M. Wing (Eds.), *The psychology of human movement* (pp. 83–117). London: Academic Press.

Stark, L. (1968). *Neurological control systems.* New York: Plenum Press.

Todorov, E. (2004). Optimality principles in sensorimotor control. *Nature Neuroscience, 7,* 907–915.

Tolman, C. E. (1948). Cognitive maps in rats and man. *Psychological Review, 55,* 189–208.

Turvey, M. T. (1990). Coordination. *American Psychologist, 45,* 938–953.

Tversky, A. (1972). A theory of choice: Elimination by aspects. *Psychological Review, 79,* 281–299.

Vaughan, J., Rosenbaum, D. A., & Meulenbroek, R. G. J. (2001). Planning reaching and grasping movements: The problem of obstacle avoidance. *Motor Control, 5,* 116–135.

Vaughan, J., Rosenbaum, D. A., & Meulenbroek, R. J. G. (2006, May 31–June 3). *Modeling reaching and manipulating in 2- and 3-D workspaces: The posture-based model.* Proceedings of the Fifth International Conference on Learning and Development, Bloomington, IN.

How the Mind Moves the Body: Lessons From Apraxia

Georg Goldenberg

Abstract

This chapter examines the concept of apraxia. It argues that apraxia was developed to bridge the gap separating the immaterial mind from the material body, and that the desire to bridge this cleavage continues to shape modern accounts of apraxia. Ideomotor apraxia and ideational apraxia are discussed.

Keywords: action control, ideomotor apraxia, ideational apraxia, gestures, pantomime, Liepmann

Cognitive science today gets increasingly interested in the embodiment of human perception, thinking, and action. Abstract information processing models are no longer accepted as satisfactory accounts of the human mind. Interest has shifted to interactions between the material human body and its surroundings and to the way in which such interactions shape the mind. Proponents of this approach have expressed the hope that it will ultimately dissolve the Cartesian divide between the immaterial mind and the material existence of human beings (Damasio, 1994; Gallagher, 2005). A topic that seems particularly promising for providing a bridge across the mind–body cleavage is the study of bodily actions, which are neither reflexive reactions to external stimuli nor indications of mental states, which have only arbitrary relationships to the motor features of the action (e.g., pressing a button for making a choice response). The shape, timing, and effects of such actions are inseparable from their meaning. One might say that they are loaded with mental content, which cannot be appreciated other than by studying their material features. Imitation, communicative gesturing, and tool use are examples of these kinds of actions.

The new turn of cognitive science meets an old tradition in clinical neuropsychology, which recognizes disturbances of imitation, production of communicative gestures, and tool use as manifestations of apraxia resulting mainly from lesions of the left hemisphere. In this chapter, I argue that the concept of apraxia has been developed with the explicit aim to bridge the border separating the immaterial mind from the material body and that the desire to bridge this cleavage continues to shape modern accounts of apraxia.

Apraxia and the Conversion of Ideas Into Action

The foundations for the neuropsychological concept of apraxia were elaborated at the beginning of the 20th century by the German psychiatrist Hugo Liepmann (1900, 1908; Goldenberg, 2003). Liepmann, who had acquired a doctoral degree in philosophy before he turned to medicine, was well aware that localizing functions in the brain constitutes an assault on the Cartesian heritage of an insurmountable border between the spatially extended part of the body, which is the brain, and the immaterial mind. As he put it cogently, the purpose of cerebral localization of function is to "look for the culprit not in the spaceless qualities of the soul but in definite places of the brain" (Liepmann, 1905, p. 38). He accepted the existence of "intrapsychic" processes, which depend on activity of the whole cortex and cannot be localized, but thought that the principle of localization could be advanced into their realm by analyzing the conversion of ideas into motor commands because motor commands are known to arise from a strictly circumscribed area of the brain: the motor cortex. He depicted this conversion in a famous diagram (Figure 7.1) showing how the idea of a movement produced by the whole cortex is transferred to the motor cortex, where motor commands to the muscles are issued. This is a hierarchical and serial model where a "higher-order" idea of the movement is converted into "lower-order" motor commands. In this model, apraxia, which is the defective control of motor actions, could arise either from deficiency of the idea itself—ideational apraxia—or from interruption of its transfer into motor command—ideokinetic apraxia.[1]

A Posterior-to-Anterior Stream of Action Control

Liepmann designated the idea of the movement as a "movement formula." He insisted that this formula does not specify motor actions but reasoned that, rather than being completely abstract, it appears

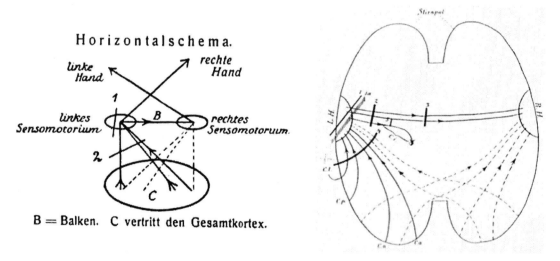

Fig. 7.1 Two versions of Liepmann's horizontal schema. The diagrams show the conversion of the "movement formula" into motor commands. This conversion is accomplished mainly in the left hemisphere, as indicated by the solid lines leading to the left sensorimotor cortex ("Sensomotorium"). Interruption of this flow ("2" in the left diagram and corresponding line in the right) leads to "ideokinetic apraxia." Whereas in the earlier diagram, shown on the left side, the movement formula is a nonlocalizable product of the whole cortex ("C vertritt den Gesamtkortex" means "C represents the entire cortex"), the solid lines in the later version, shown on the right side, originate from posterior regions of the left hemisphere, indicating a dominance of the left hemisphere already for the initial stage of movement control (Goldenberg, 2003).

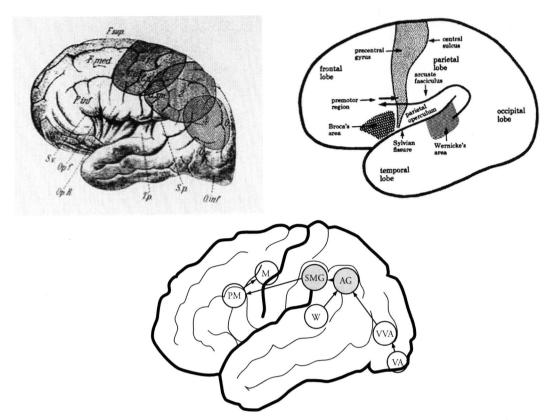

Fig. 7.2 Different models of the posterior-to-anterior processing stream and of the crucial role of left parietal regions for apraxia.

Top Left: Liepmann's "vertical schema" demonstrating three serially ordered stages of movement control (Liepmann, 1925). Lesions in location 1 cause ideational apraxia, lesions in location 2 ideokinetic apraxia. Lesions in location 3 cause "limb-kinetic" apraxia, which affects only the deftness of the opposite hand. Liepmann insisted that parietal lesions cause ideokinetic apraxia because they sever fibers traveling below the parietal cortex from the visual cortex (location 1) to the sensorimotor cortex (location 3). He explicitly refused the existence of a "praxis center" in the parietal lobe (Liepmann, 1908).

Top Right: Liepmann's ideas had fallen into discredit in the middle of the 20th century when nonlocalizationist and psychodynamic interpretations of cognitive brain functions prevailed and the classical localizing approaches were despised as "diagram making." An outstanding proponent of their revival was Boston neurologist Norman Geschwind. His schema of the praxis system follows Liepmann quite closely (Geschwind, 1975). Geschwind particularly emphasized defective performance of meaningful gestures to verbal command as a core symptom of apraxia. He placed the origin of the posterior-to-anterior stream into Wernicke's area, which is supposed to be responsible for language comprehension. Furthermore, he inserted a relay in the premotor cortex before the stream of action control reaches the primary motor cortex.

Bottom: In contrast to Liepmann and Geschwind, Heilman and Rothi (1993) postulate that "time-space motor representations" or "praxicons," which are equivalent to Liepmann's "movement formula," are stored in the left inferior parietal lobe (SMG = supramarginal gyrus; AG = angular gyrus). When gestures are performed to verbal command, these representations are activated from Wernicke's area (W), where speech is comprehended. When they are imitated, their activation comes from visual areas (VA = primary visual cortex; VVA = visual association cortex). In accord with Geschwind, further flow is assumed to pass via premotor regions (PM) to the primary motor cortex (M). Other than in Liepmann's and Geschwind's models, parietal lesions are assumed to exert their influence by the destruction of action representations rather than by the interruption of fiber paths. This idea has been very influential and has found various elaborations by other authors (e.g., Buxbaum, Johnson-Frey, & Bartlett-Williams, 2005; Sirigu et al., 1996).

as a mental image in one sensory modality. Most frequently, it will be a visual image of the intended action, but in some cases it may also be an auditory image directing, for example, the manipulation of musical instruments. As mental images were thought to be produced near the primary sensory cortex devoted to their modality, the movement formula ceased to be a nonlocalizable product of the whole cortex. For the majority of actions directed by visual images, it was a product of the occipital areas near the visual cortex. From this origin, the flow of action control traveled through the parietal lobe to the motor cortex (Figure 7.2). Thus, the origin of action control had been brought down from a nonlocalizable intrapsychic process to localized parts of the brain.

Hemisphere Dominance for Action Control

The empirical observation that defective production of meaningful gestures on command as well as defective imitation occur predominantly in patients with left hemisphere damage led Liepmann to introduce a second hierarchy of motor control in addition to the governance of anterior by posterior brain regions. He thought that only the left hemisphere can complete the conversion of the movement formula into motor commands, and in later accounts he went even further to suggest that the movement formula itself is a product predominantly of the left hemisphere (Figure 7.1). He thought that these exclusive contributions of the left hemisphere to the control of actions are particularly important for imitation of gestures and for demonstration of communicative gestures, as these motor acts must be performed "wholly from memory," without a guidance provided by interactions with external objects. The conditions that bring forward most clearly

left hemisphere motor dominance are thus characterized by a predominance of mental plans over material circumstances, a relationship that betrays its origin in the governance of the material body by the immaterial mind.

Liepmann's Heritage

Figure 7.2 shows influential modern adaptations of Liepmann's posterior-to-anterior schema of movement control. These adaptations agree with Liepmann that there is a distinct and unique "praxis system" and that different manifestations of apraxia can be accounted for by disturbances at different stages of this unified system. They further agree that this system is located in the left hemisphere and is organized in a serial processing stream from posterior to anterior regions of the brain in which parietal regions occupy a central position.

After this outline of general principles of apraxia, the following sections of this chapter analyze empirical findings and theoretical accounts for each of the manifestations of apraxia separately. Recurrent topics in these discussions are the importance of left hemisphere and particularly left parietal lesions and the distinction between abstract cognitive processes and the material body.

Ideomotor Apraxia

As outlined previously, Liepmann combined defective imitation of gestures and defective demonstration of meaningful gestures on command to "ideokinetic" apraxia, which was later renamed "ideomotor apraxia." This combination was based on the belief that both kinds of actions require guidance of movements without support from interaction with external objects. The unification of imitation and communicative gestures is in conflict with unequivocal evidence of double dissociations between them. There are patients with left parietal brain damage in whom severely defective imitation of gestures contrasts with intact performance of communicative gestures, such as pantomiming the use of objects or conveying messages by emblematic gestures like "okay" or "be quiet" (Goldenberg & Hagmann, 1997; Mehler, 1987; Peigneux et al., 2000). Conversely, there are aphasic patients who are unable to pantomime the use of objects or to demonstrate emblematic gestures but improve considerably and may even reach perfect performance when asked to imitate gestures (Barbieri & De Renzi, 1988; Cubelli, Marchetti, Boscolo, & Della Sala, 2000). If, as postulated by the theory, the conversion of the concept or idea of the movement into appropriate motor commands were deficient, one would expect such deficiency to affect gestures retrieved from knowledge about the use of tools and objects as well as gestures demonstrated by the examiner.

Obviously, at least partly different mechanisms are required for imitation of gestures than for demonstration of gestures on command.

Imitation of Gestures

In order to clearly distinguish imitation from the production of communicative gestures, it must be probed for meaningless and novel gestures. If the examiner demonstrates a meaningful and familiar gesture, patients may understand the meaning and reproduce the gesture out of their repertoire of meaningful gestures stored in long-term memory rather than copying the shape of the gesture.

Defective imitation is an easily demonstrable and impressive symptom of unilateral brain damage. Even if patients are severely aphasic, they usually understand the instruction to imitate and obviously strain to copy the gesture made by the examiner; although they use the otherwise normally skillful hand ipsilateral to their

brain lesion, they produce insecure, hesitant, and searching movements that end up in positions grossly different from those demonstrated. The deficit is particularly conspicuous when imitation is probed for simple postures of the hand or the fingers that do not pose any serious difficulty to healthy persons (see Figure 7.3).

Two proposals have been made to account for selective deficits of imitation. Both abandon the assumption that imitation probes the conversion of the mental image of the gesture into motor commands. The "direct mapping" hypothesis postulates that experience with seeing one's own movements has led to direct neuronal associations between sensory areas specialized for visual perception of body configurations and motor regions sending efferent signals to the muscles of one's own body (Brass & Heyes, 2005; Iacoboni et al., 1999; Keysers & Perrett, 2004). This theory owes much of its attractiveness to the detection of "mirror neurons" in the premotor cortex of monkeys (Rizzolatti & Craighero, 2004), which fire both when the monkey sees a human or conspecific subject perform an action and when it executes the same action. It should be noted, however, that these neurons are tuned to familiar and biologically significant actions like manipulation of food, whereas the imitation deficit of brain-lesioned patients concerns meaningless and novel gestures. Within the dichotomy between immaterial mind and material body, the direct mapping hypothesis could be classified as abandoning the role of mental processes. Sensory areas of the brain are directly connected to motor areas, and there is no interpolated stage of cognitive mediation.

By contrast, the hypothesis of "body part coding" looks for the crucial difficulties of imitation of novel gestures in a stage of cognitive mediation that facilitates the matching between visual perception of other subjects' body configurations and motor execution of corresponding own

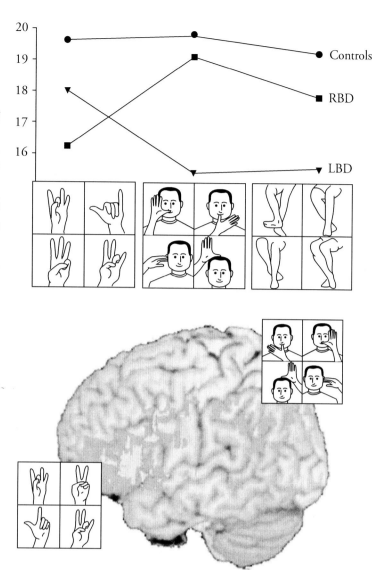

Fig. 7.3 Body part specificity of defective imitation.

Upper part: Mean scores (maximum = 20) of healthy controls and patients with either left (LBD) or right (RBD) brain damage on imitation of meaningless postures of fingers, hand, and foot (Goldenberg & Strauss, 2002). There were 10 postures of each kind. Note that although LBD patients fare generally better with finger than with hand postures, they are as a group nonetheless much worse than controls also for them.

Lower part: There are dissociations between finger and hand postures within the group of LBD patients.

The image shows the result of magnetic resonance imaging lesion subtraction: Lesions of patients with defective hand but normal finger imitation were subtracted from those with the reverse dissociation: Whereas defective imitation of hand postures is bound to lesions of inferior parietal regions and the temporo-parieto-occipital junction, defective imitation of finger postures is associated with inferior frontal lesions (Goldenberg & Karnath, 2006).

body configurations. This hypothesis posits that coding of the demonstrated gesture with reference to a classification of body parts is interpolated between perception and replication of meaningless gestures. Body part coding reduces the multiple visual features of the demonstrated gesture to simple relationships between a limited set of body parts and produces an equivalence between demonstration and imitation that is independent of the different modalities and perspectives of perceiving one's own and other persons' bodies. Body part coding requires knowledge about the division of the body in distinct parts and about the defining features and limits of these parts. Such knowledge is acquired during childhood. Verbal naming of body parts presumably plays a major role in its acquisition, but once it is acquired, subjects usually do not bother to explicitly name the body parts involved in a gesture. Children reach complete adult proficiency in imitating simple hand and finger postures like those shown in Figure 7.3 only at around the age of 7, which it should be noted is also the age at which they reach adult proficiency in naming body parts (Aouka, Goldenberg, & Nadel, 2003; Poeck & Orgass, 1964).

In favor of this cognitive account of imitation and against the direct mapping hypothesis are experimental studies that demonstrated that patients who commit errors when imitating gestures have similar problems when trying to replicate these gestures on a manikin or to match photographs of gestures made by different persons and seen under different angles of view (Goldenberg, 1995b, 1999). The motor actions of manipulating a manikin or pointing to pictures are fundamentally different from those of making the gesture itself. The observation that the deficit shows up with motor actions different from those that are to be imitated is difficult to reconcile with a direct mapping from sensory to motor representations based on structural similarity between observed and executed gestures.

BODY PART SPECIFICITY OF DEFECTIVE IMITATION

Imitation disorders following localized brain damage can be restricted to only parts of the body. The evidence collected in this line of research puts further difficulties for direct matching and helps to refine the account of body part coding. It also addresses the issues of left hemisphere dominance and of the posterior-to-anterior processing stream for imitation.

Dissociations have been documented between gestures of the fingers, the whole hand, and the foot (see Figure 7.3). Patients with left brain damage have difficulties with the imitation of hand and foot postures, while imitation of finger postures is less compromised and can even be completely normal. By contrast, patients with right brain damage have severe difficulties with finger postures and some difficulties with foot postures but imitate hand postures nearly as perfectly as normal controls (Goldenberg, 1996, 1999; Goldenberg & Strauss, 2002).

In patients with left brain damage, imitation of hand or finger postures depends on different locations within the hemisphere. Whereas defective imitation of hand postures is quite strictly bound to parietal lesions, the center of lesion overlap in patients with defective imitation of finger postures lies in the inferior frontal lobe extending into adjacent portions of the anterior insula, the precentral gyrus, and underlying white matter (Goldenberg & Karnath, 2006; Haaland, Harrington, & Knight, 2000). This distribution of regions responsible for control of hand and finger postures does not correspond to any known somatotopic representation of body parts in sensory or motor regions of the brain, which are, however, the only possible source for body part specificity of defective imitation if imitation were accomplished by direct mapping from sensory to motor regions of the brain (Buccino et al., 2001). Alternatively, it can be reconciled with the hypothesis of body part coding. Body part coding poses different kinds of difficulty for imitation of hand and of finger postures. Positions of the hand relative to parts of the head are combinations of several hand orientations with a multitude of body parts, such as the chin, lips, back and tip of the nose, cheek, or ears. The body parts involved differ from each other in many structural features. By contrast, finger configurations are composed of a very limited set of uniform elements, the fingers, which differ only in their serial position. The resulting similarity between different finger configurations makes them vulnerable to interference and renders selection of the currently correct one difficult. The main difficulty of hand postures thus resides in the complexity of structural information that has to be classified and maintained from perception to motor replication of gestures, whereas the main difficulty of finger postures concerns selection from a very restricted range of very similar configurations. One might say that the specification of hand postures has more degrees of freedom than that of finger postures (see Chapter 6).

This task analysis is compatible with known functions of the regions whose integrity appears to be necessary for correct imitation. Selection between closely related and hence competing alternatives has been recognized as a main function of inferior frontal lobes (Jung-Beeman, 2005; Rowe, Toni, Josephs, Frackowiak, & Passingham, 2000; Thompson-Schill, 2003; Zhang, Feng, Fox, Gao, & Tan, 2004). Lesions of the posterior portion of the left inferior parietal lobe are a regular finding in patients suffering from autotopagnosia, that is, the inability to locate body parts either on their own or on other person's bodies. Errors occur independently of whether body parts are designated verbally or by visual demonstration. Apparently, these patients cannot access the knowledge about the classification and boundaries of body parts that would also be needed for decomposing gestures into simple relationships between a limited number of defined body parts (Goldenberg, 2002). Interestingly, identification of single fingers can be preserved in patients with autotopagnosia (Assal & Butters, 1973; De Renzi & Scotti, 1970; Poncet, Pellissier, Sebahoun, & Nasser, 1971).

Communicative Gestures on Command

Although early studies emphasized plumpness and incomprehensibility of aphasic patients' spontaneous gestures (Broca, 1861; Finkelnburg, 1870), further research has concentrated mostly on the production of such gestures in response to a command specifying the content of the required gesture. This restriction may have practical reasons: The documentation and evaluation of spontaneous gestures is cumbersome. It is vulnerable to confounding effects of accompanying defects of verbal expression because the meaning of spontaneous gestures normally unfolds in conjunction with accompanying speech. Paucity of speech may render the gestures incomprehensible and feign a deficit of gestural expression when in fact only verbal expression is compromised. The command to produce a specific gesture evokes a template for evaluating the shortcomings of the aphasic patients' gestures, but the neglect of spontaneous gestures has given rise to the concern that the examination probes the ability to produce gestures out of their natural context rather than revealing the patients' full repertoire of communicative gestures (De Renzi, 1990).

There are two kinds of gestures that can be unequivocally specified by verbal commands and are hence suited for clinical examinations: emblematic gestures, which express a culturally defined message, such as a thumbs up for "okay" or the hand on the temple for a "military salute," and pantomimes of object use, where a demonstration of the hand movements made when using an object signifies both the object and its use. Many clinicians and the majority of scientific studies concentrate on pantomime of object use. Again, one reason for this selection may be the possible influence of accompanying aphasia: The instruction to pretend to use an object can be illustrated by demonstrations of pantomimes, and once the general instruction is understood, comprehension of the name of the object whose use should be mimed can be facilitated by showing a picture of that object. Such nonverbal support for comprehension of the verbal commands reduces the danger that aphasic patients fail to produce the correct gesture because of insufficient comprehension of the command. By contrast, comprehension of the message that should be conveyed by an emblematic gesture can hardly be supported by nonverbal means.

There may, however, be motives for the preference of pantomime of object use that go beyond the practical difficulties of examining aphasic patients and relate to a distinction between abstract representations of meaning and material interaction with objects. Whereas the shape of emblematic gestures is determined by cultural conventions, that of pantomime derives from actual object use. As pantomimes indicate actions rather than actually executing them (the pantomime of toothbrushing does not clean your teeth), they are essentially communicative, but their shape replicates material interaction between body actions and objects. This double-faced nature promises to open another window into the embodiment of mental processes.

Pantomime of Object Use

Comprehension of the instruction to pantomime remains dubious in severely aphasic patients who in response to the command to pantomime the use of an object try to grasp the object for actual use, try to name or describe it ("verbal overflow"; Goodglass & Kaplan, 1963), or outline with the finger a more or less recognizable shape on the table. Independence of apraxic errors from language comprehension becomes obvious when patients make searching movements for the correct grip or movement or when their pantomime displays some but not all distinctive features of the intended pantomime (e.g., pantomiming drinking from a glass with a narrow grip not accommodated to the width of the pretended glass). In severe cases, patients may produce stereotyped circling or swaying movements of the hand that might be taken to indicate but not specify movement of the object in peripersonal space.

Even after excluding patients whose comprehension of the instruction is questionable, defective pantomime can be found in a majority of patients with aphasia (Barbieri & De Renzi, 1988; Goldenberg, Hartmann, & Schlott, 2003; Goodglass & Kaplan, 1963; Roy, Black, Blair, & Dimeck, 1998). By contrast, its occurrence after right brain damage and without aphasia is confined to left-handed patients (see the discussion later in this chapter). In aphasic patients, defective pantomime of tool use is at least twice as frequent as defective use of the same tools (De Renzi, Faglioni, & Sorgato, 1982; Goldenberg & Hagmann, 1998).

Two opposing views on the roles of communicative abilities and of motor control in defective pantomime have been formulated. One of them posits that defective pantomime is only one of several manifestations of general "asymbolia," that is, the inability to create and use communicative signs (Bay, 1962; Duffy & Duffy, 1981; Duffy, Watt, & Duffy, 1994; Finkelnburg, 1870; Hughlings-Jackson, 1878). A related idea is that patients lack the "abstract attitude" necessary for producing communicative gestures outside their natural context and without emotional or material needs demanding expression (Goldstein, 1948). Proponents of this view insist that at least some symptoms of aphasia are themselves manifestations of general asymbolia and emphasize that many aphasic patients have difficulties also with the production of other nonverbal symbolic representations. For example, their drawings of objects lack crucial details and are undifferentiated and often unrecognizable (Bay, 1962; Gainotti, Silveri, Villa, & Caltagirone, 1983; Goldenberg et al., 2003; Swindell, Holland, Fromm, & Greenhouse, 1988), and they select aberrant hues for coloring them (De Renzi, Faglioni, Scotti, & Spinnler, 1972; Goldenberg, 1995a).

The alternative view considers defective pantomime as a manifestation of ideomotor apraxia (see the previous discussion). The crucial difficulty of pantomime is located in the execution of the motor action of object use without guidance by the manipulated objects. The withdrawal of external support unmasks any weakness in the route leading from higher-order representations of the intended action to the motor commands sent to the muscular effectors. There are several elaborations of this basic proposal. All of them agree that defective pantomime can result from partial or complete destruction of neural representations of hand shapes and movement trajectories for object use (Barbieri & De Renzi, 1988; Heilman, Rothie, & Valenstein, 1982; Sirigu et al., 1995), but some postulate that defective pantomime can also result from a disconnection between these motor representations and those motor regions that send efferences to muscular effectors (Barbieri & De Renzi, 1988; Heilman et al., 1982).

Whereas the proponents of asymbolia look for the source of errors in the realm of cognitive processing and disregard the motor mechanisms necessary for expressing its results, those of apraxia emphasize the origin of pantomime from real tool use and pay little attention to cognitive and communicative demands transcending the motor replication of actual tool use. Proponents of the competing accounts see pantomime from opposite sides of the mind–body dichotomy. The difficulty in deciding whose view is more appropriate illustrates the ambiguous position of apraxia at the interface of cognition and motor control.

Analysis of the location of lesions causing defective pantomime can help to bring down the debate from principled philosophical stances to testable predictions. I first discuss the laterality of responsible lesions and then their intrahemispheric location.

DEFECTIVE PANTOMIME IN LEFT-HANDED PATIENTS

In right-handed patients, defective pantomime is bound to left hemisphere damage and is always associated with aphasia. In left-handed patients, linguistic competence may be located either in the right hemisphere, which controls the more skillful hand, or, as in right-handers, in the left hemisphere. There are a few cases on record in whom quite extensive right brain damage did not cause any aphasia but definitely impaired pantomime (Archibald, 1987; Heilman, Coyle, Gonyea, & Geschwind, 1973; Margolin, 1980; Verstichel, Cambier, Masson, Masson, & Robine, 1994). Obviously, these patients have language located in the left hemisphere, but their pantomime depends on the right. The dissociation between the laterality of language and of pantomime poses problems for the asymbolia account. Although proponents of this theory accept that factors other than asymbolia can contribute to aphasia, the absence of any trace of aphasia in patients who have another symptom of general asymbolia cannot easily be accommodated by the theory.

PARIETAL AND INFERIOR FRONTAL CONTRIBUTIONS TO PANTOMIME

A central tenet of the apraxia theory of defective pantomime is the crucial role of inferior parietal lesions, be it as a bottleneck through which information from occipital or superior temporal regions must pass on its way to motor regions or as the site where functional knowledge specifying hand–object interactions is stored (see Figure 7.2). Empirical support for this claim is weak. Systematic group studies exploring the neural substrate of apraxia either tested imitation rather than pantomime (Basso, Capitani, Della Sala, Laiacona, & Spinnler, 1987; Basso, Faglioni, & Luzzatti, 1985; Haaland et al., 2000; Kolb & Milner, 1981) or used compound scores of imitation and pantomime: Patients who failed production of pantomime to command were asked to imitate the same gesture and were given full credit when imitation succeeded, or an average score was computed from pantomime and imitation (Buxbaum, Kyle, & Menon, 2005). An influence of parietal lesions on such scores could derive from the confounding impact of defective imitation rather than reflecting the necessity of parietal regions for pantomime itself. Nor do clinical observations of patients with parietal lobe damage and defective pantomime prove the necessity of parietal lesions for impaired pantomime, as lesions usually extend beyond the parietal lobe and affect other possibly responsible regions. Indeed, lesions strictly confined to the left parietal lobe are a regular finding in patients with a dissociation between defective imitation and preserved pantomime (Goldenberg & Hagmann, 1997; Peigneux et al., 2000).

In a recent study, Goldenberg, Hermsdörfer, Glindemann, Rorden, and Karnath (2007) subtracted the magnetic resonance imaging–documented lesions of left brain-damaged, aphasic patients with normal pantomime from those of patients with defective pantomime. The highest difference of lesion density between patients with defective and normal pantomime was found in the opercular part of the inferior frontal gyrus and adjacent portions of the insula and precentral gyrus, whereas there were no differences in parietal or temporal regions. Obviously, pantomime of object use depends on the integrity of the left frontal but not parietal regions. This finding constitutes a challenge to the apraxia theory of defective pantomime.

A NEW LOOK ON PANTOMIME

I have argued that pantomimes are relevant for elucidating the implantation of mental processes in body actions because their shape replicates material interaction between body actions and objects, but on closer look the faithfulness of this replication becomes questionable. Both actual use and pantomime are based on knowledge about objects and their function. In actual use, this knowledge influences selection of motor programs that control the interactions between manual movements and object properties. For example, when grasping a glass, scaling of grip width to the width of the glass is achieved by first opening the hand in proportion to but wider than the visually perceived width of the glass and then closing it around the glass. Opening and closing are precisely synchronized with the transport movement of the whole hand (Jeannerod, 1988), and the strength of the final grip is finely adapted to surface friction and the estimated weight of the glass (Johansson & Westling, 1984). In pantomime, knowledge about objects and their functions is transformed into motor actions that demonstrate the distinctive features of the object and its use. Thus, when miming to grasp a glass, normal subjects open their hand to the approximate width of the pretended glass at the start of the transport movement and stop the transport at its pretended location without further changing the aperture of their grip (Goodale, Jakobson, & Keillor, 1994; Laimgruber, Goldenberg, & Hermsdörfer, 2005). The width of the aperture demonstrates the width of the glass, and stopping the transport movement suffices for indicating grasping. Pantomime neglects features of object use that are important for manipulation but have little value for discriminating the object, whereas it specifies features that in actual use are determined by the manipulated object. For example, consider ironing: The distance of the hand to the table is determined by the height of the iron, but when ironing is mimed, a distance must be chosen without external support. If this distance falls outside the usual range of iron heights, the pantomime will become unrecognizable. The need to demonstrate features of the action that are hardly attended to in actual use makes pantomime a nonroutine task even when tested for tools that are frequently used in daily living. A further difficulty for selection of appropriate manual actions is posed by the restriction to manual actions that also occur in actual tool use. For example, it is not permitted to indicate the size and shape of the iron by drawing its outline in the air rather than by demonstrating the manner of use.

Going back to the initial question of whether pantomime of tool use should better be understood as a communicative gesture or as a variant of tool use, I suggest that the particular difficulty of pantomime concerns the conversion of knowledge about object use into communicative gestures. This conversion necessitates the selection of distinctive features of actual use while permitting one to neglect properties of the motor programs that adapt the hand to the material objects.

The crucial role of the left inferior frontal lobe for pantomime can be understood in a similar way as its role in imitation of finger postures (see the previous discussion). Functional imaging studies have consistently shown activation of the left inferior frontal lobe in tasks demanding active retrieval of information from semantic memory as, for example, generation of words belonging to a particular semantic category (Cabeza & Nyberg, 2000; Cappa & Perani, 2006; Thompson-Schill, 2003). Pantomime of tool use can be conceived as one instance of active retrieval from semantic memory. On this view, the vulnerability of pantomime to lesions of the left inferior frontal lobe is due to the high demands on selection of a very restrained range of features out of the many features that may come to mind when imagining the actual use of the object.

Ideational Apraxia

When using real tools and objects, the mental plan of the intended action finds expression only within the constraints given by mechanical interactions between body and external objects. One might imagine that the interplay between intentions and mechanical constraints lends itself to be analyzed within the dichotomy of mental concept and motor execution of actions or, in the nomenclature of the apraxia tradition, between ideational and ideomotor apraxia. Curiously enough, such an approach to the analysis of disturbances of object use has rarely been pursued. With very few exceptions (Poeck, 1982; Zangwill, 1960), authors are unanimous in classifying defective use of real objects as ideational apraxia and hence ascribing it to insufficiency of the mental plan of action rather than to an inability to transform that plan into bodily interactions with objects. Nevertheless, the dichotomy between the nonlocalizable psychic processes and localized brain function shows up as an opposition between two possible causes of ideational apraxia. The first descriptions of ideational apraxia conceptualized it as one out of many manifestations of "general mental insufficiency" bound to extensive brain damage rather than to narrowly circumscribed lesions (Liepmann, 1929; Pick, 1905). By contrast, later authors interpreted ideational apraxia as loss of the specific intellectual function to know and recognize how objects should be used. This function was linked to the left parietal lobe (De Renzi & Lucchelli, 1988; Morlaas, 1928). In the modern literature, the second view prevails (Buxbaum & Saffran, 2002; De Renzi & Lucchelli, 1988; Rothi, Ochipa, & Heilman, 1997), but recently the original emphasis on more general mental aptitudes has been revamped by accounts that seek the source of errors in a lack of "attentional resources" (Humphreys & Forde, 1998; Schwartz, 1995; Schwartz et al., 1999) or in a weakness of "executive functions" (Humphreys & Forde, 1998; Rumiati, Zanini, Vorano, & Shallice, 2001).

When reviewing the evidence in favor of either of these interpretations, it is important to make a distinction between use of single tools (e.g., hammering in a nail) and multistep actions involving several tools and objects (e.g., framing a picture and fixing it to the wall).

Use of Single Tools

Only patients with left brain lesions and aphasia commit errors when presented with single tools and their corresponding objects and asked to demonstrate their use (De Renzi, Pieczuro, & Vignolo, 1968; Goldenberg & Hagmann, 1998). These patients may try to cut paper with closed scissors, write with the wrong end of the pencil, press the knife into the loaf without moving it to and fro, press the hammer on the nail without hitting it, or close the paper punch on top of the sheet without inserting the sheet. The proportion of left brain–damaged patients who fail on tests of single tool use is distinctly lower than that of patients with defective imitation or defective pantomime (De Renzi et al., 1982; Goldenberg, Hentze, & Hermsdörfer, 2004; Hermsdörfer, Hentze, & Goldenberg, 2006). Afflicted patients usually have severe aphasia and large lesions that involve but are never restricted to the parietal lobes (Goldenberg & Hagmann, 1998). As many of these patients have right-sided hemiplegia, one may be inclined to ascribe their errors to the ineptness of the nondominant left hand, but it is easy to convince oneself of their pathological nature by observing healthy persons using the tools with the nondominant hand or doing so oneself.

Conventional tools like hammers, screwdrivers, knives, or scissors have in common that they are familiar to most persons and that their function is based on transparent mechanical relationships between tool and object. It has been proposed that knowledge about their correct use can be based on either of these properties. As the tools are familiar, knowledge about their prototypical use is stored in semantic memory. Such knowledge presumably specifies the typical purpose of the tool, the object it is associated with, and the motor action of its use. As their function is based on transparent mechanical relationships, possible functions can also be deduced directly from structural properties (Povinelli, 2000; Sirigu, Duhamel, & Poncet, 1991; Vaina & Jaulent, 1991). Other than retrieval of knowledge from semantic memory, direct inference of function from structure permits one to detect nonprototypical uses of familiar tools and to find out possible uses of novel tools. For example, when there is no hammer for driving in a nail, one may use pliers because they have a flat and rigid surface that can transmit the power of the beat on the nail.

The observation that only patients with extensive left brain damage fail use of single conventional tools has led to the conclusion that both sources of knowledge about their correct use are based on left hemisphere function (Goldenberg & Hagmann, 1998). This conclusion is corroborated by experimental studies that tested integrity of each of the alternative sources. Knowledge about prototypical tool use is a prerequisite for pantomime of tool use (see the previous discussion). The observation that pantomime is intact in patients with right brain damage thus indicates that the right hemisphere does not contribute to its retrieval. Likewise, only left brain–damaged patients commit errors when shown the picture of a tool and asked to select in multiple choice the object that is typically associated with the tool or another tool that serves the same purpose (De Renzi, Scotti, & Spinnler, 1969; Hartmann, Goldenberg, Daumüller, & Hermsdörfer, 2005). Evidence that the capacity to infer possible function from structure is also bound to left hemisphere integrity comes from studies that required patients to detect the function of novel tools or to select an alternative tool when the tool typically used for a task is absent, as, for example, a coin for screwing a screw when there is no screwdriver (Goldenberg & Hagmann, 1998; Heilman et al., 1997; Roy & Square, 1985). Again, patients with left but not with right hemisphere damage have difficulties.

The fact that both sources of correct use of single familiar objects depend on the left hemisphere implies neither that they are expressions of one and the same basic function nor that they are based on the same regions within the left hemisphere. Indeed, striking dissociations have been documented between patients with two different degenerative diseases: corticobasal degeneration and semantic dementia. Whereas the bulk of cortical pathology affects the parietal and superior frontal lobes in corticobasal degeneration, it is concentrated on the temporal and inferior frontal lobes in semantic dementia. Patients with corticobasal degeneration fail completely when asked to find out the use of novel tools but can associate familiar tools with their corresponding object or another tool serving the same purpose. By contrast, patients with semantic dementia who have lost any knowledge about the purpose and prototypical use of common tools can be astonishingly good in inferring possible functions from examination of the structure of the tool. For example, they may find out that a nail clipper can be used for cutting but not that it is used for cutting nails (Hodges, Bozeat, Lambon Ralph, Patterson, & Spatt, 2000; Hodges, Spatt, & Patterson, 1999; Spatt, Bak, Bozeat, Patterson, & Hodges, 2002).

Summing up so far, the interpretation of deficient tool use as being due to a specific loss of functional knowledge specifying the appropriate use of tools appears adequate for use of single tools. There is also convincing evidence for a prominent role of the left hemisphere. Within the left hemisphere, parietal lobe integrity seems to be necessary for direct inference of function from structure, which is only one source of such functional knowledge. The other source, which is retrieval of knowledge about their prototypical use from semantic memory, does not seem to depend on parietal function.

Multistep Actions With Multiple Tools and Objects

In daily life, one is rarely handed a tool and asked to perform its prototypical action on an adequately prepared recipient. Usually, the use of the single tool is embedded in a chain of actions involving several tools and objects, frequently including technical devices, and aiming at a superordinate goal transgressing and modulating the purposes of each single action step. Furthermore, daily life may require the parallel completion of two or more multistep actions, as, for example, when preparing the components of a meal.

Such multistep actions tax mental capacities beyond retrieval of knowledge about the use of single tools. They require maintenance of the ultimate goal of the whole action as well as of a record of already completed and outstanding action steps. The completion of steps must be monitored to secure that the next step is not initiated before the previous is completed. The order in which outstanding steps are initiated may necessitate preplanning for consideration of sequential constraints.

The capacities necessary for coping with these additional difficulties of multistep actions have been conceptualized within different theoretical frameworks that are not mutually exclusive. They have been characterized as attentional resources (Hartmann et al., 2005; Pick, 1905; Schwartz et al., 1999), as executive functions (Cooper, 2007; Cooper & Shallice, 2000; Forde, Humphreys, & Remoundou, 2004; Humphreys & Forde, 1998; Rumiati et al., 2001), or as demands on working memory (Goldenberg, Hartmann-Schmid, Sürer, Daumüller, & Hermsdörfer, 2007). These approaches have in common that they refer to cognitive functions that are not specifically devoted to the use of tools and objects.

In contrast to the exclusive association of defective use of single familiar tools with left brain damage, multistep actions are affected also by lesions of the right hemisphere, by diffuse brain damage, and by frontal lobe damage (Buxbaum, Schwartz, & Montgomery, 1998; Forde & Humphreys, 2004; Giovannetti, Libon, Buxbaum, & Schwartz, 2002; Goldenberg, Hartmann-Schmid, et al., 2007; Hartmann et al., 2005; Humphreys & Forde, 1998; Schwartz et al., 1998). This lack of localizing specificity seems to fit well with the involvement of rather ill-localizable functions, such as attention, executive function, or working memory capacity. Alternatively, it might indicate that the cognitive complexity of multistep actions renders them vulnerable to multiple cognitive deficiencies and that failure on multistep actions has different causes in different patient groups (Hartmann et al., 2005; Rumiati, 2005).

In sum, analysis of deficient multistep actions with multiple tools and objects seems to support the original conception of ideational apraxia as a manifestation of a "general mental insufficiency" bound to extensive brain damage rather than to narrowly circumscribed lesions (Liepmann, 1929; Pick, 1905), but there is the possibility that this apparent nonspecificity reflects insufficient dissection of different impairments linked to different kinds of brain damage rather than the involvement of superordinate, nonlocalizable, cognitive functions.

Conclusions

Analysis of the various manifestations of apraxia reveals considerable heterogeneity of their cognitive and neuronal underpinning. Figure 7.4 gives a tentative overview of lesion localization associated with defective imitation, defective pantomime, and defective tool use. Some of these symptoms are bound to left hemisphere damage, and very few are strictly related to left parietal lobe damage. I cannot see any plausible way to reconcile these anatomical findings either with a general left hemisphere dominance for action control or with any variant of a serial "praxis system" running from posterior to anterior brain regions, as depicted in Figure 7.2. None of the fundamental properties of the "praxis system" outlined in the introduction is supported by the empirical data. There obviously is no such thing as a "praxis system."

At the beginning of this chapter, I argued that Liepmann's concepts of apraxia developed from the attempt to bridge the cleavage between nonlocalizable intrapsychic processes and the material body. It is interesting to note that this dichotomy recurs in later and contemporary debates of apraxia. In this chapter, the dichotomy appeared for imitation of gestures between direct perceptual-motor mapping and body part coding, for pantomime of tool use between asymbolia and apraxia, and for actual tool use between "general mental insufficiency" and specific loss of knowledge about tool use. It might be speculated that this dichotomy constitutes the communality between the various symptoms that are usually classified as "apraxia." They do not result from

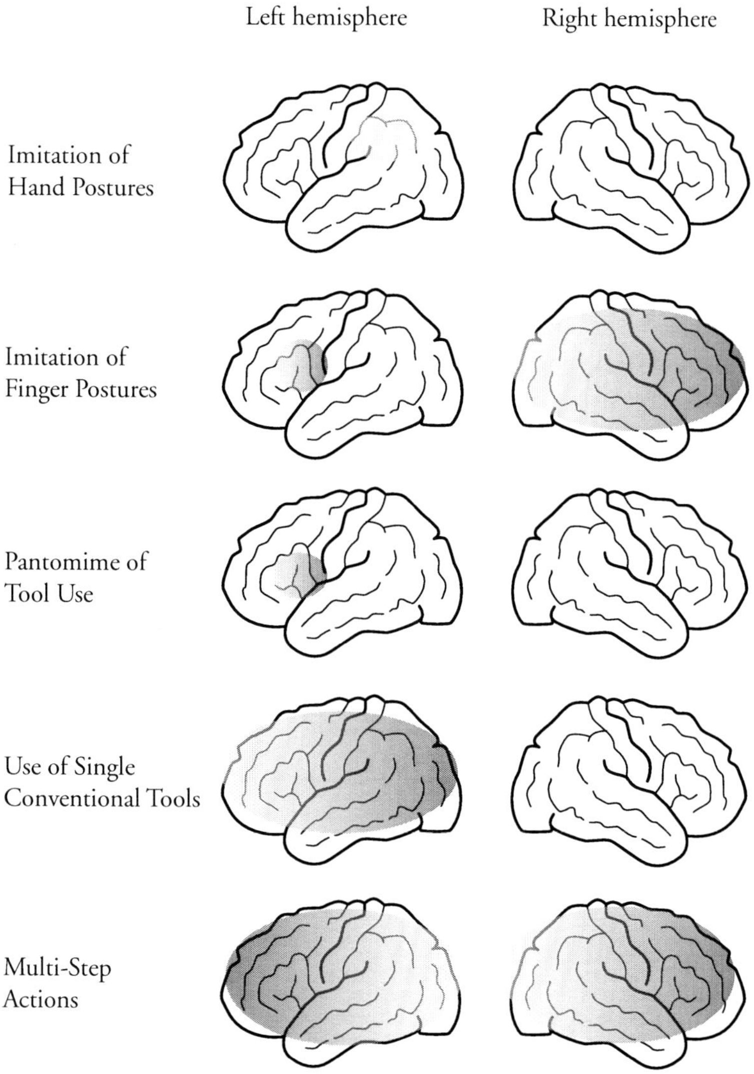

Left hemisphere   Right hemisphere

Imitation of Hand Postures

Imitation of Finger Postures

Pantomime of Tool Use

Use of Single Conventional Tools

Multi-Step Actions

Fig. 7.4 Locations of lesions associated with the different manifestations of apraxia. The figures show tentative locations of lesions responsible for defective imitation, pantomime of tool use, and actual use of tools and objects. The intrahemispheric location is indicated only when there is solid empirical evidence for it. Otherwise, the whole hemisphere is shaded to indicate the laterality of responsible lesions. Concerning the use of single tools, evidence for differential involvement of parietal and temporal lobes in different components is discussed in the text, but, as it stems from patients with diffuse degenerative damage rather than strictly circumscribed lesions, it was not considered reliable enough to be included in the figure.

damage to different parts of one unitary "praxis system." Their communality resides in their theoretical position at the interface between cognition and motor control. Each of them illuminates another aspect of this interface. In the end, contemporary scientists' interest in apraxia is nourished by the same desire that motivated Liepmann 100 years ago: to diminish and perhaps ultimately dissolve the cleavage between the immaterial soul and the material body.

Note

1. Later authors have retained the gist of this distinction but rebaptized ideokinetic to "ideomotor" apraxia, a term that Liepmann himself used synonymously with "ideational apraxia."

References

Aouka, N., Goldenberg, G., & Nadel, J. (2003). Exploring children's body knowledge via imitation of meaningless gestures. *XIth European Conference on Developmental Psychology*, 17-3, 259.

Archibald, Y. M. (1987). Persisting apraxia in two left-handed, aphasic patients with right-hemisphere lesions. *Brain and Cognition, 6*, 412–428.

Assal, G., & Butters, J. (1973). Troubles du schéma corporel lors des atteintes hémisphériques gauches. *Schweizer Medizinische Rundschau, 62*, 172–179.

Barbieri, C., & De Renzi, E. (1988). The executive and ideational components of apraxia. *Cortex, 24*, 535–544.

Basso, A., Capitani, E., Della Sala, S., Laiacona, M., & Spinnler, H. (1987). Recovery from ideomotor apraxia—A study on acute stroke patients. *Brain, 110*, 747–760.

Basso, A., Faglioni, P., & Luzzatti, C. (1985). Methods in neuroanatomical research and an experimental study of limb apraxia. In E. A. Roy (Ed.), *Neuropsychological studies of apraxia and related disorders* (pp. 179–202). Amsterdam: North-Holland.

Bay, E. (1962). Aphasia and non-verbal disorders of language. *Brain, 85,* 411–426.

Brass, M., & Heyes, C. (2005). Imitation: Is cognitive neuroscience solving the correspondence problem? *Trends in Cognitive Sciences, 9,* 489–495.

Broca, P. (1861). Perte de la parole, ramollissement chronique et destruction partielle du lobe antérieur gauche du cerveau. *Communication Société d'Anthropologie, Séance du 18 avril 1861.*

Buccino, G., Binkowski, F., Fink, G. R., Fadiga, L., Fogassi, L., Gallese, V., et al. (2001). Action observation activates premotor and parietal areas in a somatotopic manner: An fMRI study. *European Journal of Neuroscience, 13,* 400–404.

Buxbaum, L. J., Johnson-Frey, S. H., & Bartlett-Williams, M. (2005). Deficient internal models for planning hand-object interactions in apraxia. *Neuropsychologia, 43,* 917–929.

Buxbaum, L. J., Kyle, K. M., & Menon, R. (2005). On beyond mirror neurons: Internal representations subserving imitation and recognition of skilled object-related actions in humans. *Cognitive Brain Research, 25,* 226–239.

Buxbaum, L. J., & Saffran, E. M. (2002). Knowledge of object manipulation and object function: Dissociations in apraxic and nonapraxic patients. *Brain and Language, 82,* 179–199.

Buxbaum, L. J., Schwartz, M. F., & Montgomery, M. W. (1998). Ideational apraxia and naturalistic action. *Cognitive Neuropsychology, 15,* 617–644.

Cabeza, R., & Nyberg, L. (2000). Imagining cognition II: An empirical review of 275 PET and fMRI studies. *Journal of Cognitive Neuroscience, 12,* 1–47.

Cappa, S. F., & Perani, D. (2006). Boca's area and lexical-semantic processing. In Y. Grodzinsky & K. Amunts (Eds.), *Broca's region* (pp. 187–195). Oxford: Oxford University Press.

Cooper, R., & Shallice, T. (2000). Contention scheduling and the control of routine activities. *Cognitive Neuropsychology, 17,* 297–338.

Cooper, R. P. (2007). Tool use and related errors in ideational apraxia: The quantitative simulation of patient error profiles. *Cortex, 43,* 319–337.

Cubelli, R., Marchetti, C., Boscolo, G., & Della-Sala, S. (2000). Cognition in action: Testing a model of limb apraxia. *Brain and Cognition, 44,* 144–165.

Damasio, A. R. (1994). *Descartes' error—Emotion, reason and the human brain.* New York: G. P. Putnam's Sons.

De Renzi, E. (1990). Apraxia. In F. Boller & J. Grafman (Eds.), *Handbook of clinical neuropsychology* (Vol. 2, pp. 245–263). Amsterdam: Elsevier.

De Renzi, E., Faglioni, P., Scotti, G., & Spinnler, H. (1972). Impairment in associating colour to form concomitant with aphasia. *Brain, 95,* 293–304.

De Renzi, E., Faglioni, P., & Sorgato, P. (1982). Modality-specific and supramodal mechanisms of apraxia. *Brain, 105,* 301–312.

De Renzi, E., & Lucchelli, F. (1988). Ideational apraxia. *Brain, 111,* 1173–1185.

De Renzi, E., Pieczuro, A., & Vignolo, L. A. (1968). Ideational apraxia: A quantitative study. *Neuropsychologia, 6,* 41–55.

De Renzi, E., & Scotti, G. (1970). Autotopagnosia: Fiction or reality? *Archives of Neurology, 23,* 221–227.

De Renzi, E., Scotti, G., & Spinnler, H. (1969). Perceptual and associative disorders of visual recognition. *Neurology, 19,* 634–642.

Duffy, R. J., & Duffy, J. R. (1981). Three studies of deficits in pantomimic expression and pantomimic recognition in aphasia. *Journal of Speech and Hearing Research, 14,* 70–84.

Duffy, R. J., Watt, J. H., & Duffy, J. R. (1994). Testing causal theories of pantomimic deficits in aphasia using path analysis. *Aphasiology, 8,* 361–379.

Finkelnburg, F. C. (1870). Sitzung der Niederrheinischen Gesellschaft in Bonn. Medizinische Section. *Berliner Klinische Wochenschrift, 7,* 449–450, 460–462.

Forde, E. M. E., Humphreys, G. W., & Remoundou, M. (2004). Disordered knowledge of action order in action disorganisation syndrome. *Neurocase, 10,* 19–28.

Gainotti, G., Silveri, M. C., Villa, G., & Caltagirone, C. (1983). Drawing objects from memory in aphasia. *Brain, 106,* 613–622.

Gallagher, S. (2005). *How the body shapes the mind.* Oxford: Oxford University Press.

Geschwind, N. (1975). The apraxias: Neural mechanisms of disorders of learned movements. *American Scientist, 63,* 188–195.

Giovannetti, T., Libon, D. J., Buxbaum, L. J., & Schwartz, M. F. (2002). Naturalistic action impairment in dementia. *Neuropsychologia, 40,* 1220–1232.

Goldenberg, G. (1995a). Aphasic patients' knowledge about the visual appearance of objects. *Aphasiology, 9,* 50–56.

Goldenberg, G. (1995b). Imitating gestures and manipulating a mannikin—The representation of the human body in ideomotor apraxia. *Neuropsychologia, 33,* 63–72.

Goldenberg, G. (1996). Defective imitation of gestures in patients with damage in the left or right hemisphere. *Journal of Neurology, Neurosurgery, and Psychiatry, 61,* 176–180.

Goldenberg, G. (1999). Matching and imitation of hand and finger postures in patients with damage in the left or right hemisphere. *Neuropsychologia, 37,* 559–566.

Goldenberg, G. (2002). Body perception disorders. In V. S. Ramachandran (Ed.), *Encyclopedia of the human brain* (Vol. 1, pp. 443–458). San Diego, CA: Academic Press.

Goldenberg, G. (2003). Apraxia and beyond—Life and works of Hugo Karl Liepmann. *Cortex, 39,* 509–525.

Goldenberg, G., & Hagmann, S. (1997). The meaning of meaningless gestures: A study of visuo-imitative apraxia. *Neuropsychologia, 35,* 333–341.

Goldenberg, G., & Hagmann, S. (1998). Tool use and mechanical problem solving in apraxia. *Neuropsychologia, 36,* 581–589.

Goldenberg, G., Hartmann, K., & Schlott, I. (2003). Defective pantomime of object use in left brain damage: Apraxia or asymbolia? *Neuropsychologia, 41,* 1565–1573.

Goldenberg, G., Hartmann-Schmid, K., Sürer, F., Daumüller, M., & Hermsdörfer, J. (2007). The impact of dysexecutive syndrome on use of tools and technical equipment. *Cortex, 43,* 424–435.

Goldenberg, G., Hentze, S., & Hermsdörfer, J. (2004). The effect of tactile feedback on pantomime of object use in apraxia. *Neurology, 63,* 1863–1867.

Goldenberg, G., Hermsdörfer, J., Glindemann, R., Rorden, C., & Karnath, H. O. (2007). Pantomime of tool use depends on integrity of left inferior frontal cortex. *Cerebral. Cortex, 17,* 2769–2776.

Goldenberg, G., & Karnath, H. O. (2006). The neural basis of imitation is body-part specific. *Journal of Neuroscience, 26,* 6282–6287.

Goldenberg, G., & Strauss, S. (2002). Hemisphere asymmetries for imitation of novel gestures. *Neurology, 59,* 893–897.

Goldstein, K. (1948). *Language and language disturbances.* New York: Grune and Stratton.

Goodale, M. A., Jakobson, L. S., & Keillor, J. M. (1994). Differences in the visual control of pantomimed and natural grasping movements. *Neuropsychologia, 32,* 1159–1178.

Goodglass, H., & Kaplan, E. (1963). Disturbance of gesture and pantomime in aphasia. *Brain, 86,* 703–720.

Haaland, K. Y., Harrington, D. L., & Knight, R. T. (2000). Neural representations of skilled movement. *Brain, 123,* 2306–2313.

Hartmann, K., Goldenberg, G., Daumüller, M., & Hermsdörfer, J. (2005). It takes the whole brain to make a cup of coffee: The neuropsychology of naturalistic actions involving technical devices. *Neuropsychologia, 43,* 625–637.

Heilman, K. M., Coyle, J. M., Gonyea, E. F., & Geschwind, N. (1973). Apraxia and agraphia in a left-hander. *Brain, 96,* 21–28.

Heilman, K. M., Maher, L. M., Greenwald, M. L., & Rothi, L. J. G. (1997). Conceptual apraxia from lateralized lesions. *Neurology, 49,* 457–464.

Heilman, K. M., & Rothi, L. J. G. (1993). Apraxia. In K. M. Heilman & E. Valenstein (Eds.), *Clinical neuropsychology* (pp. 141–164). New York: Oxford University Press.

Heilman, K. M., Rothie, L. J., & Valenstein, E. (1982). Two forms of ideomotor apraxia. *Neurology, 32,* 342–346.

Hermsdörfer, J., Hentze, S., & Goldenberg, G. (2006). Spatial and kinematic features of apraxic movement depend on the mode of execution. *Neuropsychologia, 44,* 1642–1652.

Hodges, J. R., Bozeat, S., Lambon Ralph, M. A., Patterson, K., & Spatt, J. (2000). The role of conceptual knowledge in object use—Evidence from semantic dementia. *Brain, 123,* 1913–1925.

Hodges, J. R., Spatt, J., & Patterson, K. (1999). "What" and "how": Evidence for the dissociation of object knowledge and mechanical problem-solving skills in the human brain. *Proceedings of the National Academy of Sciences of the United States of America, 96,* 9444–9448.

Hughlings-Jackson, J. (1878). On affection of speech from disease of the brain. *Brain, 1,* 304–330.

Humphreys, G. W., & Forde, E. M. E. (1998). Disordered action schema and action disorganisation syndrome. *Cognitive Neuropsychology, 15,* 771–812.

Iacoboni, M., Woods, R. P., Brass, M., Bekkering, H., Mazziotta, J. C., & Rizzolatti, G. (1999). Cortical mechanisms of human imitation. *Science, 286,* 2526–2528.

Jeannerod, M. (1988). *The neural and behavioural organization of goal-directed movements.* Oxford: Clarendon Press.

Johansson, R. S., & Westling, G. (1984). Roles of glabrous skin receptors and sensorimotor memory control of precision grip when lifting rougher or more slippery objects. *Experimental Brain Research, 56,* 550–564.

Jung-Beeman, M. (2005). Bilateral brain processes for comprehending natural language. *Trends in Cognitive Sciences, 9,* 512–518.

Keysers, C., & Perrett, D. I. (2004). Demystifying social cognition: A Hebbian perspective. *Trends in Cognitive Sciences, 8,* 501–507.

Kolb, B., & Milner, B. (1981). Performance of complex arm and facial movements after focal brain lesions. *Neuropsychologia, 19,* 491–503.

Laimgruber, K., Goldenberg, G., & Hermsdörfer, J. (2005). Manual and hemispheric asymmetries in the execution of actual and pantomimed prehension. *Neuropsychologia, 43,* 682–692.

Liepmann, H. (1900). Das Krankheitsbild der Apraxie (motorische Asymbolie) auf Grund eines Falles von einseitiger Apraxie. *Monatschrift für Psychiatrie und Neurologie, 8,* 15–44, 102–132, 182–197.

Liepmann, H. (1905). *Ueber Störungen des Handelns bei Gehirnkranken.* Berlin: Karger.

Liepmann, H. (1908). *Drei Aufsätze aus dem Apraxiegebiet.* Berlin: Karger.

Liepmann, H. (1925). Apraktische Störungen. In H. Curschmann & F. Kramer (Eds.), *Lehrbuch der Nervenkrankheiten* (pp. 408–416). Berlin: Springer.

Liepmann, H. (1929). Klinische und psychologische Untersuchung und anatomischer Befund bei einem Fall von Dyspraxie und Agraphie. *Monatschrift für Psychiatrie und Neurologie, 71,* 169–214.

Margolin, D. I. (1980). Right hemisphere dominance for praxis and left hemisphere dominance for speech in a left-hander. *Neuropsychologia, 18,* 715–719.

Mehler, M. F. (1987). Visuo-imitative apraxia. *Neurology, 37*(Suppl. 1), 129.

Morlaas, J. (1928). *Contribution à l'étude de l'apraxie.* Paris: Amédée Legrand.

Peigneux, P., Van der Linden, M., Andres-Benito, P., Sadzot, B., Franck, G., & Salmon, E. (2000). Exploration neuropsychologique et par imagerie fonctionelle cérébrale d'une apraxie visuo-imitative. *Revue Neurologique, 156,* 459–472.

Pick, A. (1905). *Studien zur motorischen Apraxia und ihr nahestende Erscheinungen; ihre Bedeutung in der Symptomatologie psychopathischer Symptomenkomplexe.* Leipzig: Franz Deuticke.

Poeck, K. (1982). The two types of motor apraxia. *Archives Italiennes de Biologie, 120,* 361–369.

Poeck, K., & Orgass, B. (1964). Die Entwicklung des Körperschemas bei Kindern im Alter von 4–10 Jahren. *Neuropsychologia, 2,* 109–130.

Poncet, M., Pellissier, J. F., Sebahoun, M., & Nasser, C. J. (1971). A propos d'un cas d'autotopagnosie secondaire à une lésion pariéto-occipitale de l'hémisphère majeur. *Encéphale, 61,* 1–14.

Povinelli, D. J. (2000). *Folk physics for apes—The chimpanzee's theory of how the world works.* Oxford: Oxford University Press.

Rizzolatti, G., & Craighero, L. (2004). The mirror-neuron system. *Annual Review of Neurosciences, 27,* 169–192.

Rothi, L. J. G., Ochipa, C., & Heilman, K. M. (1997). A cognitive neuropsychological model of limb praxis and apraxia. In L. J. G. Rothi & K. M. Heilman (Eds.), *Apraxia—The neuropsychology of action* (pp. 29–50). Hove: Psychology Press.

Rowe, J. B., Toni, I., Josephs, O., Frackowiak, R. S. J., & Passingham, R. E. (2000). The prefrontal cortex: Response selection or maintenance within working memory? *Science, 288,* 1656–1660.

Roy, E. A., Black, S. E., Blair, N., & Dimeck, P. T. (1998). Analysis of deficits in gestural pantomime. *Journal of Clinical and Experimental Neuropsychology, 20,* 628–643.

Roy, E. A., & Square, P. A. (1985). Common considerations in the study of limb, verbal and oral apraxia. In E. A. Roy (Ed.), *Neuropsychological studies of apraxia and related disorders* (pp. 111–162). Amsterdam: North-Holland.

Rumiati, R. I. (2005). Right, left, or both? Brain hemispheres and apraxia of naturalistic actions. *Trends in Cognitive Sciences, 9,* 167–169.

Rumiati, R. I., Zanini, S., Vorano, L., & Shallice, T. (2001). A form of ideational apraxia as a selective deficit of contention scheduling. *Cognitive Neuropsychology, 18,* 617–642.

Schwartz, M. F. (1995). Re-examining the role of executive functions in routine action production. *Annals of the New York Academy of Sciences, 769,* 321–335.

Schwartz, M. F., Buxbaum, L. J., Montgomery, M. W., Fitzpatrick-DeSalme, E. J., Hart, T., Ferraro, M., et al. (1999). Naturalistic action production following right hemisphere stroke. *Neuropsychologia, 37,* 51–66.

Schwartz, M. F., Lee, S. S., Coslett, H. B., Montgomery, M. W., Buxbaum, L. J., Carew, T. G., et al. (1998). Naturalistic action impairment in closed head injury. *Neuropsychology, 12,* 13–28.

Sirigu, A., Cohen, L., Duhamel, J. R., Pillon, B., Dubois, B., & Agid, Y. (1995). A selective impairment of hand posture for object utilization in apraxia. *Cortex, 31,* 41–56.

Sirigu, A., Duhamel, J. R., Cohen, L., Pillon, B., Dubois, B., & Agid, Y. (1996). The mental representation of hand movements after parietal lobe damage. *Science, 273,* 1564–1568.

Sirigu, A., Duhamel, J. R., & Poncet, M. (1991). The role of sensorimotor experience in object recognition—A case of multimodal agnosia. *Brain, 114,* 2555–2573.

Spatt, J., Bak, T., Bozeat, S., Patterson, K., & Hodges, J. R. (2002). Apraxia, mechanical problem solving and semantic knowledge—Contributions to object usage in corticobasal degeneration. *Journal of Neurology, 249,* 601–608.

Swindell, C. S., Holland, A. L., Fromm, D., & Greenhouse, J. B. (1988). Characteristics of recovery of drawing ability in left and right brain damaged patients. *Brain and Cognition, 7,* 16–30.

Thompson-Schill, S. L. (2003). Neuroimaging studies of semantic memory: Inferring "how" from "where." *Neuropsychologia, 41,* 280–292.

Vaina, L. M., & Jaulent, M. C. (1991). Object structure and action requirements: A compatibility model for functional recognition. *International Journal of Intelligent Systems, 6,* 313–336.

Verstichel, P., Cambier, J., Masson, C., Masson, M., & Robine, B. (1994). Apraxie et autotopagnosie sans aphasie ni agraphie, mais avec activité compulsive de langage au cours d'une lésion hémisphérique droite. *Revue Neurologique, 150,* 274–281.

Zangwill, O. L. (1960). Le probleme de l'apraxie ideatoire. *Revue Neurologique, 102,* 595–633.

Zhang, J. X., Feng, C. M., Fox, P. T., Gao, J. H., & Tan, L. H. (2004). Is left inferior frontal gyrus a general mechanism for selection? *Neuroimage, 23,* 596–603.

Speech Errors and the Implicit Learning of Phonological Sequences

Gary S. Dell, Jill A. Warker, *and* Christine A. Whalen

Abstract

This chapter describes several experiments investigating implicit learning in the speech production system. It shows that speech errors reveal the implicit learning of artificial phonotactic constraints. The learning is implicit; that is, it is independent of the speakers' awareness and intentions. The learning also seems to be more than just priming of recent associations between consonants and positions because second-order constraints, in which such positioning is contingent on something else, can be learned as well, albeit more slowly. Moreover, some people can learn sequential constraints defining syllables that are illegal in their native language. These findings are discussed in the context of a model of learning based on connectionist principles.

Keywords: speech production, language acquisition, action sequences, speech errors, connectionist principles

All complex human behaviors are, to a considerable extent, learned. We were not born knowing how to sing and dance, to play five-card hold 'em poker, or to use word processing software. And, despite the emphasis of the past 50 years of linguistic research on an innate endowment for language, no one questions that human linguistic abilities are very much the product of experience.

People learn to produce speech and other rapid action sequences implicitly. That is, learning occurs simply by doing. There is no intention to learn and little conscious awareness of the knowledge that is gained. In this chapter, we describe several experiments investigating this kind of learning in the speech production system. Participants

are required to produce strings of syllables that, unbeknownst to them, follow rules such as /f/ *must be onset* (i.e., /f/ must appear in the initial part of the syllable and never at the end, or coda, part) throughout the experiment. The speakers' implicit acquisition of these rules is revealed, paradoxically, in their speech errors, or "slips of the tongue." As they learn, their slips become more likely to follow than to violate the rules. We then use these data to make some claims about language acquisition and describe a general approach to implicit learning of action sequences.

Implicit learning is typically studied in experiments that emphasize perception and cognition rather than action. For example, the first such studies used the artificial-grammar-learning task. Reber (1969) asked participants to memorize strings of letters, such as BSSXPVE, which had been derived from a finite-state grammar. After memorization, it was found that participants could judge whether novel strings conformed to the grammar. So, even though there was no intention to learn the grammar, the judgments indicated some acquisition of the system. A related procedure, the serial reaction-time paradigm, also uses stimuli that follow a set of rules (e.g., Cleeremans, 1993; Cohen, Ivry, & Keele, 1990; Nissen & Bullemer, 1987). The stimuli, though, are, for example, sequences of lights that appear in particular spatial positions, with the rules dictating the order of the positions. Participants must respond to each light by pressing a spatially congruent key as quickly as possible. As experience with rule-governed sequences increases, response times decrease, even though participants profess little awareness of the rules generating the patterns. Although action is required, in the form of the response-key presses, accounts of the task (e.g., Cleeremans, 1993) associate the learning largely with the perceptual anticipation of the next light's location based on recent memory for the sequence.

Speech Errors and Implicit Learning in Production

It has long been known that speech errors reflect the speaker's implicit knowledge of their language's grammar—the syntactic patterns that define allowable word combinations, the morphological patterns that govern word formation, and the phonological patterns that inhabit pronunciations (e.g., Dell, 1986; Garrett, 1975; Nooteboom, 1969; Stemberger, 1985). The classic example of this reflection is the *phonotactic regularity effect*: Slips rarely disobey the phonotactic constraints that determine how speech sounds combine to

make syllables and words (Wells, 1951). For example, in English, /ng/ is an illegal syllable onset but a common syllable coda. Consequently, a slip such as "singing in the raing" would be quite possible, while "singing in the ngain" would be extremely unlikely. When a speech sound, or phoneme, moves in an error, it just about always lands in a spot that is phonotactically legal. Error adherence to phonotactics has been taken as evidence that these constraints are represented and actively consulted during speech production (Fromkin, 1971).

If slips reflect knowledge of linguistic patterns as that knowledge is expressed in production, we ought to be able to use them to study how this knowledge changes, that is, to study implicit learning within the production system. Dell, Reed, Adams, and Meyer (2000) asked speakers to recite, in time with a metronome, strings of four consonant-vowel-consonant syllables, such as "hes meng ken feg." Naturally, speakers often made errors, such as "hes **h**eng . . ." instead of "hes **m**eng . . . ," and nearly every error involved the substitution of one consonant with another consonant also from the string. We refer to the substituted consonant (e.g., /m/) as the target consonant and the substituting consonant (e.g., /h/) as the moving or "slipping" consonant. Two of the eight target consonants in each string were /h/ and /ng/. These are unusual consonants in that they are *language restricted*: The phonotactic constraints of English demand that /h/ always be a syllable onset and that /ng/ always appear in coda position. Other languages allow coda /h/'s (e.g., Finnish) and onset /ng/'s (e.g., Burmese), but English does not. In accordance with the phonotactic regularity effect, every slip of /h/ and /ng/ in Dell et al.'s experiments—there were over 1,000 of these slips—was "legal"; that is, /h/-onsets moved only to other onset positions, and /ng/-codas moved only to other coda positions. You never get "heng mek..." spoken as "heng **ng**ek" or "heng me**h**." Four of the other consonants in the string were *unrestricted;* that is, during the experiment, they appeared half the time as onsets and half the time as codas. For example, in the previously mentioned string, /k/ is an onset, but on the next string in the experiment, it could appear in the syllable "gek." In Dell et al.'s experiment 1, /k/, /g/, /m/, and /n/ were the unrestricted consonants. When these consonants slipped, they behaved quite differently than the language-restricted ones. The slips of unrestricted consonants were legal—they retained their syllable positions—only 68% of the time. So, for example, if /k/ is an onset in a string, there is a reasonable chance that if it slips, it will emerge in a coda position. Thus, the contrast between the 100% legal slips of the language-restricted consonants and the 68% legal slips of the unrestricted ones illustrates how linguistic knowledge is revealed in the errors.

The key part of the experiment involved the remaining two consonants, which were called *experiment restricted.* For example in Dell et al.'s (2000) experiment 1, for half the participants, /f/ occurred only as an onset and /s/ only as a coda throughout the entire experiment. The other half of the participants experienced /f/ only as a coda and /s/ only as an onset. These restrictions are artificial because English allows /f/ and /s/ to be both onsets and codas. If the participants learn these restrictions as they go through the experiment, their errors should reflect this. Movements of /f/ and /s/ should stick to their syllable positions more than those of the unrestricted consonants. This was indeed the finding. Slips of /f/ and /s/ were legal (position maintaining) 98% of the time, far greater than the legality rate of 68% for the unrestricted /k/, /g/, /m/, and /n/ slips. A replication of this experiment with /k/ and /g/ as the restricted consonants

and /f/, /s/, /m/, and /n/ as the unrestricted controls found that 95% of the restricted slips were legal compared to only 77% of the unrestricted ones.

The participants' experience with the restricted distribution of the consonants changed their error patterns. In some sense, they *learned* the distribution. This learning has three key properties: It is rapid, it is implicit, and it is sensitive to phonological similarity. Rapid learning is apparent from how quickly the error pattern comes to track the distribution of the restricted consonants. Dell et al.'s (2000) experiments were actually multiday studies with participants reciting 96 sequences four times on each of 4 separate days. In the study with /f/ and /s/ being restricted, the proportion of legal slips of these consonants was 98% on the first day, which was the same rate as for the remaining days. The legality proportion on the first day of the study using /k/ and /g/ was 93%, comparable to that of the remaining days, which was 95%. Clearly, the high legality of slips of restricted consonants was established quite early in the study. Exactly how quickly the learning occurs was shown in a study by Taylor and Houghton (2005). They used a similar set of restricted and unrestricted consonants but "flipped" the constraint on the restricted consonants in the middle of the experimental session. For example, participants might start out the session with /f/ as an onset and /s/ as a coda, and the /f/ and /s/ errors would reflect that constraint. Then the stimuli would be changed so that /f/ was always a coda and /s/ an onset. After the change, it took around nine trials on average for the error pattern to turn around to favor the reverse constraint. Thus, nine instances of a restricted sound consistently appearing in the same syllable position were enough to both eliminate the original error pattern and establish the new one.

Not only is the learning rapid, but it is also implicit. In the studies of Dell et al. (2000) and Taylor and Houghton (2005), half the participants were informed about the distribution of the restricted consonants. They were told, for example, "when you see an 'f,' it will always be at the beginning of a syllable, and when you see an 's,' it will always be at the end." The informed participants' error patterns were indistinguishable from those generated by uninformed participants, demonstrating that awareness of the distribution is irrelevant to the distribution's effect on errors. (Participants who were not informed exhibited no awareness of the distribution of restricted consonants as assessed by a post-experimental query). The implicit nature of the distribution's influence on errors is further supported by the simple fact that the data that are revealing of the knowledge are *errors,* and one does not intend to err.

The third key property of learning in the speech-error paradigm concerns the representations over which the learning occurs. In principle, participants could be learning things about particular syllables (e.g., the syllable /fes/ occurs but not the syllable /sef/), phonemes (e.g., the consonant /f/ occurs only in onset position), or even phonological features (e.g., the labial-dental place of articulation occurs only in onset position). Goldrick (2004) demonstrated that the learning involves the featural as well as the phonemic levels. His participants recited syllable strings in which the voiceless, labial-dental fricative /f/ was restricted to onset position and found that slips of /f/ retained their positions 97% of the time, while unrestricted consonants maintained their positions 73% of the time. This replicates previous findings. However, Goldrick also showed that if the syllables to be recited included the *voiced* labial-dental fricative /v/ and the /v/'s occurred both as onsets and as codas, the tendency of slips of the similar but restricted sound /f/ to maintain their position was reduced significantly to 90%. These results suggest that participants are learning the restrictions or lack thereof at the level of both the phoneme and the feature. The fact that unrestricted /v/'s diminished the effect of restriction of /f/ suggests that at least some of the learning involves constraints at the featural level (e.g., the constraint that labial-dental fricatives can occur as codas). The phoneme level also seems to play a role insofar as the slips of /f/ still maintained their positions at a higher rate than unrestricted consonant slips, even when the features of /f/ were by themselves unrestricted. Thus, the system is at least keeping track of specific combinations of features.

We have characterized the sensitivity of slips to experiment-wide distributions in this speech-error paradigm as learning. During the experiment, participants learn that, for example, /f/ is always an onset. An important issue concerns the relation between this kind of learning and language learning in general. From one perspective, they are similar. Just as our everyday slips obey language-wide phonotactic constraints, such as the requirement that /h/ be an onset in English, the experimental slips obey the experiment-wide constraints. At least on the surface, these are similar phenomena. But there is reason to be skeptical as well. Knowledge of phonotactic constraints arises in infancy (e.g., Jusczyk, Friederici, Wessels, Svenkerud, & Juszcyk, 1993) and is gradually learned in early childhood. The sensitivity of slips to experiment-wide constraints was demonstrated in adults—who have presumably finished with their acquisition of phonology—and was acquired very rapidly rather than gradually. This seems quite different from children learning the phonotactics of their native language. Because of these differences, Taylor and Houghton (2005) suggested that the experimental work illustrates a priming of existing knowledge rather than the learning of a new constraint. For example, it can be assumed that native English speakers already have a piece of knowledge that allows /f/'s to be syllable onsets. Perhaps when one produces several examples of /f/-onset syllables, that simply strengthens this knowledge. On this view, there is no new learning aside from the repetition priming of existing phonotactic constraints (e.g., /f/ is an allowable syllable onset in English). In the remainder of this chapter, we report studies testing the limits of implicit learning in the production system. By exploring these limits, we can paint a clearer picture of the nature of the learning and its possible relations with language acquisition.

First- Versus Second-Order Experiment-Wide Constraints

The experiments of Dell et al. (2000), Taylor and Houghton (2005), and Goldrick (2004) tested for the learning of artificial *first-order* constraints. In a first-order constraint, the positioning of a consonant in a syllable does not depend on any other property of the syllable. A *second-order* constraint conditionalizes this positioning in some way; for example, *if the vowel is /ae/, /k/ must be an onset, but if the vowel is /I/, /k/ must be a coda.* Real phonotactic constraints sometimes involve contingencies between vowels and consonant positions. For instance, in English, if the vowel is the diphthong /yuw/, there are only a few consonants that can occur as onsets (the consonant /f/ as in *few* being one possibility). Most English consonants, however, can occur in both onset and coda position regardless of the vowel, so the vowel-contingent constraint on the positioning of /k/ described previously is clearly artificial. If this kind of constraint can be implicitly learned and influence speech errors, it would show that the learning system is more powerful than one that only allowed for priming of existing first-order positional possibilities for consonants.

Second-Order Contingencies Between Consonants and Adjacent Vowels

Warker and Dell (2006) used the speech-error paradigm to investigate the acquisition of the vowel-contingent constraint: *If the vowel is /ae/, /k/ must be an onset and /g/ must be a coda; if the vowel is /I/, /g/ must be an onset and /k/ must be a coda.* Half their speakers recited sequences that obeyed this constraint, and half experienced sequences with the opposite association of the /k/ and /g/ positions to the vowels. The four-syllable sequences to be produced alternated between sequences with /ae/ as the vowel (e.g., "hag kam fan sang") and those with /I/ (e.g., "fis ging min hik"). Hence, the restricted consonants /k/ and /g/ were experienced as both onsets and codas during the experiment. Any tendency for slips of these consonants to stick to their positions to a greater extent than slips of unrestricted consonants (here, /f/, /s/, /m/, and /n/) would thus illustrate sensitivity to the second-order contingency.

In Warker and Dell's study, the vowel-contingent constraint was learned as evidenced by a significantly greater proportion of position-maintaining legal slips of the restricted consonants than for the unrestricted control slips. The data, however, were different from that seen in the first-order experiments of Dell et al. (2000) in two respects. First, the second-order effects were smaller in magnitude. The average difference in legality rates between restricted and unrestricted consonants for the first-order experiments was 24%. In the second-order experiment with the restricted /k/'s and /g/'s, it was only 8%, and in a replication with restricted /m/ and /n/ instead of /k/ and /g/, it was 14%. Second and more important, the second-order learning was

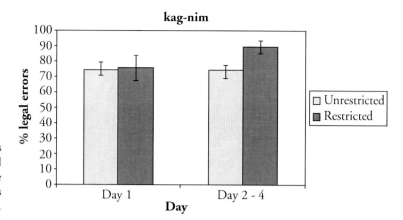

kag-nim

Fig. 8.1 Legality proportions of errors for second-order vowel contingent experiments for the first day and subsequent days of testing.

slow. There was no difference between restricted and unrestricted consonants on the first day of testing. Figure 8.1 presents the legality proportions for the second-order vowel contingent experiments separately for the first and subsequent days. In both studies, there was a robust difference only after day 1.

The findings of second-order vowel contingent learning in the speech-error paradigm allow us to conclude that implicit learning of sound distributions in production is not limited to the priming of particular onsets and codas that are already allowed in English. The slowness of the learning, though, does suggest a learning process that is not just the priming of existing knowledge. As we will see, this slow learning happens with other constraints as well.

Second-Order Contingencies Between Nonadjacent Consonants

Although most phonotactic constraints in the world's languages are either first-order or involve second-order contingencies between adjacent phonological units, the phonological structure of many languages admits contingencies between distant elements. The classic example is vowel harmony. In Finnish, for example, a word can have all its vowels from one group (a, u, and o, e.g., *talo,* "house") or all its vowels from another group (ä, y, ö, e.g., tyttö, "girl"), but the

groups cannot mix in the same word. Thus, *tylo* is phonotactically illegal in Finnish just as *ngo* is illegal in English. Notice that the contingency is between vowels that are typically separated by one or more consonants, and hence it is a nonadjacent second-order constraint.

Warker and Dell (2006) used the speech-error paradigm to test whether a nonadjacent consonant-contingent constraint could be acquired. This was done by expanding the syllables in the sequences to disyllables (CVCVC) and developing constraints in which whether a particular consonant was an onset or a coda depended on the identity of the medial consonant. For example, *if the medial consonant is /r/, /k/ is an onset and /g/ is a coda, but if the medial consonant is /l/, /g/ is an onset and /k/ is a coda.* Using the same procedure as previous studies, speakers came in for 4 days and recited sequences following this constraint or, for half the speakers, a parallel constraint with the reverse assignment of /k/ and /g/. The four-disyllable sequences in the study alternated between sequences with "ere," pronounced /ɛrə/, in the middle of the disyllable (e.g., kerem fereg sereng heren) or "ele," pronounced /ɛlə/, in the middle (e.g., helem gereng selek nelef). Overall, speakers produced more legal errors with the restricted consonants (/k/ and /g/) than with the unrestricted consonants (/m/, /n/, /f/, and /s/). However, the pattern of legality in the errors echoed that of the vowel-contingent constraint study in that learning did not show up until the second day of testing. A replication of this study using /f/ and /s/ as the restricted consonants yielded the same pattern. Figure 8.2 presents the legality proportions of restricted and unrestricted consonants on day 1 and on subsequent days averaged over the /k/-/g/ and /f/-/s/ versions of the experiment. In both studies, there was no difference between errors involving restricted and unrestricted consonants on the first day of testing. But, on subsequent days, restricted consonants moved reliably more often to legal positions in an error than unrestricted consonants did.

Warker and Dell took these results as evidence that speakers implicitly learned the consonant-contingent constraint and that this learning was slower than first-order constraint learning. However, they were hesitant to characterize the constraint as nonadjacent because the medial consonants chosen for this study (/r/ and /l/) greatly color the pronunciation of the initial vowel in the syllable. Thus, it is possible that speakers were learning an association between the syllable position and adjacent vowel rather than between the syllable position and the nonadjacent medial consonant. To address this adjacency issue, Warker, Dell, Whalen, and Gereg (in press) replicated the medial /r/-/l/ studies replacing the /r/ and /l/ with /v/ and /b/. These medial consonants do not differentially interact with the vowels the way that /r/ and /l/ do. Thus, any constraint between the initial (or final) consonant of the disyllable and the medial /v/ or /b/ is truly a nonadjacent consonant-contingent constraint.

The results of the /v/-/b/ study replicated those of the /r/-/l/ study in all respects (see Figure 8.3). On the first day of testing, the slips of restricted consonants stuck to their positions as often as the slips of unrestricted consonants did. The average difference in legality rates between the restricted and unrestricted consonants was 2.4% in the wrong direction. But on the remaining 3 days of testing, restricted consonants slipped to legal positions reliably more often than unrestricted consonants did (by 6.8%).

Taken together, the results from these studies suggest that more distant phonotactic constraints can be implicitly learned from recent production experience. However, like the adjacent second-order constraints, the nonadjacent constraints require a longer learning period than first-order constraints do. The results further support the hypothesis that a learning process is occurring as participants implicitly pick up on the association between a consonant's position and other aspects of utterance in which it is placed.

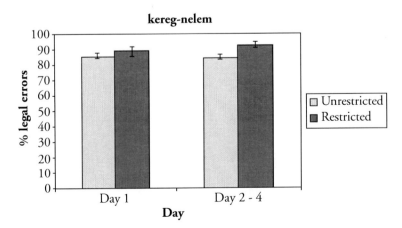

Fig. 8.2 Legality proportions of errors for /ere/-/ele/ consonant-contingent experiments for the first day and subsequent days of testing.

Learning of Constraints That Create Illegal Sequences?

In all the studies described thus far, the set of phonological forms experienced by the speakers is more restricted than those of English. Another way to say this is that the experiment-wide constraints cause some legal English forms to be illegal in the context of the experiment, but they do not do the reverse—making some illegal English forms legal for the experiment. Given this, one can hypothesize that the learning consists solely in emphasizing existing (English) phonological properties and deemphasizing others. We know from the studies of second-order learning that such a process must be more powerful than simply emphasizing/deemphasizing first-order positional constraints. But it remains a possibility that learning is limited to tinkering within the system that defines language-wide legality.

There is some evidence, though, that implicit learning can step outside the system. In a preliminary study (Whalen & Dell, 2006), we taught people to produce syllables with *onset* /ng/'s and then showed that their intended /ng/'s would sometimes slip to onset positions. To do this, we first trained five participants (in one of our studies) to produce /ng/'s as onsets by giving them words with medial /ng/'s, such as *longing* and *winged* (the two-syllable poetic pronunciation), and asking them to separate them into syllables as "lo-nging" and "wi-nged." Then they practiced on single syllables beginning with /ng/, with the experimenter constantly providing feedback and examples of correct pronunciations. Not everyone can learn to do this easily; one participant could not.

After this initial training, the participants did a 1-day version of the speech-error paradigm, where the 96 strings to be recited included /ng/'s as onsets and codas an equal number of times. Thus, strings such as "hek nem nges feg" would be included along with those such as "seng mef heg ken." The resulting data provided evidence that the speakers had acquired the constraint */ng/ is an onset*. First of all, the participants correctly produced target onset /ng/'s 95% of the time, showing at least that they can do it when they try. More important, though, onset /ng/'s emerged even when unintended in errors. In 54 cases of /ng/ as the slipping consonant, the /ng/ moved to onset position 42% of the time. Even when the target /ng/ was a coda, it slipped to onset position on seven occasions. Notice that, in all previous experiments where /ng/ was experienced only as a coda, there were zero slips of /ng/ to onset position, so the experience within the current experiment (either the training, the experiment proper, or both) is the cause of the /ng/ onset slips. Thus, recent experience with /ng/ onsets, a structure that is clearly outside English phonology, led to /ng/-onset slips, suggesting that this constraint has been temporarily added to the set of phonotactic constraints that control production.

First- and Second-Order Constraints in Perception

We have seen how artificial first- and second-order constraints affect the output of the production system. What about the perceptual system? Several studies with adults have found the learning of artificial constraints in perceptual tasks. For example, Onishi, Chambers, and Fisher (2002) asked adults to listen to syllables that followed first-order constraints on consonant positions. Then they listened to and repeated test syllables as quickly as they could. The test syllables could be either from the original list of studied syllables (old legal), new syllables that nonetheless followed the constraints (novel legal), or new syllables that violated the constraints (novel illegal). Legal syllables (both novel and old) were repeated more quickly than illegal ones, demonstrating learning of the constraint. Infants also learn these constraints simply by listening. Using the head-turn preference paradigm, Chambers, Onishi, and Fisher (2003) familiarized 16.5-month-old infants to syllables exhibiting the same first-order constraints that Onishi et al. tested with adults. Afterward, the infants showed a preference for listening to novel illegal syllables over novel legal ones, demonstrating that they discriminated the items on the basis of the experimentally imposed constraint.

Second-order constraints appear to be learned in perception as well. In the study in which adults listened to constrained syllables, Onishi et al. (2002) found that a second-order vowel contingency on consonant position could be acquired as well as a first-order one. Even infants can learn this constraint. Chambers (2004) found that 16.5-month-old infants, after exposure to a number of syllables obeying a second-order vowel-contingent constraint, discriminated novel legal from novel illegal syllables. Crucially, though, the infants' discrimination was demonstrated by a preference for the *illegal* syllables over the legal syllables. This is the opposite preference to that shown in Chambers et al.'s (2003) first-order study. On the assumption that the novelty preference found for first-order constraints illustrates more complete learning than the familiarity preference in the second-order case (Chambers, 2004), this result shows that infants learned the second-order constraint more slowly than the first-order one.

Can Any Second-Order Constraint Be Learned?

We have reviewed studies showing that adults and infants can learn first- and second-order constraints on consonant positions and that this learning can occur within both the production and the perceptual systems. Moreover, the learnable second-order constraints include contingencies between nonadjacent elements. These facts suggest that the implicit learning of phonotactic-like patterns is a powerful and general process. But can *any* constraint be learned? Of course not. One can define all sorts of contingencies that one would not expect people to be able to learn. For example, *if the vowel of the second syllable in a list of 12 CVC syllables is /a/ and if the onset of the seventh consonant is /f/, the coda of the twelfth syllable must be /k/.* To learn this third-order long-distance dependency, not only must one retain a lot of syllables in working memory, but one must also keep track, in principle, of the distributions of phonemes in the possible sets of three of the 36 phoneme slots in the list. That's 7,140 sets! Clearly human memory and processing capacities are going to limit learning, not to mention preexisting biases as to what kinds of contingencies are likely. So we should phrase the question differently: Are there limitations on learning simple second-order contingencies between information sources that are clearly jointly available within working memory (e.g., the vowels and consonants within a syllable)?

One such limitation was suggested by the results of Onishi et al. (2002). In their study of phonotactic learning within the perceptual system by adults, they examined a peculiar kind of second-order constraint. Whether a consonant was an onset or a coda was made to depend on whether the syllable was spoken by a male or female voice. (There were only two voices used in the study.) Unlike their study of the second-order vowel-contingency, Onishi et al. found no learning of the second-order speaker-identity contingency. They hypothesized that the learning mechanism was limited to detecting contingencies between representational elements that are naturally part of the phonological processing system, such as the identities and positions of the vowels and consonants. Although a speaker's voice has a large influence on how syllables sound, one can hypothesize that the system responsible for identifying speech sounds and words abstracts away from speaker identity. Informally, there are two different "boxes," or modules, one concerned with linguistic categories and another with extralinguistic ones, such as speaker identity. If we simply hypothesize that implicit learning is a module-internal process, second-order contingencies can be detected only if the contingent representational elements are in the same module. In the remainder of this chapter, we flesh out this idea. First, we present another test of whether contingencies between linguistic and extralinguistic information can be detected. But this time, it involves the production system and the speech-error paradigm. Then we describe a computational model of the implicit learning process, one that explains the different rates of first- and second-order learning and attempts to clarify the notion of a module-internal implicit learning process.

Testing a Second-Order Constraint Involving Speech Rate and Consonant Position

Onishi et al. (2002) failed to find learning of a contingency between a speaker's voice and consonant position in perception. Can we test for an analogous effect in production? We need some factor that clearly affects production but is extralinguistic in the sense that it does not involve linguistic categories. We thus chose to test whether speakers could implicitly learn a contingency between speech rate and consonant position. Using the speech-error paradigm, participants did trials at both fast (2.67 syllables per second) and slow (1.87 syllables per second) rates, with fast and slow trials alternating. The materials exhibited the second order constraint: *If the rate is fast, /f/ is an onset and /s/ is a coda, and if the rate is slow, /s/ is an onset and /f/ is a coda* (and the reverse for half the participants).

The errors produced by the speakers failed to show any evidence of learning on *any* of the 4 days of testing. That is, the rate of legal errors with restricted consonants and unrestricted consonants did not differ. To verify this null result, a replication was run using /k/ and /g/ as the restricted consonants in place of /f/ and /s/. The results again were null. Figure 8.4 shows the average data. On the first day of testing, the results were actually in the wrong direction by 9%, although not reliably so. On days 2 to 4, that average difference in legality narrowed to 0.5%. In neither study did the errors exhibit greater legality for restricted consonants, suggesting that a contingency between the extralinguistic factor of speech rate and consonant position is not easily learnable. This finding supports the perception results of Onishi et al. (2002) as well as their hypothesis that the implicit learning shown in these studies is limited to contingencies between elements that are natural components of the phonological processing system. In the following section, we make this hypothesis concrete with a computational model.

A Model of Implicit Learning of Phonotactic Constraints

Many models of implicit learning employ connectionist learning and processing mechanisms. For example, Cleeremans (1993) and Gupta and Cohen (2002) accounted for the results of implicit sequence learning experiments using models with layers of quasi-neural units, including an input layer representing incoming stimuli, an output layer for responses, and one or more "hidden" layers that mediate between stimuli and responses. As each new input comes in, the model makes a prediction about what the next input will be (e.g., in the serial reaction time paradigm, which stimulus light will appear next). The predicted output is generated by activation spreading along weighted connections from the input

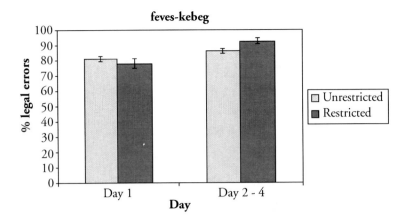

Fig. 8.3 Legality proportions of errors for /eve/-/ebe/ consonant-contingent experiments for the first day and subsequent days of testing.

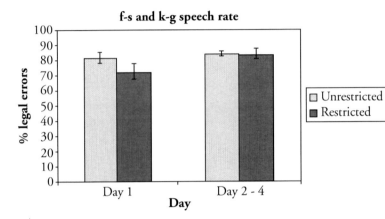

Fig. 8.4 Legality proportions of errors for speech rate-contingent experiments for the first day and subsequent days of testing.

to the hidden units and from there to the output units. The rules inherent in the experimental sequences are learned by gradually modifying the strengths or "weights" of the connections. Weight modification occurs to the extent that predicted outputs are erroneous. An error-driven learning algorithm, the generalized delta rule, or back propagation (Rumelhart, Hinton, & Williams, 1986) changes the weights after each stimulus so as to decrease the likelihood of error in the future. Knowledge of the rules of the grammar inherent in the sequences then comes to inhabit the weights. The models give a good account of the rate with which people's response times become sensitive to the rules. Over time, the model's prediction error decreases for stimuli that are rule consistent compared to those that are violations, thus demonstrating learning.

Some connectionist learning models have been applied to linguistic sequences (Chang, Dell, & Bock, 2006; Dell, Juliano, & Govindjee, 1993; Elman, 1993; MacDonald & Christianson, 2002), but these were not specifically designed to explain the implicit learning of such sequences in experimental settings. Here we describe the model of Warker and Dell (2006), an attempt to simulate the findings of experiments investigating the acquisition of first- and second-order experimental phonotactic constraints.

The architecture of the model is presented in Figure 8.5. As with the other models just described, there are input, output, and hidden layers, with feed-forward connections between adjacent levels that are learnable. The model is designed to produce single CVC syllables, specifically to engage in "syllabification," the process of assigning

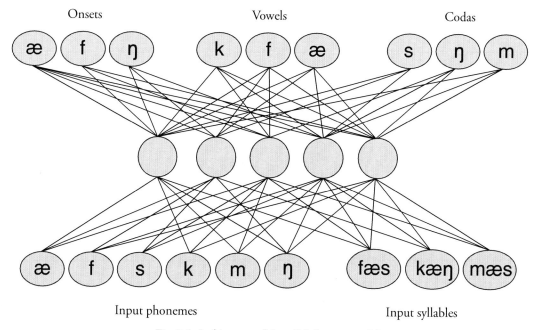

Onsets   Vowels   Codas

Input phonemes   Input syllables

Fig. 8.5 Architecture of the syllabification model.

retrieved phonemes to syllable positions (e.g., Levelt, Roelofs, & Meyer, 1999). Its input consists of units for each intended phoneme and one unit standing for the entire syllable. For example, for the intended syllable "fas," activated input units would include one for the whole syllable "fas" and one each for /f/, /ae/, and /s/. The intended output assigns, or "binds," these phonemes to syllable positions. The output layer has units for all possible bindings, that is, the phonemes used in the experiments (in the implementation, h, ng, f, s, k, g, m, n, ae, and I) crossed with each syllable position (onset, vowel, and coda). Thus, there are 30 output units, including units for bindings that are illegal for English (e.g., /ng/-onset, /f/-vowel), as well as legal ones (f/-onset, /ae/-vowel). The inclusion of units for all possible bindings is the model's way of starting life with relatively little phonotactic knowledge. Here all it starts with is the notion that syllables consist of three slots but does not make assumptions about the kinds of sounds that inhabit these slots.

Warker and Dell first trained the model to simulate acquisition of the phonotactic knowledge that their participants brought to the experiment, that is, their knowledge of English syllables. All 98 legal English CVC syllables that can be formed of the model's phonemes were presented to the model, 5,000 times each, each training instance being followed by adaptive weight change. After training, the model produced the correct output for all syllables; that is, the activation of the correct bindings, for example, for "fas," /f/-onset, /ae/-vowel, and /s/-coda, was about 0.9 and that of incorrect bindings was less than 0.1. The activation of phonotactic illegal bindings such as /h/-coda or /ng/-onset was invariably close to zero regardless of the intended syllable (around 0.005), illustrating that the model had learned that these are not allowed.

After this initial training, the model was used to simulate both first- and second-order experiments. For each kind of experiment, the model experienced only those syllables that were presented to the experimental participants, and tests of the model's tendencies to make legal errors for restricted and unrestricted consonants were conducted after 100, 500, and 1,000 repetitions of each trained syllable. We can measure the model's likelihood for making errors that move from one syllable position to another (illegal errors) by examining the activation of potential erroneous bindings. For example, suppose that the model is trained on the first-order constraint that /f/ is always an onset. We can use the activation of the coda-/f/ output unit when a syllable such as "fak" is the target to index the model's propensity to make the illegal slip "faf." After the 5,000 trials of training on all syllables but before any training for the first-order constraint, the activation of coda-/f/ for the target "fak" was 0.05. This level reduced to 0.02 after 100 simulated trials of first-order training and was down to 0.01 after 500 trials, showing clear learning. This learning contrasts with that for unrestricted consonants, such as /k/. If we look at the activation of onset-/k/ for the same target syllable

(i.e., the potential for the slip "kak"), there was less reduction over trials. Before experimental training, this activation was 0.05, the same as for /f/-coda. An additional 100 trials of training reduced the activation, but only to 0.04, and 500 trials got it down to 0.03. Thus, the difference between restricted (0.02) and unrestricted (0.04) consonants showed up after only 100 trials.

The contrast between the activations of illegal errors for restricted and unrestricted consonants was far less dramatic when the training simulated a second-order experiment. For the example syllable "fak," 1,000 trials of second-order training led to activations of 0.02 and 0.03 for restricted ("faf") and unrestricted ("kak") slips, respectively. Figure 8.6 summarizes the main model findings showing activation for illegal bindings averaged over two replications of the model, each simulating five potential slips for each condition: language restricted, experimentally restricted, and unrestricted. Clearly, the restricted–unrestricted difference is smaller and takes more trials to develop for second-order training.

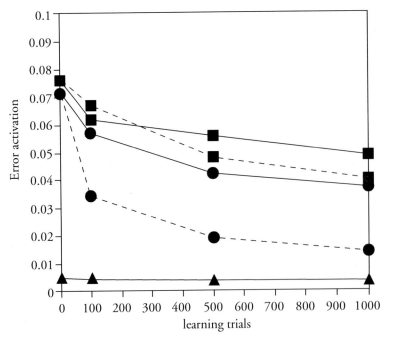

Fig. 8.6 Model simulations showing activation of illegal bindings. Circles, squares, and triangles represent experimentally restricted, unrestricted, and language-restricted consonants, respectively. The dotted lines represent first-order simulations, and the solid lines represent second-order simulations. The first- and second-order simulations led to identical results for language-restricted consonants, and hence there is just one line.

Why is learning the second-order constraint harder for the model? It has to do with the *self-interfering* nature of second-order constraints, according to Warker and Dell (2006). In the model, a first-order constraint such as /f/ always being an onset constitutes a consistent mapping between the /f/ input unit and the onset-/f/ output unit. A second-order constraint such as /f/ being an onset when the vowel is /ae/ but a coda when it is /I/ lacks this consistency. A trial with an /f/ in the input when the vowel is /I/ will interfere with, that is, overwrite, weight changes that were suitable for trials with /f/ when the vowel is /ae/. The second-order mapping comes to be learned eventually by the model when its hidden units learn to represent conjunctions of consonants and vowels. But this takes time. The model suggests that the key factor is number of trials. An alternative that is worth noting is that the passage of time rather than additional training trials is required for the necessary conjunctive representations to develop. Moreover, we speculate that this happens particularly during sleep. Performance on motor sequence learning tasks is found to jump after sleep and can be predicted by amount of light non-REM sleep that the learner experiences after acquisition (e.g., Walker, Brakefield, Morgan, Hobson, & Stickgold, 2002). In all the previously described experiments that exhibited second-order learning, the learning was present and statistically significant on the second day of the experiment, that is, after one night's sleep. It was never present during the first day.

The hidden units are the key to the learning of second-order constraints. If the connections ran straight from input to output, the model would only be able to learn first-order constraints (e.g., by strengthening links from /f/-input to onset-/f/). Thus, we hypothesize that the language production system contains "hidden units" that can learn conjunctions of speech sounds, including, at minimum, adjacent consonant-vowel sequences and nonadjacent consonant-consonant combinations. The experiments of Warker and Dell demonstrated implicit learning of second-order constraints in which a consonant's location was contingent on an adjacent vowel or a nonadjacent consonant. According to the model, that means that hidden units with the potential to detect these contingencies were available to the implicit learning system. More generally, we speculate that any second-order contingency involving salient phonological properties of syllables or disyllables should be learnable in this domain. In other words, there are hidden units for registering conjunctions of the consonants, vowels, and their properties when they are reasonably close together in time.

But what about the failures to find second-order learning with contingencies based on extralinguistic information, such as speech rate or speaker's voice? Informally, we accounted for this failure by saying that speech rate and speaker's voice were not in the "same module" as the one that held information about the vowels and consonants. Using the model, we can now state this more precisely: We claim that there are no hidden units for conjunctions between information sources that do not inhabit the same modules. So, as illustrated in Figure 8.7, there are no hidden units that can detect that the linguistic element /f/-onset is predicted by the nonlinguistic element of a fast speech rate. The existence of hidden units for conjunctions of elements formalizes the claim that those elements are isomodular. These hidden units enable the implicit learning of second-order constraints in which the positioning of one element depends on the value of another. In this way, implicit learning through the speech-error paradigm provides an experimental window into the organization of the speech-production system.

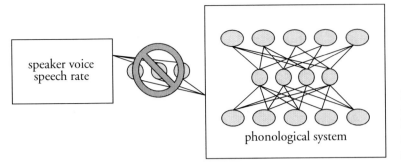

Fig. 8.7 There are no hidden units, or conjunction detectors, between extralinguistic attributes and the phonological processing system.

It is important to qualify our claim. We are not stating that people cannot learn or conceive of conjunctions of elements from different modules. If we told participants to pay close attention to the differences in the syllables, such as the syllables that begin with /f/, as a function of speech rate, we suspect that they could discover the constraint that /f/ is an onset if there is a fast speech rate. This discovery process, however, is not implicit learning—learning that occurs as a natural result of performing a task. Rather, it is the result of a conscious rule-discovery process. We have the ability to represent, in one form or another, contingencies between any dimensions that we can conceive of. Our conceptual and linguistic systems certainly allow us to imagine, say, that purple cows eat foods beginning with /f/, while green cows eat those starting with /s/ or even more complex and bizarre contingencies. The implicit learning system that is tapped by rapid recitation of syllables in the speech-error paradigm, though, cannot do this. It is limited by its structure, that is, which elements belong to the same module.

Summary and Conclusions

We reviewed evidence that speech errors reveal the implicit learning of artificial phonotactic constraints. First-order constraints on the positioning of consonants in the syllables are quickly learned. The learning is implicit; that is, it is independent of the speakers' awareness and intentions.

The learning also seems to be more than just priming of recent associations between consonants and positions because second-order constraints, in which such positioning is contingent on something else, can be learned as well, albeit more slowly. Moreover, some people can learn sequential constraints defining syllables that are illegal in their native language, as we saw in the study that showed that training with onset-/ng/'s led to slips of /ng/'s to onset position.

These findings were discussed in the context of a model of learning based on connectionist principles. From the model's perspective, language-wide and experiment-wide constraints are the same thing. It is just that language-wide constraints were learned earlier and to a much greater extent. Slips of /h/ always move to onset position because of a lifetime of experience with /h/-onsets and no experience with /h/-codas. When /f/ is experienced only as an onset during the experiment, this happens on a smaller scale. The model was able to explain why second-order constraints are learned more slowly by pointing to the self-interfering nature of these constraints and the necessity for the recruitment of hidden units to represent conjunctions of elements. We speculated that conjunctions of linguistic and extralinguistic elements, such as speech rate or speaker voice, however, are not detected in implicit learning experiments because the linguistic and extralinguistic elements inhabit different modules, which implies that there are no hidden units that can be (implicitly) recruited to represent the conjunctions.

Ultimately, the limitations on what can be detected during sequence learning may provide insight into the nature of language—a product of human biological and cultural evolution—as well as that of structured action sequences. We view the experiments described in this chapter as studies of language acquisition, even though what is being learned is artificial and the participants are adults who long ago acquired their native language. Our view is that language learning never stops. Throughout our lives, we continually adapt our linguistic processing systems to suit present circumstances, even when those circumstances are linguistically artificial. Thus, what can and cannot be learned in these studies may tell us about how the language production system deals with real phonological patterns. We have already noted that the learning of nonadjacent dependencies in the experimental work has a counterpart in actual phonologies, such as the Finnish vowel-harmony example. Real phonologies do not, however, have different phonotactic constraints for male and female speakers or for fast and slow speech. Thus, the failure to find implicit learning for second-order contingencies involving these extralinguistic properties also aligns with linguistic facts.

But there are important unanswered questions. Are the artificial phonotactic constraints investigated in the speech-error studies easily learned precisely because they are similar to those in the participants' native language or, even more interestingly, because they reflect the kind of innate *universal* grammar hypothesized in most linguistic (e.g., Jackendoff, 2002) and many psycholinguistic (e.g., Pinker, 1994) theories? Or are the universal properties of the world's languages determined largely by the adaptability of the cognitive, perceptual,

and action systems? In short, does language determine what is learnable, or does what is learnable determine what is in language? Addressing such questions will most certainly require investigation of the mechanisms by which action sequences, linguistic or otherwise, are learned. In that sense, the study of language production is part and parcel of the study of action.

Acknowledgments

This research was supported by NIH grants HD-44458 and DC-000191.

References

Chambers, K. E. (2004). *Phonological development: Mechanisms and representations.* Unpublished doctoral dissertation, University of Illinois at Urbana–Champaign.

Chambers, K. E., Onishi, K. H., & Fisher, C. (2003). Infants learn phonotactic regularities from brief auditory experience. *Cognition, 87,* 69–77.

Chang, F., Dell, G. S., & Bock, K. (2006). Becoming syntactic. *Psychological Review, 113,* 234–272.

Cleeremans, A. (1993). *Mechanisms of implicit learning: Connectionist models of sequence processing.* Cambridge, MA: MIT Press.

Cohen, A., Ivry, R. I., & Keele, S. W. (1990). Attention and structure in sequence learning. *Journal of Experimental Psychology: Learning, Memory, and Cognition, 16,* 17–30.

Dell, G. S. (1986). A spreading activation theory of retrieval in sentence production. *Psychological Review, 93,* 283–321.

Dell, G. S., Juliano, C., & Govindjee, A. (1993). Structure and content in language production: A theory of frame constraints in phonological speech errors. *Cognitive Science, 17,* 149–195.

Dell, G. S., Reed, K. D., Adams, D. R., & Meyer, A. S. (2000). Speech errors, phonotactic constraints, and implicit learning: A study of the role of experience in language production. *Journal of Experimental Psychology: Learning, Memory, and Cognition, 26,* 1355–1367.

Elman, J. L. (1993). Learning and development in neural networks: The importance of starting small. *Cognition, 48,* 71–99.

Fromkin, V. A. (1971). The non-anomalous nature of anomalous utterances. *Language, 47,* 27–52.

Garrett, M. F. (1975). The analysis of sentence production. In G. H. Bower (Ed.), *The psychol-*

ogy of learning and motivation (pp. 133–175). San Diego, CA: Academic Press.

Goldrick, M. (2004). Phonological features and phonotactic constraints in speech production. *Journal of Memory and Language, 51,* 586–603.

Gupta, P., & Cohen, N. J. (2002). Theoretical and computational analysis of skill learning, repetition priming, and procedural memory. *Psychological Review, 109,* 401–448.

Jackendoff, R. (2002). *Foundations of language.* New York: Oxford University Press.

Jusczyk, P. W., Friederici, A. D., Wessels, J. M., Svenkerud, V. Y., & Jusczyk, A. M. (1993). Infants' sensitivity to the sound patterns of native language words. *Journal of Memory and Language, 32,* 402–420.

Levelt, W. J. M., Roelofs, A., & Meyer, A. S. (1999). A theory of lexical access in speech production. *Behavioral and Brain Science, 21,* 1–38.

MacDonald, M. C., & Christianson, M. H. (2002). Reassessing working memory: A comment on Just & Carpenter (1992) and Waters & Caplan (1996). *Psychological Review, 109,* 35–54.

Nissen, M. J., & Bullemer, P. (1987). Attentional requirements of learning: Evidence from performance measures. *Cognitive Psychology, 19,* 1–32.

Nooteboom, S. G. (1969). The tongue slips into patterns. In A. G. Sciarone, A. J. van Essen, & A. A. Van Raad (Eds.), *Leyden studies in linguistics and phonetics* (pp. 114–132). The Hague: Mouton.

Onishi, K. H., Chambers, K. E., & Fisher, C. (2002). Learning phonotactic constraints from brief auditory experience. *Cognition, 83,* 13–23.

Pinker, S. (1994). *The language instinct: How the mind creates language.* New York: HarperCollins.

Reber, A. S. (1969). Transfer of syntactic structure in synthetic languages. *Journal of Experimental Psychology, 81,* 855–863.

Rumelhart, D. E., Hinton, G., & Williams, R. (1986). Learning internal representations by error propagation. In D. E. Rumelhart & J. L. McClelland (Eds.), *Parallel distributed processing: Explorations in the microstructure of cognition: Vol. 1. Foundations* (pp. 318–362). Cambridge, MA: MIT Press.

Stemberger, J. P. (1985). An interactive activation model of language production. In A. W. Ellis (Ed.), *Progress in the psychology of language* (Vol. 1, pp. 143–186). Hillsdale, NJ: Lawrence Erlbaum Associates.

Taylor, C. F., & Houghton, G. (2005). Learning artificial phonotactic constraints—Time course, durability, and relationship to natural constraints. *Journal of Experimental Psychology: Learning, Memory, and Cognition, 31,* 1398–1416.

Walker, M. P., Brakefield, T., Morgan, A., Hobson, J. A., & Stickgold, R. (2002). Practice with sleep makes perfect: Sleep-dependent motor skill learning. *Neuron, 35,* 205–211.

Warker, J. A., & Dell, G. S. (2006). Speech errors reflect newly learned phonotactic constraints. *Journal of Experimental Psychology: Learning, Memory, and Cognition 32,* 387–398.

Warker, J. A., Dell, G. S., Whalen, C. A., & Gereg, S. (in press). Limits on learning phonotactic constraints from recent production experience *Journal of Experimental Psychology: Learning, Memory, and Cognition.*

Wells, R. (1951). Predicting slips of the tongue. *Yale Scientific Magazine, 3,* 9–30.

Whalen, C. A., & Dell, G. S. (2006). Speaking outside the box: Learning of non-native phonotactic constraints is revealed in speech errors. In R. Sun (Ed.), *Proceedings of the Cognitive Science Society Meeting* (pp. 2371-2374). Mahwah, NJ: Erlbaum.

What Do We Prime? On Distinguishing Between Semantic Priming, Procedural Priming, and Goal Priming

Jens Förster, Nira Liberman, *and* Ronald S. Friedman

Abstract

This chapter examines how the various effects of priming differ from one another. It describes different types of priming—priming of semantic constructs, priming of procedures, and priming of behaviors and goals—then proposes ways of distinguishing between them. Primed goals differ from primed procedures and primed semantic constructs in a number of ways. First, goals have a different pattern of persistence and decay (or deactivation) than both procedures and semantic constructs. Second, effects of primed goals should be sensitive to expectancy and value, whereas the effects of primed semantic constructs and primed procedures should not show such sensitivity. Third, means-ends associations, which constitute the goal system, do not always correspond to semantic or overlearned associations. As a result, patterns of lateral inhibition and asymmetries in spreading activation (i.e., the fan effect) differ between goal systems and semantic associations.

Keywords: semantic constructs, procedures, behaviors, goals, persistence, decay, deactivation

In 1977, Higgins, Rholes, and Jones reported the results of the first priming study in social psychology. They demonstrated that an ambiguous target person was perceived in accordance with constructs that were activated via completion of an ostensibly unrelated earlier task. Since then, priming has been not only replicated a great number of times but also extended to domains beyond person perception to include priming of procedures as well as priming of goals (for reviews, see Förster & Liberman, 2007b; Higgins, 1996). Priming is currently used extensively in social psychological research to activate diverse constructs, states, and behaviors, including stereotypes, motivational orientations, processing styles (e.g., global versus local), mental representations of significant others, contingencies of self-worth, and egalitarian goals. Thirty years after Higgins et al.'s (1977) seminal priming experiment, it seems that nothing is left that cannot be primed.

By now, there is no doubt that priming works—it has an impact on affect, behavior, and cognition. Priming may activate cognitive constructs, goals, and procedures. However, a question that has been much less frequently posed is how these various effects of priming differ from one another. This chapter is aimed at closing this theoretical void. We first briefly describe different types of priming—priming of semantic constructs, priming of procedures, and priming of behaviors and goals—and then move on to propose ways of distinguishing between them. We hope that this discussion, even if it fails to yield firm conclusions, will help elucidate basic issues regarding the link between motivation and cognition.

Semantic Priming

Research on *semantic priming* demonstrated that priming of concepts increases their accessibility, facilitating processing of meaningfully related constructs (see Neely, 1977). For example, after reading the word "lamp," people may become faster at reading the word "light" than without priming.[1] Increased semantic activation due to priming may also engender perceptual assimilation, especially of ambiguous or vague targets. For instance, if participants are exposed to aggression-related concepts by unscrambling sentences such as "leg her break he" (Srull & Wyer, 1979), they may use this activated knowledge in rendering judgments of ambiguously aggressive target individuals such that these targets come to be viewed as more hostile.[2]

Subsequent research has used stereotypes (e.g., Devine, 1989), contextual cues (Gilovich, 1981), and labels (Darley & Gross, 1983) as primes. Social psychologists have been interested mainly in the effects of priming on disambiguation and the consequences of these effects. For example, classic studies on priming of stereotypes demonstrated that priming a person with the black stereotype enhanced the proclivity to perceive an ambiguous person as hostile (Devine, 1989) and also enhanced the tendency to perceive an ambiguous object as a gun and the corresponding decision to shoot a video game figure presumed to be holding this object (Correll, Park, Judd, & Wittenbrink, 2002).

How does priming work? It is beyond the scope of this chapter to present in detail models of priming (for a summary, see Förster & Liberman, 2007b; Higgins, 1996). For the present purposes, suffice it to say that these models assume a semantic network along which activation spreads. They also assume that accessing a construct increases its activation potential, thereby increasing its likelihood of being used. Priming activates a construct, and the activation spreads along the semantic network to constructs to which it is linked, thereby increasing their activation potential (to give just some examples, Collins & Loftus, 1975; Higgins, 1996; Neely, 1991; Wyer, 2004, in press).

Procedural Priming

Procedural priming refers to priming of procedures (e.g., strategies, ways of processing, encoding, or remembering): At the priming phase, people perform an action, and then (facilitating) carryover effects on the performance of subsequent actions are examined. For example, solving addition problems facilitates solving other such problems (Luchins, 1942). Notably, experimental demonstration of procedural priming does not involve learning because the action performed at the priming stage is overlearned to such an extent that a few more instances of practice make virtually no difference (e.g., adding numbers or inferring traits from behavior). Most important, as Gollwitzer's work demonstrates (Gollwitzer & Heckhausen, 1987), procedures are free of semantic content. For example, priming the procedure of "opening up one's attentional span" does not facilitate task-relevant contents (e.g., information semantically related to "opening up") but rather facilitates attention to peripheral information regardless of its content (see also Gollwitzer, 1990). The distinction between semantic priming and procedural priming is best exemplified in a study by Smith and Branscombe (1987), who replicated a classic study on the effect of priming on disambiguation (Srull & Wyer, 1979). In addition to the original priming group, in which participants unscrambled sentences describing hostile behaviors (e.g., leg her break he), they added a procedural priming condition in which participants were presented with the same sentences in an unscrambled form and chose the matching trait (e.g., "hostile"). Note that inferring traits from behavior was in fact the procedure people engaged in when judging the vaguely aggressive target person in the second phase—after either 15 seconds or 15 minutes, participants rated the aggressiveness of a description of a vaguely aggressive behavior. Priming traits (i.e., unscrambling sentences) had an assimilative effect only after a short delay, but procedural priming continued to have this effect after a longer delay. It seems that participants practiced the procedure of extracting traits from behavior and that making this procedural knowledge accessible facilitated making such inferences at the test stage. Moreover, it seems that the effect of procedural priming is more enduring than the typical accessibility effect resulting from priming concepts. Interestingly, in addition to these content-specific effects, there seem to be smaller but reliable *general* effects of procedural priming in that after matching traits to behaviors, people are faster with these same traits and in matching other behaviors to *different* traits (Smith, 1989; Smith, Branscombe, & Bormann, 1988).

Social psychological research provides many examples of priming of very general procedures, such as abstract (versus concrete) thinking, applying a broad (versus a narrow) perspective, or promotion-focused (versus prevention-focused) decision making. These priming procedures, which differ somewhat from the original examples of priming-specific procedures (e.g., addition or inferring traits from specific behaviors) are sometimes referred to as manipulations of mind-sets. For example, action phase theory (Gollwitzer, 1990; Heckhausen, 1991) distinguishes between a predecisional stage, characterized by a deliberative mind state in which one contemplates alternatives, and a postdecisional state, characterized by an implemental mind-set in which attention is focused on "doing" rather than on "contemplating" (see Chapter 29). Gollwitzer, Heckhausen, and Steller (1990) induced a deliberative mind-set by making people contemplate personal change or an implemental mind-set by making participants mentally prepare the execution of a personal plan in detail. Participants then were asked to write the remaining part of fairy tales that began with a description of a character with a decision conflict. Analysis revealed that deliberative mind-set participants ascribed more deliberative and fewer implementational efforts to the character than implemental mind-set participants (for additional effects of implemental and deliberative mind-sets, see Taylor & Gollwitzer, 1995). Thus, thinking in an implemental or a deliberative way "carried over" to an unrelated task or, in other words, primed the procedure of thinking about a situation in a corresponding way. According to Gollwitzer (1990), such procedural carryover effects are free from semantic content. As he states,

> Deliberative and implemental mind-sets make any knowledge that helps to solve the respective task more accessible. Part of this knowledge is categorical or episodic and relates to the specific problem at hand (i.e., the decision to be made or the project to be planned). The other part is procedural and relates to how wishes are deliberated (deliberative mind-set) or how projects are planned (implemental mind-set) in general. It is this latter part that we found to transfer to subsequent, unrelated tasks. (p. 83)

In construal level theory (Liberman, Trope, & Stephan, 2007), high level versus low level reasoning may be manipulated through a mind-set. For example, Fujita, Trope, Liberman, and Levin-Sagi (2006) had participants think of *why* they would like to maintain social contacts (a high-level construal mind-set) or *how* they would maintain social contacts (a low-level construal mind-set) and then examined performance on an unrelated self-control task that involved squeezing a handgrip in order to obtain self-diagnostic information. Fujita et al. reasoned that self-control problems involve a conflict between a behavioral tendency that stems from a high-level construal of the situation ("I would like to be fit" or "This is one of the temptations that await me on the way to fitness") and a low level construal of the situation ("This is a unique situation" or "This is only a small piece of chocolate that cannot do much harm but has good taste"). Accordingly, Fujita et al. (2006) suggested that self-control would be facilitated by a high-level construal of the situation and thus would be enhanced by procedurally priming participants with high-level construals. Consistent with this prediction, it has been found that a high-level construal mind-set enhanced self-control relative to the low-level construal mind-set (for an additional demonstration of high-level versus low-level mind-set manipulation, see Wakslak, Trope, & Liberman, 2006).

Sometimes, the same procedure may apply to both a conceptual and a perceptual domain. For example, it is possible to apply local, detailed processing to both percepts (e.g., looking at the details of a map) and to concepts (e.g., thinking in detail about a theory). The effects of procedural priming appear to cut across both perceptual and conceptual domains—priming a perceptual procedure may affect conceptual performance and vice versa. A particularly pertinent example is Friedman and Förster's demonstration of procedural priming effects on creativity (e.g., Förster, Friedman,

Özelsel, & Denzler, 2006; for a review, see Friedman & Förster, 2008). In one study, for example, Friedman, Fishbach, Förster, and Werth (2003) asked participants to complete visual tasks that forced them to focus perceptual attention on either a broad or a narrow visual area. In an ostensibly unrelated task, participants were then asked to perform a creative generation task (e.g., find as many creative ways to use a brick as possible). Participants primed with a broad focus produced more creative solutions than participants primed with a narrow focus. It was reasoned that the procedural priming expanded (or constricted) the focus of perceptual attention, a procedure that was carried over to the semantic network, and thereby improved (or diminished) creativity because creative generation profits from a broad conceptual scope (Isen & Daubman, 1984).

How does procedural priming work? It appears that mentally representing an action facilitates its performance. For example, athletic performance is enhanced if people imagine themselves performing the activity before the competition (see Feltz & Landers, 1983). It is quite possible, then, that procedural priming facilitates performance by activating mental representations of the activities in questions. An explanation along these lines for procedural priming is offered by *processing shift theory*, in which a "processing shift" is defined as an event in which cognitive procedures activated in the course of engaging in one task remain active and are carried over, or "transferred," to subsequent tasks (Schooler, 2002; Schooler, Fiore, & Brandimonte, 1997). *Transfer-appropriate* processing shifts result when the activated procedures are beneficial for subsequent processing, whereas *transfer-inappropriate* shifts result when the procedures at hand impair subsequent processing. In this view, procedural priming works in a way similar to semantic priming via spreading activation, with the sole difference being that procedures rather than semantic constructs are activated (see also Smith & Branscombe, 1987).

Although the relative endurance of procedural priming may distinguish it from concept priming, it is not always easy to distinguish between these two types of priming. Smith (1990, 1994) argued that in some priming tasks, the process in the first priming phase is both conceptually and procedurally similar to the test phase. For example, if people translate behavioral information into traits in the first phase and then have to judge a target's aggressiveness (a trait) on the basis of her described behavior, the priming task might confound procedural and concept priming. It seems that activation of semantic and procedural knowledge may occur simultaneously and might have independent effects on information processing.

Priming of Behavior and Performance

Priming may also affect behavior. The empirical finding that may have been most seminal in advancing the notion of automatic behavior activation is that of Bargh, Chen, and Burrows (1996; experiment 2), who demonstrated that participants primed with concepts related to the elderly stereotype (e.g., "Florida," "old," or "lonely") walked more slowly down a hallway compared to those primed with control words (e.g., "thirsty," "clean," or "private"). In another influential experiment, Bargh et al. (1996; experiment 1) showed that priming "rude" versus "polite" (by exposing participants to trait-related words) resulted in participants interrupting an experimenter sooner or later, respectively. Yet another pivotal finding (Bargh et al., 1996; experiment 3) was that subliminal priming of a young African American male face led participants to respond with more hostility (a stereotypic behavior associated with

this social category) to provocation by the experimenter as compared to priming with a White face.

Other researchers have demonstrated behavioral effects of priming trait constructs. For example, priming the trait "helpful" facilitates helpful behaviors (Macrae & Johnston, 1998), priming the trait "conformity" increases consensus (Epley & Gilovich, 1999), priming the trait "intelligent" leads to more correct responses on general knowledge questions (compared to priming "stupid"; Dijksterhuis & van Knippenberg, 1998), and priming the concept of "flexibility" reduces perseverance on the Wisconsin Card Sorting Task (Hassin, Bargh, & Zimerman, in press), to name a few. Finally, exposing participants to actual behaviors also has led to similar findings in that the observed behavior tends to be imitated (Chartrand & Bargh, 1999; Lakin & Chartrand, 2003).

There is little doubt that exposure to specific trait constructs, actual behaviors, or social group members (whose stereotypes contain trait and behavioral constructs) can result in activating a corresponding behavior. With important exceptions (e.g., Dijksterhuis et al., 1998; Mussweiler & Förster, 2000), priming a trait, a stereotype, or a behavior results in an increased likelihood that individuals will perform the primed behavior (i.e., a behavioral assimilation effect).[3]

Assimilation effects have been shown not only to alter behaviors but also to alter performance level on speed tests, intelligence tests, memory tests, creativity tests, and flexibility tests. For example, priming "elderly" increases response latencies on lexical decision tasks (Dijksterhuis, Spears, & Lépinasse, 2001; Kawakami, Young, & Dovidio, 2002) and decreases performance on memory tasks (Dijksterhuis, Aarts, Bargh, & van Knippenberg, 2000; Dijksterhuis, Bargh, & Miedema, 2000; but see Levy, 1996), priming "professor" leads to more correct responses to general knowledge questions, whereas priming "soccer hooligan" leads to fewer correct responses (Dijksterhuis & van Knippenberg, 1998). Priming "politician" results in participants producing longer essays than those not primed (with "long-windedness" as an associated trait of politicians; Dijksterhuis & van Knippenberg, 2000), and priming deviant categories, such as "punk," leads to higher creativity than priming more conservative ones, such as "engineer" (Förster, Friedman, Butterbach, & Sassenberg, 2005).

How does priming affect behavior? Considerations of parsimony suggest that we should consider first an explanation similar to that of semantic priming and procedural priming. Indeed, the theory of *perception-behavior link* does exactly this (Bargh & Chartrand, 1999; Bargh et al., 1996). Specifically, it suggests that actions are directly linked to perception so that perceiving a stimulus may have a direct effect on behavior. This idea is based on James's (1890) principle of ideomotor action, suggesting that actions are directly connected to mental representations of the same actions. Prinz (1997) goes so far to suggest common codes for behavior and perception representations. Consequently, the mere act of thinking about a behavior increases the likelihood of that behavior being carried out, given an appropriate situation for the behavior to be expressed. This account shares numerous features with classic explanations for semantic priming (Collins & Loftus, 1975), which is said to occur because activation spreads in the semantic (or associative) network and increases the activation potential of connected constructs, thereby making their own activation more likely. According to these models, activation spreads from the prime to the associated *behavior*, which renders it likely to be carried out: "Perceptual inputs are translated automatically into corresponding behavioral outputs" (Dijksterhuis & Bargh, 2001, p. 1; see also Kawakami et al., 2002; Chapter 4).

We would like to suggest, however, that spreading of activation in a semantic network does not suffice to explain the effects of priming on behavior. In the remainder of this chapter, we present an alternative mechanism, which is priming of goals, and discuss how it differs from semantic priming and procedural priming.

Priming of Goals

To explain how priming affects behavior, primes have been posited to activate goals, thereby eliciting action consistent with goal attainment. For example, after processing words related to achievement, people have been found to become more competitive (Bargh, Gollwitzer, Lee-Chai, Barndollar, & Trötschel, 2001), and it has been suggested that the primes activate the goal to achieve. Inasmuch as goals can be represented in memory (see, e.g., Kruglanski, 1996; Shah, Kruglanski, & Friedman, 2003), it is possible that, for example, the verbal prime "aggressive" not only activates semantic associates of the construct of aggression but also (or instead) activates the goal to be aggressive. It is further argued that certain cues (e.g., hiking shoes) may be frequently and habitually linked to certain goals (e.g., to go on a hiking trip; see Bargh, 1997) and can automatically activate those goals. In a similar vein, people (Aarts, Gollwitzer, & Hassin, 2004; Fitzsimons & Bargh, 2003; Shah 2003), ideas (Moskowitz, Gollwitzer, Wasel, & Schaal, 1999), or contexts can remind one unconsciously or consciously of one's goals (Aarts & Dijksterhuis, 2000) and activate them.

The previous examples reflect the fact that cues may activate goals to which they are linked in long-term memory because of repeated co-occurrence. It seems, however, that cues may get connected to goals in a one-time volitional act, namely, via formation of implementation intentions (Gollwitzer, 1993, 1999). Implementation intentions are plans as to when, how, and where to perform an action, for example, a plan to start writing a chapter on Friday morning right after breakfast on the computer in the study room while having the second cup of coffee. Gollwitzer and colleagues argued and showed in an extensive research program that once an implementation intention is formed, cues of the situation that it specifies automatically activate the goal (see also Goschke & Kuhl, 1993, and their notion of *commitment markers* that can be temporarily associated with goal representations).

Activation of Goals Versus Semantic Priming

How can we distinguish between the operation of primed goals, primed semantic constructs, and primed procedures? For example, does a primed concept of elderly activate a semantic structure that directly elicits slow walking? Does it activate a procedure of walking slower or of interacting with old people? Does it activate a goal to walk slower or a related goal, such as to affiliate with old people (see Cesario, Plaks, & Higgins, 2006)? To give another example, Dijksterhuis and van Knippenberg (1998) showed that priming the construct "professor" improved performance at Trivial Pursuit. To explain this result, they suggested that the prime increased motivation to work on the task compared to a control prime (e.g., "soccer hooligan"). But how can we be sure that the prime affected motivation rather than semantic constructs? Förster, Liberman, and Higgins (2005) found that priming participants with divergent individuals (e.g., "punk") enhanced divergent thinking. They argued that a procedure of divergent thinking has been activated. But could it be that instead of procedural priming, a goal of exhibiting divergence was activated?

In the remainder of this chapter, we examine some features of goals that may help distinguish between goal priming and more nonmotivational, semantic, and procedural priming (see also Förster & Denzler, 2006). We propose three characteristics of goals that may help distinguish their operation from that of semantic or procedural priming: The first unique characteristic of goals is their *dynamic nature, their pattern of persistence and decay;* the second is their *ability to affect value;* and the third is their ability to *create ad hoc connections between constructs,* connections that do not necessarily exist in the semantic network. We turn now to discuss these unique characteristics and how they might help distinguish primed goals from primed semantic constructs and primed procedures. We sometimes review relevant empirical findings but sometimes point to the absence of such findings and suggest future studies that could help distinguish between goal, semantic, or procedural priming.

The Dynamics of Goals: Persistence and Decay
Goals Persist Until Fulfillment

It appears that rates of *decay* are different for semantic priming, goal priming, and procedural priming. Studies have shown that the effects of procedural priming can last as long as 1 week (see Smith, Stewart, & Buttram, 1992). In stark contrast, semantic priming shows much faster decay rates, dissipating within a few minutes, especially if the prime is presented only a small number of times (e.g., Smith & Branscombe, 1987; Srull & Wyer, 1979).

Like procedural priming and unlike semantic priming, goal priming produces a relatively slow decay and may even produce an increase in accessibility over time after the onset of the goal (Liberman & Förster, 2005). This is because goals create a state of tension that persists and may even build up until the goal is fulfilled (Lewin, 1951). For example, Bargh et al. (2001) showed that activation of an achievement goal by priming constructs related to achievement increased performance on an anagram task and that this effect increased over a delay.

Do goals maintain accessibility of goal-related constructs because of repeated rehearsal of these constructs? An experiment by Goschke and Kuhl (1993) suggests that rehearsal is not necessary. They made participants rehearse a series of actions and then informed them that they would either perform the actions (i.e., a goal) or observe another person performing them (i.e., a nongoal). Using a recognition test, they found higher accessibility of the actions in the goal condition than in the no-goal condition, even when rehearsal of the actions was not possible in the intervening time.

Persistence of accessibility due to active goals is not confined to memory-taxing goals. In a series of studies by Förster et al. (2005), participants had to search for a combination of pictures (glasses followed by scissors) in a series of pictures, and accessibility of goal-related concepts was measured several times with a lexical decision task (with, e.g., "reading," and "intelligent" as targets). It was shown that accessibility increased until the target combination of pictures was found.

In conclusion, we suggest that patterns of decay in construct accessibility may be used to determine whether goals have been primed. If a prime's effect on accessibility increases after priming, then it is likely that goal activation has occurred. Semantic priming and procedural priming tend to decrease in accessibility over time.

Goals Are Deactivated Upon Fulfillment

Goal-related constructs are inhibited after fulfillment. Marsh, Hicks, and Bink (1998) and Marsh, Hicks, and Bryan (1999), in an extended version of the paradigm by Goschke and Kuhl (1993) described previously, used a lexical decision task to examine the accessibility of action-related constructs both before and after completion of the action. Replicating Goschke and Kuhl (1993), they found that before completion, accessibility of intended actions was enhanced relative to nonintended (i.e., to-be observed) actions. They also found that after completing the action, accessibility of action-related constructs dropped below the level of the control, no-goal group, demonstrating postfulfillment inhibition.

In the experiments by Förster et al. (2005), participants were asked to tell the experimenter when they found the combination of scissors and glasses (for which it was their goal to search). Construct accessibility was assessed directly afterward. According to the recency principle of semantic priming (i.e., recency of priming increases accessibility), one would have expected high accessibility. However, accessibility of glasses related words was below baseline (accessibility of words unrelated to glasses) and thus seemed to reflect an important characteristic of goal-directed behavior—that motivation is reduced after goal attainment.

It is possible to contend that positive feedback signifies a completed goal, whereas negative feedback signifies an incomplete goal. Consistent with this idea, Rothermund (2003) found inhibition of goal-related constructs after success feedback and increased accessibility after failure feedback. He used an interference paradigm in which participants had to read aloud a nonprimed word that was presented together with a primed word or another nonprimed word. In this task, longer reading times of the target word indicated more interference by and therefore a higher accessibility of the nontarget word. The results indicated that accessibility of goal-related constructs was enhanced after failure feedback and inhibited after success feedback. Thus, unsuccessful performance kept the goal active and maintained accessibility at a high level, whereas successful performance signaled goal completion and led to inhibition.

Kawada, Oettingen, Gollwitzer, and Bargh (2004; experiment 3) investigated goal projection (i.e., ascribing one's own goals to others). They showed that negative feedback increased goal projection. More specifically, they primed participants with the goal to compete and asked them to perform a goal-relevant task with a partner. Half the participants received success feedback (i.e., that they had outperformed the partner), and the other half received failure feedback (i.e., that their partner outperformed them). As a measure of goal projection, participants had to predict how many competitive moves another person would make in a prisoner's dilemma task. They found that success feedback, relative to failure feedback, reduced the tendency to project competitiveness onto others. No such differences were observed in the control condition, in which no goal was primed. The authors argue that their results reflect goal projection rather than trait projection (i.e., semantic priming) because such an increase of projection after failure is typical for motivational effects (see Gollwitzer & Kirchhof, 1998) that are different from semantic priming effects.

We propose that diminution of accessibility (i.e., inhibition) after goal completion is another mechanism that distinguishes goal priming and semantic priming. From the perspective of semantic priming models (Förster & Liberman, 2007b; Higgins, 1996; Wyer, 2004), goal attainment merely constitutes activation of a goal-related construct, and therefore it should increase rather than decrease accessibility. To repeat, in the experiments by Förster et al. (2005) participants had to mention the glasses–scissors combination to the experimenter as soon as they saw it. According to traditional models of semantic priming, ongoing consideration of and search for these target objects should continually increase their activation levels, thereby increasing their accessibility to consciousness even after goal fulfillment (Higgins, 1996). Thus, the finding of post-fulfillment inhibition, as opposed to increased or merely persistent activation, may distinguish accessibility from goals from accessibility that is due to semantic priming. For example, if a researcher wishes to investigate effects from subliminal activation of goals, then she might measure accessibility of the goal after the goal has been completed. She should expect a decline of accessibility relative to baseline after goal fulfillment.

Effect of Goals Depends on Goal Strength
Expectancy and Value
THE INTERACTION OF EXPECTANCY AND VALUE

We have already mentioned the importance of the notion that goals create a state of tension that persists and may even grow in magnitude pending fulfillment. This state of tension reflects the goal's strength, which, in turn, depends on the product of the subjective expectancy that the goal will be attained and its value. This theoretical relation is assumed by expected utility theory in economics and decision making (Edwards, 1961), Atkinson's theory of achievement motivation (e.g., Atkinson, 1964), the theory of reasoned action (Fishbein & Ajzen, 1974), and Vroom's theory of motivation in organizational settings (Vroom, 1966). For example, a student's motivation to study for a math exam depends on the value of the exam (e.g., whether or not it counts toward his or her grade-point average) and the expectancy of success. Therefore, if priming "math exam" activates the goal to study for it, the extent of this effect should depend on the value and the expectancy of the exam. It should increase if the exam appears to be more important than previously thought or if success is discovered to be more feasible than previously assumed. If, however, the prime activated only the semantic construct "study" or a procedure of studying, then it should be relatively insensitive to changes in value and expectancy.

Förster et al. (2005) demonstrated that the effect of active goals on accessibility is sensitive to the interaction between expectancy and value. In their experiments, participants were instructed to search through a presented series of pictures for a target combination (glasses followed by scissors) and to report it to the experimenter. As noted before, the results reflected increased accessibility of goal-related words before the combination was found and inhibition after the combination was found. Importantly, in some studies (Förster et al., 2005; experiments 4–6), the authors manipulated the expectancy of achieving the goal (by telling participants that the target combination was present in 90% of the cases versus only in 5% of the cases), the value of the goal (by telling participants that they would receive €1.00 versus only €0.05 for finding the combination), or both expectancy and value. As predicted, accessibility of goal-related words prior to fulfillment and inhibition after fulfillment were found in the high-expectancy and high-value conditions but not in the low-expectancy and low-value conditions. The combination of high value and high expectancy enhanced the effects. Therefore, the effects of expectancy and value on goal-related accessibility and on postfulfillment inhibition were interactive (i.e., multiplicative) and similar to the effects of expectancy and value on motivation. Having discussed the joint effect of expectancy and value, we now more closely examine each of these interactive components.

EXPECTANCIES AND GOAL GRADIENTS

Motivation researchers have related expectancy to uncontrollable probability of outcomes (e.g., in bets; Edwards, 1955), task difficulty (Atkinson, 1957), controllability (Locke & Latham, 1990; Rotter, 1966), and self-efficacy (Bandura, 1982). It is perhaps noteworthy that expectancy, more than value, is inherently situation specific. Rather than being a property of the goal, it reflects the interaction between the goal, the actor, and the situation. As such, it is especially amenable to manipulation and thus especially useful in distinguishing primed goals from primed semantic constructs.

Expectancy often changes with distance from the goal. For example, when studying for an exam, studying that takes place closer to the time of the exam becomes more efficient both because studied material becomes more likely to be retained and because less time is left to compensate for failures to study (for a similar analysis of distance-based expectancies, see Liberman, Sagristano, & Trope, 2002). Possibly, the finding that motivation increases larger closer to the goal (Brown, 1948; Lewin, 1935; Miller, 1944, 1959) also reflects changes in expectancy (for a similar argument, see Förster, Higgins, & Idson, 1998). Goal gradients, too, may help distinguish primed goals from primed semantic constructs—if after priming "study" the accessibility of related constructs increases the closer one gets to the exam (and, perhaps, is sensitive to changes in the *perceived* distance of the exam), then it is most likely that goals rather than only semantic constructs have been activated.

It is also instructive to note that not only spatial or temporal distance but also other psychological distances, such as social distance, and hypotheticality may often reduce expectancy (Liberman et al., 2007). For example, people typically have less control over more socially distant individuals—we typically control others less than ourselves and strangers less than friends and relatives. As a result, we may expect successful goal attainment more for close friends than for strangers.

Psychological distance may thus decrease motivation because of changes in expectancy. For example, people may be more motivated to help a close friend than a stranger. If an effect of a prime (e.g., the word "help") on accessibility depends on the psychological distance of the target of the behavior (e.g., the social distance of the receiver of help or the temporal and spatial proximity of the helping behavior in question), then in most likelihood the prime activated a goal to help rather than only a semantic construct of helping or a procedure of helping.

VALUE

Goals have the power to construct and reconstruct value over and above (and sometimes even in opposition to) preexisting, overlearned associations between constructs and evaluations (see Ach, 1910; Lewin, 1951). For example, the construct "knife" generally has a negative valence but may acquire a positive value if on a camping trip, wanting to cut salami, one searches frantically for a knife while having a vague recollection of forgetting to pack it. In this example, not only did "knife" acquire value that it did not have before the onset of the goal, but also "knife" is not necessarily a semantic associate of "salami." More generally, this example elucidates two points: First, goals may change the value of constructs with which they connect by means of pertinence to goal fulfillment. Second, these connections reflect means–ends relations, which are not necessarily redundant with semantic associations. We elaborate

here on the first point and come back to the second point later in this chapter.

Ferguson and Bargh (2004) demonstrated that goals automatically enhance value in an affective evaluation paradigm (Fazio, 2001). Specifically, they asked thirsty and nonthirsty participants to evaluate positive or negative words that were primed either with goal-relevant words (e.g., water) or with goal-irrelevant words (e.g., chair) as quickly as possible. Thirsty participants were faster to decide that a positive word was positive if it was preceded by a goal-related word compared to both nonthirsty participants and to thirsty participants who saw the same target word preceded by a goal-irrelevant word.

Goals not only affect the value of constructs but are also affected by value. Custers and Aarts (2005) used evaluative conditioning to demonstrate that experimentally increasing the value of a construct increases the likelihood that it would become a goal. In a series of experiments they presented positive words (e.g., "nice" and "pleasant") immediately after subliminal presentation of neutral activities (e.g., writing) and then asked participants whether they wanted to do the activity. Participants were more likely to choose the activities that were linked with positive words.

Whereas Custers and Aarts (2005) looked at the effect of value on goal selection, research by Förster et al. (2005) examined the effect of value on the intensity of goal-related accessibility and postfulfillment inhibition. In one of their experiments, they gave participants either high or low rewards for finding the target combination of pictures and found that both prefulfillment accessibility of goal-related constructs and postfulfillment inhibition were enhanced in the high-value condition relative to the low-value condition.

An important prediction that follows from the close connection between value and goals is that no goal priming would occur if the goal in question were irrelevant or not valuable to a person. Therefore, if an effect of priming shows sensitivity to situational personal relevance, then in most likelihood a goal has been primed. Consider the following experiment by Aarts et al. (2004): Participants were primed with descriptions of either people who worked for money or people who volunteered to do a job. They were then told that they may earn extra cash by doing another task after they finished their current experimental task. The researchers measured the time participants continued working on the first (unpaid) task as a measure of how much they wanted to make extra money. Participants who were primed with making money were faster to finish the unpaid task but only if they, according to a previous self-report, needed money. The results show that goal priming has an effect only if the primed goal is personally relevant (for conceptually similar results with thirsty versus nonthirsty participants who were primed with a goal to drink, see Strahan, Spencer, & Zanna, 2002; see also Shah, 2003, who primed "mother" and found priming effects on achievement-related tasks only if participants liked their mother and if she valued achievement).

Cesario et al.'s (2006) study is a good example for how the principle of value dependence may be used to distinguish goal priming from semantic priming of behavior. These researchers contended that on perception of a social group member, the perceiver's motivational system prepares for an interaction with the primed target. The specific goal that is being activated, however, depends not only on the characteristics of the target ("Is the target threatening?" or "Is the target old?") but also on one's evaluation of the target ("Do I like this target?" or "Do I want to approach or avoid this target?") and the context of the interaction. The authors primed participants with words that were stereotypic for either elderly people or young people. They also assessed, in an unrelated session, participants' attitudes toward the elderly and toward young people with an implicit attitude measure (Fazio, Jackson, Dunton, & Williams, 1995). They found that participants who were primed with "elderly" walked slower the more positive was their attitude toward the elderly. Participants who were primed with the youth stereotype walked faster the more positive was their attitude toward young people.

Value may also change as a function of situation-sensitive social norms. Aarts et al. (2004) used short paragraphs on a male's wooing behavior to prime males with the goal of having casual sex. Pretests had shown that helping a woman reflects gallantry and was thus selected as a dependent measure of flirting in the lab. They found that sex-primed participants, compared to nonprimed participants, were more helpful toward a female confederate but were not more helpful toward a male confederate. In addition, they examined whether goal appropriateness would moderate the effect of priming on behavior. To manipulate goal appropriateness, in one of the studies the paragraph used for priming was about a flirting protagonist who was engaged in a serious relationship. It was assumed that in this case casual sex would be morally unacceptable to the participants. The study showed no priming effect on helping behavior in this condition, although participants gave no reports of being aware of either the effect of priming or the blocking effect of goal inappropriateness. These studies demonstrate that if the effect of priming is sensitive to changes in the value of the prime, then goals could have been primed. Semantic and procedural priming should have similar effects regardless of whether the prime's value has increased or decreased.

For example, the accessibility of Porsche relative to a Toyota should not decrease just because you learn that it is relatively more valuable. Extent of semantic priming of "drive" and "buy" by "Porsche" should depend, instead, on frequency and recency of the associations. We hasten to add that situationally induced value is more useful in distinguishing semantic priming from goal priming because chronic value may in fact affect accessibility (e.g., because people may chronically activate thoughts they like; see, e.g., Higgins, King, & Mavin, 1982).

Is it also true that if activation of a goal affects the value of associated constructs, then goals must have been activated? Remember that priming may affect disambiguation and by that may also have evaluative implications. For example, the prime "aggression" made people perceive an ambiguously aggressive target as more aggressive and therefore also as more negative. We think, however, that whereas the effect of semantic priming on evaluation is mediated by disambiguation (i.e., by choosing one of a few possible labels for a stimulus), the effects of goals on evaluation do not have to be mediated by disambiguation. When the goal "go home" is primed (e.g., by presenting the word "home"), then home and its associates would acquire more positive value without necessarily being perceived in a different way or given different labels. In case no change in labeling occurred, we believe, semantic priming should not affect value.

Goals May Create Ad Hoc Connections Between Constructs

According to goal systems theory, goals form a hierarchical network with superordinate goals associatively linked both to subordinate goals (i.e., means) and to competing or complementary goals and superordinate goals (Kruglanski et al., 2002; Shah, Kruglanski, & Friedman, 2002). These networks may or may not correspond, either partly

or fully, to semantic networks. For example, the goal of buying candles may be subordinate to a higher-level goal of getting married and superordinate to the means of driving a car to the candle store, but the semantic constructs "candles," "marriage," and "car" may be not semantically associated with each other.

According to goal systems theory, means should activate the goals they subserve, and goals should activate the means that subserve them. Indeed, Kruglanski et al. (2000) have shown, using subliminal priming, that lexical decision times for goal-related means were faster after priming goals and that lexical decision for goals were faster after means were primed. Moreover, increased accessibility of the goal due to priming of means was associated with increased task persistence and better performance (Shah & Kruglanski, 2003), reflecting the existence of a direct relationship between success in goal pursuit and the strength of the connection between means and goals. Interestingly, because of the relations between means and goals, some effects that are observed for semantic priming appear to work differently for goal priming, namely, *lateral inhibition* (for a recent review, see Förster & Liberman, 2007a) and the *fan effect* (Anderson, 1976, 1983).

Lateral Inhibition

Competing constructs can inhibit each other—for example, in linguistic processing it has been found that homonyms initially activate all the semantic meanings (e.g., the word "bank" activates both the meaning of a financial institution and the meaning of a riverside). However, after the word's meaning is disambiguated by the context, the context-irrelevant meanings become inhibited (Swinney, Prather, & Love, 2000). A similar effect has been reported in social cognition (Macrae, Bodenhausen, & Milne, 1995)—participants were exposed to targets that belonged to multiple stereotyped groups (e.g., an Asian woman). Prior to that exposure, they were subliminally primed with one of the category labels (e.g., "women" or "Chinese"). Using a lexical decision task, the study showed that priming enhanced the accessibility of the primed category and inhibited the other, nonprimed category.

Consistent with these effects, goal systems theory predicts inhibitory links between competing goals, a phenomenon labeled "goal shielding." Goal shielding should occur when alternative, potentially competing goals are inhibited by pursuit of a focal goal. Indeed, research has demonstrated that priming chronic or situation-specific goals inhibited the accessibility of conflicting goal representations as compared to priming goal-unrelated concepts (Shah, Friedman, & Kruglanski, 2002). Importantly, Shah and Kruglanski (2002) found that priming of alternative goals impedes performance on focal goals only if the two goals are perceived as competing (i.e., believed to interfere with each others' attainment). When an alternative goal is primed that is believed to be facilitative of the focal goal, performance of the focal goal is facilitated (see also Shah & Kruglanski, 2003). In a series of studies, participants completed anagrams after which they were expected to perform a "functional thinking" task in which they would have to list as many uses as possible for a box. While performing the anagram task, participants were subliminally primed with the other task by dint of a brief presentation of the words "box use" before each anagram (participants in the control condition were primed with "view it"). It was found that for participants who believed that the anagram task and the functional thinking tasks were related, priming facilitated performance (as measured by both persistence and number of solutions in the anagram task). For participants who believed that the two tasks were unrelated, priming the functional thinking task interfered with performance. These studies demonstrate that priming a nonfocal, potentially competing goal may interfere with performance if the primed goal is unrelated to the focal goal but may facilitate it if the two goals are perceived as related.

The important distinction between goal networks and semantic networks appears to lie in the ad hoc, dynamic way in which constructs come to be viewed as competing versus complementary. Whereas in semantic networks these relations seem to be overlearned, in goal systems they may be constructed and reconstructed because of circumstantial changes in goal hierarchies and in situational affordances. We believe that this more dynamic, constructive aspect of lateral inhibition may point to the operation of primed goals rather than primed semantic constructs. Goals are most likely primed if effects of priming appear to be sensitive to changing goal-subordination structures and to changing facilitative versus inhibitive relations between goals.

Asymmetric Spreading of Activation and the Fan Effect

Semantic constructs are structured in hierarchies. Higher-level, superordinate representations (e.g., "bird") are linked to lower-level, subordinate representations (e.g., "robin"). In semantic priming, it appears that lower-level representations activate their superordinate category to a lesser extent than vice versa (e.g., "robin" primes "bird" more than "bird" primes "robin"). Anderson (1983) termed this phenomenon the "fan effect." A similar effect has been observed with goals, where superordinate goals are the higher-level category and their means are the lower-level, subordinate construct. Research by Fishbach, Friedman, and Kruglanski (2003) applied this logic to goal subordination in the context of self-control. The authors argued that when situationally enticed to pursue short-term goals representing temptations (e.g., use of illegal drugs or engagement in premarital sex), people activate superordinate goals (e.g., academic achievement or adhering to religious mores) in order to aid self-control. To test their hypothesis, the authors subliminally primed temptation-related words (e.g., "drugs" and "sex") and found that participants were significantly faster to make lexical decisions about words related to the higher-order goals with which these temptations stood to interfere (e.g., "grades" and "bible") than when primed with control words associated with temptations that were irrelevant to these goals.

Critically, Fishbach et al. (2003) found important differences between the fan effect and their unconscious self-control effect. First, they showed that whereas temptation primes facilitated goal response times, suggesting that momentary allurements automatically trigger activation of overriding goals, goal primes were, if anything, found in the same designs to *inhibit* activation of temptations (thereby pointing to a "goal shielding" process; Shah, Friedman, et al., 2002). Remember that the fan effect reflects that higher-level representations should facilitate the lower-level representations to a lesser extent than vice versa (Anderson, 1976, 1983); thus, a *reduced activation* from higher-order goals to temptations could be explained by models similar to cognitive effects. However, the fact that Fishbach et al. (2003) found not only diminished facilitation but also inhibition of temptations by goals points to some more dynamic mechanism: Certainly "bird" should not *inhibit* "robin" the way that goals inhibit temptations; however, it is functional to inhibit "chocolate" when "diet" is your superordinate goal. Altogether, their work strongly suggests that automatic processes in resisting temptation, processes that are adaptive for self-regulation, may be endemic to goal systems but may not function within representational networks based solely on semantic or temporal associations. As such, documentation of the operation of such processes may provide yet another means of distinguishing automatic effects that are self-regulatory in nature from non–self-regulatory effects.

Goal hierarchies only partially reflect the associative (or, for that matter, semantic) network. For example, the fact that "diet" is connected to "chocolate" possibly reflects both a semantic association as well as a goal–network relation (i.e., between a higher-level goal and a temptation). But other examples are possible, too. For example, imagine a situation in which one needs to study but is tempted to play instead with her baby niece. The words "study" and "niece" would become associated as goal and temptation, respectively, without being necessarily semantically associated. This example suggests that the goal–temptation link, as other links in the goal system, may sometimes exist solely within the goal network system and not in the semantic network. Regardless of whether they do or do not correspond to semantic associates, goals and temptations should exhibit the pattern of mutual activation and inhibition described previously (e.g., the word "niece" should activate "study," and "study" should inhibit "niece"). If such a pattern of activation and inhibition occurs, it reflects the operation of primed goals.

Conclusion

Priming is an often-used paradigm. Social psychologists convincingly showed that it is possible to prime semantic constructs (and affect perceptual thresholds and disambiguation) as well as procedures and goals. It is unclear, however, when a prime is presented whether its effect would be best characterized as semantic priming, procedural priming, or goal priming. We suggest that primed goals differ from primed procedures and primed semantic constructs in a number of ways. First, goals have a different pattern of persistence and decay (or deactivation) than both procedures and semantic constructs. Goals may persist longer and instigate inhibition after fulfillment. Second, effects of primed goals should be sensitive to expectancy and value, whereas the effects of primed semantic constructs and primed procedures should not show such sensitivity. Third, means–ends associations, which constitute the goal system, do not always correspond to semantic or overlearned associations. As a result, patterns of lateral inhibition and asymmetries in spreading activation (i.e., the fan effect) differ between goal systems and semantic associations.

Admittedly, in our discussion of the distinction between goal priming and semantic priming, we chose a rather inflexible and mechanistic model of semantic or procedural priming and juxtaposed it to a flexible model of goal priming. It is beyond the scope of the chapter to discuss recent models of knowledge representations, including new developments in connectionist or PDP memory or modal models (see, e.g., Anderson & Rosenfeld, 1988; Barsalou, 1993; Dorman & Gaudiano, 1995; McClelland, Rumelhart, & the PDP Research Group, 1986; Read & Miller, 1998; Rumelhart, McClelland, & the PDP Research Group, 1986; Smith, 1996, 1998; Smith & DeCoster, 1998), some of which explicitly address the notion of goals. However, our current analysis shows that the dynamics or processes of goal activation—such as different decay and increase rates for semantic, procedural, and goal priming; the specific sensitivity of goals for expectancy and value; and the rather specific activation pattern observed in self-control dilemmas (e.g., "diet" inhibits "cake" but "cake" activates "diet")

as well as the functional goal-shielding patterns discussed previously—need to be simulated in such models as well. Inasmuch as current models still focus on frequency and recency as the central principles of semantic priming and do not involve these kinds of functional flexibility, they cannot explain mechanisms of goal activation.

We are optimistic that future research will discover even more distinctions between goal and semantic representations (see Förster, Liberman, & Friedman, 2007). Such research could help us understand the capacity of the human mental system to adapt flexibly to the environment. It will help us understand when priming has which effects and when and how memory is stored and altered within our mental system. The idea of memory as a "storehouse" that rather inflexibly reacts to the environment, finding and saving information without the individual involved, was abandoned long ago (see Barsalou, 1993; Koriat & Goldsmith, 1996; Strack & Förster, 1998). The research that we have summarized uniquely emphasizes that memory models must be freshly adapted to incorporate the processes involved when people activate or deactivate information in order to pursue their goals.

Acknowledgments

This research was supported by a grant from the Deutsche Forschungsgemeinschaft (FO-392/8-2) to Jens Förster. We thank Konstantin Mihov for editing the manuscript. Special thanks go to Markus Denzler for invaluable discussions.

Notes

1. Some researchers in cognitive psychology distinguish between priming due to semantic, associative, and functional relations. For example, a purely associative relation (e.g., as measured by word association norms, e.g., cradle—baby) can be distinguished from a purely semantic relation (e.g., as measured by number of shared semantic features, e.g., horse—zebra; see, e.g., Perea & Rosa, 2002). In many priming studies, associative and semantic priming are confounded (such as in nurse—doctor).

Moreover, the empirical definition of associative relations is clear, but that of a semantic relation is not. As an instance of semantic relations, some studies used members of the same semantic category (e.g., pig—horse), and others considered synonyms (e.g. work—labor). Moss, Ostrin, Tyler, Marslen-Wilson (1995) included functional relations (e.g., broom—floor) as an example of semantic relations. Even though these different relations between target and prime may involve different activation and decay rates and may follow different psychological principles, for our purposes it suffices to say that all lead to priming effects. We use the term "semantic priming" as an umbrella term to include semantic, associative, and functional relations. Let us also note that in many primes that are commonly used in social psychological research (e.g., social categories), semantic, associative and functional relations are confounded (e.g., elderly—slow).

2. Priming may also create contrast effects whereby the target is seen in terms opposite to the prime. We do not wish here to discuss contrast effects and the many moderators of assimilation versus contrast. For these issues, reviews are available, such as, for example, Förster and Liberman (2007b).

3. Like semantic priming, behavioral priming may also create contrast effects whereby the primed person adopts a behavior opposite to the prime (see Dijksterhuis et al., 1998).

References

Aarts, H., & Dijksterhuis, A. (2000). Habits as knowledge structures: Automaticity in goal-directed behavior. *Journal of Personality and Social Psychology, 78,* 53–63.

Aarts, H., Gollwitzer, P. M., & Hassin, R. R. (2004). Goal contagion: Perceiving is for pursuing. *Journal of Personality and Social Psychology, 87,* 23–37.

Ach, N. K. (1910). *Über den Willensakt und das Temperament.* Leipzig: Quelle & Meyer.

Anderson, J. (1976). *Language, memory and thought.* Hillsdale, NJ: Lawrence Erlbaum Associates.

Anderson, J. A., & Rosenfeld, E. (1988). *Neurocomputing: Foundations of research.* Cambridge, MA: MIT Press.

Anderson, J. R. (1983). *The architecture of cognition.* Cambridge, MA: Harvard University Press.

Atkinson, J. W. (1957). Motivational determinants of risk-taking behavior. *Psychological Review, 64,* 359–372.

Atkinson, J. W. (1964). *An introduction to motivation.* Princeton, NJ: Van Nostrand.

Bandura, A. (1982). Self-efficacy mechanism in human agency. *American Psychologist, 37,* 122–147.

Bargh, J. A. (1997). The automaticity of everyday life. In R. S. Wyer (Ed.), *Advances of social cognition* (pp. 1–61). Mahwah, NJ: Lawrence Erlbaum Associates.

Bargh, J. A., & Chartrand, T. L. (1999). The unbearable automaticity of being. *American Psychologist, 54,* 462–479.

Bargh, J. A., Chen, M., & Burrows, L. (1996). Automaticity of social behavior: Direct effects of trait construct and stereotype activation on action. *Journal of Experimental Social Psychology, 71,* 230–244.

Bargh, J. A., Gollwitzer, P. M., Lee-Chai, A., Barndollar, K., & Trötschel, R. (2001). The automated will: Nonconscious activation and pursuit of behavioral goals. *Journal of Personality and Social Psychology, 81,* 1014–1027.

Barsalou, L. W. (1993). Challenging assumptions about concepts. *Cognitive Development, 8,* 169–180.

Brown, J. S. (1948). Gradients of approach and avoidance responses and their relation to level of motivation. *Journal of Comparative and Physiological Psychology, 41,* 450–465.

Cesario, J., Plaks, J. E., & Higgins, E. T. (2006). Automatic social behavior as motivated preparation to interact. *Journal of Personality and Social Psychology, 90,* 893–910.

Chartrand, T. L., & Bargh, J. A. (1999). The chameleon effect: The perception-behavior link and social interaction. *Journal of Personality and Social Psychology, 71,* 893–910.

Collins, A. M., & Loftus, E. F. (1975). A spreading activation theory of semantic processing. *Psychological Review, 82,* 407–428.

Correll, J., Park, C., Judd, C. M., & Wittenbrink, B. (2002). The police officer's dilemma: Using ethnicity to disambiguate potentially threatening individuals. *Journal of Personality and Social Psychology, 83,* 1314–1329.

Custers, R., & Aarts, H. (2005). Positive affect as implicit motivator: On the nonconscious operation of behavioral goals. *Journal of Personality and Social Psychology, 89,* 129–142.

Darley, J. M., & Gross, P. H. (1983). A hypothesis confirming bias in labeling effects. *Journal of Personality and Social Psychology, 44,* 20–33.

Devine, P. G. (1989). Stereotypes and prejudice: Their automatic and controlled components. *Journal of Personality and Social Psychology, 56,* 5–18.

Dijksterhuis, A., Aarts, H., Bargh, J. A., & van Knippenberg, A. (2000). On the relation between associative strength and automatic behavior. *Journal of Experimental Social Psychology, 36,* 531–544.

Dijksterhuis, A., & Bargh, J. A. (2001). The perception-behavior expressway: Automatic effects of social perception on social behavior. In M. Zanna (Ed.), *Advances in experimental social psychology* (Vol. 33, pp. 1–40). San Diego, CA: Academic Press.

Dijksterhuis, A., Bargh, J. A., & Miedema, J. (2000). Of men and mackerels: Attention, subjective experience, and automatic social behavior. In H. Bless & J. P. Forgas (Eds.), *The message within: The role of subjective experience in social cognition and behavior* (pp. 37–51). Philadelphia: Psychology Press.

Dijksterhuis, A., Spears, R., & Lépinasse, V. (2001). Reflecting and deflecting stereotypes: Assimilation and contrast in impression formation and automatic behavior. *Journal of Experimental Social Psychology, 37,* 286–299.

Dijksterhuis, A., Spears, R., Postmes, T., Stapel, D. A., Koomen, W., Van Knippenberg, A., et al. (1998). Seeing one thing and doing another: Contrast effects in automatic behavior. *Journal of Personality and Social Psychology, 75,* 862–871.

Dijksterhuis, A., & van Knippenberg, A. (1998). The relation between perception and behavior, or how to win a game of trivial pursuit. *Journal of Personality and Social Psychology, 74,* 865–877.

Dijksterhuis, A., & van Knippenberg, A. (2000). Behavioral indecision: Effects of self-focus on automatic behavior. *Social Cognition, 18,* 55–74.

Dorman, C., & Gaudiano, P. (1995). Motivation. In M. A. Arbib (Ed.), *Handbook of brain theory and neural networks* (pp. 591–594). Cambridge, MA: MIT Press.

Edwards, W. (1955). The prediction of decision among bets. *Journal of Experimental Psychology, 50,* 201–214.

Edwards, W. (1961). Probability learning in 1000 trials. *Journal of Experimental Psychology, 62,* 385–394.

Epley, N., & Gilovich, T. (1999). Just going along: Nonconscious priming and conformity to social pressure. *Journal of Experimental Social Psychology, 35,* 578–589.

Fazio, R. H. (2001). On the automatic activation of associated evaluations: An overview. *Cognition and Emotion, 15,* 115–141.

Fazio, R. H., Jackson, J. R., Dunton, B. C., & Williams, C. J. (1995). Variability in automatic activation as an unobtrusive measure of racial attitudes: A bona fide pipeline? *Journal of Personality and Social Psychology, 69,* 1013–1027.

Feltz, D. L., & Landers, D. M. (1983). The effects of mental practice on motor skill learning and performance: A meta-analysis. *Journal of Sport Psychology, 5,* 25–57.

Ferguson, M. J., & Bargh, J. A. (2004). Liking is for doing: The effects of goal pursuit on automatic evaluation. *Journal of Personality and Social Psychology, 87,* 557–572.

Fishbach, A., Friedman, R. S., & Kruglanski, A. W., (2003). Leading us not into temptation: Momentary allurements elicit overriding goal activation. *Journal of Personality and Social Psychology, 84,* 296–309.

Fishbein, M., & Ajzen, I. (1974). Attitudes toward objects as predictors of single and multiple behavioral criteria. *Psychological Review, 81,* 59–74.

Fitzsimons, G. M., & Bargh, J. A. (2003). Thinking of you: Pursuit of interpersonal goals associated with relational partners. *Journal of Personality and Social Psychology, 84,* 148–164.

Förster, J., & Denzler, M. (2006). Selbst-Regulation. In W. Bierhoff & D. Frey (Eds.), *Handbuch der Psychologie, Band "Sozialpsychologie"* (pp. 128–132). Berlin: Hogrefe.

Förster, J., Friedman, R., Butterbach, E. M., & Sassenberg, K. (2005). Automatic effects of deviancy cues on creative cognition. *European Journal of Social Psychology, 35,* 345–360.

Förster, J., Friedman, R. S., Özelsel, A., & Denzler, M. (2006). The influence of approach and avoidance cues on the scope of perceptual and conceptual attention. *Journal of Experimental Social Psychology, 42,* 133–146.

Förster, J., Higgins, E. T., & Idson, L. C. (1998). Approach and avoidance strength during goal attainment: Regulatory focus and the "goal looms larger" effect. *Journal of Personality and Social Psychology, 75,* 1115–1131.

Förster, J., & Liberman, N. (2007a). Inhibition processes in comparisons. In D. A. Stapel & J. Suls (Eds.), *Assimilation and contrast in social psychology* (pp. 269–288). New York: Psychology Press.

Förster, J., & Liberman, N. (2007b). Knowledge activation. In E. T. Higgins & A. W. Kruglanski (Eds.), *Social psychology: Handbook of basic principles* (2nd ed., pp. 201–231). New York: Guilford Press.

Förster, J., Liberman, N., & Friedman, R. (2007). Seven principles of automatic goal pursuit: A systematic approach to distinguishing goal priming from priming of non-goal constructs. *Personality and Social Psychology Review, 11,* 211–233.

Förster, J., Liberman, N., & Higgins, E. T. (2005). Accessibility from active and fulfilled goals. *Journal of Experimental Social Psychology, 41,* 220–239.

Friedman, R., Fishbach, A., Förster, J., & Werth, L. (2003). Attentional priming effects on creativity. *Creativity Research Journal, 15,* 277–286.

Friedman, R., & Förster, J. (2008). Activation and measurement of motivational states. In A. Elliott (Ed.), *Handbook of approach and avoidance motivation* (pp. 235–246). Mahwah, NJ: Lawrence Erlbaum Associates.

Fujita, K., Trope, Y., Liberman, N., & Levin-Sagi, M. (2006). Construal levels and self-control. *Journal of Personality and Social Psychology, 90,* 351–367.

Gilovich, T. (1981). Seeing the past in the present: The effect of associations to familiar events on judgments and decisions. *Journal of Personality and Social Psychology, 40,* 797–808.

Gollwitzer, P. M. (1990). Action phases and mindsets. In E. T. Higgins & R. M. Sorrentino (Eds.), *The handbook of motivation and cognition: Foundations of social behavior* (Vol. 2, pp. 53–92). New York: Guilford Press.

Gollwitzer, P. M. (1993). Goal achievement: The role of intentions. In W. Stroebe & M. Hewstone (Eds.), *European review of social psychology* (Vol. 4, pp. 141–185). Chichester: Wiley.

Gollwitzer, P. M. (1999). Implementation intentions: Strong effects of simple plans. *American Psychologist, 54,* 493–503.

Gollwitzer, P. M., & Heckhausen, H. (1987). *Breadth of intention and the counterplea heuristic: Further evidence on the motivational and volitional mind-set distinction.* Unpublished manuscript.

Gollwitzer, P. M., Heckhausen, H., & Steller, B. (1990). Deliberative and implemental mind-sets: Cognitive tuning toward congruous thoughts and information. *Journal of Personality and Social Psychology, 59,* 1119–1127.

Gollwitzer, P. M., & Kirchhof, O. (1998). The willful pursuit of identity. In J. Heckhausen & C. S. Dweck (Eds.), *Life span perspectives on motivation and control* (pp. 361–399). New York: Guilford Press.

Goschke, T., & Kuhl, J. (1993). Representation of intentions: Persisting activation in memory. *Journal of Experimental Psychology: Learning, Memory, and Cognition, 19,* 1211–1226.

Hassin, R. R., Bargh, J. A., & Zimerman, S. (in press). Automatic and flexible: The case of nonconscious goal pursuit. *Social Cognition.*

Heckhausen, H. (1991). *Motivation and action.* Berlin: Springer.

Higgins, E. T. (1996). Knowledge activation: Accessibility, applicability and salience. In E. T. Higgins & A. W. Kruglanski (Eds.), *Social psychology: Handbook of basic principles* (pp. 133–168). New York: Guilford Press.

Higgins, E. T., King, G. A., & Mavin, G. H. (1982). Individual construct accessibility and subjective impressions and recall. *Journal of Personality and Social Psychology, 43,* 35–47.

Higgins, E. T., Rholes, W. S., & Jones, C. R. (1977). Category accessibility and impression formation. *Journal of Experimental Social Psychology, 13,* 141–154.

Isen, A. M., & Daubman, K. A. (1984). The influence of affect on categorization. *Journal of Personality and Social Psychology, 47,* 1206–1217.

James, W. (1890). *Principles of psychology.* New York: Holt.

Kawada, C. L. K., Oettingen, G., Gollwitzer, P. M., & Bargh, J. A. (2004). The projection of implicit and explicit goals. *Journal of Personality and Social Psychology, 86,* 545–559.

Kawakami, K., Young, H., & Dovidio, J. F. (2002). Automatic stereotyping: Category, trait, and behavioral activations. *Personality and Social Psychology Bulletin, 28,* 3–15.

Koriat, A., & Goldsmith, M. (1996). Memory metaphors and the real-life/laboratory controversy: Correspondence versus storehouse conceptions of memory. *Behavioral and Brain Sciences, 19,* 167–228.

Kruglanski, A. W. (1996). Motivated social cognition. Principles of the interface. In E. T. Higgins & A. W. Kruglanski (Eds.), *Social psychology: Handbook of basic principles* (pp. 493–520). New York: Guilford Press.

Kruglanski, A. W., Shah, J. Y., Fishbach, A., Friedman, R., Chun, W., & Sleeth-Keppler, D. (2002). A theory of goal systems. In M. P. Zanna (Ed.), *Advances in experimental social psychology* (Vol. 34, pp. 331–378). San Diego, CA: Academic Press.

Kruglanski, A. W., Thompson, E. P., Higgins, E. T., Atash, M. N., Pierro, A., Shah, J. Y., et al. (2000). To "do the right thing" or to "just do it": Locomotion and assessment as distinct self-regulatory imperatives. *Journal of Personality and Social Psychology, 79,* 793–815.

Lakin, J., & Chartrand, T. L. (2003). Increasing nonconscious mimicry to achieve rapport. *Psychological Science, 27,* 145–162.

Levy, B. (1996). Improving memory in old age through implicit self-stereotyping. *Journal of Personality and Social Psychology, 71,* 1092–1107.

Lewin, K. (1935). *A dynamic theory of personality.* New York: McGraw-Hill.

Lewin, K. (1951). *Field theory in social science; selected theoretical papers* (D. Cartwright, Ed.). New York: Harper & Row.

Liberman, N., & Förster, J. (2005). How goals influence what we think: Towards a motivational priming model. In J. P. Forgas, K. D. Kipling, & S. M. Laham (Eds.), *Social motivation: Conscious and unconscious processes (Sydney Symposium of Social Psychology)* (pp. 228–248). Cambridge, UK: Cambridge University Press.

Liberman, N., Sagristano, M., & Trope, Y. (2002). The effect of level of construal on temporal distance of activity enactment. *Journal of Experimental Social Psychology, 38,* 523–535.

Liberman, N., Trope, Y., & Stephan, E. (2007). Psychological distance. In E. T. Higgins & A. Kruglanski (Eds.), *Social psychology: Handbook of basic principles* (2nd ed., pp. 353–381). New York: Guilford Press.

Locke, E. W., & Latham, G. P. (1990). Work motivation and satisfaction: Light at the end of the tunnel. *Psychological Science, 1,* 240–246.

Luchins, A. S. (1942). Mechanization in problem solving. *Psychological Monographs, 54,* 1–95.

Macrae, C. N., Bodenhausen, G. V., & Milne, A. B. (1995). The dissection of selection in person perception: Inhibitory processes in social stereotyping. *Journal of Personality and Social Psychology, 69,* 397–407.

Macrae, C. N., & Johnston, L. (1998). Help, I need somebody: Automatic action and inaction. *Social Cognition, 16,* 400–417.

Marsh, R. L., Hicks, J. L., & Bink, M. L. (1998). Activation of completed, uncompleted, and partially completed intentions. *Journal of Experimental Psychology: Learning, Memory, and Cognition, 24,* 350–361.

Marsh, R. L., Hicks, J. L., & Bryan, E. S. (1999). The activation of unrelated and cancelled intentions. *Memory and Cognition, 27,* 320–327.

McClelland, J. L., Rumelhart, D. E., & the PDP Research Group (Eds.). (1986). *Parallel distributed processing* (Vol. 2). Cambridge, MA: MIT Press.

Miller, N. E. (1944). Experimental studies of conflict. In M. Hunt (Ed.), *Personality and the behavior disorders* (pp. 431–465) New York: Ronald Press.

Miller, N. E. (1959). Liberation of basic S-R concepts: Extension to conflict behavior, motivation and social learning. In S. Koch (Ed.), *Psychology: A study of a science* (Vol. 2). New York: McGraw Hill.

Moskowitz, G. B., Gollwitzer, P. M., Wasel, W., & Schaal, B. (1999). Preconscious control of stereotype activation through chronic egalitarian goals. *Journal of Personality and Social Psychology, 77,* 167–184.

Moss, H. E., Ostrin, R. K., Tyler, L. K., & Marslen-Wilson, W. D. (1995). Accessing different types of lexical semantic information. *Journal of Experimental Psychology: Learning, Memory, and Cognition, 21,* 863–883.

Mussweiler, T., & Förster, J. (2000). The sex → aggression link: A perception-behavior dissociation. *Journal of Personality and Social Psychology, 79,* 507–520.

Neely, J. H. (1977). Semantic priming and retrieval from lexical memory: Roles of inhibition less spreading activation and limited-capacity attention. *Journal of Experimental Social Psychology: General, 106,* 226–254.

Neely, J. H. (1991). Semantic priming effects in visual word recognition: A selective review of current findings and theories. In D. Besner & G. W. Humphreys (Eds.), *Basic processes in reading: Visual word recognition* (pp. 264–336). Hillsdale, NJ: Lawrence Erlbaum Associates.

Perea, M., & Rosa, E. (2002). The effects of associative and semantic priming in the lexical decision task. *Psychological Research, 66,* 180–194.

Prinz, W. (1997). Perception and action planning. *European Journal of Cognitive Psychology, 9,* 129–154.

Read, S. J., & Miller, L. C. (1998). *Connectionist models of social reasoning and social behavior.* Hillsdale, NJ: Lawrence Erlbaum Associates.

Rothermund, K. (2003). Automatic vigilance for task-related information: Perseverance after failure and inhibition after success. *Memory & Cognition, 31,* 343–352.

Rotter, J. B. (1966). Generalized expectancies for internal versus external control of reinforcement. *Psychological Monographs: General and Applied, 80,* 1–28.

Rumelhart, D. E., McClelland, J. L. & the PDP Research Group (Eds.). (1986). *Parallel distributed processing* (Vol. 1). Cambridge, MA: MIT Press.

Schooler, J. W. (2002). Verbalization produces a transfer inappropriate processing shift. *Applied Cognitive Psychology, 16,* 989–997.

Schooler, J. W., Fiore, S. M., & Brandimonte, M. A. (1997). At a loss from words: Verbal overshadowing of perceptual memories. In D. L. Medin (Ed.), *The psychology of learning and motivation* (pp. 293–334). Hillsdale, NJ: Academic Press.

Shah, J. (2003). Automatic for the people: How representations of significant others implicitly affect goal pursuit. *Journal of Personality and Social Psychology, 84,* 661–681.

Shah, J. Y., Friedman, R., & Kruglanski, A. W. (2002). Forgetting all else: On the antecedents and consequences of goal shielding. *Journal of Personality and Social Psychology, 83,* 1261–1280.

Shah, J. Y., & Kruglanski, A. W. (2002). Priming against your will: How goal pursuit is affected by accessible alternatives. *Journal of Experimental Social Psychology, 38,* 368–383.

Shah, J. Y., & Kruglanski, A. W. (2003). When opportunity knocks: Bottom-up priming of goals by means and its effects on self-regulation. *Journal of Personality and Social Psychology, 84,* 1109–1122.

Shah, J. Y., Kruglanski, A. W., & Friedman, R. (2002). A goal systems approach to self-regulation. In M. P. Zanna, J. M. Olson, & C. Seligman (Eds.), *The Ontario Symposium on Personality and Social Psychology* (pp. 247–276). Hillsdale, NJ: Lawrence Erlbaum Associates.

Shah, J. Y., Kruglanski, A. W., & Friedman, R. (2003). Goal systems theory: Integrating the cognitive and motivational aspects of self-regulation. In S. Spencer, S. Fein, & M. P. Zanna (Eds.), *Motivated social perception: The Ontario Symposium* (Vol. 9, pp. 247–276). Hillsdale, NJ: Lawrence Erlbaum Associates.

Smith, E. R. (1989). Procedural efficiency: General and specific components and effects on social judgment. *Journal of Experimental Social Psychology, 25,* 500–523.

Smith, E. R. (1990). Content and process specificity in the effects of prior experiences. In T. K. Srull & R. S. Wyer (Eds.), *Advances in social cognition* (Vol. 3, pp. 1–60). Hillsdale, NJ: Lawrence Erlbaum Associates.

Smith, E. R. (1994). Procedural knowledge and processing strategies in social cognition. In R. S. Wyer & T. K. Srull (Eds.), *Handbook of social cognition* (2nd ed., Vol. 1, pp. 99–151). Hillsdale, NJ: Lawrence Erlbaum Associates.

Smith, E. R. (1996). What do connectionism and social psychology offer each other? *Journal of Personality and Social Psychology, 70,* 893–912.

Smith, E. R. (1998). Mental representation and memory. In D. T. Gilbert, S. T. Fiske, & G. Lindzey (Eds.), *The handbook of social psychology* (pp. 391–445). New York: McGraw-Hill.

Smith, E. R., & Branscombe, N. R. (1987). Procedurally mediated social inferences: The case of category accessibility effects. *Journal of Experimental Social Psychology, 23,* 361–382.

Smith, E. R., Branscombe, N. R., & Bormann, C. (1988). Generality of the effects of practice on social judgement tasks. *Journal of Personality and Social Psychology, 54,* 385–395.

Smith, E. R., & DeCoster, J. (1998). Knowledge acquisition, accessibility, and use in person perception and stereotyping: Simulation with a recurrent connectionist network. *Journal of Personality and Social Psychology, 74,* 21–35.

Smith, E. R., Stewart, T. L., & Buttram, R. T. (1992). Inferring a trait from a behavior has long-term, highly specific effects. *Journal of Personality and Social Psychology, 62,* 753–759.

Srull, T. K., & Wyer, R. S., Jr. (1979). The role of category accessibility in the interpretation of information about persons: Some determinants and implications. *Journal of Personality and Social Psychology, 37,* 1660–1672.

Strack, F., & Förster, J. (1998). Self-reflection and recognition: The role of metacognitive knowledge in the attribution of recollective experience. *Personality and Social Psychology Review, 2,* 111–123.

Strahan, E. J., Spencer, S. J., & Zanna, M. P. (2002). Subliminal priming and persuasion: Striking while the iron is hot. *Journal of Experimental Social Psychology, 38,* 556–568.

Swinney, D., Prather, P., & Love, T. (2000). The time-course of lexical access and the role of context: Converging evidence from normal and aphasic processing. In Y. Grodzinsky, L. P. Shapiro, & D. A. Swinney (Eds.), *Language and the brain: Representation and processing* (pp. 273–294). New York: Academic Press.

Taylor, S. E., & Gollwitzer, P. N. (1995). Effects of mindset on positive illusions. *Journal of Personality and Social Psychology, 69,* 213–226.

Vroom, V. H. (1966). Organizational choice: A study of pre- and post-decision processes. *Organizational Behavior and Human Performance, 1,* 212–225.

Wakslak, C. J., Trope, Y., & Liberman, N. (2006). Transcending the now: Time as a dimension of psychological distance. In J. Glicksohn & M. S. Myslobodsky (Eds.), *Timing the future: The case for a time-based prospective memory* (pp. 171–189). River Edge, NJ: World Scientific Publishing.

Wyer, R. S. (2004). *Social comprehension and judgment: The role of situation models, narratives, and implicit theories.* Mahwah, NJ: Lawrence Erlbaum Associates.

Wyer, S. R. (in press). The role of knowledge accessibility in cognition and behavior: Implications for consumer information processing. In C. Haugvedt, F. R. Kardes, & P. M. Herr (Eds.), *Handbook of consumer research.* Mahwah, NJ: Erlbaum.

PART 3

Action and Mental Representation

The Prefrontal Cortex Stores Structured Event Complexes That Are the Representational Basis for Cognitively Derived Actions

Jordan Grafman *and* Frank Krueger

Abstract

This chapter focuses on actions at the level of cognitive event execution—whether the person is engaged in the action or making a judgment about a perceived action. It presents studies of events that make up so-called structured event complexes (SECs). SECs contain parsed and recognizable events that fall into a structured sequence. Evidence is presented that the human prefrontal cortex (PFC) stores SECs. It is argued that SECs are the key to understanding the human ability to build and execute daily life activities. Such knowledge, when stored as memories, provides a link between past, current, and future activities.

Keywords: actions, judgment, events, event execution, SECs, PFC

This book is about action. Action can be conceived of as doing something in order to achieve a purpose, although at times it can simply describe a random movement or doing something without apparent purpose. This chapter focuses on actions at the level of cognitive event execution—whether the person is engaged in the action or making a judgment about a perceived action. We study events that make up what we have called structured event complexes (SECs). SECs contain parsed and recognizable events that fall into a structured sequence. They also represent information about activities of daily life. Retrieving stored event sequences is essential for action planning and performing daily life activities. Clinical observations suggest that the prefrontal cortex (PFC) is crucial for goal-directed behavior such as

carrying out plans, controlling a course of actions, or organizing everyday life routines (Eslinger & Damasio, 1985; Fuster, 1980; Janowsky, Shimamura, & Squire, 1989; Milner, Petrides, & Smith, 1985; Shallice, 1982; Shallice & Burgess, 1991; Stuss & Benson, 1984).

Researchers have proposed a number of theories of PFC function, many of which center around the processes that are mediated by the PFC. The "processing" approach takes the view that cognition in the PFC can be described in terms of performance without thoroughly specifying the representation that underlies these "processes" (e.g., see Duncan, 2001; Fuster, 1991; Miller & Cohen, 2001; Shallice & Burgess, 1998). In this view, processes such as switching, maintenance, and inhibitory control are computational procedures or algorithms that are independent of the nature or modality of the stimulus being processed and that operate on knowledge stored in posterior parts of the brain.

In our opinion, the "processing" approach to PFC function is a fundamental shift away from how cognitive neuroscientists have previously tried to understand information storage in memory. It further implies that the PFC is minimally committed to long-term storage of knowledge as compared to the temporal, parietal, and occipital lobes. Rather than adapt the processing view, we, instead, propose a "representational" approach to PFC function that assumes that (a) the PFC stores long-term memories of event knowledge associated with action and (b) seeks to establish the format and domains according to which such information is stored (Huey, Krueger, & Grafman, 2006; Moll, Zahn, de Oliveira-Souza, Krueger, & Grafman, 2005; Wood & Grafman, 2003; see Chapter 19). In our view, representations are memories localized in neural networks that, when activated, enable implementation of the stored information. Therefore, in contrast to what other investigators have coined as processes, we consider such activity, instead, as a set of representations that remain activated over a period of time and that compete with activation of different sets of representations by facilitation or inhibition of neural activity. In our opinion, this approach is much more compatible with how neuroscience seeks to understand the functions of posterior cortical regions such as motor and visual representations than the process approach.

In this chapter, we present evidence that the human PFC stores SECs. As noted previously, SECs are representations composed of goal-oriented sequences of events that are involved in executing, planning, and monitoring of actions (Grafman, 1995, 2002; Wood & Grafman, 2003). We first briefly summarize the key elements of the biology and structure of the PFC and argue that the SEC framework is consistent with what is known about its structure, connectivity, development, neurophysiology, and evolution. Then we describe the characteristics and principles of the SEC framework. Finally, we review the different lines of evidence supporting the SEC framework, focusing on the effects of PFC lesions on event knowledge and on functional neuroimaging experiments that reveal specific patterns of regional PFC activation associated with different aspects of event knowledge. Events, by definition, imply action, and therefore by focusing on the cognitive aspects of event knowledge, we are directly addressing issues related to action knowledge and execution. Our assumption is that by storing the cognitive aspects of action via event knowledge, humans are able to use that knowledge to both motivate their own actions and recognize the reason for action in others.

Properties of the Human PFC

As stated previously, we believe that a representational approach is key to understanding the cognitive functions of the PFC (e.g., Wood & Grafman, 2003). Given our view that SECs are goal-oriented event sequences whose unique cognitive characteristics are stored as a separate domain of knowledge from other forms of knowledge, the PFC is the strongest candidate region to store such representational knowledge. Therefore, before we detail the principles of the SEC framework, we briefly summarize the key elements of the biology and structure of the PFC and argue for a rationale that specifies why there must be representational knowledge intimately concerned with action stored in the PFC.

Structure

The PFC occupies approximately one-third of the entire human cerebral cortex and has a columnar design like other cortical regions. Some regions of the PFC have a total of six layers; other regions are agranular (without a granular cell layer). The PFC can be subdivided into lateral, medial, and orbitofrontal regions. Brodmann's areas (8–11, 23–25, 32, and 44–47) provide crude boundaries for the cytoarchitectonic subdivision within each of these gross regions (Barbas, 2000; Brodmann, 1912). The medial and lateral PFC belong to two distinct architectonic trends within the human PFC (Pandya & Yeterian, 1996). The medial trend is phylogenetically and ontogenetically older than the lateral trend, which is especially well developed in humans (Stuss & Benson, 1986). Comparing the human with the primate PFC, it has been claimed that the human PFC (and Brodmann's area 10 in particular) is proportionally larger compared to the rest of the cerebral cortex (Rilling & Insel, 1999; Semendeferi, Armstrong, Schleicher, Zilles, & van Hoesen, 2001; Semendeferi, Lu, Schenker, & Damasio, 2002). On the other hand, functional arguments suggest that, rather than the relative size of the human PFC, its advantage in humans must be due to a more sophisticated and differentially organized neural architecture (Chiavaras, LeGoualher, Evans, Petrides, 2001; Elston, 2000; Elston & Rosa, 2000).

Connectivity

All PFC regions are interconnected with other areas of the brain, and almost all these pathways are reciprocal. There exist at least five distinct PFC regions concerned with action implementation, each of which is independently involved in separate corticostriatal loops (Alexander, Crutcher, & DeLong, 1990; Masterman & Cummings, 1997). The PFC also has strong limbic system connections via its medial and orbital efferent connections that terminate in the amygdala, thalamus, and parahippocampal regions (Groenewegen & Uylings, 2000;

Price, 1999) and long pathway connections to association cortices in the temporal, parietal, and occipital lobes. Within the PFC and particularly in the most anterior regions of the PFC, the interregional connectivity is dense and may supersede the connectivity between the PFC and other regions. This could allow a certain kind of cognitive insularity to occur, providing some protection for the time required for cognitive deliberation before action.

Development

The PFC undergoes relatively late development during ontogenesis compared to other cortical association areas (Conel, 1939; Flechsig, 1920; Huttenlocher, 1990; Huttenlocher & Dabholkar, 1997). Imaging studies indicate that the PFC does not fully mature until early adulthood (Chugani, Phelps, & Mazziotta, 1987; Diamond, 1991; Durston et al., 2001; Giedd et al., 1999; Paus et al., 1999; Sowell, Thompson, Holmes, Jernigan, & Toga, 1999), and research on primates suggests that PFC lesions occurring early in development do not affect performance on tasks presumably subserved by the PFC until the monkey's PFC matures (Diamond, 1991; Goldman-Rakic, 1987, 1992). In addition, there is evidence that some PFC regions show structural and functional declines earlier than other brain regions in the aging human (Giedd et al., 1999).

Neurophysiology

A key principle of neurons in the PFC of monkeys and humans is their ability to fire during an interval between a stimulus and a delayed probe (Levy & Goldman-Rakic, 2000). Besides the property of sustained firing, a unique structural feature of neurons in the PFC has recently been found (Elston, 2000; Elston & Rosa, 2000). Pyramidal cells in the PFC of macaque monkeys (and presumably humans) are significantly more spinous as compared to pyramidal cells in other cortical areas, making them capable of handling a larger amount of excitatory inputs. This is just one of several possible explanation for the PFC's ability to integrate input from many sources in order to make decisions and implement actions.

Evolution

There is an evolutionary cognitive advance from primates to humans in the ability of neurons to sustain their firing and code the temporal and sequential properties of ongoing events in the environment or in mind over longer and longer periods of time (Fuster, Bodner, & Kroger, 2000). We suspect that longer-sustained firing and the ability to integrate input from many sources has enabled the human brain to code, store, and retrieve long and complex sequences of behavior, leading to the SEC form of representation we describe here (Nichelli, Clark, Hollnagel, & Grafman, 1995; Rueckert & Grafman, 1996, 1998).

In summary, the structure and connectivity of the PFC, the physiological properties of its neurons, and evolutionary principles are strongly suggestive of its role in the integration of sensory and memory information and in the representation and control of actions and behavior. Along with extended firing of neurons, specialized neural systems were developed that enabled the parsing and encoding of these behaviors into sequentially linked but individually recognizable events. The event sequence itself must be parsed as each event begins and ends in order to explicitly recognize the nature, duration, and number of events that compose the sequence (Zacks, Braver, et al., 2001; Zacks, Speer, Swallow, Braver, & Reynolds, 2007; Zacks & Tversky, 2001). These event sequences, in order to be goal oriented and to cohere, must obey a logical structure. This structure can be conceptualized as a representa-

tion, that is, a "permanent" unit of memory that, when activated, corresponds to a dynamic brain state signified by the strength and pattern of neural activity in a local brain sector. In this sense, over the course of evolution, the PFC became capable of representing knowledge of more complex behaviors or behaviors that occurred over a longer period of time that frequently are related to various forms of action. We have labeled these representational units in the PFC as SECs (Grafman, 1995).

Principles of the SEC Framework

SECs are representations composed of goal-oriented sequences of events that are involved in the planning and monitoring of cognitive-induced actions. For example, an SEC with the goal "get ready for work" would consist of a sequence of events also composed of actions such as waking up, getting out of bed, using the bathroom, taking a shower, getting dressed, eating breakfast, and so on. Event sequence knowledge has been described elsewhere as scripts or schemas (Rumelhart, 1980; Schank & Abelson, 1997; see Chapters 19 and 20). However, we use the term SEC to refer to the unique type of knowledge stored in the human PFC (Grafman, 1995) that comprises the underlying representations for cognitive structures such as plans, actions, rules, scripts, schemas, and mental models.

Sequence Structure

SECs are formed on the basis of repeated experience with events. Events within an SEC can be defined in terms of centrality, frequency of occurrence, relative position, duration, and temporal structure. Like objects that have boundaries in space, events have boundaries in time (Zacks, Tversky, & Iyer, 2001). For example, an object such as a ball takes up a certain amount of space of a certain shape. By analogy, an event such as "pitch a ball" takes place for a certain amount of time with a beginning and an end. SECs link a set of events to knowledge structures that store both the goals and the boundaries of events. Specifically, each SEC has a beginning event that specifies a setting (e.g., "wake up"), a following set of events (e.g., "take a shower" or "get dressed") that specify goals and activities to achieve these goals, and an event that signifies the setting that deactivates the SEC (e.g., "arrive at work"). Beside physical constraints, the sequential order of events obeys cultural and individual constraints. In the United States, for example, individuals generally shower on a daily basis in the morning before breakfast (cultural constraint), and some people brush their teeth twice in the morning—once before and once after eating breakfast (individual constraint).

Hierarchical Structure

Given the slow development of the PFC, during childhood, individual events are probably initially represented as independent memory units. For example, SECs associated with "kitchen," "bar," and "restaurant" cluster around the event "ingestion of food," whereas "bus," "train," "airplane," and "bicycle" cluster around the event "physically moving oneself around." Later in development, these primitive SECs expand into large multievent units based on repeated exposure and action. In addition, the boundaries of event sequences become more firmly established, leading to a well-structured SEC. Thus, in adulthood, SECs will range from specific episodes to context-free and abstract SECs within a domain. For example, the domain "eating" includes specific episodes representing evenings at a specific restaurant; SECs representing the actions and themes of how to behave at different types of restaurants, such as at a fast-food restaurant, at a coffeehouse, or on an airplane; and an abstract SEC representing actions and themes related to "eating" that are context independent. All

the SECs in a domain are connected in a hierarchy that encompasses subordinate and superordinate SECs.

Goal Orientation

Some SECs are well structured with all the cognitive and behavioral rules available for the sequence of actions to occur and a clear, definable goal. These SECs can guide one's action and expectations during the sequence. For example, individuals with a well-structured SEC about "eating in a restaurant" are quite confident that once they have been seated at a table and have read the menu, someone would appear to take their order. Other SECs are ill structured, requiring the individual to adapt to unpredictable events using analogical reasoning or similarity judgments to determine the sequence of actions online (by previously experienced events from memory integrating with novel events) as well as developing a quickly fashioned goal. For example, if someone sees that a person entering a bank is wearing a ski mask and carrying a gun and a bag in his hands, one can make sense of these events by filling in details from a "bank robbery" SEC. SECs also play a role in judgments and attitude formation, particularly about social events. In recalling details of a party one attended the night before, for example, one might use SECs representing features of "a good party" as a comparison standard to evaluate the present instance of a party.

Binding

There are multiple SECs that are activated on a typical day; therefore, it is likely that they (like events within an SEC) can be activated in sequence or additionally in a cascading or parallel manner. Event components interact and probably give rise to SECs through at least three binding mechanisms: sequential binding, proposed for linking events within structured event complexes within the PFC (Weingartner, Grafman, Boutelle, Kaye, & Martin, 1983); temporal binding among anatomically highly connected regions representing event subcomponents in the posterior cortex (Engel & Singer, 2001); and third-party binding of anatomically loosely connected regions by synchronized activity induced by the hippocampus, involved in the episodic memory (O'Reilly & Rudy, 2000; Weingartner et al., 1983). When the SEC is instantiated, the skeleton of sequential and thematic event information will be bound to a wide range of other representational networks, linking together neural assemblies in the posterior cortex with its domains of space, object features, and semantic knowledge by synchronized activity (i.e., temporal binding) of these event components.

Predictions and Evidence for the SEC Framework

Even if aspects of SECs are represented independently in the PFC, they must be simultaneously encoded and retrieved in order to incorporate an episode. The stored characteristics of the SEC representations form the bases for their strength of representation in memory and the relationships between SEC representations. The representational aspects of the SECs and their proposed localizations within the PFC are summarized in Figure 10.1.

Left Versus Right PFC

Lesion and functional magnetic resonance imaging (fMRI) data (Goel & Grafman, 2000; Huettel, Song, & McCarthy, 2005; Paulus et al., 2001) point to structural differences in the capacity of the left and right PFC for encoding and manipulating certain types of representations (Beeman & Bowden, 2000; Goldberg, Podell, & Lovell, 1994). In particular, the left PFC is more adept at constructing determinate, precise, and unambiguous representations of the world, whereas the right PFC is more adept at constructing and maintaining fluid, indeterminate, vague, and ambiguous representations of the world (Goel, 1995; Goel et al., 2006). Given this background, the SEC framework predicts different formats of representation within the left and right hemisphere. Specifically, we argue that the left PFC is specialized to activate the primary meaning of within-event information, sequential dependencies between single adjacent events, and coding for the boundaries between events. The right PFC, in contrast, is best able to activate and integrate information across events in order to obtain the theme or goal of the SEC. This dual form of coding should occur in parallel with shifting between the two, depending on environmental demands and strategic choices.

Lateral Versus Medial PFC

Medial and lateral PFC belong to two distinct architectonic trends within the PFC, with the medial trend phylogenetically and ontogenetically older than the lateral trend (Pandya & Yeterian, 1996). There is also strong evidence for a functional dissociation between medial and lateral PFC (Burgess, Scott, & Frith, 2003; Gilbert, Spengler, Simons, Frith, & Burgess, 2006; Gilbert, Spengler, Simons, Steele et al., 2006; Koechlin, Corrado, Pietrini, & Grafman, 2000). These distinctive properties suggest that the ability to carry out predictive or overlearned SECs may occur phylogenetically and ontogenetically earlier than the ability to adjust dynamically the sequential structure of ongoing SECs to new environmental demands and actions. The SEC framework predicts that the medial PFC stores predictable well-structured SECs that are rarely modified and have a predictable relationship with sensorimotor sequences, whereas the lateral PFC stores

STRUCTURED EVENT COMPLEX
PREFRONTAL CORTEX

HEMISPHERIC LATERALIZATION

Left PFC	Right PFC
Single event integration – Meaning and feature between single adjacent events to code for boundaries between events	**Across events integration** – Meaning and features across events to obtain goal of sequence

PREDICTABILITY

Lateral PFC	Medial PFC
Unpredictable partial order SECs – Frequently modified sequences that are used to adapt to special circumstances	**Predictable total order SECs** – Overlearned sequences that have clear definable goals and all behavioral rules available

CATEGORY SPECIFICITY

Dorsolateral PFC	Ventromedial PFC
Non-social SECs – Event sequences representing mechanistic plans and actions	**Social SECs** – Event sequences representing social rules and scripts

FREQUENCY

Anterior PFC	Posterior PFC
Complex SECs – Detailed information about event sequences	**Non-complex SECs** – Sparse information about event sequences

Fig. 10.1 SEC framework. The representational forms of the structured event complex (SEC) and their proposed localizations within the prefrontal cortex (PFC).

adaptive less structured SECs that are frequently modified to adapt to variable or special circumstances in the environment.

Dorsolateral Versus Ventromedial PFC

The PFC can be subdivided into the ventromedial PFC and the dorsolateral PFC. The ventromedial PFC is well situated to support functions involving the integration of information about emotions, social actions, and environmental stimuli, whereas the dorsolateral PFC supports the cognitive regulation of behavior and helps control our tendency to respond to environmental stimuli. Thus, the SEC framework predicts that different thematic domains of SECs are stored in different regions of the PFC: The dorsolateral PFC stores nonsocial SECs representing mechanistic plans and actions, whereas the ventromedial PFC stores social SECs representing social rules and attitudes.

Anterior Versus Posterior PFC

The framework predicts that SECs are long-term memory representations that can be modified by repeated exposure and that the strength of an SEC representation is dependent on how often a person enacts or observes this SEC. As an SEC becomes familiar, an economy of representation develops so that simpler representational codes can rapidly delegate to the lower-level systems (e.g., motor) that implement action sequences. The anterior PFC codes more detailed cognitive information about an SEC, whereas the posterior PFC codes sparser cognitive information about the same SEC, leading to different profiles of PFC activation, depending on the frequency of the activity the person executes. This would allow the same activity to be performed quickly (e.g., by using a heuristic based on sparser coding) or slowly (e.g., by using deliberate reflection based on detailed coding), depending on situational demands.

All these components can contribute to the formation of an SEC, with the different components being differentially weighted in importance, depending on the nature of the SEC and moment-by-moment behavioral demands. For example, the left anterior ventromedial PFC would be expected to represent a long multievent sequence of social information with specialized processing of the meaning and features of the single events within the sequence.

The SEC framework lends itself to the generation of testable predictions regarding the properties and localization of SECs in the PFC. By combining two methods of research, we strengthen the inferences we can

make in linking the processing of event sequence knowledge with specific brain areas. On the one hand, we apply lesion studies to examining deficits caused by specific brain damage in humans. On the other hand, we use functional neuroimaging, such as positron emission tomography (PET) and fMRI, to measure regional brain activity in healthy subjects while they perform behavioral tasks involving event sequence knowledge. Note that subjects are not actually involved in carrying out those behaviors during the experimental tasks. However, to solve the tasks, subjects have to access the stored SECs and their sequential organization. Therefore, it appears reasonable to assume that performing our tasks engages the same sorts of representations that are activated during planning, monitoring, and executing action sequences. We have started to investigate the differential contributions of PFC subregions to specific formats of representation and gross domains of thematic knowledge that lead to action.

Sequential Order

Longer-sustained firing and the ability to integrate input from many sources has enabled the human PFC to code, store, and retrieve long and complex sequences of behavior. These event sequences, in order to be goal oriented and cohere, must obey a logical structure.

In a lesion study, our research group found a double dissociation in performance between event sequence *ordering* and sentence syntax ordering by comparing patients with anterior PFC lesion to patients with a lesion in Broca's area (Sirigu et al., 1998). Subjects were asked to produce either a grammatically correct sentence or a logically consistent short narrative based on the temporal sequence of segments of words or actions, respectively. Although both tasks involved ordering of words, patients with anterior PFC lesions had difficulty ordering events correctly to form a logical sequence of actions but made virtually no errors in ordering words correctly in composing syntactically well-formed sentences. The opposite performance was observed in patients with Broca's aphasia. The results suggest that representation of order depends on the underlying knowledge structure being processed. For example, there exist at least two different networks within the frontal lobes for verbal sequence processing—one network for SEC syntax and another for sentence syntax. Broca's region, so closely tied to motor processing, may be better suited for handling the rapid analysis of word order in the context of online speech production, whereas anterior PFC regions are more tied to slower knowledge-linked event sequence processing.

Our research group also investigated script *generation and evaluation* in patients with lesions in prefrontal and posterior brain regions and in normal subjects (Sirigu et al., 1995, 1996). The script generation task tested access to script information, while script evaluation tested how subjects could organize and manipulate this event sequence knowledge in the process of planning an activity. Patients with PFC lesions did not differ from posterior lesion patients and normal subjects in the total number of actions evoked and mean evocation time. But the patients with PFC lesions committed more errors in generating the correct temporal sequence of actions, in generating events outside the stated script boundaries, and in failures to generate an event that would signal the end of the script or achievement of the action goal.

Furthermore, we have also used fMRI to investigate which specific PFC regions are involved in script-event compared to sentence-word processing. For the script-event order task, subjects were requested to detect an error in the order of two familiar scripts (e.g., "get dressed/take a shower"). In contrast, for the sentence-word order task, subjects had to detect an error in the sequence of words depicting a sentence (e.g., "the message twice/announced was"). Both tasks were found to activate partially overlapping areas in the left frontal, parietal, and temporal cortices, which are known to be implicated in language processing (Crozier et al., 1999). In addition, the script-event order task activated a large area in the dorsolateral PFC (Brodmann's area [BA] 6 and 8) bilaterally, left supplementary motor area, and left angular gyrus (BA 39). The results suggest that posterior prefrontal areas may be more specifically involved in the process of analyzing sequential links in the action category. In another fMRI study, we investigated the involvement of the PFC in temporal order and membership judgments of scripts (e.g., shopping) and category items (e.g., holidays) (Knutson, Wood, & Grafman, 2004). In the order task, subjects were asked to determine if the stimuli were shown in the correct sequential order and in the judgment task if the stimuli belonged to the same category. Both tasks activated the middle frontal gyrus bilaterally (BA 6 and 8), but in addition the event order task activated the right inferior frontal gyrus (BA 44, 45, and 47), while the chronological order task activated the left inferior frontal gyrus (BA 44 and 46).

Altogether, these results indicate that there exist different though largely overlapping neural substrates for event, sentence, and chronological knowledge during temporal ordering. This corroborates our view that the PFC is critical for the coding of the event sequence knowledge that underlies action.

Domain and Format Specificity

The subdivision of the PFC into ventromedial and dorsolateral sectors has led to the assumption that SECs representations are stored in the PFC on domain- and format-specific bases. In general, patients with ventral or medial PFC lesions are especially impaired in performing social and reward-related behavior (Dimitrov, Phipps, Zahn, & Grafman, 1999; Milne & Grafman, 2001), whereas patients with lesions to the DLPFC appear most impaired on mechanistic planning tasks (Burgess, Veitch, de Lacy Costello, & Shallice, 2000; Goel & Grafman, 2000).

In a PET study, our research group showed domain specificity in terms of localization of emotional versus nonemotional SEC representations within the PFC (Partiot, Grafman, Sadato, Wachs, & Hallett, 1995). For the nonemotional task, subjects were asked to "imagine silently the sequence of events and feelings concerned with preparation and dressing before (their) mother comes over for dinner." In contrast, for the emotional task, subjects were asked to "imagine silently the sequence of events and feelings concerned with preparation and dressing to go to (their) mother's funeral." Different patterns of PFC activation were revealed while the subjects generated the emotional and nonemotional scripts. The nonemotional script activated the right superior frontal gyrus (BA 8) and the bilateral middle (BA 8 and 9) and medial frontal gyri (BA 6 and 10), whereas the emotional script activated the left anterior cingulate (BA 24 and 32), bilateral medial frontal gyrus (BA 8 and 9), and anterior medial temporal lobe (BA 21).

Using fMRI, we showed further that social and nonsocial SECs have a distinctive representational topography in the PFC (Wood, Romero, Makale, & Grafman, 2003). We applied a modified go/no-go paradigm in which subjects had to classify either words (semantic: e.g., "menu" and "order") or phrases (scripts: e.g., "read the menu" and "order the food") according to category (social versus nonsocial).

Frontal activation for social activities was restricted to the left superior frontal gyrus (BA 8 and 9), whereas frontal activation for nonsocial activities was restricted to the right superior frontal gyrus (BA 8), left medial frontal gyrus (BA 6), and the bilateral anterior cingulate (BA 25). Orbitofrontal activation was not evident in that study. Visual inspection of the functional images showed a signal dropout in the orbitofrontal region and, therefore, we could not address the question of whether this region is implicated in the storage of social SECs. However, lesion data strongly support this viewpoint (Fuster, 1997; Milne & Grafman, 2001). Therefore, the fMRI findings were complemented by a lesion study in which patients with lesions of the PFC and matched controls were administered a classification task and a modified go/no-go paradigm (Wood, Knutson, & Grafman, 2005). Subjects were asked to classify events from social and nonsocial activities (e.g., read the menu and order the food) and related semantic items (e.g., menu and order) in terms of whether they belonged to a target activity. The results demonstrated that damage to the right orbitofrontal cortex results in impairment in the accessibility of script and semantic representations of social activities.

Finally, in another fMRI study we investigated the underlying psychological structure of event sequence knowledge and then used multidimensional scaling to identify its neural correlates (Wood et al., 2005). Multidimensional scaling is a qualitative statistical analysis technique that has been applied to explain the underlying structure of common representations (e.g., Halberstadt & Niedenthal, 1997; Kruskal & Wish, 1978; Taylor, Brugger, Weniger, & Regard, 1999). We applied multidimensional scaling to similarity ratings of pairs of events (e.g., "reading the menu" paired with "get the detergent" or "order the food") including events from social and nonsocial activities (Rosen, Caplan, Sheesley, Rodriguez, & Grafman, 2003). Three dimensions (engagement, social valence, and experience) were identified by regressing the dimension coordinates against ratings on preselected variables of interest (age of acquisition, frequency of performance, socialness, commonality, emotional valence, level of involvement, and rule knowledge). During the fMRI experiment, subjects were asked to decide whether events of activities were social (e.g., going out for dinner) or not (e.g., doing the laundry). Parametric analyses of event-related fMRI data were applied to establish which brain regions exhibited activation that covaried with the values for each of the three dimensions identified in the multidimensional scaling experiment. The experience dimension specifically activated the medial PFC (BA 10), the engagement dimension activated the left orbitofrontal cortex (BA 47), and the social valence dimension activated the amygdala and right orbitofrontal cortex (BA 11 and 47). The results demonstrated that the psychological structure of event sequence knowledge appears to be broadly organized along dimensions that are differentially stored across the human PFC.

In summary, these studies suggest that SECs are stored in different regions of the PFC on a category-specific basis. Specifically, nonsocial SECs are represented in the dorsolateral PFC and social SECs in the ventromedial PFC. The results are consistent with the anatomical reciprocal connectivity of these regions, with the dorsolateral PFC being connected primarily to nonemotional sensory and motor areas and the ventromedial PFC being connected non-emotional to social- and reward-related areas.

Frequency

The SEC framework predicts that the representation of an action sequence is partly dependent on how often a person enacts or observes the activity. Thus, memories for low-frequency event knowledge and high-frequency event knowledge should have differing accessibility. Furthermore, the higher the SEC frequency in use, the more resilient the SEC should be in the case of PFC damage.

There is neuropsychological evidence that supports the hypothesis that low-frequency and high-frequency event sequence knowledge is mediated by different neural substrates. Patients with anterior PFC damage show frequency effects in event knowledge tasks, with high-frequency event sequence knowledge being better preserved than low-frequency event sequence knowledge (Sirigu et al., 1995). In a recent fMRI study, our research group attempted to identify specialized regions within the PFC for different daily life activities that varied in frequency of experience (Krueger, Moll, Zahn, Heinecke, & Grafman, 2007). Daily life activities from a normative study were used in which individuals recorded their daily activities for 7 consecutive days (Rosen et al., 2003). The activities ranged along a frequency continuum from activities reported only once by a single individual during the week (e.g., going to an audition) to activities reported more than once by most or all of the individuals during the week (e.g., getting ready for work). After seeing the activity header (e.g., get ready for work) and a pair of events (e.g., wake up—get out of bed), subjects had to decide which one of the events occurred first in the chronological sequence of this activity. The results revealed a frequency gradient along the anterior-to-posterior axis of the medial PFC (MPFC), in which the anterior MPFC (BA 10) was engaged in low-frequency activities and the posterior MPFC (BA 10) in high-frequency activities. The frequency effect was independent of task difficulty as measured by response times and accuracy.

In our opinion, the anterior MPFC codes more complex cognitive information about an event sequence. As an event sequence becomes more frequently used, an economy of representation develops in which the posterior MPFC, activated in parallel with the anterior MPFC, codes sparser cognitive information about the same event sequence. This coding format leads to different profiles of MPFC activation, depending on the frequency of the event sequence the person executes. It would allow simpler representational codes to rapidly instruct lower-level systems (e.g., motor) to implement action sequences. In other words, the same activity can be performed quickly (e.g., by using a heuristic based on sparser coding) or slowly (e.g., by using deliberate reflection based on detailed coding), depending on situational demands on the stored event sequence knowledge.

Interestingly, each of the frequency-dependent MPFC regions falls onto one of the three architectonic subdivisions of human BA 10 proposed by Ongur, Ferry, and Price (2003). These subregions have a similar cellular pattern but vary in the degree of granularity and the development of cortical layer III (and layer IV), with the most prominent and well-developed layer III located in the polar area, which is not observed in nonhuman primates (Creutzfeldt, 1995). This increasing architectural complexity along the medial axis toward the fronto-polar cortex maps nicely onto our distinct activations for frequency-dependent knowledge across medial PFC subregions.

In conclusion, our results suggest that event sequence knowledge is subserved by different neural substrates within the PFC, depending on its frequency. Thus, the distributed representation of an SEC is partly dependent on how often a person enacts or observes these event sequences.

We have started to investigate the differential contributions of PFC subregions to specific formats of representation and categories of event sequence knowledge. There is positive evidence that the PFC is implicated in the storage of event knowledge that underlies cognitively induced actions. Yet many predictions of the SEC framework have not been fully explored to date and await more challenging tests. For example, what are the distinctions between predictable and unpredictable SECs in terms of their cognitive and topographical representations in the brain, or what are the precise roles of the left and right hemisphere in mediating SEC activation?

There has been little in the way of negative studies for this framework that links SECs to storage in the human PFC. One recent study reported that frontal lobe damage alone is not sufficient to cause impairment on everyday tasks (Humphreys & Forde, 1998). Another study found that a patient with frontal lobe damage was good at recalling the component actions from stored action scripts and performing these everyday tasks despite poor performance on more abstract "executive" tests. Another study reported no disruption of action representation in patients with frontal lobe lesions (Zanini, Rumiati, & Shallice, 2002). In action production and temporal sequencing tasks, these patients were as accurate as normal controls both in terms of the details reported and in terms of maintaining the temporal sequence. Despite these rare negative studies that contradict some of the findings reported previously, neuroimaging results are generally in agreement with our patient data, providing strong evidence that the PFC is critical for the storage of event sequence knowledge.

Conclusion

In this chapter, we have emphasized the idea that the human PFC stores SECs and that these SECs are the representational basis for cognitively motivated actions. We claimed that SECs are representations mediating goal-oriented sequences of events that are also required for planning and monitoring of complex behavior. The event sequence itself must be parsed as each event begins and ends in order to explicitly recognize the nature, duration, and number of events that compose this sequence (Zacks & Tversky, 2001). A broad definition of actions that are mediated by SECs includes movements from one location to another or those required to gesture or grasp as well as initiating deliberative thinking about whether a plan was effective in allowing a person to achieve a goal.

We argued for a "representational" approach of PFC function (as opposed to defining simple processes such as a controller, conflict resolver, executer, or manager as being the essence of what the PFC does) that seems to be most consistent with the structure, neurophysiology, and connectivity of the PFC as well as with a modern cognitive-neuroscience view that accepts that different locations in the brain store distinctive aspects of stimuli (e.g., the distinctive storage of orthographic, phonological, lexical, and semantic features of written words in different sectors of posterior cortex). The provided evidence for the SEC framework from neuropsychological studies of brain-injured patients and functional neuroimaging in healthy individuals confirm the importance and uniqueness of the human PFC for mediating knowledge at the level of cognitive events and action sequences. It also stresses the necessity, for designing experiments that control for a number of experimental variables, of using a representational framework.

We believe these SECs are the key to understanding the human ability to build and execute daily life activities. Such knowledge, when stored as memories, provides a link between past, current, and future activities. They allow us foresight and give us a significant cognitive advantage over other species. We argue there is now a substantial set of research results that suggest that studying the nature of the SEC is a competitive and fruitful way to additionally characterize and identify the distribution of the components of event knowledge in the human PFC. Although we will always be reminded that even knowledge stored in the PFC must coordinate with activated knowledge and processes stored in other areas of the brain leading to system-wide activations that underlie many aspects of functional behavior, the elusive scientific characterization of knowledge stores in the PFC remains the key missing part of the puzzle. We believe that the collected evidence so far has brought us one step closer to such an understanding of the contribution of the PFC to uniquely human behavior.

Acknowledgments

The authors are supported by the NINDS intramural research program.

References

Alexander, G. E., Crutcher, M. D., & DeLong, M. R. (1990). Basal ganglia-thalamocortical circuits: Parallel substrates for motor, oculomotor, "prefrontal" and "limbic" functions. *Progress in Brain Research, 85,* 119–146.

Barbas, H. (2000). Complementary roles of prefrontal cortical regions in cognition, memory, and emotion in primates. *Advances in Neurology, 84,* 87–110.

Beeman, M. J., & Bowden, E. M. (2000). The right hemisphere maintains solution-related activation for yet-to-be-solved problems. *Memory & Cognition, 28,* 1231–1241.

Brodmann, K. (1912). Neue Ergebnisse ueber die vergleichende histologische Lokalisation der Grosshirnrinde mit besonderer Beruecksichtigung des Stirnhirns. *Anatomischer Anzeiger, 41*(Suppl.), 157–216.

Burgess, P. W., Scott, S. K., & Frith, C. D. (2003). The role of the rostral frontal cortex (area 10) in prospective memory: A lateral versus medial dissociation. *Neuropsychologia, 41,* 906–918.

Burgess, P. W., Veitch, E., de Lacy Costello, A., & Shallice, T. (2000). The cognitive and neuroanatomical correlates of multitasking. *Neuropsychologia, 38,* 848–863.

Chiavaras, M. M., LeGoualher, G., Evans, A., & Petrides, M. (2001). Three-dimensional probabilistic atlas of the human orbitofrontal sulci in standardized stereotaxic space. *Neuroimage, 13,* 479–496.

Chugani, H. T., Phelps, M. E., & Mazziotta, J. C. (1987). Positron emission tomography study of human brain functional development. *Annals of Neurology, 22,* 487–497.

Conel, J. L. (1939). *The postnatal development of the human cerebral cortex* (Vols. 1–6). Cambridge, MA: Harvard University Press.

Creutzfeldt, O. (1995). *Cortex cerebri: Performance, structural and functional organization of the cortex.* Oxford, UK: Oxford University Press.

Crozier, S., Sirigu, A., Lehericy, S., van de Moortele, P. F., Pillon, B., Grafman J., et al. (1999). Distinct prefrontal activations in processing sequence at the sentence and script level: An fMRI study. *Neuropsychologia, 37,* 1469–1476.

Diamond, A. (1991). Guidelines for the study of brain-behavior relationships during development. In H. S. Levin, A. Eisenberg, & A. L. Benton (Eds.), *Frontal lobe function and dysfunction.* New York: Oxford University Press, 339–378.

Dimitrov, M., Phipps, M., Zahn, T., & Grafman, J. (1999). A thoroughly modern Gage. *Neurocase, 5,* 345–354.

Duncan, J. (2001). An adaptive coding model of neural function in prefrontal cortex. *Nature Reviews: Neuroscience, 2,* 820–829.

Durston, S., Hulshoff Pol, H. E., Casey, B. J., Giedd, J. N., Buitelaar, J. K., & van Engeland, H. (2001). Anatomical MRI of the developing human brain: What have we learned? *Journal of the American Academy of Child and Adolescent Psychiatry, 40,* 1012–1020.

Elston, G. N. (2000). Pyramidal cells of the frontal lobe: All the more spinous to think with. *Journal of Neuroscience, 20,* RC95.

Elston, G. N., & Rosa, M. G. (2000). Pyramidal cells, patches, and cortical columns: A comparative study of infragranular neurons in TEO, TE, and the superior temporal polysensory area of the macaque monkey. *Journal of Neuroscience, 20,* RC117.

Engel, A. K., & Singer, W. (2001). Temporal binding and the neural correlates of sensory awareness. *Trends in Cognitive Sciences, 5,* 16–25.

Eslinger, P. J., & Damasio, A. R. (1985). Severe disturbance of higher cognition after bilateral frontal lobe ablation: Patient EVR. *Neurology, 35,* 1731–1741.

Flechsig, P. (1920). *Anatomie des menschlichen Gehirns und Rueckenmarks auf myelogenetischer Grundlage.* Leipzig: Thieme.

Fuster, J. M. (1980). *The prefrontal cortex: Anatomy, physiology and neuropsychology of the frontal lobe.* New York: Raven Press.

Fuster, J. M. (1991). The prefrontal cortex and its relation to behavior. *Progress in Brain Research, 87,* 201–211.

Fuster, J. M., Bodner, M., & Kroger, J. K. (2000). Cross-modal and cross-temporal association in neurons of frontal cortex. *Nature, 405,* 347–351.

Giedd, J. N., Blumenthal, J., Jeffries, N. O., Castellanos, F. X., Liu, H., Zijdenbos, A., et al. (1999). Brain development during childhood and adolescence: A longitudinal MRI study. *Nature Neuroscience, 2,* 861–863.

Gilbert, S. J., Spengler, S., Simons, J. S., Frith, C. D., & Burgess, P. W. (2006). Differential functions of lateral and medial rostral prefrontal cortex (area 10) revealed by brain-behavior associations. *Cerebral Cortex, 16,* 1783–1789.

Gilbert, S. J., Spengler, S., Simons, J. S., Steele, J. D., Lawrie, S. M., Frith, C. D., et al. (2006). Functional specialization within rostral prefrontal cortex (Area 10): A meta-analysis. *Journal of Cognitive Neuroscience, 18,* 932–948.

Goel, V. (1995). *Sketches of thought.* Cambridge, MA: MIT Press.

Goel, V., & Grafman, J. (2000). The role of the right prefrontal cortex in ill-structured problem solving. *Cognitive Neuropsychology, 17,* 415–436.

Goel, V., Tierney, M., Sheesley, L., Bartolo, A., Vartanian, O., & Grafman, J. (2006). Hemispheric specialization in human prefrontal cortex for resolving certain and uncertain inferences. *Cerebral Cortex, 17,* 2245–2250.

Goldberg, E., Podell, K., & Lovell, M. (1994). Lateralization of frontal lobe functions and cognitive novelty. *Journal of Neuropsychiatry & Clinical Neuroscience, 6,* 371–378.

Goldman-Rakic, P. S. (1987). *Circuitry of primate prefrontal cortex and regulation of behavior by representational memory.* Washington, DC: American Physiological Society.

Goldman-Rakic, P. S. (1992). Working memory and the mind. *Scientific American, 267,* 110–117.

Grafman, J. (1995). Similarities and distinctions among current models of prefrontal cortical functions. In J. Grafman, K. J. Holyoak, & F. Boller (Eds.), *Structure and functions of the human prefrontal cortex* (pp. 337–368.) New York: New York Academy of Sciences.

Grafman, J. (2002). The human prefrontal cortex has evolved to represent components of structured event complexes. In J. Grafman (Ed.), *Handbook of neuropsychology* (Vol. 7, pp. 157–174). Amsterdam: Elsevier.

Groenewegen, H. J., & Uylings, H. B. (2000). The prefrontal cortex and the integration of sensory, limbic and autonomic information. *Progress in Brain Research, 126,* 3–28.

Halberstadt, J. B., & Niedenthal, P. M. (1997). Emotional state and the use of stimulus dimensions in judgment. *Journal of Personality & Social Psychology, 72,* 1017–1033.

Huettel, S. A., Song, A. W., & McCarthy, G. (2005). Decisions under uncertainty: Probabilistic context influences activation of prefrontal and parietal cortices. *Journal of Neuroscience, 25,* 3304–3311.

Huey, E. D., Krueger, F., & Grafman, J. (2006). Representations in the human prefrontal cortex. *Current Directions in Psychological Science, 15,* 167–171.

Humphreys, G. W., & Forde, E. M. (1998). Disordered action schema and action disorganization syndrome. *Cognitive Neuropsychology, 15,* 771–811.

Huttenlocher, P. R. (1990). Morphometric study of human cerebral cortex development. *Neuropsychologia, 28,* 517–527.

Huttenlocher, P. R., & Dabholkar, A. S. (1997). Regional differences in synaptogenesis in human cerebral cortex. *Journal of Comparative Neurology, 387,* 167–178.

Janowsky, J. S., Shimamura, A. P., & Squire, L. R. (1989). Source memory impairment in patients with frontal lobe lesions. *Neuropsychologia, 27,* 1043–1056.

Knutson, K. M., Wood, J. N., & Grafman, J. (2004). Brain activation in processing temporal sequence: An fMRI study. *Neuroimage, 23,* 1299–1307.

Koechlin, E., Corrado, G., Pietrini, P., & Grafman, J. (2000). Dissociating the role of the medial and lateral anterior prefrontal cortex in human planning. *Proceedings of the National Academy of Sciences of the United States of America, 97,* 7651–7656.

Krueger, F., Moll, J., Zahn, R., Heinecke, A., & Grafman, J. (2007). Event frequency modulates the processing of daily life activities in human medial prefrontal cortex. *Cerebral Cortex, 17,* 2346–2353.

Kruskal, J. B., & Wish, M. (1978). *Multidimensional scaling.* London: Sage Publications.

Levy, R., & Goldman-Rakic, P. S. (2000). Segregation of working memory functions within the dorsolateral prefrontal cortex. *Experimental Brain Research, 133,* 23–32.

Masterman, D. L., & Cummings, J. L. (1997). Frontal-subcortical circuits: The anatomic basis of executive, social and motivated behaviors. *Journal of Psychopharmacology, 11,* 107–114.

Miller, E. K., & Cohen, J. D. (2001). An integrative theory of prefrontal cortex function. *Annual Review of Neuroscience, 24,* 167–202.

Milne, E., & Grafman, J. (2001). Ventromedial prefrontal cortex lesions in humans eliminate implicit gender stereotyping. *Journal of Neuroscience, 21,* RC150 (1–6).

Milner, B., Petrides, M., & Smith, M. L. (1985). Frontal lobes and the temporal organization of memory. *Human Neurobiology, 4,* 137–142.

Moll, J., Zahn, R., de Oliveira-Souza, R., Krueger, F., & Grafman, J. (2005). Opinion: The neural basis of human moral cognition. *Nature Review Neuroscience, 6,* 799–809.

Nichelli, P., Clark, K., Hollnagel, C., & Grafman, J. (1995). Duration processing after frontal lobe lesions. *Annals of the New York Academy of Sciences, 769,* 183–190.

Ongur, D., Ferry, A. T., & Price, J. L. (2003). Architectonic subdivision of the human orbital and medial prefrontal cortex. *Journal of Comparative Neurology, 460,* 425–449.

O'Reilly, R. C., & Rudy, J. W. (2000). Computational principles of learning in the neocortex and hippocampus. *Hippocampus, 10,* 389–397.

Pandya, D. N., & Yeterian, E. H. (1996). Morphological correlations of human and monkey frontal lobe. In A. R. Damasio, H. Damasio, & Y. Christen (Eds.), *Neurobiology of decision making* (pp. 13–46). Berlin: Springer.

Partiot, A., Grafman, J., Sadato, N., Wachs, J., & Hallett, M. (1995). Brain activation during the generation of non-emotional and emotional plans. *Neuroreport, 6,* 1397–1400.

Paulus, M. P., Hozack, N., Zauscher, B., McDowell, J. E., Frank, L., Brown, G. G., et al. (2001). Prefrontal, parietal, and temporal cortex networks underlie decision-making in the presence of uncertainty. *Neuroimage, 13,* 91–100.

Paus, T., Zijdenbos, A., Worsley, K., Collins, D. L., Blumenthal, J., Giedd, J. N., et al. (1999).

Structural maturation of neural pathways in children and adolescents: In vivo study. *Science, 283,* 1908–1911.

Price, J. L. (1999). Prefrontal cortical networks related to visceral function and mood. *Annals of the New York Academy of Sciences, 877,* 383–396.

Rilling, J. K., & Insel, T. R. (1999). The primate neocortex in comparative perspective using magnetic resonance imaging. *Journal of Human Evolution, 37,* 191–223.

Rosen, V. M., Caplan, L., Sheesley, L., Rodriguez, R., & Grafman, J. (2003). An examination of daily activities and their scripts across the adult lifespan. *Behavior Research Methods, Instruments, and Computers: A Journal of the Psychonomic Society, Inc., 35,* 32–48.

Rueckert, L., & Grafman, J. (1996). Sustained attention deficits in patients with right frontal lesions. *Neuropsychologia, 34,* 953–963.

Rueckert, L., & Grafman, J. (1998). Sustained attention deficits in patients with lesions of posterior cortex. *Neuropsychologia, 36,* 653–660.

Rumelhart, D. E. (1980). Schemata: The building blocks of cognition. In R. J. Spiro, B. C. Bruce, & W. F. Brewer (Eds.), *Theoretical issues in reading comprehension: Perspectives from cognitive psychology, linguistics, artificial intelligence, and education* (pp. 33–58). Hillsdale, NJ: Lawrence Erlbaum Associates.

Schank, R., & Abelson, P. (1997). *Scripts, plans, goals and understanding.* Hillsdale, NJ: Lawrence Erlbaum Associates.

Semendeferi, K., Armstrong, E., Schleicher, A., Zilles, K., & van Hoesen, G. W. (2001). Prefrontal cortex in humans and apes: A comparative study of area 10. *American Journal of Physical Anthropology, 114,* 224–241.

Semendeferi, K., Lu, A., Schenker, N., & Damasio, H. (2002). Humans and great apes share a large frontal cortex. *Nature Neuroscience, 5,* 272–276.

Shallice, T. (1982). Specific impairments of planning. *Philosophical Transactions of the Royal Society of London. Series B, Biological Sciences, 298,* 199–209.

Shallice, T., & Burgess, P. W. (1991). Deficits in strategy application following frontal lobe damage in man. *Brain, 114*(Pt. 2), 727–741.

Shallice, T., & Burgess, P. (1998). The domain of supervisory processes and the temporal organization of behaviour. In A. C. Roberts, T. W. Robbins, & L. Weiskrantz (Eds.), *The prefrontal cortex: Executive and cognitive functions.* Oxford: Oxford University Press.

Sirigu, A., Cohen, L., Zalla, T., Pradat-Diehl, P., Van Eeckhout, P., Grafman, J., et al. (1998). Distinct frontal regions for processing sentence syntax and story grammar. *Cortex, 34,* 771–778.

Sirigu, A., Zalla, T., Pillon, B., Grafman, J., Agid, Y., & Dubois, B. (1995). Selective impairments in managerial knowledge following pre-frontal cortex damage. *Cortex, 31,* 301–316.

Sirigu, A., Zalla, T., Pillon, B., Grafman, J., Agid, Y., & Dubois B. (1996). Encoding of sequence and boundaries of scripts following prefrontal lesions. *Cortex, 32,* 297–310.

Sowell, E. R., Thompson, P. M., Holmes, C. J., Jernigan, T. L., & Toga, A. W. (1999). In vivo evidence for post-adolescent brain maturation in frontal and striatal regions. *Nature Neuroscience, 2,* 859–861.

Stuss, D. T., & Benson, D. F. (1984). Neuropsychological studies of the frontal lobes. *Psychology Bulletin, 95,* 3–28.

Stuss, D. T., & Benson, D. F. (1986). *The frontal lobes.* New York: Raven Press.

Taylor, K. I., Brugger, P., Weniger, D., & Regard, M. (1999). Qualitative hemispheric differences in semantic category matching. *Brain Language, 70,* 119–131.

Weingartner, H., Grafman, J., Boutelle, W., Kaye, W., & Martin, P. R. (1983). Forms of memory failure. *Science, 221,* 380–382.

Wood, J. N., & Grafman, J. (2003). Human prefrontal cortex: Processing and representational perspectives. *Nature Reviews: Neuroscience, 4,* 139–147.

Wood, J. N., Knutson, K. M., & Grafman, J. (2005). Psychological structure and neural correlates of event knowledge. *Cerebral Cortex, 15,* 1155–1161.

Wood, J. N., Romero, S. G., Makale, M., & Grafman, J. (2003). Category-specific representations of social and nonsocial knowledge in the human prefrontal cortex. *Journal of Cognitive Neuroscience, 15,* 236–248.

Zacks, J. M., Braver, T. S., Sheridan, M. A., Donaldson, D. I., Snyder, A. Z., Ollinger, J. M., et al. (2001). Human brain activity time-locked to perceptual event boundaries. *Nature Neuroscience, 4,* 651–655.

Zacks, J. M., Speer, N. K., Swallow, K. M., Braver, T. S., & Reynolds, J. R. (2007). Event perception: A mind-brain perspective. *Psychology Bulletin, 133,* 273–293.

Zacks, J. M., & Tversky, B. (2001). Event structure in perception and conception. *Psychology Bulletin, 127,* 3–21.

Zacks, J. M., Tversky, B., & Iyer, G. (2001). Perceiving, remembering, and communicating structure in events. *Journal of Experimental Psychology: General, 130,* 29–58.

Zanini, S., Rumiati, R. I., & Shallice T. (2002). Action sequencing deficit following frontal lobe lesion. *Neurocase, 8,* 88–99.

Interactions Between Action and Visual Objects

Rob Ellis

Abstract

This chapter examines the interactions between actions and visual objects. It is argued that represented visual objects, whether we are seeing them or recalling them in memory, propel us to act on them. If a represented object has to be ignored so that actions can be directed toward another, target object, then actions associated with the ignored object are inhibited. Our action intentions also direct us to see aspects of the world that are congruent with those intentions. Such conclusions about the relations between action and visual objects reinforce the validity of the view that perceptual systems have evolved in all species of animals solely as a means of guiding and controlling action, either present or future.

Keywords: stimulus-response, object-action compatibility, action, perception

This chapter considers the conjecture that brain states represent visual objects by virtue of their potentiating or making available an ensemble of appropriate overt behaviors or actions. A particular representational brain state is given content, or grounded, by the behaviors that it makes available.

If motor activity is partly constitutive of the representation of a visual object, it is not sufficient that there is co-occurrence between visual activity and some motor activity or other. After all, while I type this line, I have in sight a coffee mug, and the key pressing is clearly not involved in the representation of the mug. We speculate that, in this case, covert motor activity, which is associated with coffee mugs, forms part of the representation of this particular mug.

This motor activity will have been associated with the visual responses to the mug as a result of learning and is involved in object representation as well as the control of responses. Our theory has the perhaps counterintuitive implication that seeing the coffee mug may have an observable effect on my typing activities. Moreover, these effects are not dependent on my desire for a cup of coffee. The claim is that the mere sight of an object will elicit associated motor activity, and this may interact with goal-directed actions. In addition, the converse would be expected. If action codes form an intrinsic part of visual representation, performing (or preparing) an action may affect visual function. This chapter considers the behavioral evidence for both such effects.

Stimulus–Response Compatibility

So do seen objects produce behavioral effects unrelated to the current activities or goals of the viewer? This is precisely what is suggested by the so-called Simon effect. It is well established, within the extensive stimulus–response compatibility (SRC) literature (for reviews, see Alluisi & Warm, 1990; Kornblum, 1992) that congruent mappings of response to stimuli, in a choice-reaction-time experiment, produce faster and more accurate responses than incongruent mappings. A simple case is that responding with the left hand to stimuli appearing in the left visual field and with the right hand to stimuli in the right field is faster than the reverse mapping (Nicoletti, Anzola, Luppino, Rizzolatti, & Umilta, 1982). In these cases there was an explicit overlap of stimulus and response features. In the Simon effect case, similar spatial compatibility effects are observed, even when the spatial dimension of the stimulus is irrelevant to the response (Simon, 1969). For example, when colored stimuli are presented to the left or right visual field and the color cues the hand of response, responses are faster if the stimulus position corresponds to the hand of response. The traditional information-processing account of these SRC effects is in terms of the abstract response codes that are automatically generated by the presentation of a stimulus. The most precise and explicit formulation of this view is the dimensional overlap model (Kornblum, 1992; Kornblum, Hasbroucq, & Osman, 1990; Kornblum & Lee, 1995). A key concept in this is the notion of similarity between the *mental representation* of sets of stimuli and sets of response options. Similarity, physical or conceptual, may exist between the sets, and this is termed "dimensional overlap." Whenever dimensional overlap exists between, say, response sets and stimuli sets in a forced-choice task, then presentation of a stimulus property will evoke the mental representation of the corresponding response property. So a stimulus appearing on the left will evoke the mental code for a left response if the task is to respond with the left or right hand to some property of that object. In addition to this automatic activation, it is assumed that there is also a translation process that identifies the correct response for a particular stimulus property. The interaction between these two processes depends on the precise nature of the dimensional overlap and whether the dimensions are relevant to the task. In the circumstances in which the Simon effect is obtained (dimensional overlap between the response set and some task-irrelevant aspect of the stimuli), responses that are congruent with the irrelevant stimulus are facilitated in the following way. When the response code generated by the irrelevant stimulus dimension matches the response code that results from the translation mechanism, an immediate response can be initiated. In contrast, when the two codes differ, the one resulting from the irrelevant aspect of the stimuli must be inhibited or aborted and the correct response retrieved. This selection task produces an increase in response latency compared to the congruent case.

The dimensional overlap model shares with our view the assumption that stimuli may elicit response-related codes automatically. On our account, this results from the fact that the encoding of stimuli necessarily includes action-related properties. It is not just similarity that will produce SRC effects but also the relations between object properties and associated actions. Some SRC theorists have made similar claims.

Michaels (1988, 1993) has described a Gibsonian framework for explaining SRC effects. She argues that some of the benefits of compatible mappings depend not on arbitrary pairings between mental codes for aspects of a stimulus and responses but on ecological relations between visual properties and coordinated action. This approach, being Gibsonian, rejects the notion of mental representation. In contrast, Hommel (1997) has proposed the notion of the action concept, which forms the basis of intentional action (see also Greenwald, 1970; Prinz, 1990; see chapters 2 and 18). The action concept is an elaboration of the ideomotor notion of action effects. It is a representation of the sensory effects of a voluntary action and becomes associated with the motor pattern producing the effects and so forms the basis of voluntary actions. An agent can produce an intended effect by choosing an appropriate action concept that in turn selects the appropriate motor responses. Compatibility effects occur because stimulus codes may overlap with effect codes, leading to response competition in some cases.

Object–Action Compatibility

Most SRC experiments are of course profoundly nonecological. Stimuli are almost always highly abstract, and the response required of a participant is precisely that: a single response rather than a coherent action. If the ideas sketched thus far here about relations between perception and action are to be tested, new questions must be posed and appropriate experimental techniques devised. For instance, it seems important to establish that spatial location is not the only aspect of a visual object that may produce a Simon effect. The following studies were designed to answer this question. More specifically, they asked whether graspable objects potentiate reaching and grasping regardless of an explicit intention to handle the object. In all the experiments, participants viewed a real object or an image of a real object and, simultaneously or shortly afterward, made one of two responses determined by various criteria. The responses were designed to

be components of a reach-to-grasp. Three action components were investigated: (a) left- or right-handed responses, (b) clockwise or counterclockwise wrist rotations, and (c) power or precision grips.

Hand of Response

Tucker and Ellis (1998) described experiments in which participants viewed photographs of common, graspable objects. Each object was depicted in two vertical orientations—upright and inverted—and in two horizontal orientations. One of the horizontal orientations was designed to be maximally compatible with a right-handed reach-to-grasp and the other with a left-handed action. For example, a centrally placed cup with a handle to the right of the viewer would be most compatible with a right-handed reach-to-grasp, whereas the same cup with its handle to the left would be most compatible with a left-handed action of this sort. On presentation of a photograph, subjects had to decide whether the depicted object was upright or inverted and signal their decision by a speeded right- or left-handed key press. Broadly, performance was better when the hand of response was the same as the hand that would be optimal for reaching and grasping the object in its depicted orientation compared to the incompatible case. This interaction of the object compatibility with the hand of response is illustrated in Figure 11.1 and is referred to as the object–action compatibility effect.

Can the object–action compatibility effect be explained in terms of the overlap between abstract stimulus and response codes? That is, did the horizontal orientation of the objects evoke an abstract left or right stimulus code that had an effect on a left or right response code needed to make the correct key press? The possibility that this shared dimension was the source of the effect appears to be ruled out by the second experiment reported by Tucker and

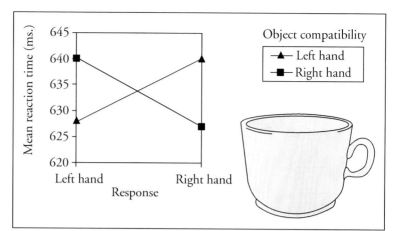

Fig. 11.1 The object–action compatibility effect, in response latency, on the hand of response when classifying objects (such as in the cup example) that are oriented so as to have an optimal hand of grasp (the right hand in the cup example).

Ellis (1998). This was in all respects identical to the first, except participants now indicated the vertical orientation of the depicted objects by key presses with the index and middle fingers of their right hand. In these circumstances, no interaction of object compatibility with finger of response was observed. This clearly suggests that the interaction observed in the first experiment depended on the relations between the horizontal orientation of the objects and the optimal effector for handling such objects. That is, it was a real *object*-to-*action* compatibility effect of the sort predicted by the action potentiation account of visual representation. A second series of experiments tend to confirm this view in that they show an analogous effect of relations between different aspects of a stimulus and a response. Moreover, the relations are between object properties (their orientation with respect to the viewer) and an aspect of a response (the direction of wrist rotation) which appear not to share a common dimension.

Direction of Wrist Rotation

In general, a reach-to-grasp action requires a wrist rotation so as to align the hand with the opposition axis of the object to be grasped (Jeannerod, 1981; Jeannerod, Paulignan, Mackenzie, & Marteniuk, 1992). Compatibility effects on this action element have also been reported

in experiments using real objects (Ellis & Tucker, 2000). Two classes of object were used. One type consisted of tall cylindrical objects, such as bottles, which required a clockwise rotation to grasp, assuming the hand started from an orientation of having the thumb at 11:00. The other sort of objects were small, such as a bottle cap, or had an elongated, horizontal major axis at right angles to the line of sight, such as a bottle laid on its side. For these objects, from the same starting position, a counterclockwise wrist rotation would be required to grasp the object.

Objects of this sort were placed singly within a device that allowed their tachistoscopic presentation. Participants were required to keep their right hand adjacent to a to-be-presented object and maintain the hand orientation so that the thumb was aligned with the 11:00 position. When the hand was so aligned (as measured by a mercury switch attached to the wrist), the object was exposed, and a short time later, a high or low tone was sounded while the object remained in view. Participants were told to remember the object for the purposes of a subsequent recognition task and signal the type of tone by a wrist rotation.

Despite the response being relevant to an entirely different, auditory stimulus, it was affected by the seen object. As in the previous hand-of-response case, a significant interaction of object compatibility and response was observed in the response latency data.

Hand Shape

A third component of reaching and grasping for which we have observed object–action compatibility effects is the hand shape needed to handle an object (Tucker & Ellis, 2001). In a first experiment, participants decided whether a briefly presented real object was organic or manufactured. They signaled their decision by either a power grip, as in squeezing a lemon, or a precision grip, as in picking up a pin. The seen objects were of two types: objects that would normally be grasped with a power grip and those that would normally be handled using a precision grip. Once again, a significant interaction of object compatibility and response type was obtained, similar in kind to that obtained for hand of response.

Taken together, the data are consistent with the idea that seeing an object potentiates actions associated with them. We term the effects microaffordance for reasons that will be discussed in a subsequent section. Related effects have been reported in participants making actual reach-to-grasp responses. Craighero, Fadiga, Rizzolatti, and Umilta (1996, 1998) demonstrated facilitation of reaching and grasping an oriented bar when a cue to respond was a picture of a bar having a similar orientation. This they termed "visuomotor priming."

Microaffordance and Remembered Objects

If action potentiation is the consequence of visual representation, it would be expected in the case of imagined or remembered objects as well as seen. Derbyshire, Ellis, and Tucker (2006) confirm that microaffordance is observed in these cases. In one experiment, effects of the orientation of remembered objects were observed. Participants viewed a rapid sequence of four images of objects, one of which was orientated to be compatible with a left- or a right-hand grasp. Each image was presented for 1 second, followed by a blank interval of 100 milliseconds, followed by a word that named an object. Participants responded with a left- or a right-hand key press according to whether such an object had appeared in the sequence of images. In these circumstances, the same object–action compatibility effect was observed as obtained in the case of seen objects. Importantly, this effect did not depend on the position of the recalled object in the presentation sequence and was not therefore the result of transient motor activation resulting from the presentation of the last image in the sequence. We conclude that microaffordance is a product of the representation of an object, whether elicited by external or by internal stimulation.

Object-Based Attention and Object-Based Ignoring

The possibility that seen objects potentiate associated actions regardless of intent poses a problem for theories of selection for action (Allport, 1987; Castiello, 1996, 1999). How do the actions on a goal-relevant object escape the competition from actions potentiated by irrelevant objects? One possibility is that the actions of ignored objects are actively inhibited. Inhibition of the visual properties of an ignored object is well established (Tipper, 1985, 1992) and is illustrated by the negative priming effect. For instance, ignoring a red letter so as to respond to a green letter will lead to a decrement in performance whenever the ignored letter appears as a target in the next trial. If, as we argue, object representations include visual *and* action properties, it should follow that action inhibition would be expected when an object has to be ignored.

A series of studies in which participants have to respond to one of two objects suggests that the actions associated with the ignored object are, indeed, inhibited (Ellis, Tucker, Symes, & Vainio, 2007). The stimuli consisted of images of abstract three-dimensional forms displayed against a realistic three-dimensional background. Each image contained two such objects drawn from a set of four: a small sphere, a small cube, a larger rectangular block, and a larger cylinder. The small objects were sized so as to be compatible with a precision grip, and the larger were compatible with a power grip. The target object was cued by its color, and participants had to signal whether it was "curved" (sphere and cylinder) or "straight" (rectangular block or cube) by making a power or precision grip.

The usual microaffordance effect was observed for the target object, with faster and more accurate responses made when compatible with the action properties of the target than when incompatible. Performance was also strongly affected by the action properties of the distractor object. Responding to a target with a grip type that was compatible with the action properties of the distractor object produced a decrement in performance relative to the incompatible cases. The effects of the selected and ignored objects were effectively the reverse of each other, as may be seen in Figure 11.2.

This outcome, a negative compatibility effect for the ignored objects, is consistent with the idea that selecting an object to act on requires inhibition of the actions associated with the nonselected objects. Moreover, the negative compatibility effect was not influenced by spatial configuration—it was observed regardless of whether the distractor was directly in front of the target (and therefore an obstacle) or behind the target (experiment 1) or when there was a wide separation between the target and distractor (experiments 2 and 4). The distractor effect therefore appears to have arisen not from physical, spatial clutter but rather from "representational clutter."

Selecting one object from several requires that the actions associated with the nonselected items be inhibited. Inhibition is not observed, however, when the location of the target is known in advance of its appearance (experiment 3 in Ellis et al., 2007). The most effective strategy in this situation would have been to allocate spatial attention, by default, to the known fixed location of the target. In these circumstances, the distractor objects did affect responses, but this did not vary according to the actions associated with them. It was their visual and spatial properties (such as size or their distance from the target object) that determined their interference effects, not whether the actions associated with them were compatible with the response being made. These data imply that microaffordance (and the consequent need to inhibit actions of nontarget objects) is an outcome of object-based attention.

There is other evidence to support the claim that microaffordance effects are a consequence of object-based attention. Vainio, Ellis, and Tucker (2007) reported data showing that some minimal level of attention to an object was required in order for it to afford action. Their participants maintained fixation on a small, central circle that was then replaced by a task-irrelevant visual object (the prime object) that was oriented for a left- or a right-hand reach-to-grasp. The fixation circle then *reappeared* superimposed on the prime object (at its center). After an unpredictable delay, a target symbol ("−" or "+") appeared very briefly within the circle, and participants responded to the target with a left- or a right-hand key press. The irrelevant prime object produced the usual object–action compatibility effects, with performance

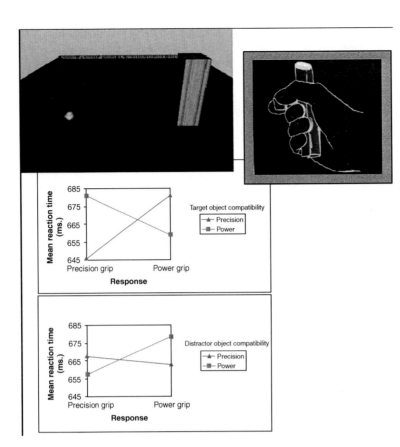

Fig. 11.2 Object–action compatibility effects, in response latency, for the target and distractor objects in two object displays (as illustrated in the example) on precision and power grip responses (made on the response device also illustrated) classifying the shape of the target object (cued by its blue-gray color).

being superior whenever the response hand was compatible with the hand that would be used to handle the prime object. This effect was entirely eliminated if the fixation circle remained throughout the presentation of the prime object. It seems that engagement with the fixation circle prevented participants noticing or coding the prime object. Although the prime object appeared at the center of the participant's visual field, we suggest that it was not represented as an object; consequently, actions associated with it were not potentiated.

Attending to an individual visual feature of an object does not appear to be sufficient to derive that object's affordance for action either. Responses to single objects show object–action compatibility effects whenever the response criterion is a relatively high-level property, such as object category membership (e.g. Tucker & Ellis, 2001). If the response criterion is a relatively low-level property, such as the object's color,

object–action compatibility effects are not observed. Symes, Ellis, and Tucker (2005) reported object–action compatibility effects when participants responded with a left- or a right-hand key press to the object category (kitchen object or garage object) of left- and right-oriented objects. When these same objects were categorized in terms of their color (green object or red object), no such effect was observed. We argue that detecting color does not entail attending to an object *as an object*, whereas categorizing an object's identity does. Microaffordance effects therefore appear to be a product of object-level attention.

That affordance is the outcome of object-level attention is consistent with theories in which selection for action depends on object-level representation (Allport, 1987; Kahneman & Treisman, 1984). It also implies that physical objects are assemblies of features that afford specific actions, with the object-level representation depending on what action is under consideration, that is, what the object is taken to be (Allport, 1987). Selection is necessary, at least in part, because of the physical limitations of the effector systems, which restrict the number of objects that can be acted on at any point in time. For these reasons, object representation, object selection, and object affordance must be tightly coupled.

Effects of Action on Perception

Were it the case that object representation, object selection, and object affordance are related in this way, then actions might be expected to have effects on perceptual processes, mirroring the effects of perceptual processes on action. Evidence is accumulating that this is indeed the case.

Wohlschläger (2000) has shown that the direction of movement of ambiguous, apparent motion displays can be influenced by rotations of the observer's hand. A counterclockwise hand rotation, for instance, will induce the perception of a counterclockwise rotation of the ambiguous display. A number of studies have suggested that action planning has a very direct effect on visual attention, with stimulus-compatible actions resulting in improved visual discrimination (e.g., Craighero, Fadiga, Rizzolatti, & Umilta, 1999; Fagioli, Hommel, & Schubotz, 2007; Pavese & Buxbaum, 2002). A recent series of experiments demonstrated this in the case of change blindness (Symes, Tucker, Ellis, & Vainio, in press). Participants viewed two alternating scenes each containing an array of fruit and vegetables. Half the items in each scene were small and would be typically grasped with a precision grip (e.g., a strawberry). The others were larger and would be graspable with a power grip (e.g., an apple). The scenes differed in that just one of the items was replaced by another fruit or vegetable of roughly the same size. When a screen flicker disrupted the interval

(150 milliseconds) between the two scenes, the usual change-blindness effect was observed. That is, the change was surprisingly difficult to detect given its dramatic nature, taking an average of 4,809 milliseconds to signal the change with a key-press response.

When, in contrast, participants signaled detection of the change by making either a precision or a power grip response, a marked compatibility benefit was observed. So when they prepared such a response given a change in a compatible object (e.g., a change in a strawberry signaled by a precision grip or a change in an apple signaled by a power grip for instance), the average time to detect that change was reduced to 4,510 milliseconds. The preparation of an action had directed or biased visual attention to action-compatible objects.

There are investigations of the influences of action on visual discrimination that, at face value, appear to contradict these data and the inferences drawn from them. They show that in some circumstances, the preparation or execution of an action can impair the discrimination of a compatible visual simile. So-called blindness to response compatible stimuli is an example. Musseler and Hommel (1997) had participants prepare a left- or a right-hand key press. Immediately prior to its execution, they were presented with a masked right- or left-pointing arrow. The likelihood of identifying the arrow was *reduced* if a compatible key press was planned during its presentation compared to the incompatible cases.[1] "Blindness" effects such as these have been accounted for in terms of a modern elaboration of ideomotor theory.

The theory of event coding (TEC) shares with the ideomotor approach the aim of accounting for the basis of purposeful action (Hommel, Musseler, Aschersleben, & Prinz, 2001). A central presumption of TEC is that perception and action share a coding system. Both a right-hand action and a right-pointing arrow will include an abstract feature code for "right" in their internal representation. A plan for an action will involve the binding together of active feature codes, and when so bound, the particular feature values will be less available for other representational purposes. Thus, if I currently intend to make a right-hand key press, this will impair my ability to encode a right-pointing arrow that appears around the same time. Thus, I will be momentarily "blind" to action-compatible stimuli. TEC accounts for the cases where action preparation facilitates visual discrimination in terms of the time course for the construction of action plans (Stoet & Hommel, 2002). During an initial, consolidation phase (of some few hundred milliseconds), the unbound features making up the action plan may prime subsequent perceptual events. Thus, whether planning an action impairs or enhances processing of a visual stimulus is determined by the temporal relations between the two events.

The Symes et al. (in press) change-blindness study suggests that a time course account of the differential effects of action planning does not account for all circumstances. Participants in these experiments had prepared their precision or power grip response 4 to 5 seconds prior to its execution, yet this fully consolidated action plan facilitated compatible perceptual objects. We *speculate* that, in fact, it is the relationship between the planned action and the perceptual object that determines the effect of the former on the latter. If the prepared action is to be made as a response to the object, then performance is enhanced by compatibility between the two (as in Symes et al., in press). If the prepared action is to be made as a response not to the object (as in Musseler & Hommel, 1997) but to some other event or stimulus, performance impairments may be observed.

Conclusions

Represented visual objects, whether we are seeing them or recalling them in memory, propel us to act on them. If a represented object has to be ignored so that actions can be directed toward another, target object, then actions associated with the ignored object are inhibited. It also appears that our action intentions direct us to see aspects of the world that are congruent with those intentions. Such conclusions about the relations between action and visual objects reinforce the validity of the view that

> perceptual systems have evolved in all species of animals solely as a means of guiding and controlling action, either present or future. Indeed, I find it difficult to get any clear conception of what "perception" might be, as a subject of scientific study, isolated from its role in the control of action. (Allport, 1987, p. 396)

Note

1. It is important to note that the response to the arrow was not the prepared key press but another action. This will be said to be significant at the end of this section.

References

Allport, D. A. (1987). Selection for action: Some behavioral and neurophysiological considerations of attention and action. In H. Heuer & F. Sanders (Eds.), *Perspectives on perception and action* (pp. 395–419). Hillsdale, NJ: Lawrence Erlbaum Associates.

Alluisi, E. A., & Warm, J. S. (1990). Things that go together: A review of stimulus-response compatibility and related effects. In R. W. Proctor & T. G. Reeve (Eds.), *Stimulus-response compatibility—An integrated perspective* (pp. 3–30). Amsterdam: North-Holland.

Castiello, U. (1996). Grasping a fruit: Selection for action. *Journal of Experimental Psychology: Human Perception and Performance, 22,* 582–603.

Castiello, U. (1999). Mechanisms of selection for the control of hand action. *Trends in Cognitive Sciences, 3,* 264–271.

Craighero, L., Fadiga, L., Rizzolatti, G., & Umilta, C. (1996). Evidence for a visuomotor priming effect. *Neuroreport, 8,* 347–349.

Craighero, L., Fadiga, L., Rizzolatti, G., & Umilta, C. (1998). Visuomotor priming. *Visual Cognition, 5,* 109–126.

Craighero, L., Fadiga, L., Rizzolatti, G., & Umilta, C. (1999). Action for perception: A motor-visual attentional effect. *Journal of Experimental Psychology: Human Perception and Performance, 25,* 1673–1692.

Derbyshire, N., Ellis, R., & Tucker, M. (2006). The potentiation of two components of the reach-to-grasp action during object categorisation in visual memory. *Acta Psychologica, 122,* 74–98.

Ellis, R., & Tucker, M. (2000). Micro-affordance: The potentiation of actions by seen objects. *British Journal of Psychology, 91,* 451–471.

Ellis, R., Tucker, M., Symes, E., & Vainio, L. (2007). Does selecting one visual object from several require inhibition of the actions associated with non-selected objects? *Journal of Experimental Psychology: Human Perception and Performance, 33,* 670–691.

Fagioli, S., Hommel, B., & Schubotz, R. I. (2007). Intentional control of attention: Action planning primes action-related stimulus dimensions. *Neuropsychologia, 14,* 3351–3355.

Greenwald, A. G. (1970). Sensory feedback mechanisms in performance control: With special reference to the ideo-motor mechanism. *Psychological Review, 77,* 73–99.

Hommel, B. (1997). Toward an action-concept model of stimulus–response compatibility. In B. Hommel & W. Prinz (Eds.), *Theoretical issues in stimulus–response compatibility* (pp. 281–320). Amsterdam: Elsevier.

Hommel, B., Musseler, J., Aschersleben, G., & Prinz, W. (2001). The theory of event coding (TEC). *Behavioural and Brain Sciences, 24,* 849–937.

Jeannerod, M. (1981). Intersegmental coordination during reaching at natural visual objects. In J. Long & A. Baddeley (Eds.), *Attention and performance IX* (pp. 153–169). Hillsdale, NJ: Lawrence Erlbaum Associates.

Jeannerod, M., Paulignan, Y., Mackenzie, C., & Marteniuk, R. M. (1992). Parallel visuomotor processing in human prehension. In R. Caminiti, P. B. Johnson, & Y. Burnod (Eds.), *Control of arm movement in space* (pp. 27–44). Berlin: Springer-Verlag.

Kahneman, D., & Treisman, A. M. (1984). Changing view of attention and automaticity. In R. Parasuraman, R. Davies, & J. Beatty (Eds.), *Varieties of attention* (pp. 29–61). New York: Academic Press.

Kornblum, S. (1992). Dimensional overlap and dimensional relevance in stimulus-response and stimulus-stimulus compatibility. In G. E. Stelmach & J. Requin (Eds.), *Tutorials in motor behaviour* (pp. 743–777). Amsterdam: North-Holland.

Kornblum, S., Hasbroucq, T., & Osman, A. (1990). Dimensional overlap: Cognitive basis for stimulus-response compatibility—A model and taxonomy. *Psychological Review, 97,* 253–270.

Kornblum, S., & Lee, J. (1995). Stimulus-response compatibility with relevant and irrelevant stimulus dimensions that do and do not overlap with the response. *Journal of Experimental Psychology: Human Perception and Performance, 21,* 855–875.

Michaels, C. F. (1988). S-R compatibility between response position and destination of apparent motion. *Journal of Experimental Psychology: Human Perception and Performance, 14,* 231–240.

Michaels, C. F. (1993). Destination compatibility, affordances, and coding rules: A reply to Proctor, Van Zandt, Lu and Weeks. *Journal of Experimental Psychology: Human Perception and Performance, 19,* 1121–1127.

Musseler, J., & Hommel, B. (1997). Blindness to response-compatible stimuli. *Journal of Experimental Psychology: Human Perception and Performance, 23,* 861–872.

Nicoletti, R., Anzola, G. P., Luppino, G., Rizzolatti, G., & Umilta, C. (1982). Spatial compatibility effects on the same side of the body midline. *Journal of Experimental Psychology: Human Perception and Performance, 8,* 664–673.

Pavese, A., & Buxbaum, L. J. (2002). Action matters: The role of action plans and object affordances in selection for action. *Visual Cognition, 9,* 559–590.

Prinz, W. (1990). A common coding approach to perception and action. In O. Neumann & W. Prinz (Eds.), *Perspectives on perception and action* (pp. 167–201). Berlin: Springer-Verlag.

Simon, J. R. (1969). Reactions toward the source of stimulation. *Journal of Experimental Psychology, 81,* 174–176.

Stoet, G., & Hommel, B. (2002). Feature integration between perception and action. In W. Prinz & B. Hommel (Eds.), *Common mechanisms in perception and action: Attention and performance* (Vol. 19, pp. 538–552). Oxford: Oxford University Press.

Symes, E., Ellis, R., & Tucker, M. (2005). Dissociating object-based and space-based affordances. *Visual Cognition, 12,* 1337–1361.

Symes, E., Tucker, M., Ellis, R., & Vainio, L. (in press). Action directed attention: planning a grasp reduces change-blindness to grasp-compatible change-objects. *Journal of Experimental Psychology: Human Perception and Performance.*

Tipper, S. P. (1985). The negative priming effect: inhibitory priming by ignored objects. *Quarterly Journal of Experimental Psychology, 37A,* 571–590.

Tipper, S. P. (1992). Selection for action: The role of inhibitory mechanisms. *Current Directions in Psychological Science, 1,* 105–109.

Tucker, M., & Ellis, R. (1998). On the relations between seen objects and components of potential actions. *Journal of Experimental Psychology: Human Perception and Performance, 24,* 830–846.

Tucker, M., & Ellis, R. (2001). Micro-affordance of grasp type in a visual categorisation task. *Visual Cognition, 8,* 769–800.

Vainio, L., Ellis, R., & Tucker, M. (2007). The role of visual attention in action priming. *Quarterly Journal of Experimental Psychology, 60,* 241–261.

Wohlschläger, A. (2000). Visual motion priming by invisible actions. *Vision Research, 40,* 925–930.

The Movement of Eye and Hand as a Window Into Language and Cognition

Michael Spivey, Daniel Richardson, *and* Rick Dale

> Man has no Body distinct from his Soul, for that called
> Body is a portion of the Soul.
>
> —*William Blake (1790)*

Abstract

This chapter reviews different studies on the influence of a person's own movements (and potential movements) in perceptual and cognitive performance. It then focuses on eye movements and reaching movements as particularly informative measures of real-time processing. Not only do eye and hand movements function as convenient indicators of continuous cognitive processes (for the experimenter), but they can also function as manipulators of those very same cognitive processes (for the subject). That is, where you look and what you touch can influence how you think. The chapter concludes with a discussion of studies that examine the cognitive processes of two people engaged in coordinated actions.

Keywords: eye movements, hand movements, perception, cognitive performance, cognitive processes

We review a variety of new results indicating that actual motor movements (not just mental representations of them) are also intimate components of linguistic and cognitive processes. Everywhere from spoken word recognition to sentence comprehension to visual memory to problem solving to video games to everyday conversation, motor movements often appear to be the very stuff of which cognitive operations are made. Rather than treating language and cognition as modular systems that are independent of perception and action, this dynamic embodied view of mental activity treats them as contiguous with the rest of the brain and body.

As William Blake suggested so long ago, "the soul," or, in today's terminology, "the mind," does indeed appear to be inextricable from the body. For example, research on the embodiment of cognition has been accumulating considerable evidence that cognitive processes routinely depend on "perceptual simulations" (e.g., Barsalou, 1999b; Pecher & Zwaan, 2005; Richardson, Spivey, Barsalou, & McRae, 2003; Zwaan, Stanfield, & Yaxley, 2002; see Chapters 1 and 13). Interestingly, decades of experimental research in the ecological psychology tradition (e.g., Gibson, 1979; Tucker & Ellis, 1998; Turvey & Carello, 1981; see Chapter 11) and in the ideomotor framework (Greenwald, 1970; Sebanz, Knoblich, & Prinz, 2003; Chapters 2 and 18) have shown that the senses themselves are inextricable from motor processing. Therefore, if cognition is entangled with the senses and the senses are entangled with motor processing, perhaps we should not be surprised to observe the mind itself inextricable from action.

Having a body plays an undeniable role in how perception and cognition function. Some have even suggested that perception and cognition could not carry out "normal processing" without a functioning body (Noë, 2005). This could perhaps be a slightly overzealous way of putting it, as it might unrealistically suggest that a man who is paralyzed has lost his intelligence (cf. Pylyshyn, 1974; see also Edelman, 2006). Nonetheless, regardless of what might be defined as "normal processing," differently abled bodies and thus differently trained motor cortices are likely to have significantly different perceptual-motor routines and therefore different "perceptual simulations" and therefore at least subtly different cognitive processes. Imagine a very tall person who is accustomed to having to duck through doorways. Such a person surely has slightly different perception–action cycles for indoor navigation compared to people of average height, and perhaps this alters the way he distributes his visual attention as he locomotes as well as his conceptualization of three-dimensional spatial layout and his use of affordances in the environment (cf. Warren & Whang, 1987; see also Bhalla & Proffitt, 1999).

The role of action in real-time cognitive processing is considerably more prominent than is generally assumed in the mainstream of the cognitive sciences. In this chapter, we review a variety of studies demonstrating the influence of a person's own movements (and potential movements) in perceptual and cognitive performance. We then focus on eye movements and reaching movements as particularly informative measures of real-time processing. Not only do eye and hand movements function as convenient *indicators* of continuous cognitive processes (for the experimenter), but they can also function as *manipulators* of those very same cognitive processes (for the subject). That is, where you look and what you touch can influence how

you think. Finally, this chapter concludes with a discussion of studies that examine the cognitive processes of two people engaged in coordinated actions. If two people's coordinated actions are describable as "joint action" and action is fundamental to cognition, does this suggest that they temporarily share, to some degree, a "joint cognition"?

Thinking and Moving

A great number of studies have shown that cognitive processes rely heavily on perceptual and motor mechanisms. From imagination relying on perceptual systems to visual recognition relying on motor systems, the literature is replete with examples of cognition not being anything like the suite of encapsulated computational modules that traditional cognitive psychology once promised. Rather than being a separate stage of information processing that takes place on its own in between perception and action, cognition appears instead to be composed of complex dynamic mixtures of anticipated percepts and prepared actions, that is, perceptual-motor simulations.

A familiar notion in cognitive psychology is that although visual imagery occurs in the absence of any sensory input, it is closely related to sensory mechanisms (Kosslyn, Behrmann, & Jeannerod, 1995; Kosslyn & Ochsner, 1994; Mellet et al., 2000). Similarly, there is evidence that motor imagery engages the same systems that control action in the world (Jeannerod, 1994). These motor systems also appear to influence how we perceive and interpret stimuli. Moreover, motor activity has a close, productive relationship to certain types of cognitive activity, such as groping for a word (Krauss, 1998) or turning something over in one's mind (de'Sperati, 2003).

For example, our tacit knowledge of physical constraints on our own limb movement influences how we perceive biological motion. When we trace a wide circle with our hand, the velocity changes as a result of the constraints of arm motion. Observers watching a moving dot will judge velocity to be constant when it is actually changing velocity in a pattern of biomechanical motion (Cohen, 1964). Viviani, Baud-Bovy, and Redolfi (1997) found that similar visual illusions hold for kinematic perception when subjects' hands are moved by a robot arm. Similarly, Babcock and Freyd (1988) found that subjects can recover information about the dynamics of the movement production from the perception of static handwritten forms. Tse and Cavanagh (2000) showed subjects' animations of Chinese characters being produced stroke by stroke. Although a whole line appeared at once, subjects perceived apparent motion: Each appeared as a line drawn from one point to another. Interestingly, subjects raised in China perceived the direction of the stroke in accordance with how they would draw the figure, whereas non-Chinese subjects, driven only by bottom-up cues, perceived apparent motion in the opposite direction.

Human observers are easily able to detect human forms in a dynamic point light display (Johansson, 1973) and even pick up gender and recognize friends (Cutting & Kozlowski, 1977). This perceptual ability employs motor control systems: We recognize biological motion via our own ability to produce it. For example, Shiffrar and Freyd (1993) looked at the apparent motion of limbs that was induced by two static photographs of human forms in slightly different postures. Usually, apparent motion is perceived along the shortest path between two locations. At rapid rates of presentation, then, subjects reported seeing a limb move from behind the back to in front of the chest, along a path that went through the body. However, as the delay between the images increased, subjects perceived motion along a biologically plausible path, around the body, as constrained by the natural movements of joints. Moreover, it has been shown that exactly at the presentation rate where subjects switch from seeing the shortest path through the body to the biologically plausible motion around the body, the motor cortex becomes activated (Stevens, Fonlupt, Shiffrar, & Decety, 2000). In this way, motor areas controlling our own bodies are involved in a specifically biological interpretation of visual input (cf. Knoblich, Thornton, Grosjean, & Shiffrar, 2005).

In fact, subtle deviations in sensory-motor experience can influence our perception of others (cf. Hamilton, Wolpert, & Frith, 2004). For example, when ballet dancers watch other ballet dancers or when capoeira dancers watch other capoeira dancers, they exhibit activation in the premotor cortex and related areas (Calvo-Merino, Glaser, Grèzes, Passingham, & Haggard, 2005). Thus, while simply watching the dancers, they seem to be generating their own motor simulations of the movements being carried out. However, when ballet dancers watch capoeira or when capoeira dancers watch ballet, this mirror system is not active. And this is not due solely to amount of visual exposure. Female ballet dancers, who are of course visually exposed to a great deal of male ballet movements but do not include many of them in their own movement repertoire, also *do not* show activation of the premotor cortex when watching male ballet dancers.

We use motor systems not just to perceive the actions of others but also to make predictions regarding perceptual events. Knoblich and Flach (2001) had participants throw darts at a dartboard and later showed them video clips of themselves and others throwing these darts (from a side-view perspective). Without being allowed to see the trajectory of the dart itself, only the dynamics of the arm movement (and in some conditions the body as well), participants were asked to predict whether each thrown dart would land in the upper third, middle, or lower third of the dartboard. Participants were reliably better at making these predictions when they were watching video clips of themselves than when they were watching video clips of others. Thus, even though these participants had never before watched themselves (from a third-person perspective) throw darts, their perceptual anticipation of action effects (such as where the dart would land) was more accurate when the observed movement had been produced by the same motor system now performing the perceptual-motor simulation.

The importance of one's own sensory-motor routines for judgments about *observed* motor movements becomes especially relevant when one considers the cases of two individuals whose somatosensory input, across the entire surface of the body (except the head), has been eliminated because of a degenerative neural disease when they were young. They are the only two such patients in the world. These gentlemen can walk, very slowly and carefully, purely because they can *watch* when each foot lands and looks stable and then can command the next leg to step and find stable footing. They get no tactile or proprioceptive feedback from their limbs as to whether the foot is evenly supported or whether the weight that is being put on it is evenly balanced or whether their fingers have adequately grasped a drinking glass before lifting it. They must rely entirely on visual feedback to tell them these things. Here are two persons whose somatosensory-motor feedback loops have been inactive for many years. Does this significant limitation in their degree of embodiment impair their ability to make cognitive judgments (or construct perceptual simulations) regarding someone else interacting physically with their environment?

Bosbach, Cole, Prinz, and Knoblich (2005) gave these two patients the task of watching an actor lift a box and judging whether the box is heavy or light depending on the actor's posture and limb dynamics. For this simple task, these two deafferented patients did as well as nonimpaired control participants. But what about when the actor occasionally lifted the box in a manner suggesting that he had been deceived as to the weight of the box? Are the postural and limb dynamics in such a case readily perceivable by an observer? Although control participants were quite good at this task, the two deafferented patients performed far worse. This result suggests that one's own perceptual-motor routines play a significant role in cognitively simulating the mental state of someone else interacting with their environment.

By mentally simulating our physical interactions with objects, motor systems take part in representing and reasoning about those objects. Our knowledge about objects—mugs, cars, or musical instruments—is clearly rich with both perceptual and motor information. We can produce (Klatzky, Pellegrino, McClosky, & Lederman, 1993) and recognize (Wang & Goodglass, 1992) mimes of objects with ease. Brain imaging has revealed not only that this information is relevant to charades and actual physical interactions with objects but also that motor representations are active when we remember or imagine objects. Functional neuroimaging has revealed somatotopically organized activation of the premotor cortex when humans observe object-related and non–object-related actions (Buccino et al., 2001). During action observation, an internal replica of that action appears to be generated in the premotor cortex. If that action involves any objects, additional activation is observed in posterior parietal regions, as if the observer himself were actually using that object.

Behavioral evidence also suggests that when we passively observe an object, there is latent activation of motor systems. Tucker and Ellis (1998) showed participants images of household objects (e.g., a mug) and asked them to judge whether they were presented in their usual orientation or were upside down. Responses were faster when they were made with the hand that was on the same side as the object's affordance (e.g., the handle of the mug). Moreover, even the shape of a person's hand, while they manually respond to visual images in an object categorization task, affects their response times as a function of the graspability of that object with that hand shape. Tucker and Ellis (2001) had participants categorize visual images of objects as natural or manufactured, either by squeezing a response handle with a full-hand power grasp in one condition or by pinching a response manipulandum with thumb-and-forefinger precision grasp in the other condition. When people were responding to the natural/manufactured task with a power grasp, larger objects (that afforded a power grasp for lifting) were categorized more quickly. When they were responding with a precision grasp, smaller objects (that afforded a precision grasp for lifting) were categorized more quickly. Thus, the cognitive task of determining the category membership of an object was automatically recruiting current manual grasping parameters and being affected by their match or mismatch to the affordances of that object.

Beyond imagined actions and thinking about objects, action representations appear to permeate all sorts of cognitive activities. Research in social psychology shows that the implicit activation of a stereotype can directly affect motor behavior. In a remarkable study that has now been replicated in several different laboratories, the concept of an elderly person was primed in participants, and they were observed leaving the laboratory (Bargh, Chen, & Burrows, 1996). In accordance with the "slow" component of the elderly stereotype, participants walked

away at a significantly slower rate than those of a control group. Here, a primed concept affected motor behavior, but the reverse direction of influence has also been demonstrated: Motor actions can affect cognitive judgments. Cacioppo, Priester, and Berntson (1993) instructed participants to view and evaluate various ideographs while using their hands and forearms to pull toward themselves or while using their hands and forearms to push away from themselves. The pulling-toward-the-self motion was hypothesized to unconsciously activate a concept of affiliation or acceptance. The pushing-away motion was hypothesized to unconsciously activate a concept of avoidance or rejection. When later reviewing the same images, these participants were instructed to rate the ideographs on a likability scale. The images that had been viewed during a pulling motion received significantly higher ratings than those that had been viewed during a pushing motion. In these ways, both motor actions and cognitive processes appear to influence each other.

Such arguments are compelling for these "perceptiony" skills, such as making judgments about visual objects and events. However, for many theorists, the prime example of a *disembodied* cognitive activity, which should be encapsulated from perceptual and motor processes, is language. A key property of language is that it can describe things that are not present and that have never been seen or done by the speaker or listener. Yet in a range of linguistic tasks, we nonetheless find motor participation. Even relatively high-level linguistic and conceptual representations appear to be deeply rooted in perceptual-motor components (e.g., Barsalou, 2002; Boroditsky & Ramscar, 2002; Mandler, 1992; Zwaan, Madden, Yaxley, & Aveyard, 2004). For example, activation of the motor cortex can result from just hearing an action verb (Hauk & Pulvermüller, 2004; Pulvermüller,

2005; Tettamanti et al., 2005). Electromuscular activity in the hands and feet themselves is modulated by reading sentences about hand and foot actions (Buccino et al., 2005). In fact, even the comprehension of a sentence about movement can be affected by the direction of the motoric response being used. Glenberg and Kaschak (2002) had participants push or pull a lever to respond to sentences that described away-from-self or toward-self events, and they found a reliable stimulus–response compatibility effect such that participants were faster to push (than pull) the lever in response to sentences about away-from-self events and faster to pull (than push) the lever in response to sentences about toward-self events.

Actions play a role in language *learning* as well. When 2-year-olds are learning new names for objects, they tend to associate objects that they have moved along a particular axis (vertically or horizontally) with objects that exhibit spatial elongation along that same axis (Smith, 2005). For example, if the toddler is told that a certain roundish object is a "wug" and then encouraged to move the wug up and down in space, she will associate vertical extendedness to wugs. Later, the toddler is presented with two wug-like objects, one of which is wider than it is tall and the other taller than it is wide, and asked, "Which one of these is a wug?" The toddler will tend to choose the tall thin object as the wug. Other toddlers who had moved their first wug left and right in space and are now presented with the same choice tend to choose the short and wide object as the wug.

In these examples, one can see the wide-ranging ubiquity of motor representations in cognitive and perceptual tasks. Along with Wexler, Kosslyn, and Berthoz (1998) and Goldstone and Barsalou (1998), among others, we suggest that these perceptual-motor effects on cognitive processes are not just accidental peripheral intrusions onto higher cognition but instead a crucial part of the workings of the whole cognitive system. As a result, when we measure action, we are thereby also measuring cognition. In the sections to follow, we focus particularly on hand movements and eye movements as not only *indicators* of real-time cognitive processes but also *manipulators* of cognitive processes.

The Eye Is Quicker Than the Hand

In this chapter, much of our discussion revolves around (semi)continuous measures of eye movements and hand movements as integral components of real-time cognitive processing. Eye movements have a long history of being used as an unusually informative measure of perceptual-cognitive processing in a wide range of tasks (cf. Richardson & Spivey, 2004). In contemporary cognitive psychology, eye tracking has produced important experimental findings in a variety of areas, including visual search, scene perception, visual imagery, visual memory, driving, reading, spoken-language processing, video games, chess, and problem solving (for reviews, see Rayner, 1998; Underwood, 2005).

Many of the disadvantages of outcome-based measures, such as reaction time and accuracy, are avoided when using eye-movement data as a measure of cognitive processing. As eye saccadic movements naturally occur three to four times per second, eye-movement data provide a semicontinuous record of regions of the display that are briefly considered relevant for carrying out whatever actions are at hand. Crucially, this record provides data *during* the course of cognitive processing, not merely as an *outcome* of the cognitive processing. Moreover, saccades take only about 150 to 200 milliseconds to program once the target has been selected (Matin, Shao, & Boff, 1993; Saslow, 1967), so they are a rather early measure of cognitive processing, and they tend to be resistant to strategic influences. Perhaps most important, eye movements exhibit a unique sensitivity to partially active representations that may not be detected by other experimental methods. Essentially, if one thinks of it in terms of thresholds for executing motor movement, eye movements have an exceptionally low threshold for being triggered compared to other motor movements. Since they are extremely fast, metabolically cheap, and quickly corrected, there is little cost if the eyes fixate a region of a display that turns out to be irrelevant for the actual action that is eventually chosen. Therefore, briefly partially active representations—that might never elicit reaching, speaking, or even internal monolog activity because they fade before reaching those thresholds—can nonetheless occasionally trigger an eye movement that reveals this otherwise undetectable momentary consideration of that region of the visual display as being potentially relevant for interpretation and/or action.

This early and quite sensitive semicontinuous measure of cognitive processing can also frequently be used in ways that do not interrupt task processing with requests for metacognitive reports or other overt responses that may alter what would otherwise be normal uninterrupted processing of the task. Thus, in addition to providing evidence for partially active representations throughout the course of an experimental trial and not just at it its outcome, eye tracking also allows for a certain degree of ecological validity in task performance, as the "responses" it collects are ones that naturally happen anyway.

Similarly, while moving a computer mouse toward a to-be-clicked object on a computer screen, the mouse cursor traverses intermediate regions of space that allow the trajectory to reveal spatial attraction effects that also "naturally happen anyway." Just as the eyes may occasionally fixate a distractor object before finally landing on the target object, computer mouse movements will routinely curve toward a distractor object on their way toward the target object. That said, mouse movements are a less immediate measure of cognition than eye movements for several reasons. They are initiated later than eye movements, they are slower than eye movements, and they are considerably more voluntary than eye movements. Amidst these relative drawbacks, the advantage of mouse movements over eye movements is that they are *anything but* saccadic. That is, since arm movements are often *not* ballistic, each individual movement of the mouse can reveal a graded effect of spatial attention being partially allocated to a distractor object on the screen, manifested as a trajectory that curves somewhat toward the distractor on its way to the target object. In contrast, individual saccadic movements of the eyes can only provide a dichotomous variable of whether the distractor object attracted overt spatial attention (was fixated).

Another way to describe this key advantage of computer mouse movements is that the smooth and often nonlinear movement of the arm can be sampled at 60 Hz with the mouse (faster with optical measures), and each 17-millisecond time slice carries new information about what objects in x,y space might be "attracting" the movement of the mouse cursor. Whereas with most eye-movement tasks, even when the eye tracker is sampling at 250 Hz or higher, the eye-movement pattern usually only gives new information about what objects are "attracting" attention about three to four times per second, that is, when a saccade moves the eyes to a new fixation (but, for very subtle curvatures of saccadic eye movements, cf. Doyle & Walker, 2001; Theeuwes, Olivers, & Chizk, 2005). Importantly, the commensurate strengths and weaknesses of eye tracking and mouse tracking are certainly not mutually exclusive, and the interrelation of eye and hand is a quite fertile topic of much research (e.g., Ballard, Hayhoe, & Pelz, 1995; Flanagan & Rao, 1995). To treat these two methods as adversarial would be counterproductive since they can be easily combined as simultaneous measures of real-time cognitive processing in the same task (for discussion, see Magnuson, 2005; Spivey, Grosjean, & Knoblich, 2005). Both eye movements and reaching movements provide quite special windows into the mind, often revealing continuous competition between mental representations during the course of recognizing objects, words, scenes, and sentences.

Hands and Eyes as Real-Time Indicators of Cognition

A number of studies have examined the temporal dynamics of hand movements and eye movements to provide a semicontinuous record of where in space overt visual attention has been applied over the course of 1 or 2 seconds surrounding the response to a stimulus. Substantially more informative than a reaction time collected solely at the onset of a response, these temporally drawn-out measures of oculometrics and manual kinematics can reveal aspects of cognitive processing that take place both before and after the point in time at which a reaction time is collected.

For example, Abrams and Balota (1991) reported a study in which they gave participants a lexical decision task (i.e., "is this a word or a nonword?") and had them respond with a leftward movement of a slide bar for "nonword" responses and with a rightward movement for "word" responses. (Half the subjects had the reverse regime.) Higher-frequency words elicited not only faster initiation of the rightward movement but also greater force and acceleration of the sliding movement (for related results, see also Angel, 1973; Mattes, Ulrich, & Miller, 1997). Thus, they argued that the kinematics of an entire response movement, not

just the latency of its initiation (as with reaction times), can provide rich information about real-time cognitive processes.

In addition to studying the kinematics over time of a single movement, competition between multiple-response options can also be informative. Coles, Gratton, & Donchin (1988) gave participants two response handles (dynamometers) that recorded the force and timing of the squeeze performed on them. The left handle was used for responding to one type of target stimulus and the right handle for responding to another type of target stimulus. On some trials, the target stimulus for the left handle was surrounded by irrelevant stimuli that actually corresponded to a right-handle response. On these trials, the onset of the left-handle response was delayed, not surprisingly. However, there was also a significant graded increase in force applied to the *right handle* when compared to noncompetition control trials. That is, the response competition typically purported to take place in those kinds of trials was not resolved in a cognitive stage that then issued a single lateralized movement command to the motor system. Rather, the two possible responses (squeezing the left handle and squeezing the right handle) were both partially active and competing, as indicated by bilateral activation in motor areas of the brain (from their converging electroencephalography evidence), as indicated by electrical activity in the muscles of both arms (from their converging electromyography evidence), and as indicated by the actual force that was physically applied to the handles themselves. Findings like these have sparked a long-standing debate over whether activation from perceptual and cognitive representations continuously flows into response selection and motor execution processes or whether such activation is transmitted in completed packets from isolated stage to isolated stage (e.g., Balota & Abrams, 1995; McClelland, 1979; Meyer, Osman, Irwin, & Yantis, 1988; Miller, 1988; Ratcliff, 1988; see also Gold & Shadlen, 2001).

Another way to track the real-time flow of sensory input all the way through to motor output is to record the trajectory of natural reaching movements. Goodale, Pélisson, and Prablanc (1986) instructed participants to reach for a target object and made it shift location while the arm was in motion. Even when the participant could not see their arm and even when they claimed not to have consciously perceived the target object shifting its location, the arm smoothly adjusted its trajectory mid-flight in order to arrive at the target's new location. Tipper, Howard, and Jackson (1997) extended this experimental design to cases where distractor objects were present in addition to the target object. They observed that, under various circumstances, the distractor object could either attract the movement path toward itself or repel the movement path away from itself.

This graded spatial attraction of the movement path toward distractor objects becomes particularly useful under conditions where a temporarily ambiguous stimulus could potentially be mapped onto either the target or distractor objects. For example, when a virtual reaching movement, via a computer mouse, is directed toward a target object, distractor objects with similar features can exert a kind of "pull" of the movement toward themselves. Spivey et al. (2005) presented pictures of objects on a computer screen and gave participants prerecorded spoken instructions such as "Click the carriage," and "Click the tower." With the mouse cursor starting at the bottom center of the screen and the objects displayed in the upper left and right corners, participants generally moved the mouse upward and curving leftward or rightward. Interestingly, when the distrac-

tor object's name shared phonetic features with the target object's name (e.g., a carrot opposite the carriage or a towel opposite the tower), the mouse-movement trajectory tended to be conspicuously curved. When the distractor object's name did not share phonetic features with the target object's name (e.g., a raccoon opposite the carriage or a crayon opposite the tower), there was significantly less curvature in the mouse-movement trajectory.

Figure 12.1A shows raw data from an individual trial where a participant was instructed to "Click the carriage," and the mouse-movement trajectory gravitated somewhat toward the carrot on its way to landing on the carriage. Figure 12.1B shows raw data from a different trial with a different participant but the same instruction, and the mouse-movement trajectory showed essentially no spatial attraction toward the raccoon on its way to landing on the carriage. (Related findings with saccadic eye movements were reported by Allopenna, Magnuson, & Tanenhaus, 1998, and by Spivey-Knowlton, Tanenhaus, Eberhard, & Sedivy, 1998.)

This graded spatial attraction toward a competitor object is also visible with semantic categorization tasks. Dale, Kehoe, and Spivey (2007) presented taxonomic classes as the response options at the top of the screen, such as MAMMAL and FISH, and presented the picture of an animal at the bottom of the screen (where the mouse cursor started). When the animal was a typical member of its category, such as a horse, the computer mouse trajectory was relatively direct to the correct category. In contrast, when the animal was an atypical member of its category, such as a whale, the trajectory was significantly more curved in the direction of the competing category (which shared several perceptual features with the animal). Even the very first time step of the mouse trajectory showed significantly

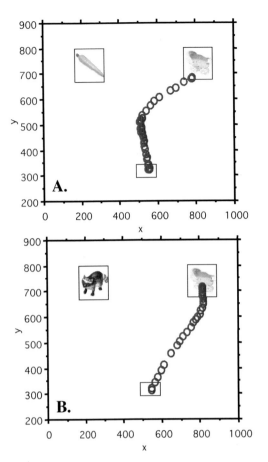

Fig. 12.1 When instructed to "click the carriage," individual computer mouse movements will often exhibit graded spatial attraction toward objects in the display whose names share some phonetic features with the spoken word (e.g., the carrot) (panel A). In control conditions, where the alternative object's name is not similar to the spoken word, movement trajectories tend to be more direct (panel B).

different angles of movement for the typical and atypical animals, indicating that the degree of feature match with the competing category was affecting the earliest portion of the movement. These results share much in common with attractor-network simulations that treat categorization as a temporally dynamic process in which the presentation of an exemplar initiates a trajectory through a high-dimensional state space that eventually settles into an attractor basin (McRae, 2004; Spivey & Dale, 2004). Thus, performance in this mouse-movement task can be thought of projecting that high-dimensional mental space

onto the two-dimensional action space of the computer screen to provide a data visualization of the trajectory in question.

In contrast to the slow curving trajectories of hand movements, most cognitive studies of eye movements examine fast ballistic saccades (but, for cognitive influences on smooth pursuit eye movements, cf. Krauzlis & Adler, 2001). Nonetheless, even saccades can, under certain circumstances, exhibit a blending of two competing movement commands. For example, Gold and Shadlen (2000) showed that a voluntary saccade based on a perceptual decision can blend with an involuntary saccade elicited by microstimulation to produce an intermediate direction of saccade. First, they had also inserted a microelectrode into the monkey's frontal eye fields, a brain area in the frontal cortex that controls saccadic eye movements, and found a region where microstimulation of those neurons would elicit an involuntary saccade in an upward direction. Then they presented displays of randomly moving dots to the monkey, which had been trained to detect small portions of coherent unidirectional (leftward or rightward) motion amidst the randomly moving dots and to respond with a voluntary saccade to a left-side or right-side response target. When only a small proportion of the dots exhibited coherent motion, the monkey would take considerable viewing time to accumulate this partial information before producing its voluntary response saccade. If the involuntary microstimulated saccade was elicited early on during this period, the resulting eye movement would be almost perfectly upward (consistent with the involuntary saccade direction). However, across numerous trials, as the involuntary microstimulated saccade was elicited later and later during that period of accumulation of perceptual information, the direction of the voluntary response saccade was more and more evident in the resulting elicited saccade. That is, with longer and longer delays between the onset of a barely leftward-moving random dot display and elicitation of the involuntary saccade, the microstimulation would produce a saccade that was less and less upward and more and more a combination of upward and leftward. Essentially, as time went by, the gradually emerging perceptual decision was coextensive with the gradually emerging voluntary saccade, and this partially active motor signal would "leak into" the saccade resulting from the microstimulation. Thus, Gold and Shadlen (2000, 2001) argued that perceptual decisions are not discretely achieved in perceptual areas of the brain and only then shunted to motor areas who wait like dumb pencil pushers to execute a unitary instruction without informed nuance. Rather, the gradual microevolution of a perceptual decision over hundreds of milliseconds continuously cascades into motor areas of the brain that are thus part and parcel of the decision process.

Although a saccadic eye movement to an empty region in between two competing objects is a rare event, it has been shown that fast *sequences* of saccades do correspond to the gradual unfolding of competing interpretations of a spoken sentence (Tanenhaus, Spivey-Knowlton, Eberhard, & Sedivy, 1995). For example, when instructed to "pick up the large red rectangle," participants often make anticipatory eye movements to a variety of large red objects in the display before the noun "rectangle" is even spoken (Eberhard, Spivey-Knowlton, Sedivy, & Tanenhaus, 1995). This finding indicates that the incrementality of spoken-language comprehension allows listeners to use adjectives to infer reference to objects in the display, even before the noun (conventionally assumed to be what performs the referencing function) is heard. Moreover, temporary misparsing of the structure of syntactically ambiguous sentences, often called "garden-path" effects, is also detectable in the real-time scan path elicited by spoken instructions. For example, eye-movement patterns have demonstrated that the motor affordances availed by the set of real objects in front of the participant immediately constrain syntactic parsing processes (Chambers, Tanenhaus, & Magnuson, 2004). Consider a display like Figure 12.2, containing a liquid egg in a bowl, another egg in a glass, an empty bowl, and a pile of flour. Eye-movement patterns revealed that a listener initially pursues different syntactic parses of the temporarily ambiguous instruction "pour the egg in the bowl onto the flour," depending on whether the alternative egg in a glass is also in liquid form or in shell form. When the alternative egg is in liquid form (Figure 12.2A), listeners immediately parse "in the bowl" as discriminating which egg is being referenced and therefore pursue the correct syntactic structure. However, when the alternative egg is in shell form (Figure 12.2B) and thus does not afford *pouring,* "in the bowl" is not naturally interpreted as distinguishing which egg is being referenced. Instead, scan paths indicate that listeners briefly consider "in the bowl" as denoting the goal of the pouring event; that is, participants briefly look at the empty bowl as though it may be where the egg is to be poured.

Interestingly, these kinds of eye movements in response to spoken-language input can even be informative when what's being "looked at" isn't really there. Richardson and Matlock (2007) presented static drawings of scenes with various kinds of paths, roads, and fences and played prerecorded stories that included sentences like "The fence is next to the coastline" and "The fence follows the coastline." Although these two sentences essentially convey the

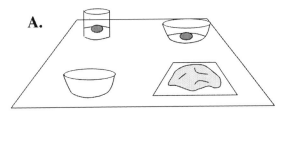

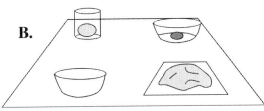

Fig. 12.2 Although each display contains two eggs, in the instruction "Pour the egg in the bowl onto the flour," a referential ambiguity occurs only in panel A, since panel B's alternative egg is not pourable. As a result, the visual context in panel A encourages listeners to initially parse "in the bowl" as discriminating between the two eggs, producing a correct syntactic analysis of the sentence. In panel B, however, "Pour the egg," can clearly refer only to the upper right egg, and therefore listeners often initially parse "in the bowl" as denoting the goal of the pouring event (and thus briefly, incorrectly, look at the other bowl).

same information, the latter of the two carries with it an implicit form of metaphorical movement, called fictive motion. Richardson and Matlock found that, while participants viewed these static scenes, fictive motion sentences induced more eye movements along the length of the fence (or path or road) than did the meaning-equivalent literal sentences. In fact, when a context sentence described the terrain as rocky or otherwise difficult to traverse, participants looked even longer at the fence (or path or road) when the target sentence exhibited fictive motion, as if the fence's "following" of the coastline involved movement that the eyes could actually pursue. These results are consistent with the claim that the understanding of motion events (even metaphorical motion) involves a mental animation of visual representations (cf. Zwaan et al., 2004; see also Hegarty, 1992; Kourtzi

& Kanwisher, 2000; Rozenblit, Spivey, & Wojslawowicz, 2002).

In fact, even when the visual display is completely blank, eye movements to different blank regions can reveal structure in the mental representations being constructed during spoken-language comprehension and during memory. Participants who thought the eye tracker had been turned off during a putative "break" between experiments listened to stories about a skyscraper and about a canyon and spontaneously made eye movements on a blank wall in the (upward or downward) direction of the verbally described motion (Spivey & Geng, 2001; for related findings, see also Altmann & Kamide, 2004). And in memory tasks, people tend to treat the location in space where information was delivered as a kind of spatial marker for memory retrieval, even when that information is obviously no longer there. For example, when four talking faces deliver arbitrary facts from four corners of the display and then disappear and then the participant is presented with a statement to verify with respect to those facts, he or she will often spontaneously look at the original location in space (now empty) that used to contain the talking face that delivered the fact in question (Richardson & Spivey, 2000; see also Richardson & Kirkham, 2004). Thus, although there may be certain selected tasks that fail to show a reliable link between eye movements and memory (Anderson, Bothell, & Douglass, 2004), a variety of findings have consistently demonstrated that, in general, the control of visual imagery and visual working memory is coextensive with the control of eye movements (e.g., Brandt & Stark, 1997; de'Sperati, 2003; Laeng & Teodorescu, 2002; Postle, Idzikowski, Della Sala, Logie, & Baddeley, 2006; Spivey, Richardson, & Fitneva, 2004). The particular point being made by Richardson and colleagues (inspired by Ballard, Hayhoe, Pook, & Rao, 1997) is that the spatial environment is so routinely relied on as an external memory that indexes to locations in space are called on, via eye movements, even when the information once held in that region is long gone.

Across these many examples of eye movements and hand movements revealing the real-time processes of cognition, the common observation that rings true throughout this section is that perceptual systems appear to continuously transmit their evolving representations to motor systems. When a partially active perceptual representation is associated with a particular motor representation, the resulting partially active motor representation will often find a way to influence or control behavior. Thus, rather than imagining that there may be some intermediate cognitive system that functions in a stage-based manner independently of perception and action, cognition itself may be better conceived of as a set of emergent properties that result from the continuous interaction between perceptual processes and motor processes (Kelso, 1995; Port & Van Gelder, 1995; Spivey, 2007).

Hands and Eyes as Real-Time Manipulators of Cognition

In their memory task, Richardson and Spivey (2000) did not find improved memory on trials where participants fixated the original location compared to trials where participants did not fixate the original location. However, this could have been due to participants occasionally producing the correct answer before needing to make any eye movements at all. When eye position is converted into an independent variable (instead of a dependent variable), with participants being allowed to look at the original location or being explicitly instructed to look elsewhere, looking at

the original location improves memory for the now-absent information by about 20% (Laeng & Teodorescu, 2002; see also Postle et al., 2006; Sacks & Hollingworth, 2005). Thus, movements of the eyes to particular locations in space not only *provide a measure* of cognitive processing but also *influence* cognitive processing.

But the eyes are not the only effectors that treat the external environment as a place where cognitive operations can take place. In the case of mental rotation tasks, Kirsh and Maglio (1994) demonstrated that expert Tetris video game players relied far more on actual external rotations of objects on the screen (elicited by button presses) than on mental rotations of internal representations of those objects. Essentially, in these experts, the motor cortex had learned to take up the job of overtly carrying out the rotations of objects for determining their fit into slots at the bottom of the display, as it was faster and more accurate than trusting cognitive processes to perform those rotations covertly.

In fact, there is extensive behavioral and neurological evidence that motor representations naturally assist in mental rotation tasks. Wohlschläger and Wohlschläger (1998) demonstrated that when subjects mentally rotated a three-dimensional object, performance was better if the manual response used a rotational motor action that was in the same direction to the mental rotation. Transcranial magnetic stimulation of the primary motor cortex disrupts mental rotation (Ganis, Keenan, Kosslyn, & Pascual-Leone, 2000), neuroimaging reveals activation of motor areas when humans perform a mental rotation task (Richter et al., 2000), and gradual angular translations of neuronal population vectors in the motor cortex are observed when monkeys perform mental rotation tasks (Georgopoulos, Lurito, Petrides, Schwartz, & Massey, 1989). This should not be surprising given that there are basically two ways to find out what an object will look like at a different orientation: physically rotate the object or mentally rotate an internal image of the object. Wexler et al. (1998) contend that these two strategies are linked, that *mental* rotation is a perceptual-motor simulation of *manual* rotation.

Manual gestures during conversation are another case where hand movements not only *reveal* something about cognition (McNeill, 1992) but also *influence* the gesturer's cognitive processes. Sometimes gestures appear to be part of the communicative signal, intended to aid the listener's comprehension (for a review, see Kendon, 1994). However, there are other circumstances where they appear to be used to aid the speaker's own speech-production processes (Krauss, 1998). In either case, they clearly contain informational content. For example, gestures are more common when the speaker is trying to retrieve lexical items that are spatial, concrete, and imageable. In fact, electromyography measures even show greater amplitude of electromuscular activity in the dominant arm during gestures co-occurring with the retrieval of lexical items that are more spatial and more concrete (Morsella & Krauss, 2005). It may very well be that, during a laborious lexical retrieval event, recruiting manual motor processes to act out some of the semantic properties of that not-yet-found lexical item facilitates the pattern completion process of retrieval.

This physically externalized "acting-out" process is also helpful for spatial reasoning tasks. Schwartz and Black (1999) presented evidence that, in some cases, human subjects can more successfully carry out a reasoning task if they physically simulate perceptual and motor experiences rather than "thinking it through." (Note, if the reader has not come across this particular reasoning problem before, then it might be instruc-

tive to try to solve the problem "rationally" or "mathematically" first.) The question was this: There are two glasses of the same height, filled to an equal height with water. One glass is narrow, and one is wide. Which glass would have to be tilted to a greater angle for the water to pour out? It was found that most subjects gave the incorrect answer, replying that the wider glass would have to be tilted more. However, Schwartz and Black asked another group of subjects to mime holding either a narrow or a wide glass filled to a certain level and slowly to tilt their hands, stopping when they imagined water would start pouring. It was found that subjects tilted the narrow glass to a greater degree. In this case, then, an externalized perception–action simulation gave a more accurate judgment than cognitive reasoning did on its own.

Even *accidental* "actings out" can have fortuitous results for cognitive reasoning. Glucksberg (1964) carefully watched participants as they attempted to solve Duncker's (1945) candle problem. With the real objects in front of them (a candle, a box of tacks, and a book of matches), participants were given the task of mounting the candle on the wall using only those objects. Glucksberg recorded how many times they touched the cardboard box of tacks (which solves the problem by being emptied and tacked to the wall as the mounting platform itself) and found that participants who managed to come up with the correct solution happened to touch the box, well before their "Aha!" moment, more times than those who did not solve the problem. This suggests that, before their seemingly instantaneous insight to use the box as the solution, something inside their nervous system was paying a little extra attention to the box. Moreover, right before that "Aha!" moment, the object that these participants had most recently touched was always the box—and in most cases that touch had been adventitious and nonpurposeful. It is almost as if the participant's *hands* suspected that the box itself would be useful before the participant *himself* knew.

A related example of perceptual-motor subsystems partially suspecting the correct solution to an insight problem, well before the explicit language subsystems have managed to verbalize it to themselves, comes from a study by Grant and Spivey (2003). Eye movements were recorded while participants attempted to solve a diagram-based version of Duncker's (1945) classic tumor-and-lasers radiation problem. "Given a human being with an inoperable stomach tumor and lasers that destroy organic tissue at sufficient intensity, how can one cure the person with these lasers and, at the same time, avoid harming the healthy tissue that surrounds the tumor?" A schematic diagram was provided, composed simply of a filled oval, representing the tumor, with a circumscribing oval representing the stomach lining (which must not be injured). Nothing else in Duncker's problem description was depicted in the schematic diagram. As this problem is a very difficult insight problem, only a third of the participants solved it without needing hints. Although the eye-movement patterns were very similar for successful and unsuccessful solvers, one difference stood out. During the 30 seconds before encountering their "Aha!' moment, successful solvers tended to look at the stomach lining, the circumscribing oval, more than unsuccessful solvers did (during the corresponding 30 seconds just before they gave up and requested a hint). A bit like Glucksberg's (1964) successful candle-problem solvers idly touching the box before discovering its usefulness, Grant and Spivey's successful solvers were making frequent eye movements inward toward the tumor and back outward again, stopping regularly on the stomach lining, almost *sketching* the solu-

tion (of multiple low-energy lasers converging on the tumor) with their scan path. Thus, the eye-movement patterns in Grant and Spivey's first experiment provided an *indicator* of the parts of the diagram that seemed to be associated with achieving the correct solution. In a second experiment, Grant and Spivey tested whether attracting attention (and eye movements) to that part could *manipulate* cognition into achieving the insight necessary for solving the problem.

In the second experiment, the schematic diagram was animated (with a single-pixel increase in diameter pulsating at 3 Hz) to subtly increase the perceptual salience of the stomach lining in one condition or the tumor in a control condition. A second control condition had no animation at all. In the two control conditions, one-third of the participants solved the problem without hints, as expected. However, in the pulsating stomach lining condition, *two-thirds* of the participants solved the problem without hints. Grant and Spivey (2003) hypothesized that the increased perceptual salience of the stomach lining helped elicit patterns of eye movements and attention that were conducive to developing a *perceptual simulation* (Barsalou, 1999b) of the correct solution, involving multiple weak lasers passing harmlessly through the stomach lining at different locations and converging their energies at the tumor. Thus, a perceptual-motor process—an eye-movement pattern characterized by saccades into and back out of the stomach region, including a conspicuous proportion of fixations of stomach lining itself—appears to play an important role in high-level cognition.

Clearly, eye movements and hand movements are more than just convenient indicators of real-time cognition to be used by an experimenter for measuring cognitive processes. Eye movements and hand movements are also real-time manipulators of cognition used by the individual to perform cognitive operations on objects in the environment via the perception–action cycle (cf. Neisser, 1976). And, to be sure, these are not the only kinds of movements that can perform this "jump-starting" of cognitive processes. In fact, when people are instructed to imagine various smells, they tend to spontaneously sniff the air (though odor free), and they do so longer when they are imagining a pleasant scent than when they are imagining an unpleasant scent (Bensafi, Pouliot, & Sobel, 2005). Apparently, *all* our effectors can participate in cognition. The many motor actions available to us are not just the feed-forward results of perceptual and cognitive processing; sometimes perceptual and cognitive processes are the results of motor actions.

Coupled Action

In the previous section, we reviewed evidence that action does not just *reflect* cognitive and perceptual processes but appears to *influence* them as well. This suggests a rich dynamic between perception–action systems on the one hand and cognitive processes on the other. So far, this review has been limited to two themes. First, each direction of influence, whether from or to action, has been considered separately. Second, such influence has been considered only within an individual person. The perspective that perception, cognition, and action interact suggests an extension on each of these themes. As for the first, these interacting systems generate a closed loop in which there is continuous interplay between them, suggesting that a rich dynamic emerges from their functioning. Numerous researchers have thus explored dynamic *coordination* between perception, cognition, and action. As for the second theme, we may depart from focusing on the individual. If perception and action are coordinated within an individual, then perhaps perceptual feedback from others in the context of one's actions can lead to coordinative dynamics between multiple individuals.

Coordination within persons has been extensively studied. Well-known research on manual action demonstrates this dynamic perception–action interplay. For example, work on bimanual coordination shows that rhythmic, stable action patterns emerge within an individual. Yaminishi, Kawato, and Suzuki (1980) showed that bimanual finger tapping tends toward in-phase patterns where the muscles for the two index fingers are moving in the same way at the same time. Even when the fingers start out in nonmatching phases, especially if they are moved rapidly, they involuntarily transition into this stable coordinative pattern. Haken, Kelso, and Bunz (1985) famously showed that a dynamical systems model perfectly predicts this behavior by employing the notion of an attractor landscape (for a review, see Kelso, 1995). The dynamic visuohaptic information during action produces a closed-loop system that engenders stable attractors—regions in the space of possible movement patterns that are highly stable. While the previous sections show cognition and perception flowing into action or action influencing perception and cognition, this coordination reveals the dynamic interplay between the two systems—producing, as a consequence, stable, coordinative behavioral sequences.

Interestingly, this perception–action coordination occurs between individuals as well. Schmidt, Carello, and Turvey (1990) showed that the same dynamical description of Haken et al. (1985), predictive of within-person coordination in such stable manual action shown by Yaminishi et al. (1980), also describes coordination that emerges between the leg movements of two individuals. Two participants sat side by side, and each swung one leg to the left and right. Participants viewed each other's movements, and leg movements between the individuals exhibited all the hallmark characteristics of the perception–action dynamic of within-person coordination: stable, in-phase attractors. This result reveals that the flow of perceptual information during continuous leg movement creates a coupled system *between individuals,* producing similarly coordinative behavior. Perception–action cycles therefore extend from the cognitive system of one individual to behavior in two or more cognitive systems.

It turns out that *perceiving* actions of others is not the only means by which two individuals may become a coupled perception–action system. In fact, the ability to process *potential* actions by a task partner can come to influence one's actions. Sebanz et al. (2003) show that the action of one person can be influenced by perceiving an irrelevant stimulus that cues a possible action by her partner. In stimulus-compatibility experiments, they had participants respond to one color with a left button or another color with a right button. Participants were placed in individual or joint conditions. When alone, participants had either a two-choice or go/no-go task in which they responded with right and left buttons appropriately or in the go/no-go condition just to one of the colors. In the joint condition, with a partner, each participant would be responsible for responding to one color. An irrelevant stimulus was included with the color cues. As in other stimulus-compatibility tasks, the irrelevant stimulus could potentially impede responding: The color cue was presented as a ring on a pointing finger. This pointing finger, while having a color cue for participant A, may be directed toward participant B. This irrelevant stimulus may be processed as a potential cued action for the task partner.

As evidence that participants were indeed actively processing their partner's possible actions, reaction times were significantly influenced by the incompatible finger direction. These results were similar to two-choice incompatibility effects observed *within one* participant.

How might this influence of a partner's actions come into play in a coordinative task between two people? In a study by Knoblich and Jordan (2003), individuals or pairs of participants had to actively keep a tracking stimulus on top of a moving target as the target moved back and forth across the computer screen. In the paired condition, one participant controlled leftward changes in tracking velocity, and the other controlled the rightward changes. In order to perform the task well, participants would have to compensate and anticipate changes in the target's movement—for example, the reliable prediction that the target would begin to move to the left, then stop at the edge of the display, and proceed to move across to the right, and so on. Some pairs of participants received auditory feedback about the key presses of their partners, and some did not. Pairs of participants who received feedback about the action of their partner gradually came to resemble individual participants in their ability to follow target movement with the tracking stimulus. These results reveal that environmental cues that help participants process their partner's actions permit the development of anticipatory control strategies: They were able to actively coordinate their key presses with their partner's.

These studies show that the perception–action cycle reveals very similar coordination patterns when occurring between two people as when occurring within one person. How does the individual cognitive system succeed at this cross-individual coordination? One suggestion is that we engage in perceptual-motor simulation (Barsalou,

1999b) or prediction (Wolpert & Flanagan, 2001): When watching a motor action, we implicitly generate the action internally. As recent evidence for this, Flanagan and Johansson (2003) had participants perform or observe a sequential manual action of stacking blocks. Participants who observed the action did not passively follow the movements but rather seemed to "simulate" the motor activity itself with anticipatory eye movements that in fact matched the eye movements of the actor. The authors suggest that the cognitive system actively predicts and simulates action even when just observing the actions of others.

This perspective on motor simulation and prediction resonates with the recent discoveries of a mirror neuron system (Decety & Grèzes, 1999; Rizzolatti, Fadiga, Gallese, & Fogassi, 1996). A subset of neurons in both nonhuman primate and human premotor cortex seems to fire *both* when performing an action and when observing others perform the same action (for a review, see Rizzolatti & Craighero, 2004). This shared mechanism for perceiving and predicting action may be an important component for coordinating one's behavior with others.

These examples of perception–action coordination across individuals in fact resonate with a wide variety of findings in even higher-order cognition, such as language. Language behavior induces coupling of various processes, including eye movements (Richardson & Dale, 2005), posture (Shockley, Santana, & Fowler, 2003), and language structures (Dale & Spivey, 2006; see also Bernieri & Rosenthal, 1991; Bock, 1986; Branigan, Pickering, & Cleland, 2000; Sokolov, 1993), actively coordinated in dialogue. These various processes together likely guide the complex conversational behavior we exhibit, such as maintaining common ground (H. Clark, 1996). Coordinative patterns in conversation can also come in seemingly irrelevant forms. For example, in social cognition research, seemingly pointless gesticulations and movements are often unknowingly adopted by task partners (for a review, see Bargh & Chartrand, 1999).

These variables influencing coordination of perceptual-motor processes, from fingers wagging to legs swinging to shared syntactic structures to social cognitive influences, all may interact across multiple time scales. As a result, one becomes tempted to describe cognition not in terms of domain-specific mental operations taking place in an individual's brain but instead in terms of domain-general interactions that emerge between individuals during their coordinated actions. Rather than continue searching for various "boxes in the head" (Bechtel, 1998), cognitive scientists may need to start searching for the "shared manifold of intersubjectivity" (Gallese, 2003; see also Spivey et al., 2004).

From "Cognition *for* Action" to "Cognition *as* Action"

From this broad array of examples, it should be abundantly clear that action plays a fundamental role in our understanding of cognition and language. Action is no longer seen as the lonely caboose at the end of a train of sequential modular stages, as once assumed by the traditional information-processing approach in cognitive psychology. Action, in its simulated, preparatory, and executed forms, is coextensive with a wide variety of real-time cognitive processes, including visual object recognition, biological motion perception, language comprehension, semantic categorization, and natural conversation. As argued by ecological psychologists (e.g., Gibson, 1979; Turvey, 1992), part of understanding a visual scene necessarily involves mapping one's potential behaviors onto the actions afforded to your body by that environment. And, as argued by proponents of embodied cognition (Barsalou, 1999a; Glenberg & Kaschak, 2002), part of understanding a sentence necessarily involves perceptual-motor simulations of the events described in that sentence.

Essentially, our brains cannot help but *act out,* at least implicitly, what we are thinking. And when those thoughts are multifarious or mixed because of temporary uncertainty or ambiguity, the "acting out" that manifests itself is likewise multifarious or mixed. For example, we reach initially toward the midpoint of two competing objects (Spivey et al., 2005), or we look at multiple objects in quick succession (Tanenhaus et al., 1995). The flow of information from cognitive processes to motor processes is sufficiently continuous and unabated that evidence for simultaneously active and competing interpretations of perceptual input can be observed not only in the activation of the motor cortex and of peripheral muscles (Coles et al., 1988) but even in the actual motor output that is executed (Dale et al., 2007; Gold & Shadlen, 2000).

Given this inseparability of cognition from action, certain bodily movements in the environment can begin to be seen as performing cognitive functions themselves (Kirsh, 1995). The fluidity of the perception–action cycle allows physical manipulations of the environment, such as manually rotating a real object, to proxy for certain neural processes, such as mentally rotating the visual representation of that object. The result is a blurring of the line between body-internal cognitive processes and body-external cognitive processes, which in turn makes for a particularly interesting treatment of joint action between two coordinated agents (for a review, see Sebanz, Bekkering, & Knoblich, 2006). From your automatic anticipation of your partner's movements, coupled with the planning of your own movements, emerges a dance of concepts and actions that appears at times to no longer harbor any concern for which body they belong to.

The future of cognitive psychology is being profoundly influenced by the mountains of evidence (of which we have barely scratched the surface in this review) against the putative separation of action from cognition. In fact, just as the accumulation of evidence for the role of motivation in perceptual processing reinvigorates the "new look" in perception (Bruner & Goodman, 1947) every couple of decades (Erdelyi, 1974; Niedenthal & Kitayama, 1994), a similar accumulation of evidence for the role of action in cognitive processing regularly bolsters the embodied view of cognition (e.g., Barsalou, 1999b; A. Clark, 1997; Dreyfus, 1972; Gibbs, 2006; Lakoff & Johnson, 1980; Ryle, 1949; Steels & Brooks, 1995; Wilson, 2002). The field of cognitive psychology can no longer go about its business treating its favorite dependent measures as though they were tapping pure cognition without any influence from the motor component in the task. Even just the act of pressing a button carries with it dynamic kinematic properties that can reveal more cognitive complexity than the mere reaction time does by itself (cf. Mattes et al., 1997). If this dynamic embodied cognition (that is also embedded in the environment and entrained with other agents by way of a continuous perception–action cycle) continues to reshape the way we view how the mind works and even what the mind *is,* then this dramatic makeover will not only give cognitive psychology a brand "new look" but also give it a brand new body.

Acknowledgments

Effort on this chapter was supported by NIMH grant R01-63961 to MJS and by a Paller-Dallenbach Fellowship to RD.

References

Abrams, R., & Balota, D. (1991). Mental chronometry: Beyond reaction time. *Psychological Science, 2,* 153–157.

Allopenna, P. D., Magnuson, J. S., & Tanenhaus, M. K. (1998). Tracking the time course of spoken word recognition using eye movements: Evidence for continuous mapping models. *Journal of Memory and Language, 38,* 419–439.

Altmann, G., & Kamide, Y. (2004). Now you see it, now you don't: Mediating the mapping between language and the visual world. In J. Henderson & F. Ferreira (Eds.), *The interface of language, vision, and action: Eye movements and the visual world* (pp. 347–386). New York: Psychology Press.

Anderson, J. R., Bothell, D., & Douglass, S. (2004). Eye movements do not reflect retrieval processes: Limits of the eye-mind hypothesis. *Psychological Science, 15,* 225–231.

Angel, A. (1973). Input-output relations in simple reaction time experiments. *Quarterly Journal of Experimental Psychology, 25,* 193–200.

Babcock, M. K., & Freyd, J. J. (1988). Perception of dynamic information in static handwritten forms. *American Journal of Psychology, 101,* 111–130.

Ballard, D., Hayhoe, M., & Pelz, J. (1995). Memory representations in natural tasks. *Journal of Cognitive Neuroscience, 7,* 66–80.

Ballard, D., Hayhoe, M., Pook, P., & Rao, R. (1997). Deictic codes for the embodiment of cognition. *Behavioral and Brain Sciences, 20,* 723–767.

Balota, D., & Abrams, R. (1995). Mental chronometry: Beyond onset latencies in the lexical decision task. *Journal of Experimental Psychology: Learning, Memory, and Cognition, 21,* 1289–1302.

Bargh, J. A., & Chartrand, T. L. (1999). The unbearable automaticity of being. *American Psychologist, 54,* 462–479.

Bargh, J. A., Chen, M., & Burrows, L. (1996). Automaticity of social behavior: Direct effects of trait construct and stereotype activation on action. *Journal of Personality and Social Psychology, 71,* 230–244.

Barsalou, L. (1999a). Language comprehension: Archival memory or preparation for situated action. *Discourse Processes, 28,* 61–80.

Barsalou, L. (1999b). Perceptual symbol systems. *Behavioral and Brain Sciences, 22,* 577–660.

Barsalou, L. (2002). Being there conceptually: Simulating categories in preparation for situated action. In N. L. Stein, P. J. Bauer, & M. Rabinowitz (Eds.), *Representation, memory, and development: Essays in honor of Jean Mandler* (pp. 1–15). Mahwah, NJ: Lawrence Erlbaum Associates.

Bechtel, W. (1998). Representations and cognitive explanations: Assessing the dynamicist's challenge in cognitive science. *Cognitive Science, 22,* 295–318.

Bensafi, M., Pouliot, S., & Sobel, N. (2005). Odorant-specific patterns of sniffing during imagery distinguish "bad" and "good" olfactory imagers. *Chemical Senses, 30,* 521–529.

Bernieri, F. J., & Rosenthal, R. (1991). Interpersonal coordination: Behavior matching and interactional synchrony. In R. S. Feldman & B. Rime (Eds.), *Fundamentals of nonverbal behavior* (pp. 401–432). Cambridge: Cambridge University Press.

Bhalla, M., & Proffitt, D. (1999). Visual-motor recalibration in geographical slant perception. *Journal of Experimental Psychology: Human Perception and Performance, 25,* 1076–1096.

Blake, W. (1790). *The marriage of heaven and hell.* Pierpont Morgan Library (electronic edition).

Bock, J. (1986). Syntactic persistence in language production. *Cognitive Psychology, 18,* 355–387.

Boroditsky, L., & Ramscar, M. (2002). The roles of body and mind in abstract thought. *Psychological Science, 13,* 185–189.

Bosbach, S., Cole, J., Prinz, W., & Knoblich, G. (2005). Inferring another's expectation from action: The role of peripheral sensation. *Nature Neuroscience, 8,* 1295–1297.

Brandt, S., & Stark, L. (1997). Spontaneous eye movements during visual imagery reflect the content of the visual scene. *Journal of Cognitive Neuroscience, 9,* 27–38.

Branigan, H. P., Pickering, M. J., & Cleland, A. A. (2000). Syntactic co-ordination in dialogue. *Cognition, 75,* B13–B25.

Bruner, J., & Goodman, C. (1947). Value and need as organizing factors in perception. *Journal of Abnormal and Social Psychology, 42,* 33–44.

Buccino, G., Binkofski, F., Fink, G., Fadiga, L., Fogassi, L., Gallese, V., et al. (2001). Action observation activates premotor and parietal areas in a somatotopic manner: An fMRI study. *European Journal of Neuroscience, 13,* 400–404.

Buccino, G., Riggio, L., Melli, G., Binkofski, F., Gallese, V., & Rizzolatti, G. (2005). Listening to action-related sentences modulates the activity of the motor system: A combined TMS and behavioral study. *Cognitive Brain Research, 24,* 355–363.

Cacioppo, J., Priester, J., & Berntson, G. (1993). Rudimentary determinants of attitudes: II. Arm flexion and extension have differential effects on attitudes. *Journal of Personality and Social Psychology, 65,* 5–17.

Calvo-Merino, B., Glaser, D., Grèzes, J., Passing-ham, R., & Haggard, P. (2005). Action observation and acquired motor skills: An fMRI study with expert dancers. *Cerebral Cortex, 15,* 1243–1249.

Chambers, C., Tanenhaus, M., & Magnuson, J. (2004). Actions and affordances in syntactic ambiguity resolution. *Journal of Experimental Psychology: Learning, Memory and Cognition, 30,* 687–696.

Clark, A. (1997). *Being there: Putting brain, body and world together again.* Cambridge, MA: MIT Press.

Clark, H. (1996). *Using language.* Cambridge: Cambridge University Press

Cohen, A. L. (1964). *Problems in motion perception.* Uppsala: Lundequistska Bokhandeln.

Coles, M., Gratton, G., & Donchin, E. (1988). Detecting early communication: Using measures of movement-related potentials to illuminate human information processing. *Biological Psychology, 26,* 69–89.

Cutting, J. E., & Kozlowski, L. T. (1977). Recognizing friends by their walk: Gait perception without familiarity cues. *Bulletin of the Psychonomic Society, 9,* 353–356.

Dale, R., Kehoe, C., & Spivey, M. (2007). Graded motor responses in the time course of categorizing atypical exemplars. *Memory and Cognition, 35,* 15–28.

Dale, R., & Spivey, M. (2006). Unraveling the dyad: Using recurrence analysis to explore patterns of syntactic coordination between children and caregivers in conversation. *Language Learning, 56,* 391–430.

Decety, J., & Grèzes, J. (1999). Neural mechanisms subserving the perception of human actions. *Trends in Cognitive Sciences, 3,* 172–178.

de'Sperati, C. (2003). Precise oculomotor correlates of visuospatial mental rotation and circular motion imagery. *Journal of Cognitive Neuroscience, 15,* 1244–1259.

Doyle, M., & Walker, R. (2001). Curved saccade trajectories: Voluntary and reflexive saccades curve away from irrelevant distractors. *Experimental Brain Research, 139,* 333–344.

Dreyfus, H. (1972). *What computers can't do: A critique of artificial reason.* New York: Harper & Row.

Duncker, K. (1945). On problem solving. *Psychological Monographs, 58*(5, Whole No. 270).

Eberhard, K., Spivey-Knowlton, M., Sedivy, J., & Tanenhaus, M. (1995). Eye movements as a window into real-time spoken language comprehension in natural contexts. *Journal of Psycholinguistic Research, 24,* 409–436.

Edelman, S. (2006). Mostly harmless: Book review of Noë's "Action in Perception." *Artificial Life, 12,* 183–186.

Erdelyi, M. (1974). A new look at the new look: Perceptual defense and vigilance. *Psychological Review, 81,* 1–25.

Flanagan, J. R., & Johansson, R. S. (2003). Action plans used in action observations. *Nature, 424,* 769–771.

Flanagan, J., & Rao, A. (1995). Trajectory adaptation to a nonlinear visuomotor transformation: evidence of motion planning in visually perceived space. *Journal of Neurophysiology, 74,* 2174–2178.

Gallese, V. (2003). The manifold nature of interpersonal relations: The quest for a common mechanism. *Philosophical Transactions of the Royal Society of London. Series B, Biological Sciences, 358,* 517–528.

Ganis, G., Keenan, J. P., Kosslyn, S. M., & Pascual-Leone, A. (2000). Transcranial magnetic stimulation of primary motor cortex affects mental rotation. *Cerebral Cortex, 10,* 175–180.

Georgopoulos, A., Lurito, J., Petrides, M., Schwartz, A., & Massey, J. (1989). Mental rotation of the neuronal population vector. *Science, 243,* 234–236.

Gibbs, R. W. (2006). *Embodiment and cognitive science.* New York: Cambridge University Press.

Gibson, J. (1979). *The ecological approach to visual perception.* Boston: Houghton Mifflin.

Glenberg, A., & Kaschak, M. (2002). Grounding language in action. *Psychonomic Bulletin and Review, 9,* 558–565.

Glucksberg, S. (1964). Functional fixedness: Problem solution as a function of observing responses. *Psychonomic Science, 1,* 117–118.

Gold, J., & Shadlen, M. (2000). Representation of a perceptual decision in developing oculomotor commands. *Nature, 404,* 390–394.

Gold, J., & Shadlen, M. (2001). Neural computations that underlie decisions about sensory stimuli. *Trends in Cognitive Sciences, 5,* 10–16.

Goldstone, R., & Barsalou, L. (1998). Reuniting perception and conception. *Cognition, 65,* 231–262.

Goodale, M., Pélisson, D., & Prablanc, C. (1986). Large adjustments in visually guided reaching do not depend on vision of the hand or perception of target displacement. *Nature, 320,* 748–750.

Grant, E., & Spivey, M. (2003). Eye movements and problem solving: Guiding attention guides thought. *Psychological Science, 14,* 462–466.

Greenwald, A. (1970). A choice reaction time test of ideomotor theory. *Journal of Experimental Psychology, 86,* 20–25.

Haken, H., Kelso, J., & Bunz, H. (1985). A theoretical model of phase transitions in human hand movements. *Biological Cybernetics, 51,* 347–356.

Hamilton, A., Wolpert, D., & Frith, U. (2004). Your own action influences how you perceive another person's action. *Current Biology, 14,* 493–498.

Hauk, O., & Pulvermüller, F. (2004). Neurophysiological distinction of action words in the fronto-central cortex. *Human Brain Mapping, 21,* 191–201.

Hegarty, M. (1992). Mental animation: Inferring motion from static displays of mechanical systems. *Journal of Experimental Psychology: Learning, Memory, and Cognition, 18,* 1084–1102.

Jeannerod, M. (1994). The representing brain: Neural correlates of motor intention and imagery. *Behavioral and Brain Sciences, 17,* 187–245.

Jeannerod, M. (1995). Mental imagery in the motor context. *Neuropsychologia, 33,* 1419–1432.

Johansson, G. (1973). Visual perception of biological motion and a model for its analysis. *Perception and Psychophysics, 14,* 201–211.

Kelso, J. A. S. (1995). *Dynamic patterns: The self-organization of brain and behavior.* Cambridge, MA: MIT Press.

Kendon, A. (1994). Do gestures communicate? A review. *Research on Language and Social Interaction, 27,* 175–200.

Kirsh, D. (1995). The intelligent use of space. *Artificial Intelligence, 73,* 31–68.

Kirsh, D., & Maglio, P. (1994). On distinguishing epistemic from pragmatic action. *Cognitive Science, 18,* 513–549.

Klatzky, R. L., Pellegrino, J. W., McClosky, B. P., & Lederman, S. J. (1993). Cognitive representations of functional interactions with objects. *Memory and Cognition, 213,* 294–303.

Knoblich, G., & Flach, R. (2001). Predicting the effects of actions: Interactions of perception and action. *Psychological Science, 12,* 467–472.

Knoblich, G., & Jordan, J. (2003). Action coordination in groups and individuals: Learning anticipatory control. *Journal of Experimental Psychology: Learning, Memory, and Cognition, 29,* 1006–1016.

Knoblich, G., Thornton, I., Grosjean, M., & Shiffrar, M. (Eds.). (2005). *Human body perception from the inside out.* Oxford: Oxford University Press.

Kosslyn, S. M., Behrmann, M., & Jeannerod, M. (1995). The cognitive neuroscience of mental imagery. *Neuropsychologia, 33,* 1335–1344.

Kosslyn, S. M., & Ochsner, K. N. (1994). In search of occipital activation during visual mental imagery. *Trends in Neurosciences, 17,* 290–292.

Kourtzi, Z., & Kanwisher, N. (2000). Activation in human MT/MST by static images with implied motion. *Journal of Cognitive Neuroscience, 12,* 48–55.

Krauss, R. (1998). Why do we gesture when we speak. *Current Directions in Psychological Science, 7,* 54–59.

Krauzlis, R., & Adler, S. (2001). Effects of directional expectations on motion perception and pursuit eye movements. *Visual Neuroscience, 18,* 365–376.

Laeng, B., & Teodorescu, D. (2002). Eye scanpaths during visual imagery reenact those of perception of the same visual scene. *Cognitive Science, 26,* 207–231.

Lakoff, G., & Johnson, M. (1980). *Metaphors we live by.* Chicago: University of Chicago Press.

Magnuson, J. (2005). Moving hand reveals dynamics of thought. *Proceedings of the National Academy of Sciences, 102,* 9995–9996.

Mandler, J. (1992). How to build a baby: II. Conceptual primitives. *Psychological Review, 99,* 587–604.

Matin, E., Shao, K., & Boff, K. (1993). Saccadic overhead: Information-processing time with and without saccades. *Perception and Psychophysics, 53,* 372–380.

Mattes, S., Ulrich, R., & Miller, J. (1997). Effects of response probability on response force in simple RT. *Quarterly Journal of Experimental Psychology: A, 50,* 405–420.

McClelland, J. (1979). On the time relations of mental processes: An examination of systems of processes in cascade. *Psychological Review, 86,* 287–330.

McNeill, D. (Ed.). (1992). *Language and gesture.* Cambridge: Cambridge University Press.

McRae, K. (2004). Semantic memory: Some insights from feature-based connectionist attractor networks. In B. Ross (Ed.), *The psychology of learning and motivation: Advances in research and theory* (Vol. 45, pp. 41–86). San Diego, CA: Elsevier/Academic Press.

Mellet, E., Tzourio-Mazoyer, N., Bricogne, S., Mazoyer, B., Kosslyn, S. M., & Denis, M. (2000). Functional anatomy of high-resolution visual mental imagery. *Journal of Cognitive Neuroscience, 12,* 98–109.

Meyer, D., Osman, A., Irwin, D., & Yantis, S. (1988). Modern mental chronometry. *Biological Psychology, 26,* 3–67.

Miller, J. (1988). Discrete and continuous models of human information processing: Theoretical distinctions and empirical results. *Acta Psychologica, 67,* 191–257.

Morsella, E., & Krauss, R. (2005). Muscular activity in the arm during lexical retrieval: Implications for gesture-speech theories. *Journal of Psycholinguistic Research, 34,* 415–427.

Neisser, U. (1976). *Cognition and reality: Principles and implications of cognitive psychology.* San Francisco: Freeman.

Niedenthal, P., & Kitayama, S. (1994). *The heart's eye: Emotional influences in perception and attention.* San Diego, CA: Academic Press.

Noë, A. (2005). *Action in perception.* Cambridge, MA: MIT Press.

Pecher, D., & Zwaan, R. (Eds.). (2005). *Grounding cognition: The role of perception and action in memory, language, and thinking.* Cambridge: Cambridge University Press.

Port, R., & van Gelder, T. (Eds.). (1995). *Mind as motion: Explorations in the dynamics of cognition.* Cambridge, MA: MIT Press.

Postle, B., Idzikowski, C., Della Sala, S., Logie, R., & Baddeley, A. (2006). The selective disruption of spatial working memory by eye movements. *Quarterly Journal of Experimental Psychology, 59,* 100–120.

Pulvermüller, F. (2005). Brain mechanisms linking language and action. *Nature Reviews Neuroscience, 6,* 576–582.

Pylyshyn, Z. (1974). Minds, machines and phenomenology: Some reflections on Dreyfus' "What computers can't do." *Cognition, 3,* 57–77.

Ratcliff, R. (1988). Continuous versus discrete information processing: Modeling accumulation of partial information. *Psychological Review, 95,* 238–255.

Rayner, K. (1998). Eye movements in reading and information processing: 20 years of research. *Psychological Bulletin, 124,* 372–422.

Richardson, D. C., & Dale, R. (2005). Looking to understanding: The coupling between speakers' and listeners' eye movements and its relationship to discourse comprehension. *Cognitive Science, 29,* 39–54.

Richardson, D., & Kirkham, N. (2004). Multimodal events and moving locations: Eye movements of adults and 6-month-olds reveal dynamic spatial indexing. *Journal of Experimental Psychology: General, 133,* 46–62.

Richardson, D., & Matlock, T. (2007). The integration of figurative language and static depictions: An eye movement study of fictive motion. *Cognition, 102,* 129–138.

Richardson, D., & Spivey, M. (2000). Representation, space and Hollywood Squares: Looking at things that aren't there anymore. *Cognition, 76,* 269–295.

Richardson, D., & Spivey, M. (2004). Eye tracking: Research areas and applications. In G. Wnek & G. Bowlin (Eds.), *Encyclopedia of biomaterials and biomedical engineering* (pp. 573–582). New York: Marcel Dekker.

Richardson, D., Spivey, M., Barsalou, L., & McRae, K. (2003). Spatial representations activated during real-time comprehension of verbs. *Cognitive Science, 27,* 767–780.

Richter, W., Somorjai, R., Summers, R., Jarmasz, M., Menon, R., Gati, J., et al. (2000). Motor area activity during mental rotation studied by time-resolved single-trial fMRI. *Journal of Cognitive Neuroscience, 12,* 310–320.

Rizzolatti, G., & Craighero, L. (2004). The mirror neuron system. *Annual Review of Neuroscience, 27,* 169–192.

Rizzolatti, G., Fadiga, L., Gallese, V., & Fogassi, L. (1996). Premotor cortex and the recognition of motor actions. *Cognitive Brain Research, 3,* 131–141.

Rozenblit, L., Spivey, M., & Wojslawowicz, J. (2002). Mechanical reasoning about gear-and-belt systems: Do eye movements predict performance? In M. Anderson, B. Meyer, & P. Olivier (Eds.), *Diagrammatic representation and reasoning* (pp. 223–240). Berlin: Springer-Verlag.

Ryle, G. (1949). *The concept of mind.* New York: Barnes & Noble.

Sacks, D., & Hollingworth, A. (2005). Attending to original object location facilitates visual memory retrieval. *Journal of Vision, 5,* 443a.

Saslow, M. G. (1967). Effects of components of displacement-step stimuli upon latency of saccadic eye movements. *Journal of the Optical Society of America, 57,* 1024–1029.

Schmidt, R., Carello, C., & Turvey, M. (1990). Phase transitions and critical fluctuations in the visual coordination of rhythmic movements between people. *Journal of Experimental Psychology: Human Perception and Performance, 16,* 227–247.

Schwartz, D., & Black, T. (1999). Inferences through imagined actions: Knowing by simulated doing. *Journal of Experimental Psychology: Learning, Memory, and Cognition, 25,* 116–136.

Sebanz, N., Bekkering, H., & Knoblich, G. (2006). Joint action: Bodies and minds moving together. *Trends in Cognitive Science, 10,* 70–76.

Sebanz, N., Knoblich, G., & Prinz, W. (2003). Representing others' actions: Just like one's own? *Cognition, 88,* B11–B21.

Shiffrar, M., & Freyd, J. J. (1993). Timing and apparent motion path choice with human body photographs. *Psychological Science, 4,* 379–384.

Shockley, K., Santana, M. V., & Fowler, C. A. (2003). Mutual interpersonal postural constraints are involved in cooperative conversation. *Journal of Experimental Psychology: Human Perception and Performance, 29,* 326–332.

Smith, L. B. (2005). Action alters shape categories. *Cognitive Science, 29,* 665–679.

Sokolov, J. (1993). A local contingency analysis of the fine-tuning hypothesis. *Developmental Psychology, 29,* 1008–1023.

Spivey, M. (2007). *The continuity of mind.* New York: Oxford University Press.

Spivey, M., & Dale, R. (2004). On the continuity of mind: Toward a dynamical account of cognition. In B. Ross (Ed.), *The psychology of learning and motivation* (Vol. 45, pp. 87–142). San Diego, CA: Elsevier/Academic Press.

Spivey, M., & Geng, J. (2001). Oculomotor mechanisms activated by imagery and memory: Eye movements to absent objects. *Psychological Research, 65,* 235–241.

Spivey, M., Grosjean, M., & Knoblich, G. (2005). Continuous attraction toward phonological competitors. *Proceedings of the National Academy of Sciences of the United States of America, 102,* 10393–10398.

Spivey, M., Richardson, D., & Fitneva, S. (2004). Thinking outside the brain: Spatial indices to linguistic and visual information. In J. Henderson & F. Ferreira (Eds.), *The interface of vision language and action* (pp. 161–189). New York: Psychology Press.

Spivey-Knowlton, M., Tanenhaus, M., Eberhard, K., & Sedivy, J. (1998). Integration of visuospatial and linguistic information in real-time and real-space. In P. Olivier & K. Gapp (Eds.), *Representation and processing of spatial expressions* (pp. 201–214). Mahwah, NJ: Lawrence Erlbaum Associates.

Steels, L., & Brooks, R. (1995). *The artificial life route to artificial intelligence: Building embodied, situated agents.* Hillsdale, NJ: Lawrence Erlbaum Associates.

Stevens, J. A., Fonlupt, P., Shiffrar, M., & Decety, J. (2000). New aspects of motion perception: Selective neural encoding of apparent human movements. *Neuroreport: For Rapid Communication of Neuroscience Research, 11,* 109–115.

Tanenhaus, M., Spivey-Knowlton, M., Eberhard, K., & Sedivy, J. (1995). Integration of visual and linguistic information during spoken language comprehension. *Science, 268,* 1632–1634.

Tettamanti, M., Buccino, G., Saccuman, M., Gallese, V., Danna, M., Scifo, P., et al. (2005). Listening to action-related sentences activates fronto-parietal motor circuits. *Journal of Cognitive Neuroscience, 17,* 273–281.

Theeuwes, J., Olivers, C., & Chizk, C. (2005). Remembering a location makes the eyes curve away. *Psychological Science, 16,* 196–199.

Tipper, S., Howard, L., & Jackson, S. (1997). Selective reaching to grasp: Evidence for distractor interference effects. *Visual Cognition, 4,* 1–38.

Tse, P., & Cavanagh, P. (2000). Chinese and Americans see opposite apparent motions in a Chinese character. *Cognition, 74,* B27–B32.

Tucker, M., & Ellis, R. (1998). On the relations between seen objects and components of potential actions. *Journal of Experimental Psychology: Human Perception and Performance, 24,* 830–846.

Tucker, M., & Ellis, R. (2001). The potentiation of grasp types during visual object categorization. *Visual Cognition, 8,* 769–800.

Turvey, M. (1992). Affordances and prospective control: An outline of the ontology. *Ecological Psychology, 4,* 173–187.

Turvey, M., & Carello, C. (1981). Cognition: The view from ecological realism. *Cognition, 10,* 313–321.

Underwood, G. (Ed.). (2005). *Cognitive processes in eye guidance.* Oxford: Oxford University Press.

Viviani, P., Baud-Bovy, G., & Redolfi, M. (1997). Perceiving and tracking kinesthetic stimuli: Further evidence of motor-perceptual interactions. *Journal of Experimental Psychology: Human Perception and Performance, 23,* 1232–1252.

Wang, L., & Goodglass, H. (1992). Pantomime, praxis, and aphasia. *Brain and Language, 42,* 402–418.

Warren, W., & Whang, S. (1987). Visual guidance of walking through apertures: Body-scaled information for affordances. *Journal of Experimental Psychology: Human Perception and Performance, 13,* 371–383.

Wexler, M., Kosslyn, S., & Berthoz, A. (1998). Motor processes in mental rotation. *Cognition, 68,* 77–94.

Wilson, M. (2002). Six views of embodied cognition. *Psychonomic Bulletin and Review, 9,* 625–636.

Wohlschläger, S., & Wohlschläger, A. (1998). Mental and manual rotation. *Journal of Experimental Psychology: Human Perception and Performance, 24,* 397–314.

Wolpert, D. M., & Flanagan, J. R. (2001). Motor prediction. *Current Biology, 11,* R729–R732.

Yaminishi, J., Kawato, M., & Suzuki, R. (1980). Two coupled oscillators as a model for the coordinated finger tapping by both hands. *Biological Cybernetics, 37,* 219–225.

Zwaan, R., Madden, C., Yaxley, R., & Aveyard, M. (2004). Moving words: Dynamic representations in language comprehension. *Cognitive Science, 28,* 611–619.

Zwaan, R., Stanfield, R., & Yaxley, R. (2002). Language comprehenders mentally represent the shapes of objects. *Psychological Science, 13,* 168–171.

Action Representation as the Bedrock of Social Cognition: A Developmental Neuroscience Perspective

Jean Decety *and* Jessica A. Sommerville

Abstract

This chapter proposes that shared action representations provide the basic biological mechanism for social interaction. It argues that shared representations are the primary means by which we align ourselves with others, paving the road for a range of social and motor processes, including action understanding, imitation, and empathy. It also argues that the sense of agency—the awareness of oneself as an agent who is the initiator of actions, desire, thoughts, and feelings—plays an essential role in social interaction.

Keywords: social interaction, shared representations, sense of agency, perception, empathy

Recent progress in developmental and cognitive neuroscience suggests a critical role for motor representations in social interaction. A variety of evidence indicates that these representations are organized at the level of goal-directed acts. Specifically, they include information about the movement properties of an action and the typical end state that it embodies (i.e., its consequence or effect), with the latter taking precedence over the former (Prinz, 2003). Importantly, these representations subserve both action perception and production, allowing emulation or simulation of motor representations during action observation or internally via imagination. Accordingly, action representations are shared in the sense that different individuals have the same kind of representation activated for the same actions or emotions.

In this chapter, we propose that shared action representations provide the basic biological mechanism for social interaction. We argue that shared representations are the primary means by which we align ourselves with others, paving the road for a range of social and motor processes, including action understanding, imitation, and empathy. However, this is not to suggest that other perception–behavior effects do not exist and do not play a role in social cognition. Indeed, a variety of work indicates that various nonmotoric perceptual cues automatically activate trait concepts and stereotypes that subsequently lead to behavior that corresponds to or is consistent with these constructs (e.g., Bargh, Chen, & Burrows, 1996; Dijksterhuis & Bargh, 2001; Kay, Wheeler, Bargh, & Ross, 2004).

Moreover, the primary level of implicit connection between the self and others that shared representations engender cannot account for full-blown social cognition. Social cognition is not only about similarities between individuals but also about differences. This can be achieved by representations that partially overlap. We also argue that the sense of agency—the awareness of oneself as an agent who is the initiator of actions, desire, thoughts, and feelings—plays an essential role in social interaction.

Perception and Action Are Intertwined

The idea that perception and action are intimately linked is not new. For instance, William James (1890) claimed that "every mental representation of a movement awakens to some degree the actual movement which is its objects." Such a phenomenon is consistent with the idea of continuity between different aspects of motor cognition based primarily on perception–action cycles, which are the fundamental logic of the nervous system. Accordingly, these processes are functionally intertwined: perception is a means to action, and action is a means to perception. Indeed, the vertebrate brain has evolved for governing motor activity with the basic function to transform sensory patterns into patterns of motor coordination (Sperry, 1952). The metaphor of "affordance" was coined by Gibson (1966) to account for the direct link between perception and action. Affordances are the possibilities for use, intervention, and action offered by the local environment to a specific type of embodied agent. For example, a human perceives a garbage can as "affording trashing," but the affordances presented by a garbage can to a raccoon would be radically different.

Later, Shepard (1984) argued that, as a result of biological evolution and individual learning, the organism is, at any given moment, tuned to resonate to the incoming patterns that correspond to the invariants that are significant for it. These patterns have become most deeply internalized (i.e., represented), and even in the complete absence of external information, the system can be excited entirely from within (e.g., while imagining). Thus, Shepard makes explicit reference to internal representation and makes it possible to articulate the notion of resonance with that of motor representations. In addition, humans actively seek information about themselves and others. This latter aspect is compatible with contemporary theory of motor representations, which stresses the autonomy of the individual with respect to the external milieu and views his or her actions as a consequence of triggering by the environment or as a consequence of an internal process (Decety, 2009; Jeannerod, 1997).

A Common Framework for Action Production and Perception

Over the past decade, an impressive number of findings from both behavioral and cognitive neuroscience approaches strongly support a direct connection between the neural and cognitive systems involved in producing one's own action and the systems involved in perceiving the actions of others. This direct link between perception and action has several consequences (and adaptive values), including social mimicry, social facilitation, and stereotype activation, that may influence the subsequent behavior of the perceiver (e.g., Chartrand & Bargh, 1999; Chartrand, Maddux, & Lakin, 2005; Dijksterhuis & Bargh, 2001).

One influential theory, known as the common coding hypothesis, suggests that, somewhere in the chain of operation that leads from perception to action, the system generates certain derivatives of stimulation and certain antecedents of action that are commensurate in the sense that they share the same system of representational dimensions (e.g., Prinz, 2003). The core assumption of the common coding is that actions are coded in terms of the perceivable effects (i.e., the distal perceptual events) they should generate. Performing a movement leaves behind a bidirectional association between the motor pattern it was generated by and the sensory effects that it produces. Such an association can then be used backward to retrieve a movement by anticipating its effects (Hommel, 2004). These perception–action codes are also accessible during action observation, and perception activates action representations to the degree that the perceived and the represented actions are similar (Wilson & Knoblich, 2005).

Evidence From Animal Research

A variety of electrophysiological research has demonstrated that (a) motor representations are involved both in action production and in perception of others' actions and that (b) these representations are organized as goal-directed motor schema. Single-neuron recordings in the monkey have shown that two primary areas (ventral premotor cortex and superior temporal sulcus) contain cells that selectively discharge during the observation of actions executed by conspecifics. Some of these cells (called mirror neurons), in area F5 of the ventral premotor cortex, are sensorimotor neurons that fire both when the monkey executes certain kinds of actions and when the monkey perceives the same actions being performed by another (Rizzolatti, Fadiga, Gallese, & Fogassi, 1996).

Subsequent work has revealed that mirror neurons in the premotor cortex respond on the basis of the goal of an action, not merely its motor components. In nonhuman primates, a subset of mirror neurons respond when the final part of an action, crucial in triggering the response when the action is seen entirely, is hidden and can be only inferred (Ulmità et al., 2001). By automatically matching the agent's observed action onto its own motor repertoire without executing it, the firing of mirror neurons in the observer brain simulates the agent's observed action and thereby contributes to the understanding of the perceived action. Subsequent studies have shown that some neurons display mirror properties between motor and other modalities such as audition (Kohler et al., 2002), indicating that single neurons are concerned with some actions regardless of the modality through which a given action is inferred (i.e., it is the consequence of the action that seems to be represented).

Such neurons are not restricted to the premotor cortex but have also been recorded in other areas of the brain, notably in the posterior parietal cortex (area PF) in relation to actions performed with objects. A single-cell electrophysiological study with monkeys reported that inferior parietal mirror neurons, in addition to recognizing the goal of the observed motor acts, discriminate identical motor acts according to the context in which these acts are embedded, such as grasping a piece of food to eat versus grasping the same item to place (Fogassi et al., 2005). The authors further argued that because the discriminated motor act is part of a chain leading to the final goal of the action, this neuronal property allows the monkey to predict the goal of the observed action and, thus, to "read" the intention of the acting individual.

Another cortical region, the superior temporal sulcus (STS), responds to the observation of actions done by others. In the macaque monkey, Perrett et al. (1989) have found that there are neurons in the superior part of the STS that are sensitive to the sight of static and dynamic information about the body. The majorities of these cells are selective for one perspective view and are thought to provide viewer-centered descriptions that can be used in guiding behavior. For some cells in the lower bank of STS, the responses to body movements were related to the object or to the goal of the movements. Movements effective in eliciting neuron responses in this region include walking, turning the head, bending the torso, and moving the arms. A small set of STS neurons discharge also during the observation of goal-directed hand movements (Perrett et al., 1989). Moreover, a population of cells, located in the anterior part of the STS, responds selectively to the sight of reaching but only when the agent performing the action is seen attending to the target position of the reaching (Jellema, Baker, Wicker, & Perrett, 2000). In addition, the responses of a subset of these cells are modulated by the direction of attention (indicated by head and body posture of the agent performing the action). This combined analysis of direction of attention and body movements suggests a role for neural activation in the STS during the detection of intentional actions. These two regions (i.e., posterior STS and premotor cortex) are reciprocally connected via the posterior parietal cortex. Thus, in the monkey, there seems to be a circuitry composed of the STS, area PF, and F5 that codes the actions of others and maps these actions onto the motor repertoire of the observer (see Figure 13.1 for a map of the cortical areas involved in motor resonance).

This mirror mechanism may subserve different functions, including action understanding (Rizzolatti & Craighero, 2004), empathy (Decety & Jackson, 2004; Meltzoff & Decety, 2003; Preston & de Waal, 2002), imitation (Brass & Heyes, 2005), and social facilitation. This latter function is supported by direct neurophysiological evidence from a study conducted by Ferrari, Maiolini, Addessi, Fogassi, and Visalberghi (2005). The authors reported a series of single-neuron recordings in monkeys addressing observation of eating behavior. Their results indicate that such an observation significantly enhanced eating behavior in the observer even when only the sound of eating actions was played. They suggested that eating facilitation triggered by observation or listening of eating actions can rely on the mirror neuron system of ventral premotor cortex that provides a matching between the observed/listened action and the executed action.

Evidence From Human Research

In humans, a number of cognitive (e.g., Loula, Prasad, Harber, & Shiffrar, 2005) and functional imaging studies demonstrated the involvement of motor representation during the perception of action performed by others (e.g., Hamzei et al., 2003). Notably, one functional magnetic resonance imaging (fMRI) study showed that the activation pattern in the premotor cortex elicited by the observation of actions performed by another individual follows somatotopic organization (i.e., different parts of the body are represented in an orderly sequence in a number of cortical regions, such as the primary motor cortex and the somatosensory cortex) related to the observed action. Watching mouth, foot, and hand actions elicits different sites in the premotor and superior parietal cortices, which are normally involved in the actual execution of the observed actions (Buccino et al., 2001). Interestingly, when participants watched movements without objects, only the premotor cortex was activated, while when the actions observed involved objects, the parietal cortex became activated. Thus, it seems that the premotor cortex activation is not dependent on the movement having a goal.

Studies related to the phenomenon of apparent motion offer compelling evidence for the involvement of motor representation in the perception of bodily movements in humans (Shiffrar & Pinto, 2002). For instance, Stevens, Fonlupt, Shiffrar, and Decety (2000) adapted the apparent biological motion paradigm to present subjects

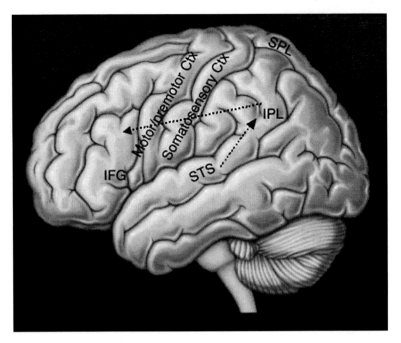

Fig. 13.1 A lateral view of a human left hemisphere. IFG = inferior frontal gyrus; STS = superior temporal sulcus; IPL = inferior parietal lobule (Brodmann's areas 39 and 40); SPL = superior parietal lobule (Brodmann's areas 5 and 7). Note that the IFG corresponds to the ventral premotor cortex in monkeys in which area F5 is located.

The premotor cortex has a central role in the selection of movements. The SPL is involved in coding space and in directing spatial attention in relation to the control of body movements. The IPL is the place where different modalities are integrated with action representations. The right temporoparietal junction seems to be critical for the sense of agency. The posterior STS and premotor cortex are reciprocally connected via the parietal cortex.

The arrows illustrate the flow of information processing across the three major cortical regions involved in the perception of others' actions. Functional neuroimaging, including fMRI and MEG studies, suggest that the sight of actions performed by others triggers neurons in the posterior portion of the STS, which provides a higher-order visual description of the observed action. This description is then fed into the frontoparietal mirror-neuron circuit, where the goal of actions and motor specification are coded.

in the scanner with a human model in different postures. Depending on the activation conditions, the subjects were shown either possible or impossible biomechanical paths of apparent motion. The left primary motor cortex and parietal lobule in both hemispheres were found to be selectively activated when the subjects perceived possible paths of right limb human movement. No activation in these areas was detected during conditions of impossible biomechanical movement paths. Thus, only the perception of actions that conform to the motor capabilities of the observer evokes motor representations in the observer.

Further evidence suggests that activation of the mirror system is mediated not

only by whether the actions are motorically plausible for the observer but also by the observer's level of expertise performing the action. For instance, one fMRI study demonstrated that expert ballet dancers show stronger activation of premotor and parietal cortices when watching other ballet dancers than do novices. The extent of premotor and parietal activation in these areas is greatest when dancers observe their own style of dance versus another kinematically similar dance style (Calvo-Merino, Glaser, Grèzes, Passingham, & Haggard, 2005). Interestingly, this finding—less activation in novices than in experts—cannot be interpreted in terms of neural efficiency because this latter interpretation would predict exactly the opposite pattern of results. Indeed, neural efficiency assumes that higher ability in a cognitive task is associated with more efficient neuronal processing of this task. Such efficiency is reflected in decrease in neural work (e.g., glucose metabolic rate). For instance, Lamm, Bauer, Vitouch, & Gstättner (1999) documented significant event-related potential differences between good and poor performers in a visuospatial task. The poor performers showed higher activity in the posterior parietal region, and their topography was more extended into the frontocentral regions. Thus, the greater activation of the frontoparietal circuit during the perception of dancing movements by experts fits neatly with the involvement of motor representations during observation of action when there is congruence between subjects' own motor repertoire and perceived actions performed by others.

The effect of similarity between the observer's motor repertoire and the perceived action was also demonstrated in one fMRI study during which participants were shown video clips of themselves and of others lifting a box and had to judge the beliefs of the actors about the weight of the box. Results demonstrated activity in a number of cortical regions involved in motor control, namely, the dorsal premotor cortex, left parietal cortex, and right cerebellum, when participants made judgments about their own actions as well as those of others (Grèzes, Frith, & Passingham, 2004).

Interestingly, there is some evidence that the motor resonance system is present not only in adult brains but also in young children. An electroencephalographic study with intracranial recordings on a 36-month-old child showed that corresponding areas of the sensorimotor cortex were activated when the child watched another person drawing with his right hand and when the child drew with her own right hand (Fecteau et al., 2004).

Recent work suggests that the functional relation between action production and action perception has its roots in infancy. One recent study conducted by Longo and Bertenthal (2006) tested 9-month-old infants on an object search task ("A not B" task). In this task, infants watch while an experimenter hides a toy at one location (location A) and then are given the opportunity to search for the hidden object. After infants successfully search at location A on multiple trials, the experimenter hides the object (while the infant watches) at a second location (location B). Previous research suggests that infants of this age typically revert to searching at location A rather than searching correctly at location B ("A not B error"), presumably because the motor memory of searching at the location A persists and influences subsequent reaches (Marcovitch & Zelazo, 1999; Smith, Thelen, Titzer, & McLin, 1999; Thelen, Shoner, Scheier, & Smith, 2001). Longo and Bertenthal (2006) tested infants on two versions of the task: a canonical version (as described previously) and a looking-only version. The looking-only version was identical to the canonical version with one critical difference: On A trials, infants merely watched the experimenter hide the object at location A and retrieve it (they were never allowed to actively search at A). On B trials, infants in both conditions watched the experimenter hide the object at location B and then were allowed to search. Infants in the looking-only version were as likely to err on B trials as those in the canonical version: Both infants persisted in searching at location A. Moreover, this bias was enhanced by increasing the number of A trials, occurred only for reaches that infants themselves were able to perform (e.g., ipsilateral but not contralateral reaches), and disappeared when infants watched a mechanical device hide and retrieve objects. These new findings suggest that infants motorically simulate the actions of others during action observation and that their ability to do so is heavily reliant on the extent to which these actions are represented in infants' own motor repertoire.

Taken together, these findings demonstrate that observed and executed actions rely on a common neural and computational code. Such a mechanism is present from very early in life and through social interaction constitutes a shared representational framework for self and other actions (Decety & Sommerville, 2003; Sommerville & Decety, 2006; Trevarthen, 1979).

From Resonance to Action Understanding

The fact that action representations encode both the means of an action (e.g., the motor properties) and the typical end associated with it, with the latter having precedence over the former, suggests that the mirror system might underlie our ability to identify the *goals* of particular motor acts. Indeed, many researchers have suggested that the covert simulation or emulation of one's own action representations during action observation enables us to anticipate the likely outcome of others' actions (e.g., Wilson & Knoblich, 2005).

If the mirror system assists in the identification and understanding of others' goals and intentions, then specific cortical regions should be selectively responsive to changes in the goals or intentions underlying actions. Recent neuroimaging work is consistent with this claim. One fMRI study investigated goal detection in participants who watched short movies in which an actor reached toward one of two adjacent objects and picked up the object. On subsequent trials, the goal alone, trajectory alone, neither dimensions, both dimensions, or only one dimension varied in a random fashion (Hamilton & Grafton, 2006). The authors predicted that neural

regions responsive to a change in another person's goal should show a greater response to novel goals than repeated goals but should not distinguish trajectories. They focused on three potential region of interest for goal representation: the inferior frontal gyrus (IFG), the intraparietal sulcus (IPS), and the right STS. They found that two cortical regions in the left IPS were specifically sensitive to goals. These two regions showed a greater response to a novel goal than a repeated goal, and the hemodynamic response function was reduced when the second video clip depicting the same goal was presented regardless of the trajectory taken by the hand. Thus, regions in the mirror system selectively activate to a change in goal.

Understanding actions also requires the ability to infer a forthcoming goal based on context. In another study designed to investigate the neural mechanisms mediating the understanding of the intentions of others, participants watched three kinds of stimuli: grasping hand actions without a context, context only (scenes containing objects), and grasping hand actions performed in two different contexts (Iacoboni et al., 2005). In the latter condition, the context suggested the intention associated with the grasping action (either drinking or cleaning). Actions embedded in contexts, compared with the other two conditions, yielded a significant signal increase in the posterior part of the inferior frontal gyrus and the adjacent sector of the ventral premotor cortex where hand actions are represented. These findings suggest that premotor mirror neuron areas are not only involved in action recognition but also involved in understanding the intentions of others. Additional evidence that the inferior frontal gyrus plays a crucial role in action understanding and action simulation is provided by a study by Pobric and Hamilton (2006), who demonstrated selective impairment in individuals undergoing a perceptual weight-judgment task when repetitive transcranial magnetic stimulation was applied over the inferior frontal gyrus.

Recent developmental evidence suggests a relation between infants' ability to recognize and identify action goals and their own ability to produce goal-directed actions and action sequences. One study assessed 10-month-old infants' ability to identify the goal of a simple action sequence: pulling a cloth that supported an out-of-reach toy in order to grasp the toy (Sommerville & Woodward, 2005). After infants were presented with the completed cloth-pulling sequence using a visual habituation paradigm, they saw test events in which the actor performed only the first step of the sequence (grasping the cloth). These events varied, however, in whether the actor acted toward a new goal (e.g., a new toy). Infants' sensitivity to the change in the actor's goal was related to their own expertise at solving the task. Infants who were able to readily pull the cloth to get the toy in their own actions attended to the goal change, whereas infants who were unskilled at cloth pulling did not. These findings are consistent with the idea that existing action representations can be used to identify another person's goal or intention. Expert cloth pullers, like expert ballet dancers, likely had well-established action representations for this particular action sequence that could be utilized during action observation, whereas unskilled cloth pullers did not.

Another study revealed that providing infants with motor experience enhanced their ability to identify the goal-relevant components of a simple reach-and-grasp (Sommerville, Woodward, & Needham, 2005). These researchers assessed 3.5-month-old prereaching infants' ability to perceive the reach of another person as object-directed using a visual habituation paradigm. Infants watched an actor reach for one of two toys on a puppet stage repeatedly. After infants

habituated to this event, the locations of the toys were switched, and infants saw two different types of test events. On new object events, infants saw the actor reach to a new toy in the same location that she had initially. On new side events, the actor reached to a new side of the stage for the same toy she had initially grasped. Infants who were provided with an intervention task that facilitated their ability to reach for and pick up toys prior to the habituation paradigm looked longer at the new object events than at the new side events, indicating that they represented the reach as object directed. In contrast, infants who received no action intervention prior to the habituation task looked equally to both test events. Intriguingly, these findings fit well with recent results suggesting that regions on the lateral bank of the IPS respond to a change in the goal object of a reach and not the reach trajectory and that these same regions show depressed activation following pursuit of the same goal on repeated trials (Hamilton & Grafton, 2006). Work remains to determine whether a decrease in parietal activity underlies the habituation effects found in infants or whether habituation arises from a more general, unlocalized attention mechanism.

The role of the mirror system in intention identification is further bolstered by research on children with autism. A variety of studies suggests that children with autism may have difficulty identifying or anticipating other people's goals and intentions (e.g., Carpenter, Pennington, & Rogers, 2001; Pierno, Mari, Glover, Georgiou, & Castiello, 2005). In one study, the authors used an electroencephalograph to measure *mu* responsiveness over the sensorimotor cortex in response to actual and observed hand movements in individuals with autism spectrum disorder (ASD) and control subjects (Oberman et al., 2005). Previous studies revealed mu-wave suppression during self-performed actions and observed actions, presumably due to mirror system functioning (e.g., Muthukumaraswamy, Johnson, & McNair, 2004). Oberman and colleagues found that whereas control individuals demonstrated mu suppression to both observed and self-performed hand actions, ASD participants demonstrated mu suppression only during self-performed hand actions. Another study provides converging evidence for mirror system disruption in children with autism (Théoret et al., 2005). When transcranial magnetic stimulation was applied over the primary motor cortex during the observation of intransitive, meaningless finger movements, ASD individuals showed significantly lower modulation of M1 excitability in comparison to matched controls. The authors reported that this deficit was not due to abnormalities in basic motor cortex in ASD individuals. Taken together, these results provide evidence of mirror system dysfunction in individuals with autism. This dysfunction could, in principle, contribute to a range of social impairments that are characteristic of individuals with autism.

Taken together, these findings provide evidence that the mirror system plays a critical role in goal identification and intention inference processes. To what extent does the mirror system underwrite or contribute to more sophisticated aspects of action understanding? Some authors have suggested that the mirror system may support mental state attribution via simulation (e.g., Blakemore & Decety, 2001), a proposal that is in keeping with theories in philosophy of mind that postulate that psychological state understanding is based on off-line reproduction of behavior and introspection (e.g., Goldman, 2002; Gordon, 1986; Harris, 1989). In contrast, other authors have suggested that the mirror system's primary function concerns more basic aspects of action analysis (Wilson & Knoblich, 2005). Numerous functional neuroimaging studies

investigating mental state attribution across a variety of tasks (false belief understanding, attribution of intentions, mentalistic descriptions of object motion, evaluation of other's knowledge states, and so on) have documented several cortical areas outside the mirror system that are reliably activated during mental state reasoning tasks: the right posterior STS, temporal poles, the amygdala, and the medial prefrontal cortex (for reviews, see Frith & Frith, 2003; Siegal & Varley, 2002). Moreover, studies with patients show that damage to several regions in the prefrontal cortex impairs theory of mind abilities (e.g., Happé, Brownell, & Winner, 1999). Such findings suggest that the mirror system alone cannot support mental state attribution (see also Saxe, 2005). However, questions remain regarding the potential developmental relation between the mirror system and the mentalizing system.

From Social Mirroring to Action Imitation

In everyday life, imitation is remarkably prevalent. For instance, people unconsciously mimic others' postures, vocalization, mood, and mannerisms. This tendency to automatically mimic and synchronize one's own behavior with others facilitates the smoothness of social interaction and may even foster empathy (Hassin, Uleman, & Bargh, 2005). For instance, one study demonstrated that participants who had been mimicked by the experimenter were more helpful and generous toward other people than nonmimicked participants (Van Baaren, Holland, Kawakami, & Van Knippenberg, 2004). These researchers also found that these beneficial consequences of mimicry were not restricted to behavior that was directed toward the mimicker but included behavior directed toward people not directly involved in the mimicry situation. Interestingly, autistic individuals who are profoundly impaired in social and emotional abilities do not show spontaneous mimicry of facial expressions but can do voluntary mimicry just fine (McIntosh, Reichmann-Decker, Winkielman, & Wilbarger, 2006). Such a core deficit in involuntary motor resonance may be the seed for their profound impairment in basic emotional connectedness.

Social mirroring does not require anything new to be learned or an understanding of the meaning of the imitated action. It is based on matching the current behavior of another with similar-looking actions of one's own. This matching process may rely on the mirror system. However, an important difference between monkeys and humans needs to be considered. The mirror neurons in monkeys respond only to goal-directed actions and not to movements. In contrast, interference between observation and action has been documented in subjects watching movements with no obvious goal (Brass, Bekkering, & Prinz, 2001; Kilner, Paulignan, & Blakemore, 2003). Furthermore, premotor cortex activation has been reported in humans during the observation of meaningless movements (Grèzes, Costes, & Decety, 1998). It should be noted, however, that there is no direct neuroimaging evidence in support of the neural mechanism that underpins automatic mimicry. Of the neuroimaging studies that examined action observation and imitation, each required participants to consciously attend to the stimuli and the task. Conscious attention, however, is not a component of the mimicry phenomenon, which is unconscious and vanishes as soon as the individual becomes aware of his or her mimicry. It is highly plausible that part of the mirror neuron circuitry contributes to the lower-level processing involved in mimicry. However, the functional impact of top-down, controlled processes on the mirror neuron system remains to be demonstrated. The various forms of imitation—ranging from automatic mimicry to reproducing an action intentionally off-

line—may well constitute a continuum from simple acts to complex ones for which executive functions, including attention and response selection, are at play.

Intentional Imitation

A key part of social learning is our ability to reproduce the actions of our social partners. Existing evidence suggests that the ability to do so hinges on shared motor representations of self and other actions and that such an ability emerges early in life. Imitation appears to be present at birth: Neonates can imitate facial gestures presented to them (Meltzoff & Moore, 1977). Over the course of the first year of life, infant imitation becomes increasingly sophisticated and elaborate. Infants progress from imitating facial expressions to imitating actions on objects both immediately and after a delay (Hayne, Boniface, & Barr, 2000) to reproducing the unseen goal of an action sequence (Meltzoff, 1995).

The direct perception–action coupling mechanism in the premotor/motor and posterior parietal cortices during action observation also appears to be involved in action imitation. The developmental time course of brain development is consistent with this claim. Whereas many areas of the brain continue to undergo rapid growth during the first several years of life and reach their full maturation at adolescence, the premotor/motor and posterior parietal cortices appear to be fairly well developed at birth. One study has demonstrated that the primary somatosensory motor cortex shows higher relative regional cerebral blood flow (an index of brain maturation) at birth and requires a shorter time to reach normal adult values, suggesting a more advanced maturation of the motor regions (Chiron et al., 1992). Another study assessed the volume of white matter and cortical gray matter in healthy children (Giedd et al., 1999). They found that the volume of white matter increased linearly with age and that the changes in volume of gray matter were non-linear and regionally specific. Altogether, these neuroanatomical and functional data fit neatly with the early imitative abilities in neonates. The neural substrate that underpins the mirror system seems in place early on.

However, the prefrontal cortex, which underpins executive control and notably executive inhibition, is not fully mature immediately after birth. While cytoarchitecture reaches full development before birth in humans, the myelination (i.e., the formation of myelin sheath around nerve fiber that allows efficient conduction of action potentials down the axon and dramatically increases conduction time between neurons) of prefrontal connective fibers extends long after birth, until adolescence (Fuster, 1997). This lack of inhibition of the mirror system at the beginning of childhood confers developmental benefits through neonatal imitation and motor mimicry. Then inhibitory mechanisms progressively develop in parallel with cognitive abilities (including more advanced forms of imitation such as differed imitation) for which inhibition and working memory are requisite. Indeed, some authors have suggested that early imitation of facial gestures may reflect young infants' inability to inhibit motor system activation during action observation (Bertenthal & Longo, in press; Decety, 2002b, 2006). Such compulsive imitation is also present in adults following frontal lobe lesions (Lhermitte, Pillon, & Serdaru, 1986).

Some of the first evidence for the involvement of the mirror system during imitation of simple finger movements comes from an fMRI study, in which participants were tested in two conditions: observation only and observation execution (Iacoboni et al., 1999). In the former condition, subjects were shown a moving finger, a cross on a stationary finger, or a cross on an empty background. The instruction was to observe the stimuli. In the "observation-execution" condition, the same stimuli were presented, but this time the instruction was to lift the right finger, as fast as possible, in response to them. The results showed that the activity was stronger during imitation trials than during the other motor trials in four areas: the left pars opercularis of the inferior frontal gyrus (which is considered to be homologue to F5 in the monkey), the right anterior parietal region, the right parietal operculum, and the right STS region.

Using magnetoencephalography (MEG), Nishitani and Hari (2000) investigated the cortical temporal dynamics of action representation during execution, online imitation, and observation of right-hand reaching movements that ended with a precision pinch of the tip of a manipulandum. During execution, the left inferior frontal cortex was activated first (peak around 250 milliseconds before the pinching); this activation was followed within 100 to 200 milliseconds by activation in the left primary motor area and 150 to 250 milliseconds later. During imitation and observation, the sequence was otherwise similar, but it started from the left occipital cortex. Activation was always strongest during action imitation. Only occipital activation was detected when the subject observed the experimenter reaching his hand without pinching. In a second study, neuromagnetic measures were taken in participants who observed still pictures of lip forms, online imitated them, or made similar forms in a self-paced manner (Nishitani & Hari, 2002). In all conditions and in both hemispheres, cortical activation progressed in 20- to 70-millisecond steps from the occipital cortex to the superior temporal region (where the strongest activation took place), the inferior parietal lobule and the inferior frontal lobe (Broca's area), and, finally, 50 to 140 milliseconds later, to the primary motor cortex. The signals from Broca's area and the motor cortex were significantly stronger during imitation than in other conditions.

A series of neuroimaging studies revealed that the intention to imitate exerts a top-down effect on the brain regions involved in the observation of actions. Specifically, in addition to the areas typically activated during passive action observation, observation for imitation requires additional executive demands. In the scanner, participants were instructed to carefully watch pantomimed actions performed by a human model either for later recognition or for imitation (Decety et al., 1997; Grèzes, Costes, & Decety, 1999). When conditions of observation of action were contrasted with a baseline condition, in which static postures were shown, increased activity was detected in the premotor cortex at the level of the upper limb representation, the inferior frontal gyrus (Broca's area), the posterior STS, and the parietal cortex. When subjects observed actions for later imitation, as compared with passive observation of the same actions, a specific hemodynamic increase was detected in the Supplementary Motor Area (SMA), the middle frontal gyrus, the premotor cortex, and the superior and inferior parietal cortices in both hemispheres. A different pattern of brain activation was found when subjects were observing the actions for recognition. In that case, the parahippocampal gyrus in the temporal lobe was chiefly activated. Thus, the intention to imitate requires additional processes of executive functions that are necessary to hold in working memory the actions perceived and also an inhibitory mechanism to refrain imitating during the scanning.

Another piece of evidence that imitation relies on shared representations rests on the finding that imitation in humans is selectively elicited by human stimuli and that the neural signature of imitation appears to be selective to human models. For instance,

young infants of 5 to 8 weeks old imitate tongue protrusion openings of a human model but not when an object performs this gesture (Legerstee, 1991), and older infants imitate the unseen target action of a human model but not an inanimate object (Meltzoff, 1995). Furthermore, in adults, motor priming seems to be specific to human forms. Castiello, Lusher, Mari, Edwards, and Humphreys (2002) have explored the nature and specificity of motor priming by examining behavioral responses to actions produced by a robotic arm versus that produced by a human arm. They showed a priming advantage for the latter. Cerebral correlates of this effect involved the premotor cortex and the right inferior parietal lobule as demonstrated by Perani et al. (2001). They reported greater activity in these regions when subjects observed grasping movements executed by a human hand than when the same actions were performed by a virtual hand. Subsequent work by Castiello (2003) showed priming effects even when the kinematics of a model are not available and suggests that the motor intention of conspecifics can be inferred from their gaze. In a subsequent fMRI study, the same group reported a selective activation of the left premotor cortex when participants observed a human model performing grasping actions. This activation was not evident for the observation of similar actions performed by a robot (Tai, Scherfler, Brooks, Sawamoto, & Castiello, 2004).

Not only is the tendency to imitate dependent on a human agent, but the similarity of the person to be imitated to the imitator also appears to affect the extent to which the actor's actions will be imitated and the accuracy with which they are reproduced. In one study, infants' imitation of peer versus adult actions was compared (Ryalls, Gul, & Ryalls, 2000). Fourteen- and 18-month-old infants were given the opportunity to reproduce a behavior that had previously been modeled by either a peer (a 3-year-old boy) or an adult. In both cases the modeler had been trained on how to carry out the modeled sequences. When given the opportunity to reproduce the target action, infants exposed to the peer model performed more correct target actions than infants exposed to the adult model. These findings fit nicely with the claim that activation of the motor system should be greatest when the observed actor and actions closely resemble that of the observer (Wilson & Knoblich, 2005).

Certain characteristics of imitation appear to be unique to humans. These characteristics include the ability to separate means from ends and the ability to not only imitate but also recognize when others imitate us. These human specializations may rest on key differences in either the anatomy of the mirror system across species or additional brain areas that are recruited by these aspects of imitation.

The act of imitation itself includes at least two components. One component involves reenacting the goal of the action, and the other component involves reproducing the means by which the goal is achieved. Humans have the unique ability to reproduce both the means and the goal even in the absence of the model and can do so flexibly given the context of the situation. For instance, in one study, 2-year-old children and chimpanzees watched a demonstrator use a rake-like tool to obtain a desirable out-of-reach object using one of two methods. Both groups benefited from the demonstration, but only children faithfully copied the demonstrator's methods of obtaining the toy. In contrast, although chimpanzees replicated the goal state, the methods that they used to do so were based primarily on the general functional relations of the problem and not the methods used to obtain the object (Nagell, Olguin, & Tomasello, 1993).

The ability to segregate means and goals emerges early in life. Carpenter, Call, and Tomasello (2002) engaged 12- and 18-month-old infants in an imitation game in which they watched a mouse hop across a mat either into a house or to a final location on the mat. Toddlers who saw the mouse hop into the house reproduced the final placement of the mouse but omitted the hopping action, whereas those who saw the final placement on the mat reproduced the behavioral means of the sequence. That is, both age-groups flexibly interpreted the goal of the sequence dependent on the context. Similar results have been documented in a study by Gergely, Bekkering, and Kiraly (2002). Fourteen-month-old infants saw an event in which a human actor activated a tap light using her head. If the reason that the actor failed to use her hands to activate the light was clear (e.g., she was holding a blanket around her body), toddlers imitated only the goal of the event. However, if it was not apparent why the actor used her head to activate the light, toddlers reenacted both the means and the goal (i.e., they used their head to activate the light). These results with typically developing children contrast with those of children with autism. Children with autism appear to be able to reproduce only the goal of an action sequence presented to them and not the means (Hobson & Lee, 1999). Taken together, these findings suggest that although goals and means are closely intertwined in the act of imitation, they are, to some extent, dissociable and therefore may partly tap distinct neural processes.

Support for this hypothesis comes from a neuroimaging study that examined the neural instantiation of processing the goal and the means in an imitation paradigm (Chaminade, Meltzoff, & Decety, 2002). In this experiment, participants observed a human agent (only his hand and forearm were visible) building Legos™ block constructions, and they were asked to observe and imitate either (a) the whole action performed by the experimenter (means and goal), (b) the goal only (end state of the object manipulation), or (c) the means only (the gesture without the last position). Partially overlapping clusters of activation were found in the right dorsolateral prefrontal cortex and in the cerebellum when subjects imitated either the goal or the means, suggesting that these regions are involved in processing both aspects of the action. Moreover, specific activity was detected in the medial prefrontal cortex during the imitation of the means, whereas imitating the goal was associated with increased activity in the left premotor cortex.

These findings support the idea that the means and the goal of imitation partially rely on dissociable circuits. Interestingly, the medial prefrontal region activation during imitation of the means indicates that observing the means used by another individual prompts the observer to construct/infer the goal toward which this human agent is aiming. The medial prefrontal region is known to play a critical role in inferring others' intentions and is consistently involved in mentalizing (i.e., the ability to understand that human actions are governed by mental states such as beliefs, desires, and intentions). An alternative and complementary interpretation of the implication of the medial prefrontal cortex is based on the hypothesis that it contributes to goal achievement by three processes: goal-based action selection, rapid action evaluation, and discrimination of the early steps from the final steps toward the goal (Matsumoto, Suzuki, & Tanaka, 2004). This latter aspect is present in conditions of imitation of the means without knowing the final position of the action made by the model.

Humans can also detect imitation and engage in reciprocal imitation. In one study, Agnetta and Rochat (2004) investigated infants' ability to distinguish between an actor who was imitating the infant and one who performed contingent but different actions on an identical toy. Infants discriminated between the imitating and contingent experimenter from 9 months of age. During toddlerhood, children can not only recognize that they are being imitated by another person but also begin to use mutual imitation as a communicative device (Nadel, 2002). Interestingly, children with autism appear to be impaired in their ability to recognize that they are being imitated by another person (Smith & Bryson, 1994). In adults, reciprocal imitation is associated with activation in the left STS and inferior parietal cortex with the left inferior parietal cortex selectively activated when the participant is imitating another person and the right inferior parietal cortex selectively activated when the participant is imitated by another person (Decety, Chaminade, Grèzes, & Meltzoff, 2002; Figure 13.2). Neuroscience research has provided clues to the existence of a cerebral network specifically devoted to the distinction between self- and other-generated signals. Such a distinction has been associated with the sense of agency (i.e., the feeling of being causally involved in an action). Attribution of an action to another agent has been associated with increased activity in the right parietal cortex (e.g., Chaminade & Decety, 2002; Farrer & Frith, 2002; Farrer et al., 2003; Ruby & Decety, 2001).

Overall, findings from a range of imitation studies suggest that reproducing the actions of another person relies on the common neural and cognitive framework for observed and executed actions. Action representations may be emulated either via a bottom-up process such as automatic mimicry (e.g., Chartrand & Bargh, 1999) or by a top-down process such as during intentional imitation or imagination of motor behavior (Ruby & Decety, 2001). These studies also

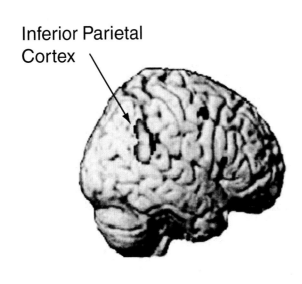

Inferior Parietal Cortex

Relative hemodynamic variation

A B C

Fig. 13.2 Right inferior parietal lobule activation at the junction of the temporal cortex superimposed on a rendered MRI. In this study, participants were scanned during a variety of object-directed actions with small objects, including self-action (A), imitation of actions performed by an experimenter (B), and observation of their actions being imitated by the experimenter (C). Note the dramatic increase in this region in this latter condition. This region plays a pivotal role in the sense of agency (adapted from Decety, Chaminade, Grèzes, & Meltzoff, 2002).

suggest that the right inferior parietal cortex plays a pivotal role in imitation, possibly in distinguishing the self from the other, an essential aspect of the sense of agency (Decety & Grèzes, 2006). It is acknowledged that agency plays a pivotal role in cognitive development, including the first stage of self-awareness (or pretheoretical experience of one's own mentality), which scaffolds theory-of-mind capacities (Rochat, 1999). Indeed, the ability to recognize oneself as the agent of a behavior is the way the self builds as an entity independent from the external world (Jeannerod, 2003).

The Role of Action Representations in Empathy

The perception–action mechanism accounts for emotion sharing and empathy (Decety, 2002b; Decety & Jackson, 2004, 2006; Preston & de Waal, 2002). This model posits that perception of emotion activates in the observer the neural mechanisms that are responsible for the generation of similar emotion. This mechanism was previously proposed to account for emotion contagion. Indeed, Hatfield, Cacioppo, and Rapson (1993) argued that people catch the emotions of others as a result of afferent feedback generated by elementary motor mimicry of others' expressive behavior, which produces a simultaneous matching emotional experience. For example, while watching someone smile, the observer activates the same facial muscles involved in producing a smile at a subthreshold level, and this would create the corresponding feeling of happiness in the observer. Indeed, viewing facial expressions triggers expressions on one's own face even in the absence of conscious recognition of the stimulus (e.g., Dimberg, Thunberg, & Elmehed, 2000). Interestingly, de Gelder, Snyder, Greve, Gerard, and Hadijkhani (2004) demonstrated that observing fearful body expressions produces increased activity not only in brain areas associated with emotional processes but also in areas linked with representation of action and movement. These results indicate that the mechanism of fear contagion automatically prepares the brain for action.

Developmental research has shown that very young infants are able to send emotional signals and to receive and detect the emotional signals sent by others. For instance, Field (1989) observed facial expressions of interest, sadness, and disgust shortly after birth in healthy infants. Likewise, discrete facial expressions of emotion have been identified in newborns, including joy, interest, disgust, and distress (Izard, 1982). These findings suggest that subcomponents of full emotional expressions are present at birth, which raises the possibility that these processes are hardwired in the brain. It has been suggested that infant arousal in response to emotions signal by others serves as an instrument for social learning, reinforcing the significance of the social exchange, which then become associated with the infant's own emotional experience (Nielsen, 2002). Consequently, infants would come to experience emotions as shared states and learn to differentiate their own states, in part, by witnessing the resonant responses they elicit in others. This automatic emotional resonance between self and other provides the basic mechanism on which empathy later develops.

Making a facial expression generates changes in the autonomic nervous system and is associated with feeling the corresponding emotion. In a series of experiments, Levenson, Ekman, and Friesen (1990) instructed participants to produce facial configurations for anger, disgust, fear, happiness, sadness, and surprise while heart rate, skin conductance, finger temperature, and somatic activity were monitored. They found that such voluntary facial activity produced significant levels of subjective experience of associated emotions as well as specific and reliable autonomic measures. Recently, an fMRI experiment confirmed and extended these findings by showing that when participants are required to observe or to imitate facial expressions of various emotions, increased neurodynamic activity is detected in the superior temporal sulcus, the anterior insula, and the amygdala, as well as areas of the premotor cortex corresponding to the facial representation (Carr, Iacoboni, Dubeau, Mazziotti, & Lenzi, 2003).

Further evidence for the involvement of the perception–action coupling mechanism has been documented in imitation of facial expressions. In one study, subjects watched movies of facial expressions and hand movements while sitting passively and under imitative and motor control conditions (Leslie, Johnson-Frey, & Grafton, 2004). The authors documented activation of the left pars opercularis, the bilateral premotor areas, right STS, bilateral SMA posterior temporo-occipital, and cerebellar areas during both hand and face imitation. Passive viewing of facial expressions selectively involved the right ventral premotor area, whereas imitation of facial expressions yielded bilateral activation.

Paired Deficits in Emotion Expression and Emotion Recognition

The finding of paired deficits between emotion production and emotion recognition also provides strong arguments in favor of the perception–action matching model. A lesion study carried out with a large number of neurological patients reported that damage within the right somatosensory related cortices (including primary and secondary somatosensory cortices, insula, and anterior supramarginal gyrus) impaired the judgment of other people's emotional states when viewing their face (Adolphs, Damasio, Tranel, Cooper, & Damasio, 2000). Another study with brain-damaged patients indicated that recognizing emotions from prosody draws on the right frontoparietal cortex (Adolphs, Damasio, & Tranel, 2002). These findings strongly support the hypothesis that the recognition of emotion in others requires the perceiver to reconstruct images of somatic and motoric components that would normally be associated with producing and experiencing the emotion signaled in the stimulus.

Moreover, there are several dramatic case studies that support the idea that the similar neural systems are involved both in the recognition and in the expression of specific emotion. For instance, Adolphs, Tranel, Damasio, and Damasio (1995) investigated S.M., a 30-year-old patient whose amygdala was bilaterally destructed by a metabolic disorder. Consistent with the prominent role of the amygdala in mediating certain negatively valenced emotions such as fear, S.M. was found to be impaired both in the recognition of fear from facial expressions and in the phenomenological experience of fear. Another case, N.M., who suffered from bilateral amygdala damage and left thalamic lesion, was found to be impaired in recognizing fear from facial expressions and exhibited an equivalent impairment of fear recognition from body postures and emotional sounds (Sprengelmeyer et al., 1999). The patient also reported reduced anger and fear in his everyday experience of emotion. There is also evidence for paired deficits for the emotion of disgust. Calder, Keane, Manes, Antoun, and Young (2000) described patient N.K., with left insula and putamen damage, who was selectively impaired at recognizing social signals of disgust from multiple modalities (facial expressions, nonverbal sounds, and emotional prosody) and who was less disgusted than controls by disgust-provoking scenarios. Further and direct support for a specific role of the left insula in both the recognition and the experience of disgust was recently provided by an fMRI study in which participants inhaled odorants producing a strong feeling of disgust and in another condition watched video clips showing the facial expression of disgust. It was found that observing such facial expressions and feelings of disgust activated the same sites in the anterior insula and anterior cingulate cortex (Wicker et al., 2003).

Sharing Pain With Others

The expression of pain provides a crucial signal that can motivate caring behaviors in others. It is thus an ecologically valid way to investigate the neural systems involved in empathy and evaluate to what extent there is an overlap between the neural response to self-experienced pain and pain perceived in others. It is already well known that a restricted number of neural regions are involved in the processing of painful stimuli, including the anterior cingulate cortex (ACC), the insula, the somatosensory cortex, the periacqueductal gray, the thalamus, and the ventral prefrontal cortex. Further, these regions are differentially involved in the sensory and affective and motivational aspects of pain processing. In one of the first fMRI studies of empathy for pain, it was demonstrated that the ACC, the anterior insula, cerebellum, and brain stem were activated when healthy participants experienced a painful stimulus as well as when they observed another person receiving a similar stimulus, but only the actual experience of pain resulted in activation in the somatosensory cortices and in subcalosal cingulate cortex (Singer et al., 2004). Similar results were also reported by Morrison, Lloyd, di Pellegrino, and Roberts (2004) from a study in which participants were scanned during a condition of feeling a moderately painful pinprick stimulus to the fingertips and another condition in which they witnessed another person's hand undergo similar stimulation. Both conditions resulted in common hemodynamic activity in a pain-related area in the right dorsal ACC. Common activity in response to noxious tactile and to visual stimulation were restricted to the right inferior Brodmann's area 24b. In contrast, the primary somatosensory cortex showed significant activations in response to noxious tactile but not visual stimuli. The different response patterns in the two areas are consistent with the ACC's role in coding the motivational-affective dimension of pain, which is associated with the preparation of behavioral responses to aversive events. These findings are supported by an fMRI study in which participants were shown still photographs depicting right hands and feet in painful or neutral everyday-life situations and asked to imagine the level of pain that these situations would produce (Jackson, Meltzoff, & Decety, 2005). Significant activation in regions involved in the affective aspect of pain processing—notably, the ACC, the thalamus, and the anterior insula—was detected but no signal change in the somatosensory cortex (Figure 13.3).

Moreover, the level of activity within the ACC was strongly correlated with subjects' mean ratings of pain attributed to the different situations.

In a follow-up fMRI study, Jackson, Brunet, Meltzoff, and Decety (2006), again using pictures of hands and feet in painful scenarios, instructed the participants to imagine and rate the level of pain perceived from two different perspectives (self versus other). Results indicated that both the self-perspective and the other perspective are associated with activation in the neural network involved in the processing of the affective aspect of pain, including the ACC and the insula. However, the self-perspective yielded higher pain ratings and recruited the pain matrix more extensively, including the secondary somatosensory

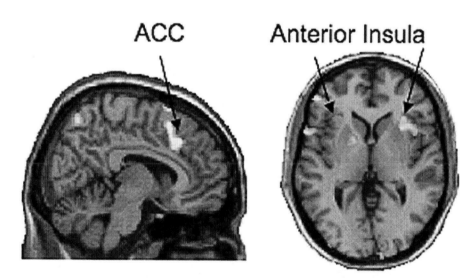

Fig. 13.3 Sagittal (on the left) and coronal (on the right) views of activated clusters in the anterior cingulate cortex (ACC) and anterior insula elicited by the perception of other individuals in painful situations superimposed on an averaged structural MR image. Physiological research in pain processing demonstrates that the ACC has a role in the affective-motivational dimension of pain, that is, related to behavioral responses associated with avoiding or escaping the nociceptive stimulus. This region interrelates attentional and evaluative functions with that of establishing emotional valence and response priorities. The insular cortex is involved in monitoring the physiological state of the body. It receives direct input from the spinothalamic pathways via the medial thalamic nuclei (the major nociceptive pathway). Interestingly, both the ACC and the anterior insula are found activated by the mere sight of pain in others (adapted from Jackson, Meltzoff, & Decety, 2005).

cortex, the midinsula, and the posterior part of the subcalosal ACC. Adopting the perspective of the other was associated with increase in the right temporoparietal junction. In addition, distinct subregions were activated within the insular cortex for the two perspectives (anterior aspect for others and more posterior for self). These neuroimaging data highlight both the similarities between self and other and self–other distinctiveness as important aspects of human empathy. The experience of one's own pain is associated with more caudal activations (within area 24), consistent with the spinothalamic nociceptive projections, while the perception of pain in others is represented in more rostral (and dorsal) regions (within area 32). A similar rostrocaudal organization is observed in the insula, which is coherent with its anatomical connectivity and electrophysiological properties. For instance, painful sensations are evoked in the posterior part of the insula (and not in the anterior part) by direct electrical stimulation of the insular cortex in neurological patients (Ostrowsky et al., 2002).

Shared circuits between emotion generation and emotion perception in others have also been documented in a positron emission tomography study that compared the neural response to externally (by watching emotional laden film clips) versus internally (by autobiographical scripts) generated emotions (Reiman et al., 1997). Both film-generated emotion and recall-generated emotion were associated with symmetrical increases in the medial prefrontal cortex and thalamus. The film condition also resulted in activation of the hypothalamus, the amygdala, the anterior temporal cortex, and the temporoparietal junction, while the recall condition was specifically associated with activation in the anterior insula and orbitofrontal cortex. Thus, there is an overlap between externally and internally produced emotions, but this overlap is partial. It should be noted that the films and recall scripts included three emotions (happiness, sadness, and disgust) that were not analyzed separately.

Altogether, shared neural circuits between self and other at the cortical level have been documented for emotion recognition and pain processing. Such a system prompts the observer to resonate with the emotional state of another individual, with the observer activating the motor representations and associated autonomic and somatic responses that stem from the observed target. This basic mechanism gives rise to shared feelings and effects between self and other on which mature empathy and moral reasoning develop.

Conclusions

We have provided evidence for shared neural circuits between perception and action, which seem biologically hardwired in the brain. The mere observation of others' behavior automatically elicits motor resonance in the self by emulating motor representations. Such a sharing has been documented for action understanding, imitation, and empathy. Importantly, the mirror system is selectively activated during the observation of human (and not nonhuman) action. This selectivity not only confers an advantage for survival (by uniquely enhancing the reproduction of species-typical behavior) but also creates a foundation for intersubjectivity because it provides a functional bridge (i.e., shared representations) between first-person information and third-person information, which allows an implicit connection between the self and the other (Decety & Sommerville, 2003). Moreover, such sharing illustrates the fundamental intersubjective nature of the self. An early dysfunction of this motor resonance mechanism during development can ultimately lead to abnormal self–other representations and reduced social interaction and prevent the development of empathic understanding.

The self, however, is not only intersubjective but also agentic. Under normal circumstances there is no complete overlap between self-representation and other representations. This would lead to confusion and chaotic social interaction. Furthermore, although the process of motor representation is largely nonconscious, the content of higher-level representations can be accessed consciously in certain conditions. By becoming aware of their intentions, actions, emotions, and desires, psychological agents are capable of action monitoring and self-regulation. And they may consciously reflect on these shared representations. Thus, self-awareness and agency play a crucial function both at the intrasubjective and intersubjective levels for navigating the social world.

References

Adolphs, R., Damasio, H., & Tranel, D. (2002). Neural systems for recognition of emotional prosody: A 3-D lesion study. *Emotion, 2,* 23–51.

Adolphs, R., Damasio, H., Tranel, D., Cooper, G., & Damasio, A. (2000). A role for the somatosensory cortices in the visual recognition of emotion as revealed by three dimensional lesion mapping. *Journal of Neuroscience, 20,* 2683–2690.

Adolphs, R., Tranel, D., Damasio, H., & Damasio, A. (1995). Fear and the human amygdala. *Journal of Neuroscience, 15,* 5879–5891.

Agnetta, B., & Rochat, P. (2004). Imitative games by 9-, 14-, and 18-month-old infants. *Infancy, 6,* 1–36.

Bargh, J. A., Chen, M., & Burrows, L. (1996). Automaticity of social behavior: Direct effects of trait construct and stereotype-activation on action. *Journal of Personality and Social Psychology, 71,* 230–244.

Bertenthal, B. I., & Longo, M. R. (in press). Two modes for the understanding of actions: A developmental perspective. In *The Carnegie Symposium on Cognition: Vol. 34. Embodiment, ego space, action.* Hillsdale, NJ: Psychology Press.

Blakemore, S.-J., & Decety, J. (2001). From the perception of action to the understanding of intention. *Nature Reviews Neuroscience, 2,* 561–567.

Brass, M., Bekkering, H., & Prinz, W. (2001). Movement observation affects movement execution in a simple response task. *Acta Psychologica, 106,* 3–22.

Brass, M., & Heyes, C. (2005). Imitation: Is cognitive neuroscience solving the correspondence problem? *Trends in Cognitive Sciences, 9,* 489–495.

Buccino, G., Binkofski, F., Fink, G. R., Fadiga, L., Fogassi, L., Gallese, V., et al. (2001). Action observation activates premotor and parietal areas in a somatotopic manner: An fMRI study. *European Journal of Neuroscience, 13,* 400–404.

Calder, A. J., Keane, J., Manes, F., Antoun, N., & Young, A. W. (2000). Impaired recognition an experience of disgust following brain injury. *Nature Neuroscience, 3,* 1077–1078.

Calvo-Merino, B., Glaser, D. E., Grèzes, J., Passingham, R. E., & Haggard, P. (2005). Action observation and acquired motor skills: An fMRI study with expert dancers. *Cerebral Cortex, 8,* 1243–1249.

Carpenter, M., Call, J., & Tomasello, M. (2002). Understanding "prior intentions" enables two-year-olds to imitatively learn a complex task. *Child Development, 73,* 1431–1441.

Carpenter, M., Pennington, B. F., & Rogers, S. J. (2001). Understanding of others' intentions in children with autism. *Journal of Autism and Developmental Disorders, 31,* 589–599.

Carr, L., Iacoboni, M., Dubeau, M. C., Mazziotta, J. C., & Lenzi, G. L. (2003). Neural mechanisms of empathy in humans: A relay from neural systems for imitation to limbic areas. *Proceedings of National Academy of Sciences of the United States of America, 100,* 5497–5502.

Castiello, U. (2003). Understanding other people's actions: Intention and attention. *Journal of Experimental Psychology: Human Perception and Performance, 29,* 416–430.

Castiello, U., Lusher, D., Mari, M., Edwards, M., & Humphreys, G. W. (2002). Observing a human or a robotic hand grasping an object: Differential motor priming effects. In W. Prinz and B. Hommel (Eds.), *Common Mechanisms in Perception and Action* (pp. 315–333). New York: Oxford University Press.

Chaminade, T., & Decety, J. (2002). Leader or follower? Involvement of the inferior parietal lobule in agency. *Neuroreport, 13,* 1975–1978.

Chaminade, T., Meltzoff, A. N., & Decety, J. (2002). Does the end justify the means? A PET exploration of the mechanisms involved in human imitation. *NeuroImage, 12,* 318–328.

Chartrand, T. L., & Bargh, J. A. (1999). The chameleon effect: The perception-behavior link and social interaction. *Journal of Personality and Social Psychology, 76,* 893–910.

Chartrand, T. L., Maddux, W. W., & Lakin, J. L. (2005). Beyond the perception-behavior link: The ubiquitous utility and motivational moderators of nonconscious mimicry. In R. R. Hassin, J. S. Uleman, & J. A. Bargh (Eds.), *The new unconscious* (pp. 334–361). New York: Oxford University Press.

Chiron, C., Raynaud, C., Mazière, B., Zilbovicius, M., Laflamme, L., Masure, M. C., et al. (1992). Changes in regional cerebral blood flow during brain maturation in children and adolescents. *Journal of Nuclear Medicine, 33,* 696–703.

Decety, J. (2002a). Is there such a thing as a functional equivalence between imagined, observed and executed actions. In A. N. Meltzoff & W. Prinz (Eds.), *The imitative mind: Development, evolution and brain bases* (pp. 291–310). Cambridge: Cambridge University Press.

Decety, J. (2002b). Naturaliser l'empathie [Empathy naturalized]. *L'Encephale, 28,* 9–20.

Decety, J. (2006). A cognitive neuroscience view of imitation. In S. Rogers & J. Williams (Eds.), *Imitation and the social mind: Autism and typical development* (pp. 251–274). New York: Guilford Press.

Decety, J., Chaminade, T., Grèzes, J., & Meltzoff, A. N. (2002). A PET Exploration of the Neural Mechanisms Involved in Reciprocal Imitation. *NeuroImage, 15,* 265–272.

Decety, J., & Grèzes, J. (2006). The power of simulation: Imagining one's own and other's behavior. *Brain Research, 1079,* 4–14.

Decety, J., Grèzes, J., Costes, N., Perani, D., Jeannerod, M., Procyk, E., et al. (1997). Brain activity during observation of action: Influence of action content and subject's strategy. *Brain, 120,* 1763–1777.

Decety, J., & Jackson, P. L. (2004). The functional architecture of human empathy. *Behavioral and Cognitive Neuroscience Reviews, 3,* 71–100.

Decety, J., & Jackson, P. L. (2006). A social-neuroscience perspective on empathy. *Current Directions in Psychological Science, 15,* 54–58.

Decety, J., & Sommerville, J. A. (2003). Shared representations between self and other: A social cognitive neuroscience view. *Trends in Cognitive Sciences, 12,* 527–533.

De Gelder, B., Snyder, J., Greve, D., Gerard, G., & Hadijkhani, N. (2004). Fear fosters flight: A mechanism for fear contagion when perceiving emotion expressed by a whole body. *Proceedings of the National Academy of Sciences of the United States of America, 47,* 16701–16706.

Dijksterhuis, A., & Bargh, J. A. (2001). The perception-behavior expressway: Automatic effects of social perception on social behavior. *Advances in Experimental Social Psychology, 33,* 1–40.

Dimberg, U., Thunberg, M., & Elmehed, K. (2000). Unconscious facial reactions to emotional facial expressions. *Psychological Science, 11,* 86–89.

Farrer, C., Franck, N., Georgieff, N., Frith, C. D., Decety, J., & Jeannerod, M. (2003). Modulating the experience of agency: A positron emission tomography study. *NeuroImage, 18,* 324–333.

Farrer, C., & Frith, C. D. (2002). Experiencing oneself vs. another person as being the cause of an action: The neural correlates of the experience of agency. *NeuroImage, 15,* 596–603.

Fecteau, S., Carmant, L., Tremblay, C., Robert, M., Bouthillier, A., & Théoret, H. (2004). A motor resonance mechanism in children? Evidence from subdural electrodes in a 36-month-old child. *Neuroreport, 15,* 2625–2627.

Ferrari, P. F., Maiolini, C., Addessi, E., Fogassi, L., & Visalberghi, E. (2005). The observation and hearing of eating actions activates motor programs related to eating in macaque monkeys. *Behavioural Brain Research 161,* 95–101.

Field, T. (1989). Individual and maturational differences in infant expressivity. In N. Eisenberg (Ed.), *Empathy and related emotional responses,* (pp. 9–23). San Francisco: Jossey-Bass.

Fogassi, L., Ferrari, P. F., Gesierich, B., Rozzi, S., Chersi, F., & Rizzolatti, G. (2005). Parietal lobe: From action organization to intention understanding. *Science, 308,* 662–667.

Frith, U., & Frith, C. D. (2003). Development and neurophysiology of mentalizing. In C. D. Frith & D. Wolpert (Eds.), *The neuroscience of social interaction* (pp. 45–75). New York: Oxford University Press.

Fuster, J. M. (1997). *The prefrontal cortex.* Philadelphia: Lippincott/Raven Press.

Gergely, G., Bekkering, H., & Kiraly, I. (2002). Rational imitation in preverbal infants. *Nature, 415,* 755.

Gibson, J. J. (1966). *The senses considered as perceptual systems.* Boston: Houghton Mifflin.

Giedd, J. N., Blumenthal, J., Jeffries, N. O., Castellanos, F. X., Liu, H., Zijdenbos, A., et al. (1999). Brain development during childhood and adolescence: A longitudinal MRI study. *Nature Neuroscience, 2,* 861–863.

Goldman, A. I. (2002). Simulation theory and mental concepts. In J. Dokic & J. Proust (Eds.),

Simulation and knowledge of action (pp. 2–19). Philadelphia: Benjamins.

Gordon, R. M. (1986). Folk psychology as simulation. *Mind and Language, 1,* 158–171.

Grèzes, J., Costes, N., & Decety, J. (1998). Top-down effect of strategy on the perception of human biological motion: A PET investigation. *Cognitive Neuropsychology, 15,* 553–582.

Grèzes, J., Costes, N., & Decety, J. (1999). The effect of learning on the neural networks engaged by the perception of meaningless actions. *Brain, 122,* 1875–1888.

Grèzes, J., Frith, C. D., & Passingham, R. E. (2004). Inferring false beliefs from the actions of oneself and others: An fMRI study. *NeuroImage, 21,* 744–750.

Hamilton, A. F. C., & Grafton, S. T. (2006). Goal representation in human anterior intraparietal sulcus. *Journal of Neuroscience, 26,* 1133–1137.

Hamzei, F., Rijntjes, M., Dettmers, C., Glauche, V., Weiller, C., & Büchel, C., (2003). The human action recognition system and its relationship to Broca's area: An fMRI study. *NeuroImage, 19,* 637–644.

Happé, F., Brownell, H., & Winner, E. (1999). Acquired "theory of mind" impairments following stroke. *Cognition, 70,* 211–240.

Harris, P. L. (1989). *Children and emotion.* Oxford: Blackwell.

Hassin, R., Uleman, J., & Bargh, J. (Eds.). (2005). *The new unconscious.* New York: Oxford University Press.

Hatfield, E., Cacioppo, J. T., & Rapson, R. L. (1993). Emotional contagion. *Current Directions in Psychological Science, 2,* 96–99.

Hayne, H., Boniface, J., & Barr, R. (2000). The development of declarative memory in human infants: Age-related changes in deferred imitation. *Behavioral Neuroscience, 114,* 77–83.

Hobson, R. P., & Lee, A. (1999). Imitation and identification in autism. *Journal of Child Psychology and Psychiatry, 40,* 649–659.

Hommel, B. (2004). Event files: Feature binding in and across perception and action. *Trends in Cognitive Sciences, 8,* 494–500.

Iacoboni, M., Molnar-Szakacs, I., Gallese, V., Buccino, G., Mazziotta, J. C., & Rizzolatti, G. (2005). Grasping the intentions of others with one's own mirror neuron system. *PLoS Biology, 3,* e79.

Iacoboni, M., Woods, R. P., Brass, M., Bekkering, H., Mazziotta, J. C., & Rizzolatti, G. (1999). Cortical mechanisms of human imitation. *Science, 286,* 2526–2528.

Izard, C. E. (1982). Measuring emotions in human development. In *Measuring emotions in infants and children* (pp. 3–20). Cambridge: Cambridge University Press.

Jackson, P. L., Brunet, E., Meltzoff, A. N., & Decety, J. (2006). Empathy and the neural mechanisms involved in imagining how I feel versus how you would feel pain: An event-related fMRI study. *Neuropsychologia, 44,* 752–761.

Jackson, P. L., Meltzoff, A. N., & Decety, J. (2005). How do we perceive the pain of others: A window into the neural processes involved in empathy. *NeuroImage, 24,* 771–779.

James, W. (1890). *Principles of psychology.* New York: Holt.

Jeannerod, M. (1997). *The cognitive neuroscience of action.* Oxford: Blackwell.

Jeannerod, M. (2003). The mechanism of self-recognition in human. *Behavioural Brain Research, 142,* 1–15.

Jellema, T., Baker, C. I., Wicker, B., & Perrett, D. I. (2000). Neural representation for the perception of the intentionality of actions. *Brain and Cognition, 44,* 280–302.

Kay, A. C., Wheeler, C., Bargh, J. A., & Ross, J. A. (2004). Material priming: The influence of mundane physical objects on situation construal and competitive behavioral choice. *Organization Behavior and Human Development Processes, 95,* 83–96.

Kilner, J. M., Paulignan, Y., & Blakemore, S. J. (2003). An interference effect of observed biological movement on action. *Current Biology, 13,* 522–525.

Kohler, E., Keysers, C., Umiltà, M. A., Fogassi, L., Gallese, V., & Rizzolatti G. (2002). Hearing sounds, understanding actions: Action representation in mirror neurons. *Science, 297,* 846–848.

Lamm, C., Bauer, H., Vitouch, O., & Gstättner, R. (1999). Differences in the ability to process a visuo-spatial task are reflected in event-related slow cortical potentials of human subjects. *Neuroscience Letters, 269,* 137–140.

Legerstee, M. (1991). The role of person and object in eliciting early imitation. *Journal of Experimental Child Psychology, 51,* 423–433.

Leslie, K. R., Johnson-Frey, S. H., & Grafton, S. T. (2004). Functional imaging of face and hand imitation: Towards a motor theory of empathy. *NeuroImage, 21,* 601–607.

Levenson, R. W., Ekman, P., & Friesen, W. V. (1990). Voluntary facial action generates emotion-specific autonomic nervous system activity. *Psychophysiology, 27,* 363–384.

Lhermitte, F., Pillon, B., & Serdaru, M. (1986). Human autonomy and the frontal lobes. Part I: Imitation and utilization behavior: A neuropsychological study of 75 patients. *Annals of Neurology, 19,* 326–334.

Longo, M. R., & Bertenthal, B. I. (2006). Common coding of observation and execution of action in 9-month-old infants. *Infancy, 10,* 43–59.

Loula, F., Prasad, S., Harber, K., & Shiffrar, M. (2005). Recognizing people from their movement. *Journal of Experimental Psychology: Human Perception and Performance, 31,* 210–220.

Marcovitch, S., & Zelazo, P. D. (1999). The A-not-B error: Results from a logistic meta-analysis. *Child Development, 70,* 1297–1313.

Matsumoto, K., Suzuki, W., & Tanaka, K. (2004). Neuronal correlates of goal-based motor selection in the prefrontal cortex. *Science, 301,* 229–232.

McIntosh, D. N., Reichmann-Decker, A., Winkielman, P., & Wilbarger, J. L. (2006). When the social mirror breaks: Deficits in automatic, but not voluntary mimicry of emotional facial expressions in autism. *Developmental Science, 9,* 295–302.

Meltzoff, A. N. (1995). Understanding the intentions of others: Re-enactment of intended acts by 18-month-old children. *Developmental Psychology, 31,* 838–850.

Meltzoff, A. N., & Decety, J. (2003). What imitation tells us about social cognition: A rapprochement between developmental psychology and cognitive neuroscience. *Philosophical Transactions of the Royal Society of London. Series B, 358,* s491–s500.

Meltzoff, A. N., & Moore, M. K. (1977). Imitation of facial and manual gestures by human neonates. *Science, 198,* 75–78.

Morrison, I., Lloyd, D., di Pellegrino, G., & Roberts, N. (2004). Vicarious responses to pain in anterior cingulate cortex: Is empathy a multisensory issue? *Cognitive, Affective, and Behavioral Neuroscience, 4,* 270–278.

Muthukumaraswamy, S. D., Johnson, B. W., & McNair, N. A. (2004). Mu-rhythm modulation during observation of an object-directed grasp. *Cognitive Brain Research, 19,* 195–201.

Nadel, J. (2002). Some reasons to link imitation and imitation recognition to theory of mind. In J. Proust & J. Dokic (Eds.), *Simulation and knowledge of action* (pp. 251–280). Amsterdam: John Benjamins.

Nagell, K., Olguin, R. S., & Tomasello, M. (1993). Processes of social learning in the tool use of chimpanzees (*Pan troglodytes*) and human children (*Homo sapiens*). *Journal of Comparative Psychology, 107,* 174–186.

Nielsen, L. (2002). The simulation of emotion experience: On the emotional foundation of theory of mind. *Phenomenology and the Cognitive Sciences, 1,* 255–286.

Nishitani, N., & Hari, R. (2000). Temporal dynamics of cortical representation for action. *Proceedings of the National Academy of Sciences the United States of America, 97,* 913–918.

Nishitani, N., & Hari, R. (2002). Viewing lip forms: Cortical dynamics. *Neuron, 36,* 1211–1220.

Oberman, L. M., Hubbard, E. M., McCleery, J. P., Altschuler, E. L., Ramachandran, V. S., & Pineda, J. A. (2005). EEF evidence for mirror neuron dysfunction in autism spectrum disorders. *Cognitive Brain Research, 24,* 190–198.

Ostrowsky, K., Magnin, M., Ryvlin, P., Isnard, J., Gueno, M., & Mauguière, F. (2002). Representation of pain and somatic sensation in the human insula: A study of responses to direct electrical cortical stimulation. *Cerebral Cortex, 12,* 376–385.

Perani, D., Fazio, F., Borghese, N. A., Tettamanti, M., Ferrari, S., Decety, J., et al. (2001). Different brain correlates for watching real and virtual hand actions. *NeuroImage, 14,* 749–758.

Perrett, D. I., Harries, M. H., Bevan, R., Thomas, S., Benson, P. J., Mistlin, A. J., et al. (1989). Frameworks of analysis for the neural representation of animate objects and actions. *Journal of Experimental Biology, 146,* 87–113.

Pierno, A. C., Mari, M., Glover, S., Georgiou, I., & Castiello, U. (2008). Failure to read motor intentions from gaze in children with autism. *Neuropsychologia, 46,* 488–454.

Pobric, G., & Hamilton, A. F. (2006). Action understanding requires the left inferior frontal cortex. *Current Biology, 16,* 524–529.

Preston, S. D., & de Waal, F. B. M. (2002). Empathy: Its ultimate and proximate bases. *Behavioral and Brain Sciences, 25,* 1–72.

Prinz, W. (2003). Experimental approaches to action. In J. Roessler & N. Eilan (Eds.), *Agency and self-awareness* (pp. 175–187). Oxford: Oxford University Press.

Reiman, E. M., Lane, R. D., Ahern, G. L., Schwartz, G. E., Davidson, R. J., Friston, K. J., et al. (1997). Neuroanatomical correlates of externally and internally generated emotion. *American Journal of Psychiatry, 154,* 918–925.

Rizzolatti, G., & Craighero, L. (2004). The mirror-neuron system. *Annual Review of Neuroscience, 27,* 169–192.

Rizzolatti, G., Fadiga, L., Gallese, V., & Fogassi, L. (1996). Premotor cortex and the recognition of motor actions. *Cognitive Brain Research, 3,* 131–141.

Rochat, P. (1999). *Early social cognition: Understanding others in the first months of life.* Mahwah, NJ: Lawrence Erlbaum Associates.

Ruby, P., & Decety, J. (2001). Effect of subjective perspective taking during simulation of action: A PET investigation of agency. *Nature Neuroscience, 4,* 546–550.

Ryalls, B. O., Gul, R. E., & Ryalls, K. R. (2000). Infant's imitation of peer and adult models: Evidence for a peer model advantage. *Merrill-Palmer Quarterly, 46,* 188–202.

Saxe, R. (2005). Against simulation: The argument from error. *Trends in Cognitive Sciences, 9,* 174–179.

Shepard, R. N. (1984). Ecological constraints on internal representation: Resonant kinematics of perceiving, imagining, thinking, and dreaming. *Psychological Review, 91,* 417–447.

Shiffrar, M., & Pinto, J. (2002). The visual analysis of bodily motion. In W. Prinz & B. Hommel (Eds.), *Common mechanisms in perception and action: Attention and performance* (Vol. 19, pp. 381–399). Oxford: Oxford University Press.

Siegal, M., & Varley, R. (2002). Neural systems involved in "theory of mind." *Nature Reviews Neuroscience, 3,* 463–471.

Singer, T., Seymour, B., O'Doherty, J., Kaube, H., Dolan, R. J., & Frith, C. D. (2004). Empathy for pain involves the affective but not sensory components of pain. *Science, 303,* 1157–1161.

Smith, I. M., & Bryson, S. E. (1994). Imitation and action in autism: A critical review. *Psychological Bulletin, 116,* 259–273.

Smith, L. B., Thelen, E., Titzer, R., & McLin, D. (1999). Knowing in the context of acting: The task dynamics of the A-not-B error. *Psychological Review, 106,* 235–260.

Sommerville, J. A., & Decety, J. (2006). Weaving the fabric of social interaction: Articulating developmental psychology and cognitive neuroscience in the domain of motor cognition. *Psychonomic Bulletin and Review, 13,* 179–200.

Sommerville, J. A., & Woodward, A. L. (2005). Pulling out the structure of intentional action: The relation between action processing and production in infancy. *Cognition, 95,* 1–30.

Sommerville, J. A., Woodward, A. L., & Needham, A. (2005). Action experience alters 3-month-old infants' perception of others' actions. *Cognition, 96,* B1–B11.

Sperry, R. W. (1952). Neurology and the mind-body problem. *American Scientist, 40,* 291–312.

Sprengelmeyer, R., Young, A. W., Schroeder, U., Grossenbacher, P. G., Federlein, J., Buttner, T., et al. (1999). Knowing no fear. *Proceedings of the Royal Society of London. Series B, Biology, 266,* 2451–2456.

Stevens, J. A., Fonlupt, P., Shiffrar, M. A., & Decety, J. (2000). New aspects of motion perception: Selective neural encoding of apparent human movements. *Neuroreport, 11,* 109–115.

Tai, Y. F., Scherfler, C., Brooks, D. J., Sawamoto, N., & Castiello, U. (2004). The human premotor cortex is mirror only for biological actions. *Current Biology, 14,* 117–120.

Thelen, E., Schoner, G., Scheier, C., & Smith, L. B. (2001). The dynamics of embodiment: A field theory of infant perseverative reaching. *Behavioral and Brain Sciences, 24,* 1–86.

Théoret, H., Halligan, E., Kobayashi, M., Fregni, F., Tager-Flusberg, H., & Pascual-Leone, A. (2005). Impaired motor facilitation during action observation in individuals with autism spectrum disorder. *Current Biology, 15,* R84–R85.

Trevarthen, C. (1979). Communication and cooperation in early infancy: A description of primary intersubjectivity. In M. Bullowa (Ed.), *Before speech: The beginning of human communication* (pp. 321–347). New York: Cambridge University Press.

Ulmità, M. A., Kohler, E., Gallese, V., Fogassi, L., Fadiga, L., Keysers, C., et al. (2001). I know what you are doing: A neurophysiological study. *Neuron, 31,* 155–165.

Van Baaren, R. B., Holland, R. W., Kawakami, K., & Va Knippenberg, A. (2004). Mimicry and prosocial behavior. *Psychological Science, 15,* 71–74.

Wicker, B., Keysers, C., Plailly, J., Royet, J. P., Gallese, V., & Rizzolatti, G. (2003). Both of us disgusted in my insula: The common neural basis of seeing and feeling disgust. *Neuron, 40,* 655–664.

Wilson, M., & Knoblich, G. (2005). The case of motor involvement in perceiving conspecifics. *Psychological Bulletin, 131,* 460–473.

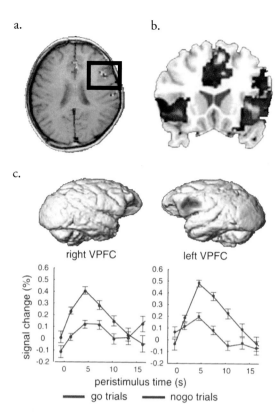

Fig. 3.7 Functional magnetic resonance imaging of GO/NO-GO task performance. a. Subtracting activation during NO-GO performance from GO performance yields activation in right inferior frontal gyrus (Konishi et al., 1998). b. Subtracting activation during STOP from GO trials on a stop-signal task yields activation that is greater in right compared to left inferior frontal gyrus (Aron & Poldrack, 2006). c. A homologous frontal cortical area in the monkey has recently been identified with fMRI (Morita et al., 2004). Although a bilateral response is found, it is larger in the left hemisphere, contralateral to the hand used for responding.

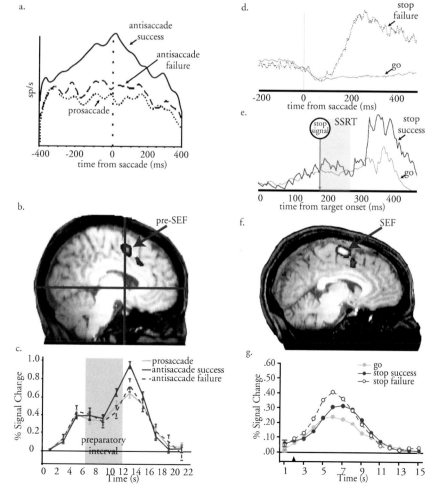

Fig. 3.8 Performance monitoring in the SEF. a. The firing rate of SEF neurons is greater prior to antisaccades than prosaccades and antisaccade failures (Schlag-Rey et al., 1997). a. and b. Activity in an area just anterior to the human SEF shows greater activity just prior to antisaccades compared to prosaccades and antisaccade failures (Curtis & D'Esposito, 2003). d. Some monkey SEF neurons show a burst of activity following errors on STOP trials of a stop-signal task and e. some show a burst of activity following successfully cancelled STOP trials (Stuphorn et al., 2000). f. and g. Similarly in humans, the SEF shows increased activation related to success and failures of inhibition (Curtis et al., 2005).

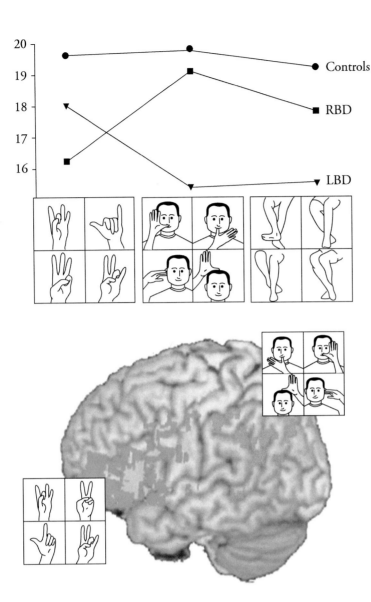

Fig. 7.3 Body part specificity of defective imitation. Upper part: Mean scores (maximum = 20) of healthy controls and patients with either left (LBD) or right (RBD) brain damage on imitation of meaningless postures of fingers, hand, and foot (Goldenberg & Strauss, 2002). There were 10 postures of each kind. Note that although LBD patients fare generally better with finger than with hand postures, they are as a group nonetheless much worse than controls also for them. Lower part: There are dissociations between finger and hand postures within the group of LBD patients. The image shows the result of magnetic resonance imaging lesion subtraction: Lesions of patients with defective hand but normal finger imitation were subtracted from those with the reverse dissociation: Whereas defective imitation of hand postures is bound to lesions of inferior parietal regions and the temporo-parieto-occipital junction, defective imitation of finger postures is associated with inferior frontal lesions (Goldenberg & Karnath, 2006).

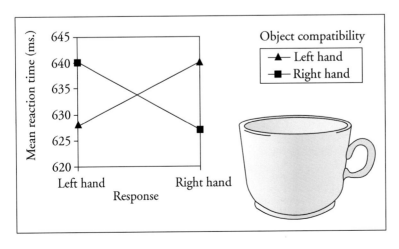

Fig. 11.1 The object–action compatibility effect, in response latency, on the hand of response when classifying objects (such as in the cup example) that are oriented so as to have an optimal hand of grasp (the right hand in the cup example).

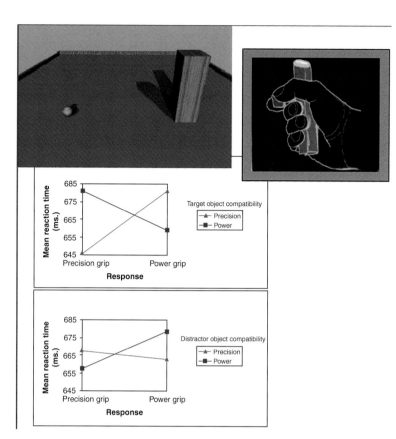

Fig. 11.2 Object-action compatibility effects, in response latency, for the target and distractor objects in two object displays (as illustrated in the example) on precision and power grip responses (made on the response device also illustrated) classifying the shape of the target object (cued by its blue-gray color).

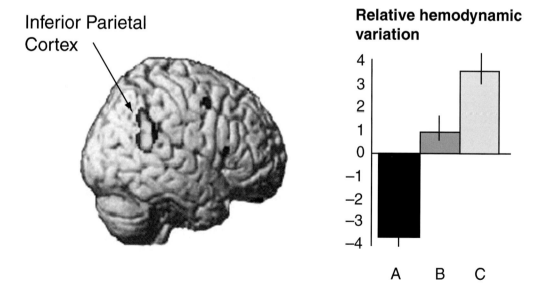

Fig. 13.2 Right inferior parietal lobule activation at the junction of the temporal cortex superimposed on a rendered MRI. In this study, participants were scanned during a variety of object-directed actions with small objects, including self-action (A), imitation of actions performed by an experimenter (B), and observation of their actions being imitated by the experimenter (C). Note the dramatic increase in this region in this latter condition. This region plays a pivotal role in the sense of agency (adapted from Decety, Chaminade, Grèzes, & Meltzoff, 2002).

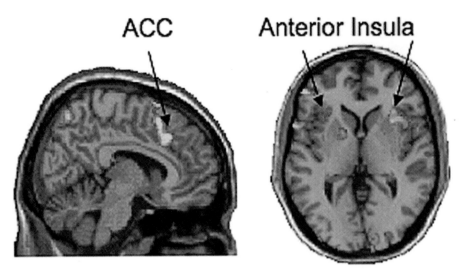

Fig. 13.3 Sagittal (on the left) and coronal (on the right) views of activated clusters in the anterior cingulate cortex (ACC) and anterior insula elicited by the perception of other individuals in painful situations superimposed on an averaged structural MR image. Physiological research in pain processing demonstrates that the ACC has a role in the affective-motivational dimension of pain, that is, related to behavioral responses associated with avoiding or escaping the nociceptive stimulus. This region interrelates attentional and evaluative functions with that of establishing emotional valence and response priorities. The insular cortex is involved in monitoring the physiological state of the body. It receives direct input from the spinothalamic pathways via the medial thalamic nuclei (the major nociceptive pathway). Interestingly, both the ACC and the anterior insula are found activated by the mere sight of pain in others (adapted from Jackson, Meltzoff, & Decety, 2005).

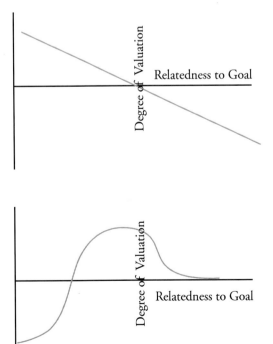

Fig. 16.1 Two patterns of valuation and devaluation. The top pattern was obtained with consumption products as items. The bottom panel was obtained with concerns as items. More positive values on the y-axis correspond to greater preference for products and to greater concerns.

Positive Hedonic 'liking'

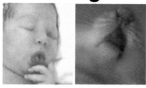

Negative Aversive 'disliking'

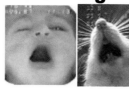

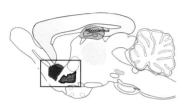

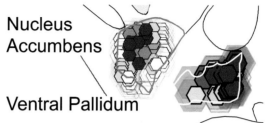

Nucleus Accumbens

Ventral Pallidum

Opioid Hedonic Hotspots

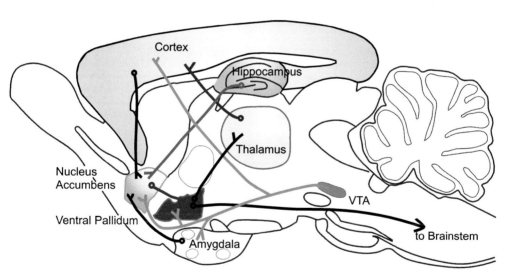

Fig. 24.1 "Liking" reactions and brain hedonic hot spots. Top: Positive hedonic "liking" reactions are elicited by sucrose taste from human infant and adult rat (e.g., rhythmic tongue protrusion). By contrast, negative aversive "disliking" reactions are elicited by bitter quinine taste. Below: Forebrain hedonic hot spots in limbic structures where mu opioid activation causes a brighter pleasure gloss to be painted on sweet sensation. Red/yellow shows hot spots in nucleus accumbens and ventral pallidum where opioid microinjections caused the biggest increases in the number of sweet-elicited "liking" reactions. Based on Peciña and Berridge (2005), Smith and Berridge (2005), and Peciña, Smith, and Berridge (2006).

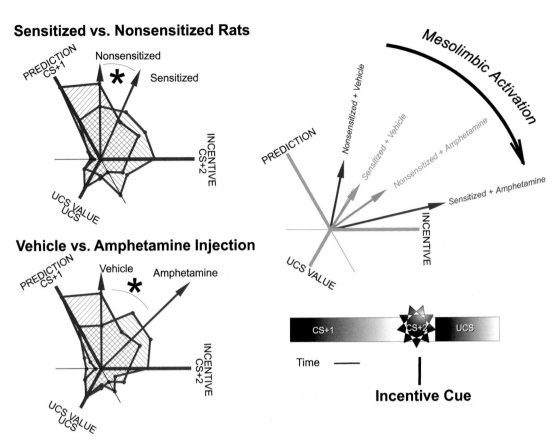

Fig. 24.3 Mesolimbic activation magnifies decision utility coding by neuron firing in ventral pallidum. Population profile vector shifts toward incentive coding with mesolimbic activation. Profile analysis shows stimulus preference coded in firing for all 524 ventral pallidum neurons. Ordinarily, neurons prefer to code predicted utility (firing maximally to CS+1 tone). Sensitization and amphetamine administration each shift neuronal coding preference toward decision utility (firing maximally to the CS+2 click) and away from predicted utility of CS+1 (without altering signal for experienced utility of the sugar UCS). Combination of sensitization with amphetamine shifts ventral pallidum coding profiles even further toward the signal for pure decision utility or incentive salience. Thus, as mesolimbic activation increases, ventral pallidum neurons increasingly carry coded signals for decision utility (relative to predicted utility and experienced utility signals). Entire populations are shown by shaded areas. Arrows shows the maximal averaged response of the population under each treatment. Based on Tindell, Berridge, Zhang, Peciña, and Aldridge (2005, pp. 2628 and 2629, figs. 6 and 7).

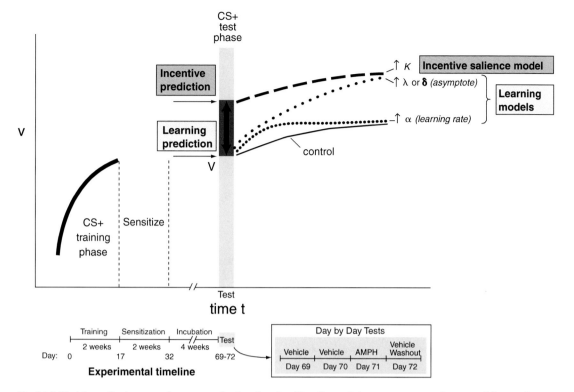

Fig. 24.4 Decision utility increment happens too fast for relearning. Time line and alternative outcomes for neuronal firing coding of reward cue after mesolimbic activation of sensitization and/or amphetamine in ventral pallidum recording experiment (Tindell, Berridge, Zhang, Peciña, & Aldridge, 2005). The incentive salience model predicts that mesolimbic activation dynamically increases the decision utility of a previously learned CS+. The increased incentive salience coding is visible the first time the already-learned cue is presented in the activated mesolimbic state. Learning models by contrast require relearning to elevate learned predicted utilities. They predict merely gradual acceleration if mesolimbic activation increases rate parameters of learning and gradual acceleration plus asymptote elevation if mesolimbic activation increases prediction errors. Actual data support the incentive salience model. Based on data from Tindell et al. (2005).

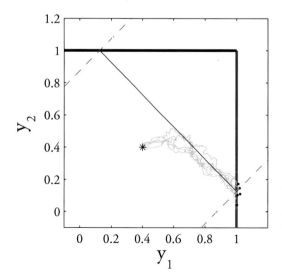

Fig. 25.3 Typical sample paths in the linearized leaky accumulator model illustrating convergence to an attracting line. The thick lines are the thresholds $y_i = 0$, the thin solid line is the attracting line, the dashed lines are the thresholds for the DD process x, the star is the initial condition, and dots are the final states following threshold crossing. Parameter values are $g(t) \equiv 1$, $\alpha = \beta = 4$, $a_1 = 5$, $a_2 = 4$, $\theta = 1$, and $\sigma = 0.1$. Adapted from McMillen and Holmes (2006).

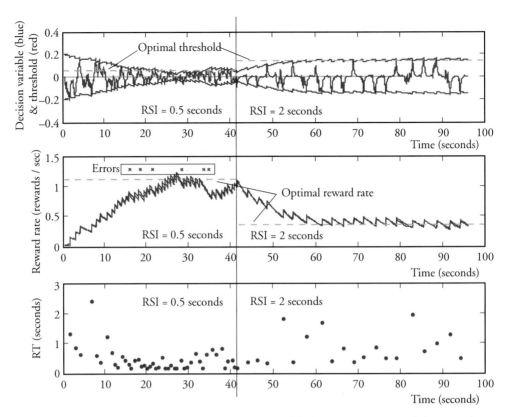

Fig. 25.7 Numerical simulations of the continuous time computational model of Equations22 to 28. Panels from top to bottom, respectively, show thresholds as envelopes with DD solutions inside and optimal thresholds dashed; running reward rate estimate with errors indicated by x's and optimal reward rates dashed; and reaction times. Parameter values are noted in text.

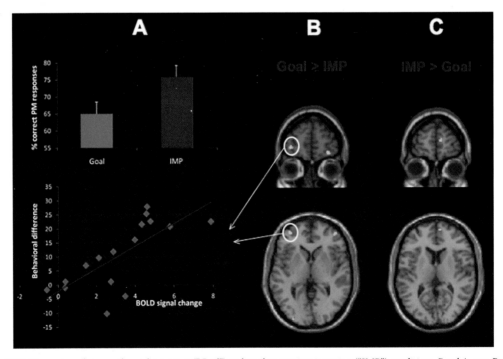

Fig. 29.2 Comparisons between the goal-intention ("Goal") and implementation-intention ("IMP") conditions. Panel A, top: Percentage of correctly detected prospective memory (PM) targets in the two conditions. Panel A, bottom: Correlation between the difference in BOLD signal in left lateral BA 10 elicited by correctly detected PM targets in the two conditions (horizontal axis) and the behavioral difference between the two conditions (vertical axis). Panel B: Brain regions showing greater target-related activity in the goal-intention condition compared with the implementation-intention condition, plotted on coronal (y = 56) and axial (z = 2) slices of a normalized T1-weighted scan. Panel C: Brain regions showing greater target-related activity during the implementation-intention condition compared with the goal-intention condition (plotted at y = 60 and z = 10).

Affect, Goals, and Motivation

14 Affect and Action Control

Deidre L. Reis *and* Jeremy R. Gray

> Action readiness change is the major feature of
> emotion; . . . the defining feature.
>
> —N. H. Frijda, *The Emotions* (1986, p. 469)

Abstract

This chapter discusses the relation between emotion and action control. It tries to show that emotion-cognition interactions exist at all levels of the action control hierarchy from attention to decision making and planning. The influences of emotion on memory, decision making, reasoning, attention, and emotion regulation are considered. These are related to action control within an established model of emotion in which the major end point is change in action readiness (Frijda, 1986). Our aim is to show that affect is integral to action control in a strong sense: pervasively so and at effectively all levels of the action control hierarchy.

Keywords: emotion, cognition, interaction, memory, decision-making reasoning, emotion regulation

The word *emotion* suggests a conceptual link between affect and action control: Etymologically, *emotion* is from the Latin *ex* (away, out) and *movere* (to move). Empirically, a link between at least some emotions and some actions is unequivocal—in facial expressions of joy, fear, and sadness, for example. Emotion theorists have long posited a major role for affect in the control of behavior more generally (e.g., Carver, Sutton, & Scheier, 2000; Frijda, 1986; Lang, Bradley, & Cuthbert, 1990; Schneirla, 1959). Action control theorists have equally noted the relevance of affect for action control, including motivation and volition (Gollwitzer, 1999; see Chapters 15, 17, and 29). Our aim in this chapter is to show that affect is integral to action control not just in obvious ex- amples but in a strong sense: pervasively so and at effectively all levels of the action control hierarchy from attention to decision making and planning. An exhaustive review would require a book; we provide a selective review, elaborating an integrated view of affect and action control, especially through a consideration of the influences of emotion on memory, decision making, reasoning, attention, and emotion regulation. We relate them to action control within an established model of emotion in which a major end point is action readiness (Frijda, 1986). That is, for expository purposes in this chapter, we take Frijda's model of the process of emotion and refer to it as a rough-and-ready model of action control, light on detail (see other chapters in this section) but useful for the big picture.

We review evidence suggesting that emotion and cognition interact in many ways, as revealed in behavioral, psychophysiological, and neural measures. Separate circuits and structures are responsible for more emotional versus more cognitive functions (LeDoux, 2000; LeDoux & Armony, 1999; Panksepp, 1998). This distinction is critical for understanding psychological and emotional disorders as well as the fundamentals of healthy functioning and the nature of their interaction. We do not propose that emotion and cognition should be "blended beyond distinction" (Panksepp, 1994) but do hold to a view that they are "integrated" in the sense of being only partly—but not completely—separable (Gray, Braver, & Raichle, 2002). The existence of multilevel emotion–cognition interactions suggests that these two systems are tightly integrated, and constantly interacting. By biasing memory, decision-making and choice behavior, reasoning, attention, and physiology, emotions influence action and action readiness in ways both strong and subtle.

But What Is Emotion?
Contemporary Views

How to understand or even simply define emotions has been debated by psychologists, neuroscientists, and philosophers over centuries (Ekman & Davidson, 1994). Ancient Greek philosophers viewed emotions as pernicious influences on judgment—and so emotions need to be controlled by the rational mind. However, a wealth of contemporary research in emotion suggests that affect is not categorically disruptive and in fact is best understood as adaptive, that is, functional, on balance. There are many situations where emotion may benefit cognition and decision making by favoring choices that encourage goal attainment, by coordinating social interactions and relationships to address problems (Keltner & Haidt, 1999), and possibly by helping to resolve conflict between control dilemmas more generally (Gray, Schaefer, Braver, & Most, 2005).

Researchers have used the term *emotion* in many different senses without a widely adopted definition (Larsen & Fredrickson, 1999). Nonetheless, action control is not merely a consistent but a central, even defining, theme in many leading accounts of emotion. Functional accounts of emotions characterize them as likely to occur in situations in which adaptive action is necessary and preceded by events that occur quickly and without warning (Davidson, 1994). According to this view, emotions are usually accompanied by autonomic activity that supports the action occurring alongside the emotion. Frijda (1986) defines emotional phenomena in terms of action readiness: "noninstrumental behaviors and noninstrumental features of behavior, physiological changes, and evaluative, subject-related experiences, as evoked by external or mental events, and primarily by the significance of such events" (p. 4). Action control is also central to emotion as characterized by Lang (1995), who defines emotions as "action dispositions—states of vigilant readiness that vary widely in reported affect, physiology, and behavior" (p. 372) that are driven by either appetitive or aversive motivation. Russell and Feldman Barrett (1999) distinguish "prototypical emotional episodes" from "core affect" by delineating specific, defining characteristics of each. A prototypical emotional episode involves a set of actions focused on an object (which can be a person, thing, or event) and at a minimum must include core affect, appropriate behavior, attention toward the object of the episode, and the experience of having an emotion. Furthermore, emotional episodes must have a beginning and end point and a specific duration. In contrast, core affect is much more general and includes basic feelings of which one may be conscious but does not need to be directed at any particular object. These views are summarized in Table 14.1. Other definitions of emotion could be included here; we provide these summaries only as a basic overview of the variety of conceptions of emotion in the literature and to point to some consensus on the importance of the control of actions.

In subsequent sections, we relate emotion–cognition interactions to components of Frijda's (1986) model, from a stimulus event and ending with action readiness (Figure 14.1). The structure of this model—that it is in effect a skeleton or outline rather than a fully specified model—is particularly well suited to our exposition of how emotion–cognition interactions are directly relevant to action control in terms of memory, decision making, reasoning, attention, and emotion regulation. In Frijda's outline of the process of emotion (pp. 453–473; see Figure 14.1), the natural and useful starting point for expository purposes is the eliciting stimulus, especially as it is initially interpreted or classified by the subject's nervous system (the "analyzer"). The next stage ("comparator") computes the relevance of the stimulus for the subject, especially in terms of implications for hedonic experience. These first two stages can be influenced by attentional and perceptual biases toward or away from classes of stimuli. The third stage ("diagnoser") further evaluates the stimulus in terms of its relevance given the current context, including the ability to cope with that stimulus. In this stage, long-term memory and aspects of decision making are important. The fourth stage ("evaluator") integrates prior information about relevance and results in an overall assessment about control precedence—the urgency, difficulty, and seriousness of the event in light of one's concerns, current situation, and ability to respond. On this basis, the next stage ("action proposer") generates an action plan or change in readiness for action, leading to both physiological changes (especially arousal) and action generation. Throughout these stages, regulatory processes interact with processing at each stage. The process

Table 14.1 Selected Definitions of Emotion, Many Explicitly Noting a Role for Emotion in the Control of Action

Researcher	Definition of Emotion
Davidson (1994)	–Functional account: response to a situation where adaptive action is necessary –Situation is usually preceded by events that occur quickly & without warning –Accompanied by physiological activity that may support action
Frijda (1986)	–Noninstrumental behaviors and features of behavior, physiological changes, and evaluative, subject-related experiences –Evoked by external or mental events (primarily by the significance of those events)
Izard (1994)	–Feeling or motivational state driven by neurochemical substrates –May occur without cognition
Lang (1995)	–Action disposition—involves a state of readiness –May vary with respect to affect, physiology, and behavior –Driven by appetitive or aversive motivations
Russell & Feldman Barrett (1999)	–A set of actions focused on an object –Includes core affect, appropriate behavior, attention toward the object of focus, and the experience of having the emotion –Have clear beginning and end points, and specific duration

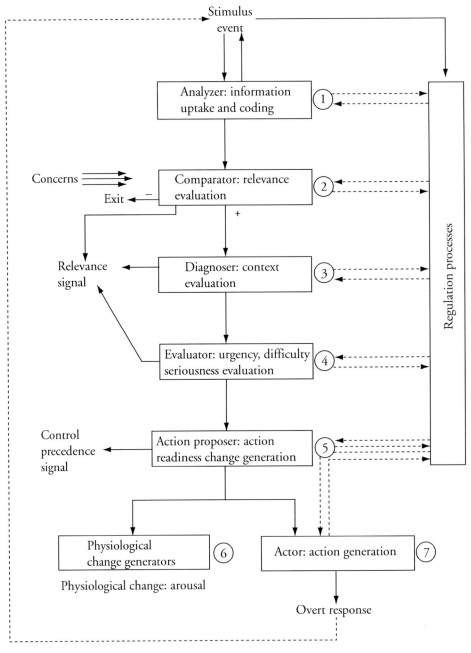

Fig. 14.1 Frijda's model of the emotion process (1986, p. 454), which for expository purposes we refer to as a model of action control. Reprinted with the permission of Cambridge University Press.

does not end there—the actions taken (and not taken) in turn influence the context and the original instigating stimulus (see Chapter 15 for a control system view). Thus, Frijda's model of the emotion process also constitutes a rough-and-ready model of the process of action control. In this way, the model provides a useful framework for understanding the integrated nature of emotion and action control (cf. Gray, 2001).

Emotion–Cognition Interactions in the Service of Action Control

In our view, both cognition and emotion function as control systems that regulate behavior. That is, the function of both cognition and emotion is ultimately expressed through the control of action; the functions are adaptive to the extent that the behaviors so controlled are adaptive. Contemporary studies using behavioral, psychophysiological, and neuroimaging methods have shed light on how and when emotion and cognition interact (Dalgleish & Power, 1999; Drevets & Raichle, 1998). Emotion–cognition interactions occur at multiple levels of processing and across many different types of emotional circumstances and cognitive tasks. We review studies that operationalize emotion through mood inductions, emotional priming, and the use of stimuli with overtly emotional content. The cognitive paradigms utilized measure effects on memory, decision making, reasoning, and attention. To illustrate the bidirectionality of the emotion–cognition relation, we also review emotion regulation. Emotion regulation is a factor at all stages of Frijda's model that influences the ultimate action(s) taken (or not taken). The pervasiveness of emotion–cognition interactions at multiple levels of processing suggests that emotion and cognition are not completely separable but instead are, in a word, integrated (Gray, 2004).

Interactions Revealed in Performance

In this section we review results from studies in which subjects deliberate about task-relevant content during the course of the experiment with the intention of coming to some sort of conclusion or decision, as reflected overtly in some performance measure, with particular attention to how emotion may interact with that process. Emotion–cognition interactions are seen in many cases where conflicting inputs from emotional and cognitive systems lead to conflicts that must be resolved before a decision can be made. Here we will review evidence at the information-processing level from studies of memory, emotion regulation,

decision making, and logical reasoning to demonstrate that emotion–cognition interactions influence action control.

Memory

Memory is potentially relevant to action control in several ways. Long-term memory would influence the early stages (Figure 14.1), particularly by influencing how a stimulus is categorized or evaluated (Chapter 5). Research on phenomena such as flashbulb memories, recovered memory, and mood-dependent memory has demonstrated that emotion often has a profound impact on memory—though the direction and nature of the influence may vary (Bohannon, 1988; Bower, 1981; Brown & Kulik, 1977; Christianson, 1992; Loftus, 1993). Behavioral conditioning paradigms using electric shock or food reward can also be construed, in cognitive terms, as emotional learning and memory.

Not only does the emotional content of a stimulus influence how it is processed and remembered, but ongoing mood at the time of processing may play a major role in how information is stored and later utilized. For example, positive and negative mood inductions can lead to differential rates of false memory (Storbeck & Clore, 2005). Using the Deese–Roediger–McDermott paradigm (Roediger & McDermott, 1995), participants were instructed to memorize a list of words centered on a particular concept (e.g., bed, pillow, or rest). The common concept word (in this case, sleep) is closely related in semantic meaning but is never actually presented and is thus a "lure" to test false memory. Participants who were in a pleasant mood showed higher rates of false memory for lures, while those in a negative mood state demonstrated lower lure rates. In a follow-up study, the authors determined that the affective influence occurred at the stage of encoding rather than recall. The same paradigm was used, but during recall participants were asked to also list any related words that came to mind but were not presented in the original list. There was no interaction between recall instruction (presented versus non-presented lures) and mood group, signifying that the effect of inclusion instruction did not differ across mood groups in the production of critical lures (e.g., the differences between mood groups did not disappear with the instruction to include any words that came to mind). These results suggest that the reduced false memory rate of the negative mood group is due to a more item-specific processing strategy during encoding that made them less likely to access lures at retrieval; similarly, positive moods encouraged a more global, relational information-processing strategy, increasing the false memory effect. The authors propose that these results support the affect-as-information hypothesis, such that affective cues act as feedback and help determine the information-processing strategy (item specific or global/relational) the individual will use during task performance. In this case, affective state influenced cognitive information processing, biasing encoding strategies in a selective, specific way with clear effects on memory.

Affective states also influence working memory in a variety of ways relevant to action control, especially as influencing later stages in Frijda's model (Figure 14.1). The ability to consider context, inhibit prepotent responses, and engage in on-the-spot problem solving and reasoning would all depend to some degree on working memory and would be especially relevant in the diagnosis and evaluation stages; we review effects of emotion on reasoning here. Studies examining the effect of mood on working memory–related tasks have found differential influences of positive versus negative moods and suggest a possible hemispheric basis for the direction of effects (Bartolic,

Basso, Schefft, Glauser, & Titanic-Schefft, 1999; Heller & Nitschke, 1997). In a study examining the influence of emotion on cognitive control, Gray (2001) found evidence for a double dissociation of verbal and spatial working memory. After viewing videos intended to induce approach, neutral, or withdrawal states, participants completed a series of *n*-back working memory tasks with letters as stimuli (the task was to recall either the letter's identity or location). Approach states improved verbal working memory but impaired spatial working memory, while withdrawal states yielded the opposite pattern of results. One interpretation of these results is that cognitive control is modulated on a hemispheric basis in the brain. Given the body of evidence linking both approach states and maintenance of verbal information with left hemisphere activation as well as that associating withdrawal states and maintenance of spatial information with right hemisphere activation, this interpretation seems most parsimonious and plausible. These results demonstrate affective state interacts with cognitive processing in a selective way, leading to specific behavioral outcomes in which some cognitive abilities are improved and others impaired, depending on the characteristics of the emotion induced.

Decision Making

The role of affect in decision making (both the process of considering competing options as well as enacting that decision through behavior) has been of considerable research interest. Such influences of emotion on action control are strongly relevant to action control (Figure 14.1) as influencing evaluations of relevance, urgency, and value. Intriguing evidence for emotion–cognition interactions as an influence on these processes comes from patients with damage to prefrontal regions known to be involved in decision making and emotional processing (Chapter 10). Using the Iowa Gambling Task (IGT), Bechara, Damasio, Damasio, and Anderson (1994) examined the decision-making behavior of patients with damage to the ventromedial prefrontal cortex (VMPFC). In the IGT, four decks of cards are presented to participants. Two of the decks offer small rewards and similarly small penalties (the "safe" decks), while the other two decks offer large rewards but also large penalties ("risky" decks). Participants are told that the game involves choosing cards from any of these decks until they are told to stop (they do not know how many selections they will be given). In the long run, the advantageous strategy is to choose from the safe decks to wind up with a net gain. Patients with VMPFC damage chose greater numbers of cards from the risky decks, while controls chose more from the safe decks. The authors suggest that because of their brain damage, these patients lack mechanisms of emotion-related feedback that healthy participants use to adaptively bias the choices they make in the IGT. Hence, in the case of VMPFC patients, it appears that their decision-making abilities are impaired because of their lack of appropriate affective basis on which adaptive choices could be made.

Mood states differentially influenced decision making related to the *endowment effect*, or the tendency for an individual's selling price for a given object to exceed the buying price of the same object (Lerner, Small, & Loewenstein, 2004). This effect is thought to reflect the increased value attributed to an item once an individual has had it in their possession. Half the individuals were given an item at the beginning of an experiment (in this case, a highlighter set) and told to hold on to it for later use. At the conclusion of the experiment, participants are asked how much they would accept to sell their item (their "sell price"). The other participants

are shown the item at the beginning of the experiment, but it is not given to them. At the end of the study, they are asked how much money they would have to receive to forfeit the item (their "choice price"), which presumably estimates how much they value the item.

Lerner et al. (2004) induced negative mood states in participants to determine how such states would influence decision-making behavior in a situation that normally produces an endowment effect. Participants viewed either a sad, disgusting, or neutral movie and were then asked for their sell or choice prices for the highlighter set. Following a sadness induction, individuals were willing to sell their items for less money and pay more money to obtain a different item (thought to reflect a tendency to change one's circumstances however possible when in a depressed mood). After a disgust mood induction, participants were willing to sell their items for less and would pay less to acquire new items (thought to reflect the desire to push away things when in a state of disgust). Individuals in the neutral condition replicated the robust endowment effect, showing higher sell prices than choice prices. Thus emotion selectively interacts with cognitive decision making while individuals are processing information (here, considering their valuation of a product), such that different negatively valenced moods elicit distinct action tendencies. Of note, these emotional influences were global mood inductions unrelated to the task, suggesting a strong carryover effect of emotional information.

Other studies have found similarly powerful effects of affective content on decision making. In particular, the introduction of emotionally relevant cues can cause people to view economic choices in a *scope insensitive* manner. In several studies, Hsee and Rottenstreich (2004) found that exposure to emotional stimuli influenced how participants judged the value of a range of items. Participants were primed with either an affective (feeling-based) or computational (i.e., analytical) mind-set by completing a questionnaire before being asked to state how much they valued an object. In the affective priming condition, participants were asked to describe how they felt when hearing trigger words such as *George W. Bush* or *baby;* while in the computational condition, they were asked to complete mathematical word problems. Following the priming manipulation, subjects were asked how much they would be willing to pay for a set of 5 versus 10 popular music compact discs (CDs). If participants were scope sensitive, they would calculate their willingness to pay based on multiplying the number of discs available by an amount reflective of the cost of a single disc, with their value of 10 CDs being roughly double their value of five CDs. Yet participants primed with an emotional mind-set showed scope insensitivity such that their value for 10 CDs did not increase proportionally over the value ascribed to five CDs. One possible reason for this is that the affective prime encouraged participants to focus on the feelings engendered by the CDs and their desire to have the CDs instead of focusing on the number and value of the CDs they could obtain. In contrast, participants primed with an analytical mind-set showed a much more scope-sensitive pattern of valuation evidenced by a more linear, proportional slope of estimated values. In a second study, an affect-rich object (a music book that participants were asked to imagine they would enjoy a great deal) similarly elicited scope-insensitive valuations in contrast to an affect-poor object (the amount of cash the book was worth). Additionally, when participants were asked to indicate the amount they would give to a charitable cause, affective stimuli (here, photographs of endangered panda bears) again elicited

scope insensitivity. Subjects saw either one or four pandas represented as photographs or dots on a graph and were asked how much they would donate to help the pandas. Participants who saw affect-rich photographs showed scope insensitivity in the amount they were willing to donate (e.g., donating comparable amounts for one versus four pandas) versus participants in the affect-poor condition who donated proportionally larger amounts for four pandas versus one. Here, affective content influenced valuation judgments and the choices made by participants. In sum, by eliciting emotional responses, affective stimuli have the potential to change the types of economic decisions people make.

Reasoning

Reasoning is very relevant to action control, especially during evaluation stages when faced with unfamiliar and complex circumstances, such as contingencies that differ by context, during simulation of the consequences of potential action plans, and during emotion regulation. Emotionally relevant semantic content appears to have a variable effect on reasoning abilities. In a study using classic "If *p* then *q*" logical reasoning (e.g., syllogisms involving *modus ponens* and *modus tollens*), participants performed worse when the content of such statements contained emotionally valenced words (e.g., "If someone is in a tragic situation, then she cries") as compared to performance with neutral words (Blanchette & Richards, 2004). Participants also performed worse on statements including neutral words that had been classically conditioned to be more emotionally negative than words that had been conditioned to remain neutral. In other words, emotional words impaired logical reasoning.

In contrast, it is also the case that emotion is not always detrimental. A study using emotional recall prior to a reasoning task illustrates a facilitating role for affect in reasoning (Chang & Wilson, 2004). The reasoning task used was a version of the Wason card selection task involving the detection of potential cheaters. In the Wason task, participants are given a rule and asked to evaluate a sequence of cards concerning rule conditions. One commonly used variant of the task is a rule that involves a potential instance of an individual cheating others. Participants in the study were asked to write an autobiographical recollection of a time when they had been cheated by someone, then were asked whether writing about the event successfully evoked the feeling they described in their story. Participants who answered affirmatively performed significantly better on this version of the task than individuals who recalled an instance of being happy or benefiting from someone's altruism, suggesting that in recalling and writing about the event, participants probably experienced emotions that adaptively biased responses such that people had an easier time detecting potential cheaters.

The apparent contradiction between these findings underscores the important distinction between *task-relevant* versus *task-irrelevant* affect in shaping action tendencies. Blanchette and Richards (2004) utilized emotional words with no connection to the reasoning problems, and as such the words likely served as distracters from the reasoning task and shifted attention away from the goal at hand. In contrast, the emotion induced by Chang and Wilson was directly applicable to the task, priming participants with emotion in a way that adaptively biased performance by facilitating action tendencies toward successful performance of the subsequent reasoning task.

Finally, affective individual differences also influence performance reasoning tasks, revealing emotion–cognition interaction. Reis et al. (2007) found that higher harm avoidance (HA; the degree to which an individual is cautious or careful in his or her daily life) predicted faster performance on a reasoning task in which participants made judgments about statements related to avoiding danger. Similarly, higher emotional intelligence (EI; the ability to monitor one's own and others' emotions and to use the information to guide thinking and actions) predicted faster performance on a social reasoning task in which participants were asked to identify situations where cheating might take place (similar to the reasoning task used by Chang & Wilson, 2004). In both cases, individuals with higher ratings of the affective individual difference measures performed the related reasoning problems faster, with no loss of accuracy. The relationships between HA and precautionary reasoning as well as between EI and social reasoning were both selective and specific, indicating a double dissociation. While affective individual differences are not equivalent to emotion inductions, these results illustrate that the interaction of emotionally relevant personality measures with the cognitive reasoning processes biases behavior adaptively and facilitates performance. Beyond the specific example here, affective individual differences could potentially play a role in many stages of Frijda's model (Figure 14.1), especially early stages of stimulus detection, classification, and relevance as well as emotion regulation.

Emotion Regulation

The process of managing one's emotional reactions has a more indirect relationship to action control than memory, decision making, or reasoning but is no less important. Emotion regulation refers to the set of processes used in response to emotional experiences and how we express our reactions to emotions (Gross, 1999). How one regulates one's emotions influences how those emotions can subsequently influence action tendencies—in fact, some forms of emotion regulation are focused on regulating specific behaviors rather than reducing the intensity of the emotion itself. Emotion regulation strategies have a reciprocal relationship with all stages of processing in the model of emotion/action control (Figure 14.1) and can determine how information, relevance, context, and urgency are evaluated. The strategies employed by individuals to interpret incoming emotional information have a substantial impact on one's experience, including memory for the information and subjective feelings. Gross's process model provides a useful framework for understanding how emotion regulation strategies may operate. One antecedent-focused cognitive strategy is *reappraisal,* where one decides in advance to interpret an emotional situation in a nonemotional framework. For example, one might choose to think about giving a talk as an opportunity to get feedback from peers instead of as a time to be evaluated, or when viewing aversive images, one might determine to take the perspective of a medical doctor trying to discern the extent of an injury. (Such antecedent-focused strategies would likely fit into the "analyzer" stage of Frijda's model.) In contrast, *suppression* is a response-focused strategy where one inhibits emotionally expressive behavior after the emotion itself is experienced. An example of suppression might involve trying to conceal the anxiety one feels while giving a talk or putting on a "game face" or a "poker face." Suppression would be integrated into several stages of the model, including the "diagnoser" stage, in which context is evaluated (here, the context being a situation where one wants to inhibit behavior), as well as the "action proposer" stage, in which action readiness changes are generated because the strategy of sup-

pression dictates one's behavior. These strategies of emotion regulation have important implications, as they yield different behavioral, cognitive, and physiological results. Hence, emotion regulation strategies are important forms of emotion-cognition interactions that are highly relevant to action control.

Richards and Gross (2000) explored the influence of emotion regulation strategy on memory and subjective emotional experience. Individuals were explicitly instructed to either suppress or reappraise a negative emotional experience while viewing either a sad film or aversive images. Those in the suppression condition demonstrated poorer subsequent memory for the verbal details accompanying the stimuli in comparison with reappraisers and those in the neutral condition. Only those who were instructed to reappraise reported significantly less negative of an emotional experience. Thus, the cognitive strategy employed for dealing with emotional stimuli influenced memory as well as subjective emotional experience. Because suppressors' memory was impaired only for verbal information, it is possible that suppression occurred through verbal processes (e.g., participants silently reminding themselves not to show emotion and to continue monitoring their behavior). Furthermore, reappraisers showed better nonverbal memory than other participants, although the reasons for this enhancement are unclear (for a review, see also Richards, 2004). Emotion regulation paradigms also demonstrate emotion–cognition interactions at the physiological and neural level, as described in later sections.

To recap, emotion can have varied influences on different aspects of cognition, including memory, decision and choice, and reasoning. In cases where the affective components are task relevant, performance may be enhanced, yet when affect is task irrelevant, it may distract action control from the goal at hand. In this section, we reviewed influences on performance—that is, as revealed in overt action. In the next section, we review influences of emotion on covert responses and changes that potentially, albeit less directly, also influence action control.

Interactions Revealed in Psychophysiological Responses

The interactive nature of the relationship between emotion and cognition is also evident in psychophysiological changes. In many instances, cognitive strategies bias physiological responses to emotional information. Physiological responses are also a critical component of Frijda's model of emotion, in which the end result of the evaluation and change in action readiness are both a physiological change and the generation of action (Figure 14.1). Several methods are employed to assess physiological changes, with skin conductance, startle reflexes, and muscle corrugator activity among the most widely used techniques. Skin conductance responses (SCRs) are used to measure somatic state activation through an electrode adhered to the surface of the finger. The magnitude of an SCR consistently covaries with arousal levels, with greater magnitude during higher arousal. Although SCRs do not map onto pleasantness ratings, they do correlate with both interest ratings and the duration of time spent viewing a stimulus (Lang, Greenwald, Bradley, & Hamm, 1993). The startle response is elicited by a sudden, unexpected stimulus, such as a burst of white noise, and is assessed by the degree of contraction of a muscle around the eye (*orbicularis oculi*) similar to a blink. It has been well documented that the startle blink magnitude is a sensitive index of affective modulation (Lang, Bradley, & Cuthbert, 1998; Lang et al., 1993). That is, the blink magnitude is larger when the

response is elicited while the participant is subjected to a negative stimulus and smaller when the stimulus is positive. This is likely a consequence of the fact that an unpleasant stimulus drives an aversive, more tense behavioral state (heightening the startle response), while a pleasant stimulus activates an approach-oriented state that attenuates the startle response (Lang, 1995). Similarly, electromyogram corrugator activity, measured from a facial muscle, has been consistently found to increase in a negative emotional context and decrease in pleasant conditions (Bradley, Cuthbert, & Lang, 1990). These psychophysiological methods provide additional measurements of affective state that are more accurate and time sensitive than self-report and therefore are useful tools with which to study emotion–cognition interactions. In this section, we review evidence from studies using memory, decision making, and emotion regulation.

Memory

In a memory paradigm, SCR activity during an encoding period predicted how well information would be recalled at a later time (Bradley, Greenwald, Petry, & Lang, 1992). Subjects were shown a series of unpleasant or pleasant photographs that were ranked either high or low in arousal while SCRs were recorded. After a 15-minute interval, subjects were given an incidental speeded recall test and were asked to rank photographs for interest and emotion. Participants responded more quickly to slides that had been seen before and were rated high in arousal, but when slides had not been seen before, response times were significantly longer for arousing pictures (presumably because of stronger attentional capture). Participants had SCRs of greater magnitude in response to high-arousal versus low-arousal slides and a similar pattern for unpleasant versus pleasant slides, a finding consistent with other studies. Thus, the authors propose that the psychophysiological response accompanying the emotion–cognition interaction of encoding arousing pictures into memory may have a facilitating role in later recall since the SCR represents a component of the original event associated with the stimulus.

Decision Making

The IGT has been also used to determine whether patients with VMPFC damage experienced normal physiological reactions (i.e., increased skin conductance while deliberating on and making risky choices) during a decision-making task. SCRs were measured while subjects performed the IGT (Bechara, Damasio, Tranel, & Damasio, 1997). Interestingly, during the task, normal participants generated anticipatory SCRs prior to choosing a card from a risky deck throughout the experiment, even before they expressed conscious knowledge of what the pattern of decks signified (but see Maia & McClelland, 2004). At this stage of preconscious awareness, normal participants still chose from the advantageous decks, though they could not explain why. However, not only did patients with VMPFC damage fail to generate anticipatory SCRs prior to choosing from the risky decks, but they also continued to choose from the risky decks even at a later stage of the task when several expressed conscious knowledge of the game strategy. The generation of SCRs in anticipation to choosing from risky decks thus correlated with the ability to choose an advantageous strategy in the IGT. The intriguing finding that SCRs correlated with decision-making behavior is interpreted by the authors as evidence for "somatic markers"—nonconscious, physiological biases elicited by emotion that can guide behavior even before conscious knowledge does (Bechara et al., 1997). The system proposed includes the generation of affective responses within the amygdala, the output of which is sent to the VMPFC, which then integrates the somatic information with information about current circumstances and goals (Bechara, Damasio, Damasio, & Lee, 1999). Similarly, the authors postulate that the VMPFC communicates with the amygdala when one is faced with a decision; the amygdala then sends feedback regarding somatic "markers" from previous experiences with the decision at hand (here, the deck being contemplated).

Advocates of the somatic marker hypothesis contend that VMPFC patients are unable to use emotion to guide behavior (despite being able to experience emotion), whereas amygdala patients are incapable of having a sufficiently robust emotional experience during the IGT, precluding them from experiencing the type of somatic state related to the task at hand (Bechara et al., 1999). While VMPFC patients generated SCRs in response to reward and punishment during the IGT, amygdala patients did not. Neither group demonstrated SCRs in anticipation of choosing from the risky deck. The authors interpret this finding as evidence for the amygdala's role in generating *informative affective states* and the VMPFC's role in *integrating somatic information* with cognitive knowledge of the task. The physiological responses from the lesion patient groups in conjunction with their behavioral responses indicate there is substantial integration of emotional and cognitive information during the decision-making task and support the idea of discrete roles for the amygdala and VMPFC in each of these processes. Furthermore, these responses seem to have a functional role in shaping action tendencies since their presence or absence prior to the action is directly predictive of the type of behavior in which the individual engages.

One possible explanation is that patients with damage to the VMPFC are insensitive to future consequences, which drives them to choose options with immediate benefits despite possible negative outcomes later (Bechara et al., 1994, 1997). Numerous alternative interpretations have been posited to explain these tendencies. The risky and safe decks have different characteristics, as the risky decks have greater negative consequences—thus, patients may be more risk seeking (Sanfey, Hastie, Colvin, & Grafman, 2003). Another explanation is that patients are less able to inhibit prepotent responses driving them to choose the risky deck. Alternatives to the somatic marker hypothesis are plausible, but the role of the VMPFC in guiding decision-making behavior has robust empirical support. Whether or not this region actually provides unconscious biases, it seems essential for successful choice behavior—the ability to enact an advantageous decision. The behavior of VMPFC-damaged patients is consistently characterized by impairments in both emotion and feeling in addition to decision making (Damasio, 1994); hence, this area is also likely to be integrally involved with emotion–cognition interactions that help guide action control and behavior.

Emotion Regulation

Paradigms where emotional responses must be managed provide evidence for emotion–cognition interactions as revealed in physiological measures. Gross (1998) reported that instructions to suppress emotional responding led to subjective estimations of emotional experience comparable to similar judgments from subjects instructed to just watch the film. Importantly, however, the suppressor group demonstrated greater physiological activation in the sympathetic nervous system as measured by skin conductance, finger pulse amplitude, and finger temperature. Those instructed to reappraise showed patterns comparable to those in the watch condition in contrast

with the prediction that their physiological responses would be decreased (as were their subjective ratings of disgust). One possibility is that as a response-focused strategy (in which one must regulate a response that has already occurred), suppression was simply a more effortful strategy to pursue and placed additional demand on participants, which was manifested in physiological outcomes. However, evidence from neuroimaging discussed later in this chapter seems to suggest that reappraisal is a comparably demanding cognitive strategy (Ochsner, Bunge, Gross, & Gabrieli, 2002).

In a related study of emotion regulation, Jackson, Malmstadt, Larson, and Davidson (2000) used different techniques to examine the consequences of regulation strategies on physiological responses. Eyeblink startle magnitude and corrugator activity were assessed at several intervals while aversive stimuli were presented. Unlike Gross (1998), Jackson et al. allowed subjects to regulate using whatever strategy they found most appropriate instead of giving them explicit instructions. Participants were presented with aversive or neutral photographs for 8 seconds. Four seconds after the onset of the photo, they were given a verbal instruction to suppress, enhance, or maintain (though no specific strategies were offered regarding how to do so). Physiological measures were taken at several points: following presentation but before instruction, after instruction, and after the photograph was removed. In this way, the paradigm examined the initial emotional response to the stimulus, the effect of the cognitive strategy utilized to regulate emotion, and the consequence of the recovery period strategy. The key finding was that instructions to suppress emotional responding led to smaller startle blink magnitudes and decreased corrugator activity relative to the maintain condition. In contrast, instructions to enhance responses led to larger startle magnitudes and increased corrugator activity relative to maintain instructions. At first glance, these findings seem to contradict evidence by Gross (1998), who found that suppression instructions increased skin conductance yet decreased heart rate and that reappraisal did not change skin conductance. However, these researchers used different instructions that most likely influenced how participants responded. While Gross characterized suppression as behaving in a way that an observer would not know one was feeling anything, Jackson et al. told participants that, when suppressing, "we would like you to decrease the intensity of disgust you feel."

Physiological changes in response to emotion–cognition interactions appear to be closely linked to generating action tendencies, as outlined in the emotion-process model (Frijda, 1986). In the case of memory and decision-making tasks, the generation of SCRs is linked to subsequent performance on the task, with this correlation suggesting the possibility that the physiological response works to bias action control by bolstering the preparatory state of the action system itself. SCR magnitude predicted subsequent recall on a memory task, and the generation of SCRs in a decision-making task predicted the likelihood of using an advantageous strategy. Furthermore, when instructed to suppress emotional reactions, participants demonstrated startle responses of lesser magnitude, again suggesting that physiological responses are closely tied to action tendencies and may even signal a readiness for action.

Interactions Revealed in Neural Measures

Neuroimaging studies complement performance-based, psychophysiological, and patient-based research to suggest there may be distinct neural mechanisms involved with emotion–cognition integration. Furthermore, based on reciprocal suppression of specific brain regions involved with cognitive and emotional processing (Drevets & Raichle, 1998; Gray et al., 2002), it is likely that areas engaged with these processes are tightly integrated. Responses to emotional information may also show different neural correlates depending on the cognitive strategies implemented. Here we review evidence from studies of memory, decision making, attention, and emotion regulation.

Memory

A functional magnetic resonance imaging (fMRI) study of emotion inductions and subsequent working memory performance demonstrated that emotion is integrated with higher cognition (Gray et al., 2002). That is, emotion can interact with cognition in a selective, specific way. Participants viewed positive, negative, or neutral films intended to induce brief emotional states and were then scanned while performing an *n*-back task using either faces or words to test spatial or verbal working memory. As in previous work (Gray, 2001), mild anxiety enhanced spatial working memory while impairing verbal working memory (for an independent replication, see Beilock, Rydell, & McConnell, 2007), with an opposite pattern holding for induced amusement. In addition, a region of the lateral prefrontal cortex (PFC) showed strongest activation for face-pleasant and word-unpleasant conditions (which were behaviorally the most difficult). This area showed intermediate activity for neutral conditions and lowest activity for the easiest conditions (face unpleasant and word pleasant), suggesting it is sensitive to emotion–cognition integration. Moreover, because activity in this region correlated with behavioral performance, it is possible that this region might directly support cognitive–emotional integration.

The influence of emotion on the process of refreshing a word stored in memory reflects another instance of emotion–cognition interactions biasing action tendencies. In a study examining "mental rubbernecking," the process by which emotional stimuli tend to draw attention away from other cognitive processes, participants refreshed emotionally valenced words from memory faster than neutral words (Johnson et al., 2005). In addition, refreshing a neutral word that had been presented in a set with an emotional word took longer than refreshing a neutral word in a set of neutral words or an emotional word in a mixed set, supporting the idea that the presence of an emotional word distracted attention from the task at hand. The interaction between the emotional response to the word and the refresh process biases action tendencies such that attention is briefly drawn away from the more cognitive task in order to pay attention to a potentially relevant emotional stimulus. Johnson et al. followed up this behavioral observation with an fMRI study of the process of refreshing emotionally salient words in memory and found that activity in the anterior orbitofrontal cortex (OFC) was greater when participants refreshed neutral versus emotional items, and when items were repeated, activity was greater for refreshing emotional items. These findings support the idea that the OFC region may be involved in exerting control over potentially disruptive emotional responses. In this way, the OFC may influence action tendencies as it allows the individual to direct attention to the cognitive task at hand.

Decision Making

In a study of decision making, different neural responses were observed in response to fair versus unfair offers during the ultimatum game (Sanfey, Rilling, Aronson, Nystrom, & Cohen, 2003). In the ultimatum game, participants are told their partner (here, a computerized algorithm—though participants believed they were playing against real people) is given $10 and must propose an offer to divide the $10 between them. The partner is allowed to make only one offer, and if the participant accepts, each receives the amount proposed, but if the participant rejects the offer, neither individual receives anything. Normatively, there is no reason to reject any offer since receiving any amount is preferable to receiving none. Yet participants show a reliable tendency to reject offers they believe are unfair (where the proposer receives $8 or $9 and the participant receives only $2 or $1), presumably to punish the unfair proposer.

When Sanfey et al. (2003) scanned participants during the ultimatum game, they determined that unfair offers activated areas known for involvement in both emotion (anterior insula) and cognition (dorsolateral PFC). Interestingly, activation in the anterior insula increased for rejected offers, suggesting that in those cases emotion "overruled" cognitive processes and biased action tendencies toward a response driven by emotion more than cognition (since the decision to reject is not rational by normative standards). Of note, the response in the right anterior insula was stronger for unfair offers from a human versus unfair computer opponents, suggesting that a slight by a real person is more emotionally upsetting than one by a computer. While at face value these results might suggest emotion is a hindrance to advantageous decision making, the tendency to punish an unfair partner is in some sense an appropriate choice. Although participants were told that their interactions with each individual were isolated interactions, punishing a perceived wrong is of significant consequence because it has several consequences. First, it establishes one's social identity and maintains one's reputation; research also indicates that individuals feel satisfaction from punishing those who violate social norms—even when punishment comes with an economic cost to the punisher (deQuervain, Fischbacher, Treyer, Schellhammer, & Schnyder, 2005; Fehr & Fischbacher, 2004). These tendencies indicate that emotion–cognition interactions can influence action tendencies and behavior in adaptive ways, particularly with respect to social interactions (Keltner & Haidt, 1999).

Emotion Regulation

At the neural level, emotion–cognition interactions are observable during periods of emotion regulation. In an fMRI study of regulation, participants viewed a series of emotionally evocative pictures with instructions to either reappraise or simply attend to their emotional response (Ochsner et al., 2002). Reappraisal (in contrast to attending) activated areas including the dorsal and ventral left PFC and the dorsal medial PFC. The anterior cingulate cortex showed a positive correlation between activation and self-reported success of reappraisal strategy. Attending versus reappraising activated the left medial OFC. Furthermore, the ventrolateral PFC showed a correlation between activation during reappraisal and reappraisal-related decrease in activation in the amygdala. One possible explanation for these results is that the lateral PFC may modulate amygdala activity through the OFC, which is plausible because the OFC has reciprocal connections with both areas. In addition, the prefrontal region may modulate perceptual and semantic inputs to the amygdala from occipital and parietal regions—such that when holding a reappraisal goal constant in working memory, inputs may be recognized as aversive and thus be gated from registering with the amygdala or medial OFC.

Attention

Even tasks as basic as attentional matching paradigms illustrate neural mechanisms reflecting interactions between emotion and cognition. An fMRI study of attention to threat-related stimuli and anxiety revealed interesting interactions between emotion, cognitive control, and individual differences (Bishop, Duncan, Brett, & Lawrence, 2004). Participants were scanned while performing a simple matching task: they were shown a set of four photos, including two houses and two scenes, and were asked to decide whether the houses were identical. The two conditions were frequent- versus infrequent-threat-distracters (referring to how often the faces presented exhibited fearful expressions). Within each block, the first three stimuli ("start" trials) indicated whether the frequent distracter would be fearful or neutral in order to establish expectancy in that block. The rostral anterior cingulate cortex (rACC) showed greater activation during infrequent-threat-distracters compared with neutral distracters. Of note, no significant rACC activation was observed when participants were instructed to match faces instead of houses, suggesting that rACC plays a role in processing task-irrelevant emotional information.

Further support for emotion–cognition interactions at the neural level is seen in the relationship between state anxiety (an affective mood) and neural activity. Scores of state anxiety negatively correlated with activity during left dorsolateral PFC and ventrolateral PFC during the start trials of frequent-threat-distracter blocks (e.g., higher anxiety predicted less activity), suggesting that affective state may reduce activity in two areas known to be involved with attentional control. Hence, negative affect may decrease cognitive ability and reduce action control tendencies supporting the underlying goal of attending to stimuli. Furthermore, higher anxiety ratings were correlated with decreased rACC activity during all types of trials—which the authors posit may explain why PFC activity is decreased in response to threat-related distracters (e.g., a decreased signal from rACC may prevent the PFC from decreasing its response to threatening stimuli, thus making the response more fear related and distracting from the task). Given the extensive association of the rACC with emotional processing and regulation and its connections with the amygdala, insula, and OFC (Bush, Luu, & Posner, 2000), it is plausibly involved in emotion–cognition interactions within the brain.

Top-down modulation of attention is another instance where emotion–cognition interactions clearly bias action tendencies. A number of studies have demonstrated that even when fearful faces are masked such that participants do not report conscious awareness of seeing the faces, the amygdala shows a heightened response to the stimulus (Morris, Öhman, & Dolan, 1998; Whalen et al., 1998). Such evidence has been interpreted to signify that detection of fearful stimuli by the amygdala is automatic and does not rely on cognitive processing to occur. However, other studies have found that without attention, the amygdala may not respond to fearful stimuli. Pessoa, McKenna, Gutierrez, and Ungerleider (2002) conducted an fMRI study with the hypothesis that masking techniques utilized in earlier studies had failed to fully engage attentional resources and thus did not prove the amygdala detection of fearful faces was truly independent of top-down processing. To engage attention away from the faces, participants were asked to determine whether bars in the periphery of the screen were of similar spatial orientation while a face appeared in the center of the screen. Analyses indicated that the amygdala did not respond to fearful stimuli in the unattended condition—in both the left and the right amygdala, responses were identical across stimulus types, and there was no effect of valence on activation. They conclude the amygdala response is thus not automatic but rather dependent on top-down attentional control—thus, the neural response to fearful stimuli involves an emotion–cognition interaction at the level of neural processing that biases action tendencies to pay heightened attention to the appropriate stimulus.

An elegant study examining individual differences in anxiety in relation to amygdala activation to unattended, fearful stimuli adds an additional dimension to this debate—the role of individual differences in neural activity (Bishop, Duncan, & Lawrence, 2004). During an attentional matching task, the key questions were (a) whether amygdala activation to fearful versus neutral faces was modulated by attention and (b) whether state anxiety plays a role in the neural response. The authors found that while the left amygdala showed greater activation to attended versus unattended fearful faces, the overall amygdala response to fearful, unattended stimuli was dependent on state anxiety, an affectively relevant individual difference measure. Individuals with high state anxiety showed stronger activation in the amygdala to fearful faces when they were either attended or unattended; those with low state anxiety showed activation only to faces that were attended. As Bishop et al. point out, if one considers only the high-anxiety participants, one concludes that the amygdala responds to fearful stimuli independent of attention, and yet if one examines only the low-anxiety participants, it appears that the amygdala is sensitive to top-down attentional modulation. The ability of this study to resolve two conflicting findings underscores the importance of considering affective individual differences when interpreting emotion–cognition interactions.

Finally, the effects of emotion–cognition interactions on behavior were illustrated in an fMRI study of attention, emotion, and working memory (Dolcos & McCarthy, 2006). In a delayed-response working memory task, participants were shown a set of faces, followed by two distracters, then asked to determine whether a subsequent face was part of the initial set. The distracters were either emotional, neutral, or scrambled emotional images. Performance on the working memory task at a behavioral level was significantly impaired with emotional distracters in comparison to neutral and scrambled distracters, indicating that the emotional stimuli interfered with the cognitive working memory process by shifting attention to the distracter. At a neural level, activity during the distracter period varied depending on the type of distracter. Emotional distracters activated ventral regions involved in emotion processing, including the amygdala, ventrolateral PFC, and medial PFC. In addition, emotional distracters deactivated areas involved with executive functions, such as the dorsolateral PFC, lateral PFC, and posterior cingulate cortex. Of note, participants who showed strongest activity in response to emotional distracters in the ventrolateral PFC rated the distracters as less emotional and less distracting, suggesting that the ventrolateral PFC is involved in inhibiting distracting emotions. This interpretation is consistent with the idea of the emotion–cognition interaction in this region biasing action tendencies such that cognitive resources are dedicated to inhibiting emotional responses while resources are steered away from the cognitive working memory task.

Conclusions

A relation between emotion and action control is evident not only in examples that must be true almost by definition, such as facial expression, but also exists throughout the action control hierarchy. In fact, the relationship is so pervasive and direct that, as a reference model of action control, it is possible to view a model of the emotion process (Frijda, 1986) as a model of action control for expository purposes. The consequences of emotion—while typically adaptive on the whole—range from the beneficial (e.g., in many social interactions) to profoundly detrimental (e.g., suicide), depending on the combination of circumstances giving rise to the stimuli, the actor's response, and the subsequent action tendencies that are elicited. We reviewed evidence for diverse emotion–cognition interactions, including memory, reasoning, decision making, and emotion regulation, with particular attention to the implications for understanding action tendencies and overt behavior. Emotion–cognition interactions are ubiquitous—they exist in many forms and under a multitude of circumstances. Emotion and cognition are both powerful control systems—with action tendencies being the ultimate target of control.

References

Bartolic, E. I., Basso, M. R., Schefft, B. K., Glauser, T., & Titanic-Schefft, M. (1999). Effects of experimentally-induced emotional states on frontal lobe cognitive task performance. *Neuropsychologia, 37*, 677–683.

Bechara, A., Damasio, A., Damasio, H., & Anderson, S. W. (1994). Insensitivity to future consequences following damage to human prefrontal cortex. *Cognition, 50*, 7–15.

Bechara, A., Damasio, H., Damasio, A. R., & Lee, G. P. (1999). Different contributions of the human amygdala and ventromedial prefrontal cortex to decision-making. *Journal of Neuroscience, 19*, 5473–5481.

Bechara, A., Damasio, H., Tranel, D., & Damasio, A. R. (1997). Deciding advantageously before knowing the advantageous strategy. *Science, 275,* 1293–1295.

Beilock, S. L., Rydell, R. J., & McConnell, A. R. (2007). Stereotype threat and working memory: Mechanisms, alleviation, and spill over. *Journal of Experimental Psychology: General, 136,* 256–276.

Bishop, S. J., Duncan, J., Brett, M., & Lawrence, A. D. (2004). Prefrontal cortical function and anxiety: Controlling attention to threat-related stimuli. *Nature Neuroscience, 7,* 184–188.

Bishop, S. J., Duncan, J., & Lawrence, A. D. (2004). State anxiety modulation of the amygdala response to unattended threat-related stimuli. *Journal of Neuroscience, 24,* 10364–10368.

Blanchette, I., & Richards, A. (2004). Reasoning about emotional and neutral materials is logic affected by emotion? *Psychological Science, 15,* 745–752.

Bohannon, J. N. (1988). Flashbulb memories of the space shuttle disaster: A tale of two theories. *Cognition, 29,* 179–196.

Bower, G. H. (1981). Mood and memory. *American Psychologist, 36,* 129–148.

Bradley, M. M., Cuthbert, B. N., & Lang, P. J. (1990). Startle reflex modification: Emotion or attention? *Psychophysiology, 27,* 513–522.

Bradley, M. M., Greenwald, M. K., Petry, M. C., & Lang, P. J. (1992). Remembering pictures: Pleasure and arousal in memory. *Journal of Experimental Psychology: Learning, Memory, and Cognition, 18,* 379–390.

Brown, R., & Kulik, J. (1977). Flashbulb memories. *Cognition, 5,* 73–99.

Bush, G., Luu, P., & Posner, M. I. (2000). Cognitive and emotional influences in anterior cingulate cortex. *Trends in Cognitive Sciences, 4,* 215–222.

Carver, C. S., Sutton, S. K., & Scheier, M. F. (2000). Action, emotion, and personality: Emerging conceptual integration. *Personality and Social Psychology Bulletin, 26,* 741–751.

Chang, A., & Wilson, M. (2004). Recalling emotional experiences affects performance on reasoning problems. *Evolution and Human Behavior, 25,* 267–276.

Christianson, S. E. (1992). *The handbook of emotion and memory: Research and theory.* Hillsdale, NJ: Lawrence Erlbaum Associates.

Dalgleish, T., & Power, M. (1999). *Handbook of cognition and emotion.* New York: Wiley.

Damasio, A. R. (1994). *Descartes' error: Emotion, reason, and the human brain.* New York: HarperCollins.

Davidson, R. J. (1994). On emotion, mood, and related affective constructs. In P. Ekman & R. J. Davidson (Eds.), *The nature of emotions: Fundamental questions* (pp. 51–55). New York: Oxford University Press.

deQuervain, D. J.-F., Fischbacher, U., Treyer, V., Schellhammer, M., & Schnyder, U. (2005). The neural basis of altruistic punishment. *Science, 305,* 1254–1258.

Dolcos, F., & McCarthy, G. (2006). Brain systems mediating cognitive interference by emotional distraction. *Journal of Neuroscience, 26,* 2072–2079.

Drevets, W. C., & Raichle, M. E. (1998). Reciprocal suppression of regional cerebral blood flow during emotional versus higher cognitive processes: Implications for interactions between emotion and cognition. *Cognition and Emotion, 12,* 353–385.

Ekman, P., & Davidson, R. J. (1994). *The nature of emotion: Fundamental questions.* New York: Oxford University Press.

Fehr, E., & Fischbacher, U. (2004). Social norms and human cooperation. *Trends in Cognitive Science, 8,* 185–190.

Frijda, N. H. (1986). *The emotions.* Paris: Cambridge University Press.

Gollwitzer, P. M. (1999). Implementation intentions: Strong effects of simple plans. *American Psychologist, 54,* 493–503.

Gray, J. R. (2001). Emotional modulation of cognitive control: Approach-withdrawal states double-dissociate spatial from verbal two-back task performance. *Journal of Experimental Psychology: General, 130,* 436–452.

Gray, J. R. (2004). Integration of emotion and cognitive control. *Current Directions in Psychological Science, 13,* 46–48.

Gray, J. R., Braver, T. S., & Raichle, M. E. (2002). Integration of emotion and cognition in the lateral prefrontal cortex. *Proceedings of the National Academy of the Sciences of the United States of America, 99,* 4115–4120.

Gray, J. R., Schaefer, A., Braver, T. S., & Most, S. B. (2005). Affect and the resolution of cognitive control dilemmas. In L. Feldman Barrett, P. M. Niedenthal & P. Winkielman (Eds.), *Emotion and consciousness* (pp. 67–94). New York: Guilford Press.

Gross, J. J. (1998). Antecedent- and response-focused emotion regulation: Divergent consequences for experience, expression, and physiology. *Journal of Personality and Social Psychology, 74,* 224–237.

Gross, J. J. (1999). Emotion regulation: Past, present, future. *Cognition and Emotion, 13,* 551–573.

Heller, W., & Nitschke, J. B. (1997). Regional brain activity in emotion: A framework for understanding cognition in depression. *Cognition and Emotion, 11,* 637–661.

Hsee, C. K., & Rottenstreich, Y. (2004). Music, pandas, and muggers: On the affective psychology of value. *Journal of Experimental Psychology: General, 133,* 23–30.

Izard, C. E. (1994). Cognition is one of four types of emotion-activating systems. In P. Ekman & R. J. Davidson (Eds.), *The nature of emotion: Fundamental questions* (pp. 203–207). New York: Oxford University Press.

Jackson, D. C., Malmstadt, J. R., Larson, C. L., & Davidson, R. J. (2000). Suppression and enhancement of emotional responses to unpleasant pictures. *Psychophysiology, 37,* 515–522.

Johnson, M. K., Raye, C. L., Mitchell, K. J., Greene, E. J., Cunningham, W. A., & Sanislow, C. A. (2005). Using fMRI to investigate a component process of reflection: Prefrontal correlates of refreshing a just-activated representation. *Cognitive, Affective, and Behavioral Neuroscience, 5,* 339–361.

Keltner, D., & Haidt, J. (1999). Social functions of emotions at four levels of analysis. *Cognition and Emotion, 13,* 505–521.

Lang, P. J. (1995). The emotion probe: Studies of motivation and attention. *American Psychologist, 50,* 372–385.

Lang, P. J., Bradley, M. M., & Cuthbert, B. N. (1990). Emotion, attention, and the startle reflex. *Psychological Review, 97,* 377–395.

Lang, P. J., Bradley, M. M., & Cuthbert, B. N. (1998). Emotion and motivation: Measuring affective perception. *Journal of Clinical Neurophysiology, 15,* 397–408.

Lang, P. J., Greenwald, M. K., Bradley, M. M., & Hamm, A. O. (1993). Looking at pictures: Affective, facial, visceral, and behavioral reactions. *Psychophysiology, 30,* 261–273.

Larsen, R. J., & Fredrickson, B. L. (1999). Measurement issues in emotion research. In D. Kahneman, E. Diener, & N. Schwarz (Eds.), *Well-being: The foundations of hedonic psychology* (pp. 40–60). New York: Russell Sage Foundation.

LeDoux, J. (2000). Emotion circuits in the brain. *Annual Review of Neuroscience, 23,* 155–184.

LeDoux, J., & Armony, J. (1999). Can neurobiology tell us anything about human feelings? In D. Kahneman, E. Diener, & N. Schwarz (Eds.), *Well-being: The foundations of hedonic psychology* (pp. 489–499). New York: Russell Sage Foundation.

Lerner, J. S., Small, D. A., & Loewenstein, G. (2004). Heart strings and purse strings: Carryover effects of emotions on economic decisions. *Psychological Science, 15,* 337–341.

Loftus, E. F. (1993). Desperately seeking memories of the first few years of childhood: The reality of early memories. *Journal of Experimental Psychology: General, 122,* 274–277.

Maia, T. V., & McClelland, J. L. (2004). A reexamination of the evidence for the somatic marker hypothesis: What participants really know in the Iowa Gambling Task. *Proceedings of the National Academy of the Sciences of the United States of America, 101,* 16075–16080.

Morris, J. S., Öhman, A., & Dolan, R. J. (1998). Conscious and unconscious emotional learning in the human amygdala. *Nature, 393,* 467–470.

Ochsner, K. N., Bunge, S. A., Gross, J. J., & Gabrieli, J. D. E. (2002). Rethinking feelings: An fMRI study of the cognitive regulation of emotion. *Journal of Cognitive Neuroscience, 14,* 1215–1229.

Panksepp, J. (1994). A proper distinction between affective and cognitive process is essential for neuroscientific progress. In P. Ekman & R. J. Davidson (Eds.), *The nature of emotion* (pp. 224–226). New York: Oxford University Press.

Panksepp, J. (1998). *Affective neuroscience: The foundations of human and animal emotions.* New York: Oxford University Press.

Pessoa, L., McKenna, M., Gutierrez, E., & Ungerleider, L. G. (2002). Neural processing of emotional faces requires attention. *Proceedings of the National Academy of the Sciences of the United States of America, 99,* 11458–11463.

Reis, D. L., Brackett, M. A., Shamosh, N. A., Kiehl, K. A., Salovey, P., & Gray, J. R. (2007). Emotional intelligence predicts individual differences in social exchange reasoning. *NeuroImage, 35,* 1385–1391.

Richards, J. M. (2004). The cognitive consequences of concealing feelings. *Current Directions in Psychological Science, 13,* 131–134.

Richards, J. M., & Gross, J. J. (2000). Emotion regulation and memory: The cognitive costs of keeping one's cool. *Journal of Social and Personality Psychology, 79,* 410–424.

Roediger, H. L., & McDermott, K. B. (1995). Creating false memories: Remembering words not presented in lists. *Journal of Experimental Psy-*

chology: Learning, Memory, and Cognition, 21, 803–814.

Russell, J. A., & Feldman Barrett, L. (1999). Core affect, prototypical emotional episodes, and other things called emotion: Dissecting the elephant. *Journal of Personality and Social Psychology, 76,* 805–819.

Sanfey, A. G., Hastie, R., Colvin, M. K., & Grafman, J. (2003). Phineas gauged: Decision-making and the human prefrontal cortex. *Neuropsychologia, 41,* 1218–1229.

Sanfey, A. G., Rilling, J. K., Aronson, J. A., Nystrom, L. E., & Cohen, J. D. (2003). The neural basis of economic decision-making in the ultimatum game. *Science, 300,* 1755–1758.

Schneirla, T. C. (1959). An evolutionary and developmental theory of biphasic processes underlying approach and withdrawal. In M. R. Jones (Ed.), *Nebraska symposium on motivation.* Lincoln: University of Nebraska Press.

Storbeck, J., & Clore, G. L. (2005). With sadness comes accuracy; with happiness, false memory. *Psychological Science, 16,* 785–791.

Whalen, P. J., Rauch, S. L., Etcoff, N. L., McInerney, S. C., Lee, M. B., & Jenike, M. A. (1998). Masked presentations of emotional facial expressions modulate amygdala activity without explicit knowledge. *Journal of Neuroscience, 18,* 411–418.

Action, Affect, and Two-Mode Models of Functioning

Charles S. Carver *and* Michael F. Scheier

Abstract

This chapter examines several aspects of the management of action and affect. Starting with the idea that behavior reflects the processes of feedback control, it proposes that two layers of control manage two different aspects of behavior. These two layers operate together in a way that conserves resources and permits people to handle multiple tasks across time. Thus, simultaneous motives that bear on many different goals are transformed into a stream of actions that shifts repeatedly from one goal to another.

Keywords: behavior, feedback control, cognition, management of action, affect

In this chapter, we outline several aspects of the perspective we have taken on the management of action and affect. We begin with the idea that behavior reflects the processes of feedback control. More specifically, we propose that two layers of control manage two different aspects of behavior. We see these two layers as operating together in a way that conserves resources and permits people to handle multiple tasks across time. Thus, simultaneous motives that bear on many different goals are transformed into a stream of actions that shifts repeatedly from one goal to another. This is a view we have taken for well over 15 years. We describe its essence in the first part of this chapter.

During the past couple of decades, a variety of changes have occurred in how people view both cognition and action. Challenges have been made to the implicit assumption that behavior is generally managed in a top-down, intentional, directive fashion. Questions have been raised about the role of consciousness in the regulation of many kinds of action. Principles of connectionism and dynamic systems have been absorbed into a range of conceptual analyses of phenomena that are of interest to personality and social psychologists. Interest has grown in the idea that the mind holds implicit representations as well as explicit ones. These various ideas are helping to induce a somewhat different way of construing the diverse functions of the brain that underlie the control of action. In the later part of the chapter, we consider some aspects of this emerging view and their implications for how we view the control of action.

Before we start, a brief point about terminology: Our approach to behavior has long been identified with the term *self-regulation* (Carver & Scheier, 1981, 1990, 1998, 1999a, 1999b). This term means different things to different people. We use it to convey the sense of processes that are purposive, the sense that self-corrective adjustments are taking place (as needed) to stay on track for the purpose being served, and the sense that the corrective adjustments originate within the person. These elements converge in the view that human behavior is a continuing process of moving toward (and sometimes away from) goal values and that this process embodies the characteristics of feedback control. A number of people have ascribed to the term *self-regulation* the additional quality of overriding or restraining an impulse (see, e.g., Baumeister & Vohs, 2004). We generally do not assume that quality in our usage. We do address issues of restraint later in the chapter; when we do, we use the more restrictive term *self-control.*

Behavior as Goal Directed and Feedback Controlled

We start with control processes. The term *feedback control* can seem forbidding. An easy point of entry into its logic, however, is the goal concept, which is more intuitive. People have many goals at varying levels of abstraction and importance. Goals energize and guide activities. Most goals can be reached in many ways, leading to the potential for vast complexity in the organization of action. This is a view that is easy and familiar for most people.

Feedback Processes

We have long been interested in the idea that moving toward a goal reflects the action of feedback loops. A feedback loop has four subfunctions (MacKay, 1966; G. A. Miller, Galanter, & Pribram, 1960; Powers, 1973; Wiener, 1948): an input, a reference value, a comparison, and an output (Figure 15.1). It seems reasonable to view the input as perception. This function brings information into the system about present circumstances. A reference value can be thought of as equivalent to a goal. The input is compared to this value. A discrepancy detected in this way is often called an "error signal." The output is a response to the detected error. We treat the output here as equivalent to behavior, but sometimes the behavior is internal.

If the comparison detects no discrepancy, the output remains as it was. If a discrepancy is sensed, the effect on output depends on what kind of loop it is. In a discrepancy-reducing loop (also called negative, for negating), the output reduces or eliminates

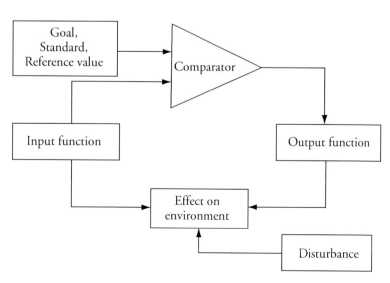

Fig. 15.1 Schematic depiction of a feedback loop, the basic unit of cybernetic control. In a discrepancy-reducing loop, a sensed value is compared to a reference value or standard, and adjustments occur in an output function (if necessary) that shift the sensed value in the direction of the standard. In a discrepancy-enlarging loop, the output function moves the sensed value away from the standard.

the discrepancy. In behavior, this means attempts to reach a valued goal, maintain a desired condition, or conform to a standard. There also are discrepancy-enlarging loops (positive feedback loops), in which the reference value is avoided rather than approached. The value in this case is a threat, or an "anti-goal." An example would be a feared or disliked possible self (Carver, Lawrence, & Scheier, 1999; Markus & Nurius, 1986; Ogilvie, 1987). Another example would be an instruction to not do something or even not think something (cf. N. E. Miller & Dollard, 1941; Wegner, 1994). A positive loop acts to enlarge the discrepancy.

The effects of discrepancy-enlarging processes in living systems are typically constrained by discrepancy-reducing processes. Put differently, acts of avoidance often lead into other acts of approach. An avoidance loop tries to escape an anti-goal. But there may be an approach goal that happens to be distant from the anti-goal. If that approach goal is adopted, the tendency to avoid the anti-goal is joined by the tendency to move toward the approach goal. The approach loop pulls the behavior into its orbit. This pattern of dual influence describes what occurs in active avoidance. An organism confronting a feared stimulus picks a relatively safe location to escape to and approaches that location.

A few more points about this description are in order. It is not hard to portray the elements of a feedback loop conceptually. In some instances of feedback control (e.g., in artificial electronic systems), it is also easy to point to the physical existence of each element. In other instances, doing that is harder. Indeed, some feedback processes have no explicit representation of a reference value. The system regulates around a value, but the value is not represented anywhere as a goal (Berridge, 2004; Carver & Scheier, 2002).

Why are we intrigued by the idea that action involves feedback loops? The answer is rather simple. Scientists in diverse disciplines see feedback processes as among the basic building blocks of nature. It was suggested many years ago, in fact, that feedback loops are embedded in many kinds of systems at many levels of abstraction (e.g., Ford, 1987; von Bertalanffy, 1968). The principle of feedback control is also used in many parts of psychology (though not so often in the parts that are most familiar to personality psychologists such as ourselves). We have been impressed by the fact that one set of functions can be used to address such an extraordinarily wide range of phenomena, and we are curious about just how far these ideas can be extended.

Before moving on, we should dispel a misconception some people have about feedback processes. A common illustration of feedback, because it is so easily understood, is homeostasis (a term meaning "same state"). Because of the wide use of this illustration, some people incorrectly infer that feedback loops can act only to create and maintain steady states. Some reference values (and goals) *are* indeed static end states. But others are dynamic and evolving (e.g., taking a month's vacation or raising children to become good citizens). In such cases, the goal for action regulation is the process of traversing the changing trajectory of the activity, not just the arrival at the end point. Feedback processes apply perfectly well to moving targets (Beer, 1995).

Levels of Abstraction

It should be apparent from the foregoing that goals vary greatly in how concrete or abstract they are. You can have the goal of being a good citizen, but you can also have the goal of recycling—a narrower goal that contributes to being a good citizen. To recycle entails other, more concrete goals: placing newspapers into containers and moving them to a pickup location. Thus it is often said that goals form a hierarchy (Carver & Scheier, 1998, 1999a, 1999b, 2003; Powers, 1973; Vallacher & Wegner, 1987). Abstract goals are attained by the process of attaining concrete goals that help define them.

Some kinds of relatively low-level goals are defined by brief sequences of action, for example, picking up a pen or walking across the room. Such sequences are relatively simple (though each could also be broken down further into subcomponents of motor control; e.g., Rosenbaum, Meulenbroek, Vaughan, & Jansen, 2001). They have something of a self-contained quality about them, and they require little monitoring once they are triggered unless they are very unfamiliar.

Such sequences can be organized into more elaborate strings of actions, which Powers (1973) called *programs*. These strings of action are more planful. They often require choices to be made at various points along the way as a function of conditions that are encountered. Programs, in turn, are sometimes enacted in the service of broader guiding *principles*. Principles are more abstract. They can provide a basis for making decisions within programs, and they can suggest that particular programs be undertaken or be refrained from. The term *principle* refers to the sorts of things that are sometimes called values (Schwartz & Bilsky, 1990; Schwartz & Rubel, 2005). What defines a principle is its abstractness and broad applicability to diverse behaviors. Just being a principle does not imply the direction in which it leads behavior. For example, different principles can lead people to support affirmative action or to oppose it (Reyna, Henry, Korfmacher, & Tucker, 2006).

Even individual values are not the end of potential complexity, though. Patterns of values can coalesce to form the essence of a person's sense of desired (and undesired) self or a person's sense of desired (and undesired) community. These are very broad goals indeed.

All these kinds of goals can be thought of as potential reference points for self-regulation. There are some potentially important differences among the various levels of abstraction, however, to which we return later.

Feedback Processes and Affect

Action control is partly about how we get from here to there. It is partly about the degree of urgency behind the action. The sense of urgency or intensity implies affect, feelings that occur in the course of experience. What is affect? Where does it come from? A truism is that affect pertains to one's desires and whether they are being met (Clore, 1994; Frijda, 1986, 1988; Ortony, Clore, & Collins, 1988). But what is the internal mechanism by which feelings arise?

Answers to these questions take several forms, ranging from neurobiological (e.g., Davidson 1992) to cognitive (Ortony et al., 1988). We have suggested an answer of our own that focuses on what appear to be some of the functional properties of affect (Carver & Scheier, 1990, 1998, 1999a, 1999b). In suggesting this answer, we used feedback control once more as an organizing principle. Now, however, the control bears on a different quality.

We have suggested that feelings arise as a consequence of a feedback loop that operates simultaneously with the behavior-guiding process and in parallel to it. We regard its operation as automatic. The easiest characterization of what this second process is doing is that it is checking on how well the first process (the behavior loop) is doing. The input for this second loop thus is the *rate of discrepancy reduction in the action system over time.* (We focus first on discrepancy reducing loops, then turn to enlarging loops.)

Consider a physical analogy. If action implies change between states, behavior is analogous to distance between those states. The action loop thus controls distance. If the affect loop assesses the action loop's progress, then the affect loop is dealing with the psychological analog of velocity, the first derivative of distance over time. To the degree that this analogy is meaningful, the perceptual input to the affect loop should be the first derivative over time of the input used by the action loop.

Input (how well you are doing) does not by itself create affect; a given rate of progress has different affective consequences in different contexts. Our argument is that this input is compared to a reference value (cf. Frijda, 1986, 1988), just as in other feedback systems. In this case, the reference is an acceptable or expected rate of behavioral discrepancy reduction. As in other feedback loops, the comparison checks for deviation from the standard. If there is a discrepancy, an error is sensed, and the output function changes.

We think the error signal in this loop is manifest phenomenologically as affect, a sense of positive or negative valence. A rate of progress below the criterion yields negative affect. A rate high enough to exceed the criterion yields positive affect. If the rate is not distinguishable from the criterion, there is no valence. In essence, the argument is that feelings with positive valence mean you are doing better at something than you need to, and feelings with negative valence mean you are doing worse than you need to (for detail, see Carver & Scheier, 1998, Chapters 8 and 9). The absence of affect means being neither ahead nor behind.

We should be clear here that we are not arguing for a deliberative thinking through of whether rate conforms to the criterion rate. We assume that the testing for error is continuous and automatic. Nor are we arguing for a deliberative thinking through of what the affective valence means. We assume that the meaning (i.e., being ahead versus behind) is intrinsic to the affect's valence.

One implication of this line of thought is that the affective valences that might potentially exist regarding any action domain should fall on a bipolar dimension. That is, it should be the case that affect can be positive, neutral, or negative for any given goal-directed action, depending on how well or poorly the action seems to be attaining the goal. This implication differentiates our view from some others, an issue we take up a bit farther along.

What determines the criterion? There undoubtedly are many influences. Further, the orientation that a person takes to an action can induce a different framing that may change the criterion (Brendl & Higgins, 1996). What is used as a criterion is probably quite flexible when the activity is unfamiliar. If the activity is very familiar, the criterion is likely to reflect the person's accumulated experience in the form of an expected rate (the more experience you have, the more you know what is reasonable to expect). Whether "desired" or "expected" or "needed" is most accurate as a depiction of the criterion rate may depend greatly on the context.

Can the criterion change? Of course. The less experience the person has in a domain, the easier it is to substitute one criterion for another. We believe, however, that change in rate criterion in a relatively familiar domain occurs relatively slowly. Continuing overshoots result automatically in an upward drift of the criterion, and continuing undershoots result in a downward drift (for greater detail, see Carver & Scheier, 2000). Thus, the system recalibrates itself over repeated experiences. A somewhat ironic consequence of such a recalibration would be to keep the balance of a person's affective experience (positive to negative, aggregated across a span of time) relatively similar even when the rate criterion changes considerably.

Doubtlessly there are limits on the ability to recalibrate and individual differences in the pace of recalibration (Diener, Lucas, & Scollon, 2006). It is unknown whether the recalibration process has costs. An interesting speculation is that, if pushed too far toward demanding pacing (and thus more potential for negative affect), this system may suffer strains similar to those posited for other physical systems of the body under the label *allostatic load* (Korte, Koolhaas, Wingfield, & McEwen, 2005; McEwen, 2004; Schulkin, 2004).

Two Kinds of Action Loops, Two Dimensions of Affect

So far we have addressed only approach loops. The view just outlined was that positive feeling exists when a behavioral system is making more than adequate progress *doing what it is organized to do*. The systems addressed so far are organized to reduce discrepancies. Yet there seems no obvious reason why the principle should not apply to systems that enlarge discrepancies. If such a system is making rapid enough progress attaining its ends, there should be positive affect. If it is doing poorly, there should be negative affect.

That affects of both valences are possible seems applicable to both approach and avoidance. That is, both approach and avoidance have the potential to induce positive feelings (by doing well), and both have the potential to induce negative feelings (by doing poorly). But doing well at *approaching an incentive* is not quite the same experience as doing well at *moving away from a threat*. Thus, there may be differences between the two positives and between the two negatives.

Drawing on the work of Higgins (e.g., 1987, 1996) and his collaborators, we have argued for two bipolar dimensions of affect, one bearing on approach and the other on avoidance (Carver, 2001; Carver & Scheier, 1998). Approach-related affect includes such positive affects as elation, eagerness, and excitement and such negative affects as frustration, anger, and sadness (Carver, 2004). Avoidance-related affect includes such positive affects as relief, serenity, and contentment and such negative affects as fear, guilt, and anxiety (for application of this reasoning to social relations, see Laurenceau, Troy, & Carver, 2005).

Affect and Action: Two Facets of One Event in Time

This two-layered viewpoint implies a natural connection between affect and action. That is, if the input function of the affect loop is a sensed rate of progress in action, the output function of the affect loop must be a change in the rate of progress in that action. Thus, the affect loop has a direct influence on what occurs in the action loop.

Some changes in rate output are straightforward. If you are lagging behind, you try harder. Some changes are less straightforward. The rates of many "behaviors" are defined not by a pace of physical action but in terms of choices among potential actions, or entire programs of action. For example, increasing your rate of progress on a project at work may mean choosing to spend a weekend working rather than playing with family and friends. Increasing your rate of being kind means choosing to do an act that reflects kindness when an opportunity arises. Thus, change in rate must often be translated into other terms, such as concentration, or allocation of time and effort.

The idea of two feedback systems functioning jointly is something we more or less stumbled into. As it happens, however, this idea is quite common in control engineering (e.g., Clark, 1996). Engineers have long recognized that having two systems functioning together—one controlling position and one controlling velocity—permits the device they control to respond in a way that is both quick and stable without overshoots and oscillations.

The combination of quickness and stability in responding is desirable in many of the devices engineers deal with. It is also desirable in people. A person with very reactive emotions is prone to overreact and oscillate behaviorally. A person who is emotionally nonreactive is slow to respond even to urgent events. A person whose reactions are between those extremes responds quickly but without overreaction and oscillation.

For biological entities, being able to respond quickly yet accurately confers a clear adaptive advantage. We believe this combination of quick and stable responding is a consequence of having both behavior-managing and affect-managing control systems. Affect causes people's responses to be quicker (because this control system is time sensitive); as long as the affective system is not overresponsive, the responses are also stable.

Our focus here is on how affects influence behavior, emphasizing the extent to which they are interwoven. However, note that the behavioral responses that are linked to the affects also lead to *reduction of the affects*. We thus would suggest that the affect system is, in a very basic sense, self-regulating (cf. Campos, Frankel, & Camras, 2004). It is undeniable that people also engage in voluntary efforts to regulate their emotions, but the affect system does a good deal of that self-regulation on its own.

Affect Issues

There are several ways in which this model differs from other theories bearing on motivation and emotion. At least two of the differences appear to have important implications.

One difference concerns the dimensional structure of affect (Carver, 2001). Some theories (though not all, e.g., Izard, 1977; Levenson, 1994, 1999) treat affects as aligned along dimensions. Our dimensional view holds that affect relating to approach has the potential to be either positive or negative and that affect relating to avoidance has the potential to be either positive or negative. Most current dimensional models of affect, however, differ in that regard.

The idea that eagerness, excitement, and elation relate to approach is intuitive. It is also intuitive that fear and anxiety relate to avoidance. Both of these relations are noted commonly (Cacioppo, Gardner, & Berntson, 1999; Watson, Wiese, Vaidya, & Tellegen, 1999). Consensus breaks down, however, on where to place other affects. For example, J. A. Gray (e.g., 1990, 1994a, 1994b) held that the system that responds to threat is engaged both by cues of punishment and by cues of frustrative nonreward. It thus relates to negative feelings that pertain to approach as well as those that pertain to avoidance. Similarly, he held that the approach system is engaged by cues of reward and cues of escape or avoidance of punishment. It thus is linked to positive feelings pertaining to avoidance as well as approach.

That view, then, is one in which each system is responsible for affect of one hedonic tone (positive in one case and negative in the other). It yields two unipolar affective dimensions (running neutral to negative and neutral to positive), each linked to the functioning of a separate behavioral system. A similar position has been taken by Lang and colleagues (e.g., Lang, 1995; Lang, Bradley, & Cuthbert, 1990), by Cacioppo and colleagues (e.g., Cacioppo & Berntson, 1994; Cacioppo et al., 1999), and by Watson and colleagues (Watson et al., 1999). In that respect, our dimensional view is quite different from those that dominate today's discussions.

Evidence of Bipolar Dimensions

Does our view have any support? Consider "doing well" at threat avoidance. In one study that bears on this question (Higgins, Shah, & Friedman, 1997, study 4), people took either an approach orientation to a laboratory task (try to attain success) or an avoidance orientation (try to avoid failing); they then experienced either goal attainment or nonattainment. After the task outcome (which was manipulated), feelings were assessed. Given an avoidance orientation, success caused elevation in calmness, and failure caused elevation in anxiety. Effects on these affects did not occur, however, among those with an approach orientation. This pattern suggests that calmness is linked to doing well at avoidance rather than doing well at approach.

A larger accumulation of evidence links certain kinds of negative affect to "doing poorly" in approaching incentives, and we review only a few sources here. One is the study by Higgins et al. (1997) just described. The conditions we described were those that led to feelings of calmness and anxiety. However, the study also provided data on sadness. Among persons with an approach orientation, failure elevated sadness, and success elevated cheerfulness. These effects did not occur among participants with an avoidance orientation. The pattern suggests a link between sadness and doing poorly at approach rather than doing poorly at avoidance.

Another source of evidence is a laboratory study (Carver, 2004) in which participants were led to believe that they could obtain a desired reward if they performed well on a task. There was no penalty for doing poorly—only an opportunity of reward for doing well. Participants had been preassessed on the sensitivity of their approach and avoidance systems (Carver & White, 1994). All received feedback that they had not done well, and they thus failed to obtain the reward. Reports of sadness and discouragement at that point related to premeasured sensitivity of the approach system but not to sensitivity of the avoidance system.

Yet another source of information is the broad literature of self-discrepancy theory. Several studies have shown that feelings of sadness relate uniquely (i.e., controlling for anxiety) to discrepancies between people's actual selves and ideal selves (for reviews, see Higgins, 1987, 1996). Ideals are qualities a person intrinsically desires: aspirations, hopes, and positive images for the self. There is evidence that pursuing an ideal is an approach process (Higgins, 1996). Thus, this literature also suggests that sadness stems from a failure of approach.

There is also evidence linking the approach system to the negative affect of anger. Harmon-Jones and Allen (1998) studied individual differences in trait anger. Higher anger related to higher left frontal activity (and to lower right frontal activity). This suggests a link between anger and the approach system because the approach system has been linked to activation of the left prefrontal cortex (e.g., Davidson, 1992). More recently, Harmon-Jones and Sigelman (2001) induced a state of anger in some persons but not others, then examined cortical activity. They found elevations in left frontal activity, suggesting that anger relates to greater engagement of the approach system (see also Harmon-Jones, Lueck, Fearn, & Harmon-Jones, 2006).

Further evidence pertaining to anger comes from research (Carver, 2004) in which people indicated the intensity of feelings they experienced in response to hypothetical events (study 2) and after the destruction of the World Trade Center (study 3). Participants had been preassessed on a self-report measure of the sensitivity of their approach and avoidance systems (Carver & White, 1994). Reports of anger related to premeasured sensitivity of the approach system, whereas reports of anxiety related instead to sensitivity of the avoidance system.

Conceptual Mechanism

Why spend so much space on this issue? This issue matters a great deal because it has implications for any attempt to identify a conceptual mechanism underlying affect. Theories that argue for two unipolar dimensions appear to assume that greater activation of a system translates directly to more affect of that valence (or more potential for affect of that valence). If the approach system relates both to positive and to negative feelings, this direct transformation of system activation to affect is not tenable.

A conceptual mechanism is needed that naturally addresses both positive and negative feelings within the approach function (and, separately, the avoidance function). One such mechanism is the one described here. There may be others, but this one has some advantages. Its mechanism fits nicely with the fact that feelings occur continuously throughout the attempt to reach an incentive, not just at the point of its attainment. Indeed, feelings rise, wane, and change valence as progress varies from time to time along the way forward.

A Counterintuitive Implication

A second issue also differentiates this model from many other views of the meaning and consequences of affect (see also Carver, 2003). Recall our argument that affect reflects the error signal from a comparison in a feedback loop. As noted, if affect reflects the error signal in a feedback loop, affect is a signal to adjust rate of progress. This would be true whether the rate is above the mark or below it—that is, whether affect is positive or negative. For negative feelings, this notion is fully intuitive. The first response to negative feelings is usually to try harder. (For now, we disregard the possibility of withdrawing effort and quitting, though that possibility clearly is important; we return to it later.) If the person tries harder—and assuming that more effort (or better effort) increases the rate of intended movement—the negative affect diminishes or ceases.

What about positive feelings? Here prediction becomes counterintuitive. In this model, positive feelings arise when things are going better than they need to. But the feelings still reflect a discrepancy (albeit a positive one), and the function of a negative feedback loop is to minimize discrepancies. Such a system is organized in such a way that it "wants" to see neither negative nor positive affect. Either quality (deviation from the standard in either direction) would represent an "error" and lead to changes in output that would eventually reduce it.

This view argues that people who exceed the criterion rate of progress (and who thus have positive feelings) will automatically tend to reduce subsequent effort in this domain. They will "coast" a little (cf. Frijda, 1994)—not necessarily stop but ease back such that subsequent rate of progress returns to the criterion. The impact on subjective affect would be that the positive feeling itself is not sustained for very long. It begins to fade.

We stress that expending greater effort to catch up when behind and coasting when ahead are both presumed to be specific to the goal domain to which the affect is attached. Usually this is the goal from which the affect arises in the first place (for exceptions, see Schwarz & Clore, 1983). We are not arguing that positive affect creates a tendency to coast *in general* but rather that it creates a tendency to coast with respect to the specific activity producing the positive feelings. We should also be clear about the time frame we are addressing. We are talking about the current, ongoing episode of action. We are emphatically *not* arguing that positive affect makes people less likely to do the behavior again later on.

This is a kind of "cruise control" model of the origins and consequences of affect. That is, a system of this sort would operate in the same way as a car's cruise control. If behavior is moving too slowly, negative affect arises. The person responds by increasing effort, trying to speed up. If the person is going faster than needed, positive affect arises, leading to coasting. A car's cruise control is very similar. Coming to a hill slows you down; the cruise control responds by giving the engine more fuel, speeding back up. If you come across the crest of a hill and roll downward too fast, the system cuts back the fuel, and the speed drags back down.

The analogy is intriguing partly because both sides have an asymmetry in the consequences of deviation from the reference point. That is, both in a car and in behavior, addressing the problem of going too slow requires adding resources. Addressing the problem of going too fast entails only cutting back on resources. The cruise control does not engage the brakes; it just reduces fuel. The car coasts back to the velocity set point. Thus, the effect of the cruise control on a high rate of speed depends in part on external circumstances. If the hill is steep, the car may exceed the cruise control's set point all the way to the valley below.

In the same fashion, people usually do not react to positive affect by actively trying to make themselves feel less good (though there are exceptions). They just ease back a little on resources devoted to the domain in which the affect has arisen. The positive feelings may be sustained for a long time (depending on circumstances) as the person coasts down the subjective analog of the hill. Eventually, though, the reduced resources would cause the positive affect to diminish. Generally, then, the system would act to prevent great amounts of pleasure as well as great amounts of pain (Carver, 2003; Carver & Scheier, 1998).

Coasting

The idea that positive affect leads to coasting, which eventually results in reduction of the positive affect, strikes some people as implausible. Some believe that pleasure is a sign to continue what one is doing or even to immerse oneself in it more deeply (cf. Fredrickson, 2001; Messinger, 2002). On the other hand, there is a logical bind in that view. If pleasure increases engagement in the activity, leading thereby to more pleasure and thus more engagement, when and why would the person ever cease that activity? When would the person ever even slow down? The only reason for slowing would be completion of the activity.

The idea that positive feelings induce coasting may seem unlikely, but we are not alone in having suggested it. In discussing joy, Izard (1977) wrote, "If the kind of problem at hand requires a great deal of persistence and hard work, *joy may put the problem aside before it is solved*. . . . If your intellectual performance, whatever it may be, leads to joy, the joy will have the effect of *slowing down performance* and removing some of the concern for problem solving. This change in pace and concern may postpone or in some cases eliminate the possibility of an intellectual or creative achievement. . . . If excitement causes the 'rushing' or 'forcing' of intellectual activity, a *joy-elicited slowing down* may be exactly what is need to improve intellectual performance and creative endeavor" (p. 257; emphasis added). More recently, Izard and

Ackerman (2000) wrote, "Periodic joy provides *respite from the activity*" (p. 258; emphasis added).

Does positive affect lead to coasting? To test the idea, a study must assess coasting with respect to the same goal as underlies the affect. Many studies have created positive affect in one context and assessed its influence on another task (e.g., Isen, 1987, 2000; Schwarz & Bohner, 1996). However, that procedure does not test this question. Suggestive evidence has been reported by Mizruchi (1991) and Louro, Pieters, and Zeelenberg (2007), but at this point the question remains relatively untested.

Coasting and Multiple Concerns

One reason for skepticism about the idea that positive affect induces coasting is that it is hard to see why a process would be built into the organism that limits positive feelings—indeed, dampens them. After all, don't people seek pleasure and avoid pain?

We believe there are at least two adaptive bases for the tendency to coast. The first lies in a basic biological principle: It is adaptive for organisms not to spend energy needlessly. Coasting prevents needless energy expenditure. The second basis stems from the fact that people have multiple simultaneous concerns (Carver, 2003; Carver & Scheier, 1998; Frijda, 1994). Given multiple concerns, people typically do not optimize their outcome on any one of them but rather "satisfice" (Simon, 1953), that is, do a good enough job on each to deal with it satisfactorily. This permits them to handle the many concerns adequately rather than just any one of them.

A tendency to coast would virtually define satisficing regarding that particular goal. That is, reduction in effort would result in an adequate rate of progress on that goal rather than the fastest rate possible. A tendency to coast could also foster satisficing of a broader set of goals. That is, if progress in one domain exceeds current needs, a tendency to coast in that domain (satisficing) would make it easy to shift to another domain at little or no cost. This would help ensure satisfactory goal attainment in the other domain and ultimately across multiple domains.

Continued pursuit of one goal without letup, in contrast, can have adverse effects. Continuing a rapid pace in one arena may sustain positive affect in that arena, but by diverting resources from other goals, it also increases the potential for problems elsewhere. This would be even more true of an effort to *intensify* the positive affect because doing that would mean further diverting resources from other goals. Indeed, a single-minded pursuit of yet-more-positive feelings in one domain can even be lethal if it causes the person to disregard threats looming elsewhere.

A pattern in which positive feelings lead to easing back and an openness to shifting focus would minimize such adverse effects. It is important to note that this view does not require that people with positive feelings shift goals. It simply holds that openness to a shift is a consequence—and a potential benefit—of the coasting tendency. This line of thought would, however, begin to account for why people do eventually turn away from what are clearly pleasurable activities.

A provocative finding in this regard is that smiling infants who are engaging in face-to-face interactions with their mothers periodically avert their gazes from their mothers, then stop smiling. Infants are more likely to do this (and to avert their gaze longer) when they are smiling intensely than when the smiles are less intense (Stifter & Moyer, 1991). This pattern hints that the experience of happiness creates an openness to shifting focus or at least a tendency to coast with respect to the interaction with mother, letting the affect diminish before returning to the interaction.

Priority Management in Self-Regulation

This line of argument implicates positive feelings in a broad function that deserves further attention. This function is the shifting from one goal to another as focal in behavior (Dreisbach & Goschke, 2004; Shallice, 1978). This basic and very important phenomenon is often overlooked. Many goals are typically under pursuit simultaneously (cf. Atkinson & Birch, 1970; Murray, 1938), but only one can have top priority at a given moment. People need to shield and maintain the intentions that are being pursued (cf. Shah, Friedman, & Kruglanski, 2002), but they also need to be able to shift flexibly among goals (Shin & Rosenbaum, 2002).

The issue of priority management was addressed very creatively many years ago by Simon (1967). He pointed out that an entity that has many goals needs a way to rank them for pursuit and a mechanism to change rankings as necessary. He reasoned as follows: Most of the goals people are pursuing are largely out of awareness at any given moment. Only the one with the highest priority has full access to consciousness. Sometimes events occur during the pursuit of that top-priority goal that create problems for another goal that now has a lower priority. Indeed, the mere passing of time can sometimes create a problem for the second goal because the passing time may be making its attainment less likely. If the second goal is also important, any emerging problem for its attainment needs to be registered and taken into account. If the situation evolves enough to seriously threaten the second goal, some mechanism is needed for changing priorities so that the second goal replaces the first one as focal.

Negative Feelings and Reprioritization

Simon (1967) reasoned that emotions are calls for reprioritization. He suggested that emotion arising with respect to a goal that is out of awareness eventually induces people to interrupt their behavior and give that goal a higher priority than it had. The stronger the emotion, the stronger is the claim being made that the unattended goal should have higher priority than the goal that is presently focal. The affect is what pulls the out-of-awareness into awareness. Simon did not address the negative affect that sometimes arises with respect to a goal that currently is focal, but the same principle seems to apply to this case as well. That is, negative affect in this case seems to be a call for an even greater investment of resources and effort in the focal goal than is now being made.

Simon's analysis applies readily to negative feelings such as anxiety and frustration. If you promised your spouse you would go to the post office this afternoon and you have been too busy working on a project to go, the creeping of the clock toward closing time can cause an increase in frustration or anxiety (or both). Neither affect would pertain to the work you are doing, however. Frustration might arise from the potentially unmet obligation (a desired outcome that is slipping away); anxiety might arise from the potentially angry spouse (a threat that is coming closer). The greater the potential loss, the greater the frustration; the greater the threat, the stronger the anxiety. The stronger the affect, the more likely it is that the goal it stems from will rise in priority until it comes fully to awareness and becomes the focal reference point for behavior.

Positive Feelings and Reprioritization

Simon's discussion of shifting priorities focused on cases in which a nonfocal goal demands a higher priority than it now has and *intrudes* on awareness. By strong implication, his discussion dealt only with negative affect. However, there is another way in which priority ordering can shift: The currently focal goal can *relinquish its place*. Simon noted this possibility obliquely. He noted that goal completion results in termination of pursuit of that goal. However, he did not address the possibility that an as-yet-unattained goal might also yield its place in line.

Consider the possibility that positive feelings pertain to reprioritization but that, rather than a call for higher priority, they are a sign of *reduction* in the priority of the goal to which the feeling pertains. This appears consistent with the sense of Simon's analysis. It simply suggests that the function he asserted for affect is relevant to affects of both valences. Positive affect regarding an avoidance act (relief or tranquility) indicates that a threat has dissipated, no longer requires as much attention as it did, and can now assume a lower priority. Positive feelings regarding approach (happiness or joy) indicate that an incentive is being attained. If it *has* been attained, effort can cease, as Simon noted. If it is not yet attained, the affect is a signal that you could temporarily put this goal aside because you are doing so well. That is, it indicates that this goal can assume a lower priority (Carver, 2003).

If a focal goal diminishes in priority, what follows? This situation is less directive than the one in which a nonfocal goal demands an increase in priority (the latter is very specific about what goal should get more attention). What happens in this case depends partly on what is waiting in line. It also depends partly on whether the context has changed in any important way while you were busy. That is, opportunities to attain incentives sometimes appear unexpectedly, and people put aside their plans to take advantage of such emergent opportunities (Hayes-Roth & Hayes-Roth, 1979;

Payton, 1990). It seems reasonable that people with positive affect should be most prone to shift goals at this point if something else needs fixing or doing (regarding a next-in-line goal or a newly emergent goal) or if an unanticipated opportunity for gain has appeared.

Sometimes the next item in line is of fairly high priority in its own right. Sometimes the situation has changed and a new goal has emerged for consideration. But sometimes neither of these conditions exists. In such a case, no change would occur because the downgrade in priority of the focal goal does not make it lower than the priorities of the alternatives. Positive affect does not *require* a change in direction. It simply sets the stage for such a change to be more likely.

Indirect support for this general line of reasoning comes from several sources. One of them is recent discussions of the circumstances under which people do and do not engage in self-esteem-protective behavior. Maintaining self-esteem is an important goal (e.g., Tesser, 1988), but people don't always take steps to enhance self-esteem (Tesser, Crepaz, Collins, Cornell, & Beach, 2000). Tesser et al. argued that self-esteem maintenance reflects a satisficing tendency. As long as the self-image is above a threshold, there is no effort to build it higher. Only if it falls below the threshold is effort engaged to prop it back up. A variety of other evidence also seems to fit the idea that positive feelings make people more open to taking up alternate goals, particularly those that seem threatened (for a review, see Carver, 2003).

Effects such as these have contributed to the emergence of the view that positive experiences represent psychological resources. Trope and Pomerantz (1998) wrote that experiences such as a success or a positive mood serve as means to other ends rather than as ends themselves. Reed and Aspinwall (1998) suggested that positive self-beliefs and self-affirmations are resources that permit people to confront problematic situations such as health threats (see also Aspinwall, 1998; Isen, 2000; for broader resource models, see Gallo & Matthews, 2003; Hobfoll, 1989, 2002; Muraven & Baumeister, 2000). This line of thought is not quite the same as the one that underlies the position taken here, but some of its connotations are similar.

The idea that positive feelings are psychological resources need not apply only to cases in which resources permit people to turn to problems. Just as secure infant attachment is seen as a resource that promotes exploration (Bowlby, 1988), Fredrickson (1998) has asserted that positive feelings promote play. The idea that positive affect serves as a resource for exploration resembles in some ways the idea that positive feelings open people to noticing and taking advantage of emergent opportunities, to being distracted into enticing alternatives—to opportunistic behavior.

This idea also has some empirical support. Kahn and Isen (1993) gave people opportunities to try out choices within a food category. Those in whom positive affect had been created switched among choices more than did controls. Isen (2000) interpreted this as indicating that positive affect promotes "enjoyment of variety and a wide range of possibilities" (p. 423), which sounds like opportunistic foraging. In the same vein, Dreisbach and Goschke (2004) found that positive affect decreased perseveration on a task strategy and increased distractibility. Both of these findings are consistent with our reasoning here.

We should be clear that we are not arguing that affect is the only source of shifts in goal reprioritization. For example, changes in context can also produce goal shifts because different contexts have been linked in the past to different goals. Our argument is simply that affect is part of the prioritization process.

Actively Preventing Automatic Functions of Affect

We have focused here on what we think are a set of automatic effects of emotions on efforts toward a focal goal and on priority management. We should note, however, that people can learn to intervene in these otherwise automatic effects. In effect, people learn to trick the system in various ways that are useful to them in certain situations.

For example, suppose you are an athlete performing in an event that takes a particular period of time. Suppose you get ahead quickly. In our view, if for that reason you feel happy, you may relax a little. But relaxing—becoming vulnerable to distraction—is undesirable in this situation. How can you prevent it from happening? A common strategy for athletes is to try to prevent feelings of pleasure from arising as the event continues. This can be done by artificially holding in mind an extremely high level of aspiration that could hardly ever be exceeded (thus no positive affect). This is similar to the idea that the best performance comes from setting a goal that is just out of reach (Locke & Latham, 1990). Another strategy is to artificially generate anger, taking the place of any pleasure in being ahead. Yet another strategy is to remind yourself that your lead is small and that you are still vulnerable or even to pretend that you are not really ahead at all.

The point more generally is that there often are ways to trick the automatic system of affective response by reframing the situation in various ways. If the affective reaction itself can be changed, the resulting impact on coasting and priority management should also change.

Priority Management and Feelings of Depression

One more aspect of priority management should be addressed here. It concerns the idea that under some circumstances, goals are not attainable and are better abandoned. We have long argued that sufficient doubt about goal attainment yields a tendency to disengage from efforts to reach the goal and even to disengage from the goal itself (Carver & Scheier, 1981, 1998, 1999a, 1999b). This is certainly a kind of priority adjustment in that the abandoned goal now receives an even lower priority than it had before. That is, no behavior is being directed to its attainment at all. How does this sort of reprioritization fit into the model described thus far?

At first glance, the idea that doubt about goal attainment (and the negative affect associated with that doubt) causes reduction in effort might seem to contradict Simon's (1967) position that negative affect is a call for higher priority. However, there is an important distinction between two negative affects associated with approach (Carver, 2003, 2004). (A parallel line of reasoning can be applied to avoidance, but we skip over that here.) Some negative affects pertaining to approach coalesce around frustration and anger. Others coalesce around sadness, depression, and dejection. The former relate to an increase in priority and the latter to a decrease.

In describing our view on affect, we said that approach-related affects exist on a dimension. However, the dimension is not a simple straight line. Theory holds that falling behind—progress below the criterion—creates negative affect as the incentive slips away. Inadequate movement forward (or no movement or reverse movement) gives rise to frustration, irritation, and anger. These feelings (or the mechanism that underlies them) function to engage effort more completely—to overcome obstacles and reverse

the inadequacy of current progress. If the situation is one in which more effort (or better effort) can improve progress, such effort allows the person to move toward the incentive at an adequate rate, and attaining the incentive seems likely. This case fits the priority management model of Simon (1967).

Sometimes, however, continued efforts do not produce adequate movement forward. Indeed, if the situation involves loss, movement forward is precluded because the incentive is gone. In a situation where failure seems (or is) ensured, the feelings are sadness, depression, despondency, dejection, grief, and hopelessness (cf. Finlay-Jones & Brown, 1981). Accompanying behaviors also differ in this case. The person tends to disengage from—give up on—further effort toward the incentive (Klinger, 1975; Wortman & Brehm, 1975; for evidence, see Lewis, Sullivan, Ramsay, & Allessandri, 1992; Mikulincer, 1988).

At least two published studies have found patterns of emotions consistent with this portrayal (Mikulincer, 1994; Pittman & Pittman, 1980). In each, participants received varying amounts of failure, and their emotional responses were assessed. In both cases, reports of anger were most intense after small amounts of failure and lower after larger amounts of failure. Reports of depression were low after small amounts of failure and intense after larger amounts of failure.

As just described, approach-related negative feelings in these two kinds of situations are presumed to link to two very different effects on ongoing action. Both effects have adaptive properties. In the first situation—when the person falls behind but the goal is not seen as lost—feelings of frustration and anger accompany an increase in effort, a struggle to gain the incentive despite setbacks. Consistent with this view, Frijda (1986) argued that anger implies having the hope that things can be set right (see also Harmon-Jones & Allen, 1998). This struggle is adaptive (thus, the affect is adaptive) because the struggle fosters goal attainment.

In the second situation—when effort appears futile—negative feelings of sadness and depression accompany *reduction* of effort. Sadness and despondency imply that things cannot be set right, that further effort is pointless. Reducing effort in this circumstance can also have adaptive functions (Carver & Scheier, 2003; Wrosch, Scheier, Carver, & Schulz, 2003; Wrosch, Scheier, Miller, Schulz, & Carver, 2003). It serves to conserve energy rather than waste it in futile pursuit of the unattainable (Nesse, 2000). If reducing effort also helps diminish commitment to the goal (Klinger, 1975), it eventually readies the person to take up pursuit of other incentives in place of this one.

The variations in effort described in the preceding paragraphs are portrayed in Figure 15.2. The left side portrays the hypothesized reduction in effort when velocity exceeds the criterion, discussed earlier. The right side portrays both the strong engagement that is implied by frustration and anger (when improvement seems possible)

and the disengagement of sadness and dejection (when improvement seems out of reach).

Two additional points about the portion of Figure 15.2 to the right of the criterion line are worth noting. First, this part of the figure has much in common with several other depictions of variations in effort when difficulty in moving toward a goal gives way to loss of the goal (for detail, see Carver & Scheier, 1998, Chapter 11). Perhaps best known is Wortman and Brehm's (1975) integration of reactance and helplessness. They described a region of threat to control, in which there is enhanced effort to regain control, and a region of loss of control, in which efforts diminish. Indeed, the figure they used to illustrate those regions greatly resembles the right side of Figure 15.2.

Another point concerns the fact that the right side of Figure 15.2 is drawn with a rather abrupt shift from frustration to sadness. The abruptness of that transition in this figure is somewhat arbitrary. There probably are cases in which the shift is abrupt and cases in which it is not. These two sets of cases may differ in the relative importance of the goals involved. Importance has been

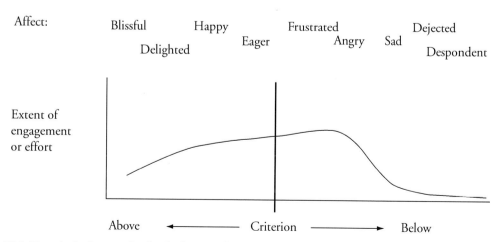

Fig. 15.2 Hypothesized approach-related affects as a function of doing well versus doing poorly compared to a criterion velocity. A second (vertical) dimension indicates the degree of behavioral engagement posited to be associated with affects at different degrees of departure from neutral. Adapted from Carver (2004).

ignored in this discussion but it obviously must play a very large role in the intensity of affective and motivational experiences (cf. Pomerantz, Saxon, & Oishi, 2000). We do not address this issue further here, but discussions can be found elsewhere (Carver & Scheier, 1998, 1999a, 1999b).

Two Modes of Functioning?

Earlier in the chapter, we distinguished between sequences of action that seem to occur more or less all at a piece when begun and programs and principles of action that appear to require more decision making and planning (Chapter 5). At that time, the boundary between the more automatic and the less automatic was noted simply as a matter of differences in level of abstraction of the action goal. Now we look at this boundary in a somewhat different way. First, however, we need to take an excursion into some additional issues that may at first seem quite unrelated to anything we have talked about thus far.

Top-Down and Bottom-Up Behavior Control

For the most part, we have written about action here as though it were controlled from the top down. That is, people form intentions and realize those intentions by making their perceptions of their actions match those intentions. So far, so good. There is evidence, however, that a good deal of behavior does not actually happen that way. Rather, it self-organizes. It falls into a pattern that was not planned or intended. Instead, the pattern emerges from the confluence of two or more other things going on at the same time (Brooks, 1999; Kelso, 1995; Newtson, 1993, 1994; Prigogene & Stengers, 1984). A common example of self-organization is the fact that gaits naturally emerge from the locomotion of quadrupeds (Turvey, 1990). Another example is how a familiar cue can cause a person to go

off track and substitute another act for the act intended (Norman, 1981).

Does this sort of evidence mean that behavior is not guided by intentions? No, not exactly. But it does mean that any view that addresses only intentions is incomplete.

We were led to think about this issue a few years ago (see Carver & Scheier, 1998, Chapter 17) from directions that were suggested by several literatures. Of particular importance was a set of arguments being made at that time in cognitive psychology. Cognitive psychology, dominated for many years by a view of cognition as sequential symbol processing, had been challenged two decades earlier by a different view, commonly called connectionism (e.g., Bechtel & Abrahamsen, 1991; McClelland, 1999). This view uses neuronal function as a metaphor for cognitive processes, assumes parallel processing as a key feature, and views representation as reflecting patterns of activation in entire networks.

Two-Mode Models

Symbolic and connectionist analyses each have advantages in different contexts. This had led a number of cognitive psychologists to conclude that cognition (in the broadest sense) employs two kinds of processes. One kind is effortful and symbolic. It had variously been termed *conscious* (Smolensky, 1988), *rule based* (Sloman, 1996), and *reflective* (Shastri & Ajjanagadde, 1993). The other kind uses connectionist processes to manage heuristic, skilled, and automatic activities. It had variously been termed *intuitive* (Smolensky, 1988), *associative* (Sloman, 1996), and *reflexive* (Shastri & Ajjanagadde, 1993). Both of these modes of functioning were assumed to operate continuously and simultaneously (see also De Neys, 2006).

A similar line of argument about two modes of functioning has also emerged in other places. In personality psychology, Epstein has long advocated an idea that is strikingly similar to this, in his cognitive-experiential self theory (Epstein, 1973, 1985, 1990, 1994). That theory begins with the premise that people experience reality through two systems. What Epstein calls the *rational* system operates mostly consciously, uses logical rules, is verbal and deliberative, and thus is fairly slow. The *experiential* system is intuitive and associative in nature. It provides a "quick and dirty" way of assessing and reacting to reality. It relies on salient information and uses shortcuts and heuristics. It functions automatically and quickly, even impulsively. It is considered to be emotional (or at least very responsive to emotions) and nonverbal.

Epstein believes the experiential system is older and more primitive. It dominates when speed is needed (as when the situation is emotionally charged). You cannot be thorough and planful when there is a need to act fast (e.g., to avoid danger). Maybe there is no time even to form an intention. The rational system evolved later, providing a more cautious, analytic, planful way of proceeding. Being able to operate in that way has some important advantages provided that there is sufficient time and freedom from pressure to think things through. Epstein believes that both systems are always at work and that they jointly determine behavior. The degree to which each is engaged varies with circumstances and also varies across persons.

A cognitive model that is very similar to Epstein's in many ways was proposed more recently by Metcalfe and Mischel (1999). This theory has very different roots, however, drawing on several decades' work on delay of gratification. In a typical study on this topic, children can have a smaller, less desired reward now or can instead wait for a while and get a larger, more desired reward later (Mischel, 1974). Delay is easier if the children mentally transform the situation (Mischel & Baker, 1975) to distract themselves from consummatory aspects of the rewards.

Drawing in part on this large body of work, Metcalfe and Mischel (1999) proposed that two systems influence levels of restraint in a wide variety of contexts. One they called a "hot" system: emotional, impulsive, and reflexive. It is said to operate in a connectionist manner. The other they called a "cool" system: strategic, flexible, slower, and unemotional. How a person responds to a difficult situation depends on which system is presently in charge. (For treatments regarding the cognitive differences between systems, see J. R. Gray, 1999; Chapter 14). Although this line of thought derived from research on delay of gratification, it obviously applies much more broadly.

There are also several two-mode theories in social psychology. Indeed, the essence of such a view has existed for a long time in the literature of persuasion (Chaiken & Trope, 1999). People sometimes process persuasive messages carefully and thoughtfully, sometimes quickly and superficially. If the message is processed in the deliberative mode, its impact depends on the quality of the arguments it contains. If the message is processed in the superficial mode, its impact depends more on the heuristic properties of the message and its context (see also Smith & DeCoster, 2000; Wilson, Lindsey, & Schooler, 2000). Hogarth (2001, 2005) has made similar arguments about intuitive and deliberate decision making.

A recent analysis of automaticity in attribution also started with the idea that there are two modes of functioning (Lieberman, Gaunt, Gilbert, & Trope, 2002). This analysis starts with the idea that when something is done effortfully over and over, it becomes automatic, and the doing of it drops out of consciousness. Lieberman et al. (2002) argued that the effortful and the automatic represent two different modes of processing. They called the automatic mode *reflexive* and the effortful mode *reflective*. They contended that the effortful and automatic versions of a given behavior (or thought) are managed by different brain areas: controlled processes by the anterior cingulate, prefrontal cortex, and hippocampus and automatic processes by the lateral temporal cortex, amygdala, and basal ganglia (see also Casey, Tottenham, & Fossella, 2002; Posner & DiGirolamo, 2000). Indeed, evidence that implicated different areas of the brain was a key reason for their assertion that there are two separate modes of functioning.

Strack and Deutsch (2004) have recently extended a similar sort of reasoning more deeply into the range of phenomena of interest to social psychologists. They pointed out that earlier work in social psychology on dual-process models tended to focus on judgments and information processing, and they noted that motives and overt behaviors also must be taken into account (see also Barrett, Tugade, & Engle, 2004). They proposed a two-mode model in which overt social behavior is a joint output of two modes of functioning that occur simultaneously and may be mutually supportive or may be in conflict. They used the terms *reflective* and *impulsive* to refer to the two modes.

Consistent with the other positions just reviewed, the latter two social psychological models (Lieberman et al., 2002; Strack & Deutsch, 2004) assume that the reflective system uses symbolic logic and is slower than the (connectionist) reflexive system. They hold that the reflexive system is attuned to pressured and emotional situations (Lieberman et al., 2002) and that it may underlie intuition (Lieberman, 2000), which had also been suggested by cognitive psychologists (Sloman, 1996; Smolensky, 1988). Strack and Deutsch (2004) added that because the reflective system requires substantial cognitive capacity, it is likely to be inefficient under high mental load, whereas the impulsive system requires little capacity and can function well under suboptimal conditions.

Strack and Deutsch (2004) proposed that these presumed differences in the two systems' operating characteristics lead to differences in behavior. The reflective system anticipates future conditions, makes decisions on the basis of those anticipations, and forms intentions. It is planful and wide ranging in its search for relevant information. It is restrained and deliberative. In contrast, the impulsive system acts spontaneously when its schemas or production systems are sufficiently activated. It acts without consideration for the future or for broader implications or consequences of the action. This depiction is very similar in many respects to the ideas of Epstein (1973, 1985, 1990, 1994) and Metcalfe and Mischel (1999).

Implicit and Explicit as Two Modes

The idea that there are two modes of functioning also seems to fit with a burgeoning literature on explicit and implicit motives, knowledge structures, and attitudes. This literature has benefited greatly from the development of a technique called the Implicit Association Test (IAT; Greenwald, McGhee, & Schwartz, 1998). The IAT provides a way to measure the strength of associations between pairs of concepts, including evaluative qualities such as "good" and "bad."

The IAT initially drew attention because it seemed a useful tool for examining such phenomena as prejudice, which many people prefer not to acknowledge explicitly, even to themselves. More recently it has been applied to a variety of other associations. These include moral judgments (Haidt, 2001), reactions to cues of stigma (Pryor, Reeder, Yeadon, & Hesson-McInnis,

2004), and links from the self to a sense of positivity versus negativity, termed *implicit self-esteem* (Greenwald et al., 2002).

The literature of studies using the IAT (and other related procedures) is growing quite rapidly (for reviews, see Fazio & Olson, 2003; Greenwald et al., 2002). That literature has also spawned several controversies, one of which stems from the fact that there often is little or no relation between explicit (self-report) measures of a construct and implicit measures of the same construct. Although it is fairly easy to see why that might be the case for prejudice (given the social desirability issues involved), it is less obvious why it would be so for such constructs as the self-concept.

Two-mode models suggest a possibility (see also Beevers, 2005; Fazio & Olson, 2003). The implicit measure is, by definition, associative. It measures only the associative link between pairs of elements. In contrast, the explicit measure is symbolic, a product of deliberative processing. Implicit knowledge presumably accrues through association learning; explicit knowledge presumably accrues through verbal, conceptual learning. Perhaps the associative and deliberative sources of knowledge about the self (or anything else) are more independent of one another than is often assumed. Thus, the two sources of experience may not agree well with each other over time, leading to different results from implicit and explicit measures. This view of the information coming by these two kinds of measures is speculative, but it would fit nicely with two-mode models of functioning.

Consistent with this line of thought, a number of studies have found that both implicit and explicit measures predict aspects of behavior but different aspects. For example, one project assessed implicit and explicit attitudes of Whites toward Blacks and examined the relations of those attitudes to behaviors that were relatively controlled or relatively spontaneous (Dovidio, Kawakami, Johnson, Johnson, & Howard, 1997). Explicit measures predicted deliberative jury decisions and evaluations of interaction partners, whereas implicit measures predicted nonverbal behaviors and primed word completions. Another, more recent project (Neumann, Hülsenbeck, & Seibt, 2004) assessed implicit and explicit attitudes toward persons with AIDS along with measures of a relatively automatic behavior and a verbal report of intentions to act. This study found that implicit attitudes predicted the automatic response but not the reported intentions and that explicit attitudes predicted the reported intentions but not the automatic response.

Although studies stimulated by the IAT have brought increasing attention to the distinction between implicit and explicit processes, this distinction is not new. It has played a key role in at least one familiar literature for a long time. Researchers in the classic motive tradition have long distinguished between implicit and self-attributed motives (McClelland, Koestner, & Weinberger, 1989) in a way that is not too dissimilar to the distinction made in the preceding sections (see Brunstein & Maier, 2005; Schultheiss, 2002). As in the newer applications, both the implicit and the explicit predict aspects of behavior, but the aspects differ.

Developmental Two-Mode Models

Another literature in which two-mode thinking has been influential is a literature in developmental psychology. Rothbart and her colleagues (e.g., Derryberry & Rothbart, 1997; Rothbart, Ahadi, & Evans, 2000; Rothbart, Ellis, Rueda, & Posner, 2003; Rothbart & Posner, 1985; see also Kochanska & Knaack, 2003; Nigg, 2000) have argued for the existence of three temperament systems: two for approach and avoidance and a third termed *effortful control.* The latter concerns attentional management and inhibitory control (the ability to suppress an approach behavior when approach is situationally inappropriate). This model assumes that effortful control is superordinate to approach and avoidance temperaments (e.g., Ahadi & Rothbart, 1994). The label *effortful* conveys the sense that this is an executive, planful activity, entailing the use of cognitive resources beyond what would be needed to react impulsively.

Rothbart (e.g., Rothbart & Bates, 1998), Eisenberg (e.g., Eisenberg et al., 2004), and Kochanska (e.g., Kochanska & Knaack, 2003) see effortful control as being grounded in cortical functions, and there is a variety of evidence from neuroimaging studies of both adults and children to support that argument (e.g., Durston, Thomas, Yang, Ulug, Zimmerman, & Casey, 2002; Durston, Thomas, Worden, Yang, & Casey, 2002). This view of effortful control has a substantial resemblance to depictions of the deliberative mode of the two-mode models outlined in previous sections.

Hierarchicality Reexamined

The preceding sections have outlined several rather distinct sources of theory that seem to fit the idea that the mind has two modes of functioning; indeed, the sources described here do not represent an exhaustive list (see Carver, 2005). These various sources appear to converge on some hypotheses that seem eminently worthy of further exploration.

All the sources promote the inference that a deliberative mode of functioning underlies action control that uses symbolic and sequential processing and thus is relatively slow. The sources also suggest that a more impulsive mode of functioning uses connectionist and associationist processing and is relatively fast. Many of the theories suggest that the two modes are semiautonomous in their functioning, competing with each other to influence actions. Indeed, many authors have suggested situational influences that influence which mode dominates at a given time (e.g., cognitive load impairs the ability to be deliberative). Some of the theoretical sources go even farther, implicating different brain regions in the two modes of functioning. Specifically, it is often suggested that the deliberative mode depends critically on specific prefrontal cortical areas and that the impulsive mode relies on other areas.

Finally, we return to our earlier discussion of self-regulation. We cautiously suggest the possibility of a correspondence between these two modes of functioning and the distinction that was made earlier in the chapter concerning levels of abstraction in action control: specifically, the split between program control and sequence control. There are several parallels between the two sets of ideas. As noted earlier, there is evidence that different parts of the brain manage effortful and automatic versions of the same behavior (Casey et al., 2002; Lieberman et al., 2002; Posner & DiGirolamo, 2000). This in itself hints that there may be an important boundary between action control that is deliberative and action sequences that are well learned enough to be spontaneous once cued. Other evidence also supports the idea that intention-based and stimulus-based actions involve different process of action initiation (Keller et al., 2006).

There are also similarities in the qualities that are ascribed to the different groups of behaviors in the two sets of ideas. We said earlier that *programs* of action entail decisions. They seem to be managed top down, using processing that is effortful. Planfulness, an element of programs, is also a typical characterization of behavior that is being managed by a prefrontal cortical system.

In contrast to this deliberative quality, well-learned *sequences* occur in a relatively automatic stream once they are triggered. Sequences may respond to cues that trigger them simply by virtue of associations in memory. Their characteristics seem more akin to those of the more basic mode of functioning.

On the other hand, there is also some evidence that does not easily fit a division based on level of abstraction. Specifically, relatively abstract goals (e.g., cooperation or performing well) that are operating out of awareness (and thus are relying on automatic functions) display several of the same operational characteristics as do consciously monitored (and thus deliberative) goals (Bargh, Gollwitzer, Lee-Chai, Barndollar, & Trötschel, 2001). Perhaps the issue here is simply how well learned the goal pursuit is rather than how abstract or concrete is the goal being pursued.

In previous discussions (e.g., Carver & Scheier, 1998, 1999b), we have often noted that the level of control that is functionally superordinate can vary with the situation (and also across persons). That is, it is possible to imagine cases in which a person is presently behaving according to a principle (e.g., a moral or ethical value), and it is possible to imagine cases in which the person is behaving according to a plan or program. It is also possible, however, to imagine cases in which the person is behaving impulsively and spontaneously without regard to either principle or plan. It is of some interest that in making this case in the past, our emphasis was typically on how sequences and programs differed from each other.

One circumstance that yields such impulsive action is ingestion of alcohol. Alcohol is known to induce a loss of self-awareness—to cause behavior to become more impulsive and responsive to cues of the moment (e.g., Hull, 1981; Hull & Slone, 2004; Steele & Josephs, 1990) and less carefully thought out (cf. Marczinsky & Fillmore, 2005). This pattern is easily interpreted as indicating that alcohol causes an effortful, planful, deliberative system to function less efficiently and to be less in control, leaving in charge an impulsive system that has only very short-term goals (Stuss, Picton, & Alexander, 2001).

Self-Control: Impulse and Restraint

The idea that there are longer- and shorter-term goals that can come into conflict with each other, is also part of a literature on self-control and self-control failure (Baumeister & Heatherton, 1996; Baumeister, Heatherton, & Tice, 1994). This literature focuses on cases in which a person is both motivated to act and motivated to restrain that action (which, interestingly enough, is essentially the case that is the focus of work on children's effortful control). In some ways, the logical structure of the cases addressed in this literature also resembles the logical structure of the delay of gratification paradigm. A difference is that in the cases now under consideration the intent often is to delay indefinitely rather than temporarily.

The literature on self-control failure tends to portray these cases as involving a relatively automatic tendency to act in one way, which is opposed by a planful and effortful tendency to restrain that act. The action that is being inhibited is often characterized as an impulse, a desire that would automatically be translated into action unless it is controlled (perhaps in part because this action is habitual, perhaps in part because it is more primal). The restraint is presumed to be effortful and to depend on limited resources. If the planful part of the mind is fully enough able to attend to the conflict, the person may be able to resist the impulse. If not, the impulse is more likely to be expressed. This portrayal seems consonant with the two-mode models of functioning (see also Carver, 2005).

Brain Function

Recent years have seen the emergence of a body of work that many people refer to with such labels as *social neuroscience* and *affective neuroscience*. This work involves the blending of ideas from personality and social psychology with ideas and methods of brain science. Of particular interest are neuroimaging techniques that permit identification of brain regions that are particularly active or inactive during specific kinds of mental activity.

It seems likely that the sorts of questions and issues that were raised in this section of the chapter will only increase the appeal of such research. Many of the theoretical models we have been discussing in the latter part of the chapter clearly argue for differential involvement in behavior of different brain areas that reflects each mode of functioning. As more and more behavioral paradigms are brought into labs to determine patterns of brain activity, more will be revealed about what properties of the central nervous system support what kinds of self-regulation.

There is also another biological literature that may similarly become important in the study of action control. This literature examines neurotransmitter functions and their relation to aspects of behavior that are relevant to the issues under discussion here. In particular, a good deal of evidence now implicates serotonin function in the behavioral dimension of impulse versus constraint (for a review, see Carver & Miller, 2006). A substantial number of studies relate low serotonin function to impulsive aggression and impulsiveness more generally. There is also evidence linking both impulsivity and aggressiveness to poorer executive (frontal lobe)

function (e.g., Dolan, Deakin, Roberts, & Anderson, 2002). The hypothesis that the impulsiveness that is associated with low serotonin function reflects poor frontal control awaits further scrutiny.

A concern that many have had about the emerging blending of brain science with other aspects of psychology is that psychological ideas may be lost in the shuffle. We believe that the issues discussed in this part of the chapter make a case that the brain science will gain as much from the psychological science as the other way around. We trust that continued conceptual developments in psychological science will continue to make that case even more forcefully.

Questions

What we have presented here is only a sketch of possibilities. Many issues remain that obviously need a good deal more thought and investigation. Here is just one set of questions that is particularly salient to us after having written that sketch. If people do, at least some of the time, form conscious intentions and take steps to meet them, there must be a way for the intentions to be realized in behavior, right down to the muscle movements that produce the necessary actions in their physical form. And yet, bottom-up self-organizations of muscle movements also appear to occur. Are the functions that control the lower-order aspects of the intention-driven behaviors (sequences on down) the same functions as would control the actions if they were newly self-organizing instead of being driven by an intention? Put differently, is the automaticity that follows from overlearning the same as the automaticity that comes from letting an action self-organize? If sequence control and even lower aspects of action control are products of a system that is connectionist and associationist, how does that lower system interact with an executive that is instructing it? As far as the lower mechanisms are concerned, is the top-down call to do those action sequences just another cue of the moment? Or does recruitment of the lower mechanisms for the execution of the higher-order action differ in some way from its spontaneous triggering by some true cue of the moment?

Acknowledgments

The first author has been supported by grants CA64710, CA78995, and CA84944 to the University of Miami; the second author has been supported by grants HL65111, HL65112, HL076852, and HL076858 to the Pittsburgh Mind-Body Center at the University of Pittsburgh and Carnegie Mellon University. Send correspondence to Charles S. Carver, Department of Psychology, University of Miami, Coral Gables, Florida 33124-0751. E-mail: Ccarver@ miami.edu.

References

Ahadi, S. A., & Rothbart, M. K. (1994). Temperament, development and the big five. In C. F. Halverson Jr., G. A. Kohnstamm, & R. P. Martin (Eds.), *The developing structure of temperament and personality from infancy to adulthood* (pp. 189–207). Hillsdale, NJ: Lawrence Erlbaum Associates.

Aspinwall, L. G. (1998). Rethinking the role of positive affect in self-regulation. *Motivation and Emotion, 22,* 1–32.

Atkinson, J. W., & Birch, D. (1970). *The dynamics of action.* New York: Wiley.

Bargh, J. A., Gollwitzer, P. M., Lee-Chai, A., Barndollar, K., & Trötschel, R. (2001). The automated will: Nonconscious activation and pursuit of behavioral goals. *Journal of Personality and Social Psychology, 81,* 1014–1027.

Barrett, L. F., Tugade, M. M., & Engle, R. W. (2004). Individual differences in working memory capacity and dual-process theories of the mind. *Psychological Bulletin, 130,* 553–573.

Baumeister, R. F., Heatherton, T. F., & Tice, D. M. (1994). *Losing control: Why people fail at self-regulation.* San Diego: Academic Press.

Baumeister, R. F., & Heatherton, T. F. (1996). Self-regulation failure: An overview. *Psychological Inquiry, 7,* 1–15.

Baumeister, R. F., & Vohs, K. D. (Eds.). (2004). *Handbook of self-regulation: Research, theory, and applications.* New York: Guilford Press.

Bechtel, W., & Abrahamsen, A. (1991). *Connectionism and the mind: An introduction to parallel processing in networks.* Cambridge, UK: Basil Blackwell.

Beer, R. D. (1995). A dynamical systems perspective on agent-environment interaction. *Artificial Intelligence, 72,* 173–215.

Beevers, C. G. (2005). Cognitive vulnerability to depression: A dual-process model. *Clinical Psychology Review, 25,* 975–1002.

Berridge, K. C. (2004). Motivation concepts in behavioral neuroscience. *Physiology and Behavior. 81,* 179–209.

Bowlby, J. (1988). *A secure base: Parent–child attachment and healthy human development.* New York: Basic Books.

Brendl, C. M., & Higgins, E. T. (1996). Principles of judging valence: What makes events positive or negative? In M. Zanna (Ed.), *Advances in experimental social psychology* (Vol. 28, pp 95–160). San Diego, CA: Academic Press.

Brooks, R. A. (1999). *Cambrian intelligence: The early history of the new AI.* Cambridge, MA: MIT Press.

Brunstein, J. C., & Maier, G. W. (2005). Implicit and self-attributed motives to achieve: Two separate but interacting needs. *Journal of Personality and Social Psychology, 89,* 205–222.

Cacioppo, J. T., & Berntson, G. G. (1994). Relationship between attitudes and evaluative space: A critical review, with emphasis on the separability of positive and negative substrates. *Psychological Bulletin, 115,* 401–423.

Cacioppo, J. T., Gardner, W. L., & Berntson, G. G. (1999). The affect system has parallel and integrative processing components: Form follows function. *Journal of Personality and Social Psychology, 76,* 839–855.

Campos, J. J., Frankel, C. B., & Camras, L. (2004). On the nature of emotion regulation. *Child Development, 75,* 377–394.

Carver, C. S. (2001). Affect and the functional bases of behavior: On the dimensional structure of affective experience. *Personality and Social Psychology Review, 5,* 345–356.

Carver, C. S. (2003). Pleasure as a sign you can attend to something else: Placing positive feelings within a general model of affect. *Cognition and Emotion, 17,* 241–261.

Carver, C. S. (2004). Negative affects deriving from the behavioral approach system. *Emotion, 4,* 3–22.

Carver, C. S. (2005). Impulse and constraint: Perspectives from personality psychology, convergence with theory in other areas, and potential for integration. *Personality and Social Psychology Review, 9,* 312–333.

Carver, C. S., Lawrence, J. W., & Scheier, M. F. (1999). Self-discrepancies and affect: Incorporating the role of feared selves. *Personality and Social Psychology Bulletin, 25,* 783–792.

Carver, C. S., & Miller, C. J. (2006). Relations of serotonin function to personality: Current views and a key methodological issue. *Psychiatry Research, 144,* 1–15.

Carver, C. S., & Scheier, M. F. (1981). *Attention and self-regulation: A control-theory approach to human behavior.* New York: Springer-Verlag.

Carver, C. S., & Scheier, M. F. (1990). Origins and functions of positive and negative affect: A control-process view. *Psychological Review, 97,* 19–35.

Carver, C. S., & Scheier, M. F. (1998). *On the self-regulation of behavior.* New York: Cambridge University Press.

Carver, C. S., & Scheier, M. F. (1999a). Several more themes, a lot more issues: Commentary on the commentaries. In R. S. Wyer Jr. (Ed.), *Advances in social cognition* (Vol. 12, pp. 261–302). Mahwah, NJ: Lawrence Erlbaum Associates.

Carver, C. S., & Scheier, M. F. (1999b). Themes and issues in the self-regulation of behavior. In R. S. Wyer Jr. (Ed.), *Advances in social cognition* (Vol. 12, pp. 1–105). Mahwah, NJ: Lawrence Erlbaum Associates.

Carver, C. S., & Scheier, M. F. (2000). Scaling back goals and recalibration of the affect system are processes in normal adaptive self-regulation: Understanding "response shift" phenomena. *Social Science and Medicine, 50,* 1715–1722.

Carver, C. S., & Scheier, M. F. (2002). Control processes and self-organization as complementary principles underlying behavior. *Personality and Social Psychology Review, 6,* 304–315.

Carver, C. S., & Scheier, M. F. (2003). Three human strengths. In L. G. Aspinwall & U. M. Staudinger (Eds.), *A psychology of human strengths: Fundamental questions and future directions for a positive psychology* (pp. 87–102). Washington, DC: American Psychological Association.

Carver, C. S., & White, T. L. (1994). Behavioral inhibition, behavioral activation, and affective responses to impending reward and punishment: The BIS/BAS scales. *Journal of Personality and Social Psychology, 67,* 319–333.

Casey, B. J., Tottenham, N., & Fossella, J. (2002). Clinical, imaging, lesion and genetic approaches toward a model of cognitive control. *Developmental Psychobiology, 40,* 237–254.

Chaiken, S. L., & Trope, Y. (Eds.). (1999). *Dual-process theories in social psychology.* New York: Guilford.

Clark, R. N. (1996). *Control system dynamics.* New York: Cambridge University Press.

Clore, G. C. (1994). Why emotions are felt. In P. Ekman & R. J. Davidson (Eds.), *The nature of emotion: Fundamental questions* (pp. 103–111). New York: Oxford University Press.

Davidson, R. J. (1992). Anterior cerebral asymmetry and the nature of emotion. *Brain and Cognition, 20,* 125–151.

De Neys, W. (2006). Dual processing in reasoning: Two systems but one reasoner. *Psychological Science, 17,* 428–433.

Derryberry, D., & Rothbart, M. K. (1997). Reactive and effortful processes in the organization of temperament. *Development and Psychopathology, 9,* 633–652.

Diener, E., Lucas, R. E., & Scollon, C. N. (2006). Beyond the hedonic treadmill: Revising the adaptation theory of well-being. *American Psychologist, 61,* 305–314.

Dolan, M. C., Deakin, J. F. W., Roberts, N., & Anderson, I. (2002). Serotonergic and cognitive impairment in impulsive aggressive personality disordered offenders: Are there implications for treatment? *Psychological Medicine, 32,* 105–117.

Dovidio, J. F., Kawakami, K., Johnson, C., Johnson, B., & Howard, A. (1997). On the nature of prejudice: Automatic and controlled processes. *Journal of Experimental Social Psychology, 33,* 510–540.

Dreisbach, G., & Goschke, T. (2004). How positive affect modulates cognitive control: Reduced perseveration at the cost of increased distractibility. *Journal of Experimental Psychology: Learning, Memory, and Cognition, 30,* 343–353.

Durston, S., Thomas, K. M., Worden, M. S., Yang, Y., & Casey, B. J. (2002). The effect of preceding context on inhibition: An event-related fMRI study. *NeuroImage, 16,* 449–453.

Durston, S., Thomas, K. M., Yang, Y., Ulug, A. M., Zimmerman, R. D., & Casey, B. J. (2002). A neural basis for the development of inhibitory control. *Developmental Science, 5,* F9–F16.

Eisenberg, N., Spinard, T. L., Fabes, R. A., Reiser, M., Cumberland, A., Shephard, S. A., Valiente, C., Losoya, S. H., Guthrie, I. K., & Thompson, M. (2004). The relations of effortful control and impulsivity to children's resiliency and adjustment. *Child Development, 75,* 25–46.

Epstein, S. (1973). The self-concept revisited: Or a theory of a theory. *American Psychologist, 28,* 404–416.

Epstein, S. (1985). The implications of cognitive–experiential self theory for research in social psychology and personality. *Journal for the Theory of Social Behavior, 15,* 283–310.

Epstein, S. (1990). Cognitive–experiential self-theory. In L. Pervin (Ed.), *Handbook of personality: Theory and research* (pp. 165–192). New York: Guilford.

Epstein, S. (1994). Integration of the cognitive and the psychodynamic unconscious. *American Psychologist, 49,* 709–724.

Fazio, R. H., & Olson, M. A. (2003). Implicit measures in social cognition research: Their meaning and use. *Annual Review of Psychology, 54,* 297–327.

Finlay-Jones, R., & Brown, G. W. (1981). Types of stressful life event and the onset of anxiety and depressive disorders. *Psychological Medicine, 11,* 803–815.

Ford, D. H. (1987). *Humans as self-constructing living systems: A developmental perspective on behavior and personality.* Hillsdale, NJ: Lawrence Erlbaum Associates.

Fredrickson, B. L. (1998). What good are positive emotions? *Review of General Psychology, 2,* 300–319.

Fredrickson, B. L. (2001). The role of positive emotions in positive psychology: The broaden-and-build theory of positive emotions. *American Psychologist, 56,* 218–226.

Frijda, N. H. (1986). *The emotions.* Cambridge: Cambridge University Press.

Frijda, N. H. (1988). The laws of emotion. *American Psychologist, 43,* 349–358.

Frijda, N. H. (1994). Emotions are functional, most of the time. In P. Ekman & R. J. Davidson (Eds.), *The nature of emotion: Fundamental questions* (pp. 112–126). New York: Oxford University Press.

Gallo, L. C., & Matthews, K. A. (2003). Understanding the association between socioeconomic status and physical health: Do negative emotions play a role? *Psychological Bulletin, 129,* 10–51.

Gray, J. A. (1990). Brain systems that mediate both emotion and cognition. *Cognition and Emotion, 4,* 269–288.

Gray, J. A. (1994a). Personality dimensions and emotion systems. In P. Ekman & R. J. Davidson (Eds.), *The nature of emotion: Fundamental questions* (pp. 329–331). New York: Oxford University Press.

Gray, J. A. (1994b). Three fundamental emotion systems. In P. Ekman & R. J. Davidson (Eds.), *The nature of emotion: Fundamental questions* (pp. 243–247). New York: Oxford University Press.

Gray, J. R. (1999). A bias toward short-term thinking in threat-related negative emotional states. *Personality and Social Psychology Bulletin, 25,* 65–75.

Greenwald, A. G., Banaji, M. R., Rudman, L. A., Farnham, S. D., Nosek, B. A., & Mellott, D. S. (2002). A unified theory of implicit attitudes, stereotypes, self-esteem, and self-concept. *Psychological Review, 109,* 3–25.

Greenwald, A. G., McGhee, D. E., & Schwartz, J. L. K. (1998). Measuring individual differences in implicit cognition: The implicit association test. *Journal of Personality and Social Psychology, 74,* 1464–1480.

Haidt, J. (2001). The emotional dog and its rational tail: A social intuitionist approach to moral judgment. *Psychological Review, 108,* 814–834.

Harmon-Jones, E., & Allen, J. J. B. (1998). Anger and frontal brain activity: Asymmetry consistent with approach motivation despite negative affective valence. *Journal of Personality and Social Psychology, 74,* 1310–1316.

Harmon-Jones, E., Lueck, L., Fearn, M., & Harmon-Jones, C. (2006). The effect of personal relevance and approach-related action expectation on relative left frontal cortical activity. *Psychological Science, 17,* 434–440.

Harmon-Jones, E., & Sigelman, J. D. (2001). State anger and prefrontal brain activity: Evidence that insult-related relative left-prefrontal activation is associated with experienced anger and aggression. *Journal of Personality and Social Psychology, 80,* 797–803.

Hayes-Roth, B., & Hayes-Roth, F. (1979). A cognitive model of planning. *Cognitive Science, 3,* 275–310.

Higgins, E. T. (1987). Self-discrepancy: A theory relating self and affect. *Psychological Review, 94,* 319–340.

Higgins, E. T. (1996). Ideals, oughts, and regulatory focus: Affect and motivation from distinct pains and pleasures. In P. M. Gollwitzer & J. A. Bargh (Eds.), *The psychology of action: Linking cognition and motivation to behavior* (pp. 91–114). New York: Guilford Press.

Higgins, E. T., Shah, J., & Friedman, R. (1997). Emotional responses to goal attainment: Strength of regulatory focus as moderator. *Journal of Personality and Social Psychology, 72,* 515–525.

Hobfoll, S. E. (1989). Conservation of resources: A new attempt at conceptualizing stress. *American Psychologist, 44,* 513–524.

Hobfoll, S. E. (2002). Social and psychological resources and adaptation. *Review of General Psychology, 6,* 307–324.

Hogarth, R. M. (2001). *Educating intuition.* Chicago: University of Chicago Press.

Hogarth, R. M. (2005). Deciding analytically or trusting your intuition? The advantages and disadvantages of analytic and intuitive thought. In T. Betsch & S. Haberstroh (Eds.), *The routines of decision making* (pp. 67–82). Mahwah, NJ: Lawrence Erlbaum Associates.

Hull, J. G. (1981). A self-awareness model of the causes and effects of alcohol consumption. *Journal of Abnormal Psychology, 90,* 586–600.

Hull, J. G., & Slone, L. B. (2004). Alcohol and self-regulation. In R. F. Baumeister & K. D. Vohs (Eds.), *Handbook of self-regulation: Research, theory, and applications* (pp. 466–491). New York: Guilford Press.

Isen, A. M. (1987). Positive affect, cognitive processes, and social behavior. In L. Berkowitz (Ed.), *Advances in experimental social psychology* (Vol. 20, pp. 203–252). San Diego, CA: Academic Press.

Isen, A. M. (2000). Positive affect and decision making. In M. Lewis & J. M. Haviland-Jones (Eds.), *Handbook of emotions* (2nd ed., pp. 417–435). New York: Guilford Press.

Izard, C. E. (1977). *Human emotions.* New York: Plenum Press.

Izard, C. E., & Ackerman, B. P. (2000). Motivational, organizational, and regulatory functions of discrete emotions. In M. Lewis & J. M. Haviland-Jones (Eds.), *Handbook of emotions* (2nd ed., pp. 253–264). New York: Guilford Press.

Kahn, B. E., & Isen, A.M. (1993). The influence of positive affect on variety-seeking among safe, enjoyable products. *Journal of Consumer Research, 20,* 257–270.

Keller, P. E., Wascher, E., Prinz, W., Waszak, F., Koch, I., & Rosenbaum, D. A. (2006). Differ-

ences between intention-based and stimulus-based actions. *Journal of Psychophysiology, 20,* 9–20.

Kelso, J. A. S. (1995). *Dynamic patterns: The self-organization of brain and behavior.* Cambridge, MA: MIT Press.

Klinger, E. (1975). Consequences of commitment to and disengagement from incentives. *Psychological Review, 82,* 1–25.

Kochanska, G., & Knaack, A. (2003). Effortful control as a personality characteristic of young children: Antecedents, correlates, and consequences. *Journal of Personality, 71,* 1087–1112.

Korte, S. M., Koolhaas, J. M., Wingfield, J. C., & McEwen, B. S. (2005). The Darwinian concept of stress: Benefits of allostasis and costs of allostatic load and the trade-offs in health and disease. *Neuroscience and Biobehavioral Reviews, 29,* 3–38.

Lang, P. J. (1995). The emotion probe: Studies of motivation and attention. *American Psychologist, 50,* 372–385.

Lang, P. J., Bradley, M. M., & Cuthbert, B. N. (1990). Emotion, attention, and the startle reflex. *Psychological Review, 97,* 377–395.

Laurenceau, J-P., Troy, A. B., & Carver, C. S. (2005). Two distinct emotional experiences in romantic relationships: Effects of perceptions regarding approach of intimacy and avoidance of conflict. *Personality and Social Psychology Bulletin, 31,* 1123–1133.

Levenson, R. W. (1994). Human emotion: A functional view. In P. Ekman & R. Davidson (Eds.), *The nature of emotions: Fundamental questions* (pp. 123–126). New York: Oxford University Press.

Levenson, R. W. (1999). The intrapersonal functions of emotion. *Cognition and Emotion, 13,* 481–504.

Lewis, M., Sullivan, M. W., Ramsay, D. S., & Allessandri, S. M. (1992). Individual differences in anger and sad expressions during extinction: Antecedents and consequences. *Infant Behavior and Development, 15,* 443–452.

Lieberman, M. D. (2000). Intuition: A social cognitive neuroscience approach. *Psychological Bulletin, 126,* 109–137.

Lieberman, M. D., Gaunt, R., Gilbert, D. T., & Trope, Y. (2002). Reflection and reflexion: A social cognitive neuroscience approach to attributional inference. In M. Zanna (Ed.), *Advances in experimental social psychology* (pp. 199–249). San Diego, CA: Academic Press.

Locke, E. A., & Latham, G. P. (1990). *A theory of goal setting and task performance.* Englewood Cliffs, NJ: Prentice Hall.

Louro, M. J., Pieters, R., & Zeelenberg, M. (2007). Dynamics of multiple-goal pursuit. *Journal of Personality and Social Psychology, 93,* 174–193.

MacKay, D. M. (1966). Cerebral organization and the conscious control of action. In J. C. Eccles (Ed.), *Brain and conscious experience* (pp. 422–445). Berlin: Springer-Verlag.

Marczinski, C. A., & Fillmore, M. T. (2005). Alcohol increases reliance on cues that signal acts of control. *Experimental and Clinical Psychopharmacology, 13,* 15–24.

Markus, H., & Nurius, P. (1986). Possible selves. *American Psychologist, 41,* 954–969.

McClelland, D. C., Koestner, R., & Weinberger, J. (1989). How do self-attributed and implicit motives differ? *Psychological Review, 96,* 690–702.

McClelland, J. L. (1999). Cognitive modeling, connectionist. In R. W. Wilson & F. C. Keil (Eds.), *The MIT encyclopedia of the cognitive sciences* (pp.137–139). Cambridge, MA: MIT Press.

McEwen, B. S. (2004). Protection and damage from acute and chronic stress: Allostasis and allostatic overload and relevance to the pathophysiology of psychiatric disorders. *Annals of the New York Academy of Sciences, 1032,* 1–7.

Messinger, D. S. (2002). Positive and negative: Infant facial expressions and emotions. *Current Directions in Psychological Science, 11,* 1–6.

Metcalfe, J., & Mischel, W. (1999). A hot/cool-system analysis of delay of gratification: Dynamics of willpower. *Psychological Review, 106,* 3–19.

Mikulincer, M. (1988). Reactance and helplessness following exposure to learned helplessness following exposure to unsolvable problems: The effects of attributional style. *Journal of Personality and Social Psychology, 54,* 679–686.

Mikulincer, M. (1994). *Human learned helplessness: A coping perspective.* New York: Plenum Press.

Miller, G. A., Galanter, E., & Pribram, K. H. (1960). *Plans and the structure of behavior.* New York: Holt, Rinehart and Winston.

Miller, N. E., & Dollard, J. (1941). *Social learning and imitation.* New Haven, CT: Yale University Press.

Mischel, W. (1974). Processes in delay of gratification. In L. Berkowitz (Ed.), *Advances in experimental social psychology* (Vol. 7, pp. 249–292). New York: Academic Press.

Mischel, W., & Baker, N. (1975). Cognitive transformations of reward objects through instructions. *Journal of Personality and Social Psychology, 31,* 254–261.

Mizruchi, M. S. (1991). Urgency, motivation, and group performance: The effect of prior success on current success among professional basketball teams. *Social Psychology Quarterly, 54,* 181–189.

Muraven, M., & Baumeister, R. F. (2000). Self-regulation and depletion of limited resources: Does self-control resemble a muscle? *Psychological Bulletin, 126,* 247–259.

Murray, H. A. (1938). *Explorations in personality.* New York: Oxford University Press.

Nesse, R. M. (2000). Is depression an adaptation? *Archives of General Psychiatry, 57,* 14–20.

Neumann, R., Hülsenbeck, K., & Seibt, B. (2004). Attitudes towards people with AIDS and avoidance behavior: Automatic and reflective bases of behavior. *Journal of Experimental Social Psychology, 40,* 543–550.

Newtson, D. (1993). The dynamics of action and interaction. In L. D. Smith & E. Thelen (Eds.), *A dynamic systems approach to development: Applications* (pp. 241–264). Cambridge, MA: MIT Press.

Newtson, D. (1994). The perception and coupling of behavioral waves. In R. R. Vallacher & A. Nowak (Eds.), *Dynamical systems in social psychology* (pp. 139–167). San Diego, CA: Academic Press.

Nigg, J. T. (2000). On inhibition/disinhibition in developmental pychopathology: Views from cognitive and personality psychology as a working inhibition taxonomy. *Psychological Bulletin, 126,* 220–246.

Norman, D. A. (1981). Categorization of action slips. *Psychological Review, 88,* 1–15.

Ogilvie, D. M. (1987). The undesired self: A neglected variable in personality research. *Journal of Personality and Social Psychology, 52,* 379–385.

Ortony, A., Clore, G. L., & Collins, A. (1988). *The cognitive structure of emotions.* New York: Cambridge University Press.

Payton, D. W. (1990). Internalized plans: A representation for action resources. In P. Maes (Ed.), *Designing autonomous agents: Theory and practice from biology to engineering and back* (pp. 89–103). Cambridge, MA: MIT Press.

Pittman, T. S., & Pittman, N. L. (1980). Deprivation of control and the attribution process. *Journal of Personality and Social Psychology, 39,* 377–389.

Pomerantz, E. M., Saxon, J. L., & Oishi, S. (2000). The psychological trade-offs of goal investment. *Journal of Personality and Social Psychology, 79,* 617–630.

Posner, M. I., & DiGirolamo, G. J. (2000). Cognitive neuroscience: Origins and promise. *Psychological Bulletin, 126,* 873–889.

Powers, W. T. (1973). *Behavior: The control of perception.* Chicago: Aldine.

Prigogene, I., & Stengers, I. (1984). *Order out of chaos.* New York: Bantam.

Pryor, J. B., Reeder, G. D., Yeadon, C., & Hesson-McInnis, M. (2004). A dual-process model of reactions to perceived stigma. *Journal of Personality and Social Psychology, 87,* 436–452.

Reed, M. B., & Aspinwall, L. G. (1998). Self-affirmation reduces biased processing of health-risk information. *Motivation and Emotion, 22,* 99–132.

Reyna, C., Henry, P. J., Korfmacher, W., & Tucker, A. (2006). Examining the principles in principled conservatism: The role of responsibility stereotypes as cues for deservingness in racial policy decisions. *Journal of Personality and Social Psychology, 90,* 109–128.

Rosenbaum, D. A., Meulenbroek, R. G. J., Vaughan, J., & Jansen, C. (2001). Posture-based motion planning: Applications to grasping. *Psychological Review, 108,* 709–734.

Rothbart, M. K., Ahadi, S. A., & Evans, D. E. (2000). Temperament and personality: Origins and outcomes. *Journal of Personality and Social Psychology, 78,* 122–135.

Rothbart, M. K., & Bates, J. E. (1998). Temperament. In W. Damon (Series Ed.) & N. Eisenberg (Vol. Ed.), *Handbook of child psychology: Vol 3. Social, emotional and personality development* (5th ed., pp. 105–176). New York: Wiley.

Rothbart, M. K., Ellis, L. K., Rueda M. R., & Posner, M. I. (2003). Developing mechanisms of temperamental effortful control. *Journal of Personality, 71,* 1113–1143.

Rothbart, M. K., & Posner, M. (1985). Temperament and the development of self-regulation. In L. C. Hartlage & C. F. Telzrow (Eds.), *The neuropsychology of individual differences: A developmental perspective* (pp. 93–123). New York: Plenum.

Schulkin, J. (Ed.). (2004). *Allostasis, homeostasis, and the costs of physiological adaptation.* New York: Cambridge University Press.

Schultheiss, O. C. (2002). An information-processing account of implicit motive arousal. In P. R. Pintrich & M. L. Maehr (Eds.), *Advances in motivation and achievement: New directions in measures and methods* (Vol. 12, pp. 1–41). Amsterdam: Elsevier.

Schwartz, S. H., & Bilsky, W. (1990). Toward a theory of the universal content and structure of values: Extensions and cross-cultural replications. *Journal of Personality and Social Psychology, 58,* 878–891.

Schwartz, S. H., & Rubel, T. (2005). Sex differences in value priorities: Cross-cultural and multi-method studies. *Journal of Personality and Social Psychology, 89,* 1010–1028.

Schwarz, N., & Bohner, G. (1996). Feelings and their motivational implications: Moods and the action sequence. In P. M. Gollwitzer & J. A. Bargh (Eds.), *The psychology of action: Linking cognition and motivation to behavior* (pp. 119–145). New York: Guilford Press.

Schwarz, N., & Clore, G. L. (1983). Mood, misattribution, and judgments of well-being: Informative and directive functions of affective states. *Journal of Personality and Social Psychology, 45,* 513–523.

Shah, J. Y., Friedman, R., & Kruglanski, A. W. (2002). Forgetting all else: On the antecedents and consequences of goal shielding. *Journal of Personality and Social Psychology, 83,* 1261–1280.

Shallice, T. (1978). The dominant action system: An information-processing approach to consciousness. In K. S. Pope & J. L. Singer (Eds.), *The stream of consciousness: Scientific investigations into the flow of human experience* (pp. 117–157). New York: Wiley.

Shastri, L., & Ajjanagadde, V. (1993). From simple associations to systematic reasoning: A connectionist representation of rules, variables, and dynamic bindings using temporal synchrony. *Behavioral and Brain Sciences, 16,* 417–494.

Shin, J. C., & Rosenbaum, D. A. (2002). Reaching while calculating: Scheduling of cognitive and perceptual-motor processes. *Journal of Experimental Psychology: General, 131,* 206–219.

Simon, H. A. (1953). *Models of man.* New York: Wiley.

Simon, H. A. (1967). Motivational and emotional controls of cognition. *Psychology Review, 74,* 29–39.

Sloman, S. A. (1996). The empirical case for two forms of reasoning. *Psychological Bulletin, 119,* 3–22.

Smith, E. R., & DeCoster, J. (2000). Dual-process models in social and cognitive psychology: Conceptual integration and links to underlying memory systems. *Personality and Social Psychology Review, 4,* 108–131.

Smolensky, P. (1988). On the proper treatment of connectionism. *Behavioral and Brain Sciences, 11,* 1–23.

Steele, C. M., & Josephs, R. A. (1990). Alcohol myopia: Its prized and dangerous effects. *American Psychologist, 45,* 921–933.

Stifter, C. A., & Moyer, D. (1991). The regulation of positive affect: Gaze aversion activity during mother-infant interaction. *Infant Behavior and Development, 14,* 111–123.

Strack, F., & Deutsch, R. (2004). Reflective and impulsive determinants of social behavior. *Personality and Social Psychology Review, 8,* 220–247.

Stuss, D. T., Picton, T. W., & Alexander, M. P. (2001). Consciousness, self-awareness, and the frontal lobes. In S. P. Salloway, P. F. Malloy, & J. D. Duffy (Eds.), *The frontal lobes and neuropsychiatric illness* (pp. 101–109). Washington, DC: American Psychiatric Publishing.

Tesser, A. (1988). Toward a self-evaluation maintenance model of social behavior. In L. Berkowitz (Ed.), *Advances in experimental social psychology* (Vol. 21, pp. 181–227). New York: Academic Press.

Tesser, A., Crepaz, N., Collins, J. C., Cornell, D., & Beach, S. R. H. (2000). Confluence of self-esteem regulation mechanisms: On integrating the self-zoo. *Personality and Social Psychology Bulletin, 26,* 1476–1489.

Trope, Y., & Pomerantz, E. M. (1998). Resolving conflicts among self-evaluative motives: Positive experiences as a resource for overcoming defensiveness. *Motivation and Emotion, 22,* 53–72.

Turvey, M. T. (1990). Coordination. *American Psychologist, 45,* 938–953.

Vallacher, R. R., & Wegner, D. M. (1987). What do people think they're doing? Action identification and human behavior. *Psychological Review, 94,* 3–15.

von Bertalanffy, L. (1968). *General systems theory.* New York: Braziller.

Watson, D., Wiese, D., Vaidya, J., & Tellegen, A. (1999). The two general activation systems of affect: Structural findings, evolutionary considerations, and psychobiological evidence. *Journal of Personality and Social Psychology, 76,* 820–838.

Wegner, D. M. (1994). Ironic process of mental control. *Psychological Review, 101,* 34–52.

Wiener, N. (1948). *Cybernetics: Control and communication in the animal and the machine.* Cambridge, MA: MIT Press.

Wilson, T. D., Lindsey, S., & Schooler, T. Y. (2000). A model of dual attitudes. *Psychological Review, 107,* 101–126.

Wortman, C. B., & Brehm, J. W. (1975). Responses to uncontrollable outcomes: An integration of reactance theory and the learned helplessness model. In L. Berkowitz (Ed.), *Advances in experimental social psychology* (Vol. 8, pp. 277–336). New York: Academic Press.

Wrosch, C., Scheier, M. F., Carver, C. S., & Schulz, R. (2003). The importance of goal disengagement in adaptive self-regulation: When giving up is beneficial. *Self and Identity, 2,* 1–20

Wrosch, C., Scheier, M. F., Miller, G. E., Schulz, R., & Carver, C. S. (2003). Adaptive self-regulation of unattainable goals: Goal disengagement, goal re-engagement, and subjective well-being. *Personality and Social Psychology Bulletin, 29,* 1494–1508.

CHAPTER 16

From Goal Activation to Action: How Does Preference and Use of Knowledge Intervene?

Arthur B. Markman, C. Miguel Brendl, *and* Kyungil Kim

Abstract

This chapter examines the influence of goals on the evaluation of goal-related items, goal-conflicting items, and goal-unrelated items. It begins by examining two factors influencing preferences: the mental representation of goals and self-regulation. It then examines how goals affect the accessibility of items as a function of goal activation and motivational state. One finding is that there are motivational factors much broader than specific action goals that affect cognition and action. To explore the generality of this finding, the chapter considers other recent research suggesting that similar broad motivational factors may play a crucial role in the explanation of a number of known cultural differences in cognitive processing.

Keywords: goals, mental representation, self-regulation, motivation, action, cognitive processing

The folk psychology of action is fairly straightforward. An agent selects a goal it wants to accomplish. It seeks actions and objects that will allow the agent to bring about the goal. The items (e.g., objects, people, and activities) that the agent represents as instrumental for satisfying the goal are called *goal-related items.* These items should be valuable to the agent. Items that block goal satisfaction are called *goal-conflicting items.* These items should be avoided by the agent and hence have negative value (Lewin, 1926). On this view, a plan of action consists of seeking goal-related items and avoiding goal-conflicting items in order to move an agent closer to goal satisfaction (e.g., Fikes & Nilsson, 1971; Miller, Galanter, & Pribram, 1960). It is noteworthy that most items that an agent encounters are neither goal related nor goal conflicting. We call this third group of items *goal-unrelated items.* From a lay perspective, an agent should neither seek nor avoid such items, and hence these items should have neither positive nor negative value.

This view implies that goals influence the value of goal-related and goal-conflicting items and in this way influence action. In this chapter, we extend this view by examining some important influences of goals on the evaluation of all three types of items. In the first part of this chapter, we begin by examining two factors influencing preferences: the mental representation of goals and self-regulation. Then we examine how goals affect the accessibility of items as a function of goal activation and motivational state. One finding is that there are motivational factors much broader than specific action goals that affect cognition and action. To explore the generality of this finding, in the second part of this chapter we turn to other recent research suggesting that similar broad motivational factors may play a crucial role in the explanation of a number of known cultural differences in cognitive processing.

Valuation and Devaluation of Items

Intuitively, we expect goals to influence our evaluations of items (e.g., objects, people, and activities). One straightforward possibility for this influence is that items will be deemed more valuable when an individual has a strongly active goal that this object will help satisfy than when the individual has a weakly active goal. We refer to this difference in preference as *valuation*. For example, habitual smokers should show a higher preference for cigarettes when they have a strong motivation to smoke than when they have a weak motivation to smoke. Not only is valuation consistent with intuition, but it is also consistent with the economic notion of utility, which (implicitly) assumes that objects are valuable to the extent that they are useful (i.e., to the extent that they allow an individual to satisfy a goal).

When we began this line of research in the mid-1990s, we found remarkably few studies that found data consistent with valuation, that is, with the idea that people's preference for an item will increase when goals that the object can satisfy are active relative to when they are inactive. As one demonstration of such a *valuation effect,* Nisbett and Kanouse (1969) found that normal (as opposed to obese) eaters purchased more food at the supermarket when they were hungry than when they were not (see also Read & van Leeuwen, 1998). Cabanac (1971) found that sensory stimuli were more pleasurable when people were deprived of that stimulus than when they were not. For example, a warm stimulus was more pleasurable when the person's internal temperature was cool than when it was warm.

In our preliminary studies, we found only weak (and statistically nonreliable) valuation effects. For example, in a study we call the "bursar bill study," we asked undergraduates how much they would be willing to pay for a raffle ticket to win a $1,000 waiver on their university bills (Brendl, Markman, & Messner, 2003). Half these students were approached while standing in line at the bursar's office to pay their bills and the other half while sitting in a cafeteria. All of them had at least $1,000 in bills to pay. Interestingly, while people were willing to pay more for this raffle ticket when standing in the bursar's office (M = $1.52) than when sitting in the cafeteria (M = 1.20), the effect was not statistically significant.

Similarly, in a second study, the same authors approached German university students after a long lecture class. Half stayed in the classroom (where they could not smoke), and half were brought outside the classroom and were allowed to smoke a cigarette. Thus, the two groups differed significantly in their need to smoke (as measured by their score on the Question naire of Smoking Urges (L. S. Cox, Tiffany, & Christin, 2001). All participants were offered the opportunity to purchase raffle tickets to win three cartons of cigarettes in a drawing to be held the following week. Participants actually purchased tickets (at a price of 25 pfennigs each). Consistent with the bursar-bill study, participants with a high need to smoke purchased only slightly (and nonsignificantly) more tickets on average (M = 1.84) than did those with a low need to smoke (M = 1.71).

Other studies of the relationship between the need to smoke and preference for cigarettes also provide inconsistent evidence for valuation effects. Sherman and colleagues (Sherman, Rose, Koch, Presson, & Chassin, 2003) used an evaluative priming procedure as well as explicit ratings to assess attitudes toward smoking. With the evaluative priming procedure, heavy smokers (those smoking more than 15 cigarettes per day) exhibited a more positive attitude when they were smoke deprived than when they had just had a cigarette (consistent with valuation). In contrast, light smokers (those smoking fewer than 15 cigarettes per day) revealed a more negative attitude toward smoking when they were smoke deprived than when they had just had a cigarette (the opposite of valuation). Furthermore, the explicit ratings did not yield any reliable effects.

Perhaps the strongest recent evidence for valuation effects comes from studies by Ferguson and Bargh (2004). They used an evaluative priming task in which the object being evaluated was flashed on a computer screen as a prime, and then people classified an adjective as positive or negative. In the presence of an active goal, goal-relevant objects primed positive and negative adjectives to different degrees. Specifically, positive adjectives were classified by respondents more quickly than were negative adjectives. The effects of goal relevance on explicit evaluations of items were less clear. In one experiment, Ferguson and Bargh found no relationship between performance on the implicit adjective priming task and a more explicit rating of preference. In another study, there were relationships between this evaluative priming and judgments of intentions to perform goal-relevant activities. This review of the literature suggests that the evidence for valuation effects is sparse and inconsistent. We interpret this data pattern as supporting the existence of valuation effects yet suggesting that there are important moderating variables that need

to be known before we can predict when evaluation effects will materialize and when they will not.

Items that hinder goal pursuit take on negative valence (e.g., Brendl & Higgins, 1996). This suggests that activating a goal (e.g., to diet) can trigger *devaluation* of items that conflict with it (e.g., attractiveness of a tempting candy) (Fishbach, Friedman, & Kruglanski, 2003). These investigators observed that a data pattern consistent with such devaluation is more likely for people who are successful at self-regulation (e.g., successful dieters) than those less successful at self-regulation (e.g., unsuccessful dieters). Specifically, successful compared to unsuccessful self-regulators find tempting vices (e.g., candy) relatively less valuable compared to nontempting virtues (e.g., fruit). For example, women who were dieting successfully were more likely to select an apple than a candy bar when primed either with the goal of dieting or with pictures of a tempting food relative to when they received no prime. These data suggest that items that actively conflict with a strongly held goal may be devalued. Note, however, that when goal activation shifts choices from vices to virtues, we cannot infer whether the goal led to devaluation of the vice and/or to valuation of the virtue. In any case, these data demonstrate how the motivational system promotes goal satisfaction.

Elucidating this motivational mechanism further, Fishbach et al. (2003) also found that successful dieters were more likely than unsuccessful dieters to activate the goal of avoiding a temptation (i.e., dieting) when presented with a tempting stimulus (e.g., candy) that primes a conflicting goal (e.g., to savor the taste). The results from Sherman et al. (2003) that we reported previously could also be interpreted from this perspective. Light smokers devalued smoking stimuli when their need to smoke increased. Maybe the tempting stimuli activated a goal to abstain from smoking. In sum, although we do not know whether devaluation of goal-conflicting items is cause or effect of successful self-control, devaluation appears to be an important mechanism involved in it.

In our research, we have found (somewhat surprising) evidence that devaluation is not limited to goal-conflicting items but extends to goal-unrelated items (e.g., Brendl et al., 2003). That is, people's preferences for items that are not directly related to the goal are reliably *lower* when their motivation to pursue the goal is high than when it is low. For example, in the bursar-bill study we described previously, a second group of participants was asked how much they would be willing to pay to win $1,000 in cash. For this raffle, participants in the bursar's office were willing to pay much less when they were standing in the bursar's office (M = $0.93) than when they were approached in a cafeteria (M = $1.73). We have since conceptually replicated this correlational field study in various experiments, such as in the smoking raffle study described previously. A second group of German university students was offered the chance to purchase raffle tickets to win a cash prize (roughly equivalent to the cost of three cartons of cigarettes). In this case, participants with a high need to smoke purchased reliably fewer tickets on average (M = 1.39) than did those participants with a low need to smoke (M = 2.40).

To investigate the mechanism behind this type of devaluation effect, in a "smoking consumption study" we not only manipulated the strength of the need to smoke in a group of habitual smokers but also had them rate their preferences this time for five different classes of consumer products that varied their relatedness to smoking (Markman, Brendl, & Kim, 2007). The items most related to smoking were brands of cigarettes and objects that are instrumentally related to smoking, such as lighters and ashtrays. The least related items were consumer products, such as DVD players and automobiles. Intermediate in relatedness were foods typically consumed while smoking (e.g., Jack Daniels) and products with cigarette brands on them (e.g., Marlboro baseball caps).

In this study, we found significant valuation for both brands of cigarettes and items instrumentally related to smoking. That is, people's preference ratings for these items were higher on average when they had a high need to smoke than when they had a low need to smoke. Replicating our previous findings, the items unrelated to smoking showed reliable devaluation (i.e., lower ratings by people with a high need to smoke than by those with a low need to smoke). What was new were the items that were intermediate in their relatedness to smoking. These showed an intermediate pattern with neither reliable valuation nor reliable devaluation. We have now obtained this pattern of valuation and devaluation for a variety of types of goals and with a variety of measures.

Ferguson and Bargh (2004) obtained a similar pattern of valuation with their evaluative priming measure. They manipulated thirst in participants and found significant evaluative priming for items that could be used to satisfy thirst directly (e.g., water and juice) but not for items that were weakly related to the active goal (e.g., beer and coffee). Interestingly, there was no devaluation effect for thirst-unrelated items (e.g., trees, talking, and so on). To show devaluation, the thirst-unrelated prime words would have to prime (i.e., speed responses to) negative adjectives the more thirsty respondents are. However, these prime words were neutral to positive. Devaluation presumably renders them less positive but not negative, and hence they may not prime negative adjectives.

These data, then, may suggest that devaluation of goal-unrelated items leads not to avoiding them but rather to approaching them less. Further, it appears that goals guide action toward goal-related items and away from goal-conflicting items, but goals do not seem to change action toward intermediately related items. These effects are relatively straightforward even if we might not have predicted all of them in advance. As we dig deeper into these phenomena, however, the patterns of data become more complex, and we begin to understand that effects that one would expect to generally occur fail to do so unless certain boundary conditions are in place.

Boundary Conditions on Valuation and Devaluation

First, we qualify the generality of the notion that activating a focal goal leads to valuation of goal-related items. The evidence for valuation effects suggests that there are numerous boundary conditions that we do not know yet. One such boundary condition is the breadth of the focal goal (Markman et al., 2007). That is, we find reliable valuation only for items that are squarely within the representation of respondents' active goal. Thus, if their goal is narrower than we might expect intuitively, we will fail to obtain valuation and instead get the intermediate pattern between valuation and devaluation observed for moderately goal-related items.

The Ferguson and Bargh study with thirst that we described earlier is consistent with the proposal that people's goals are narrowly focused on specific actions. To explore this issue further, we ran an experiment in which participants believed that they were performing a marketing study investigating their general liking of a random selection of consumer products. Unbeknownst to the participants, we were interested in a subset of these products: foods related to breakfast but not dinner (e.g., pancakes) and foods related to dinner but not breakfast (e.g., lasagna). Respondents rated product liking in general rather than desire to consume a certain food "now." We also varied time of day as an unobtrusive variable by conducting the study either in the morning or in the late afternoon. But we never pointed to that aspect explicitly. Finally, we performed an unobtrusive manipulation of need to eat. When participants arrived in the lab, they did a brief taste test in which they tasted either a small bit of bread with salted butter or a large amount of bread with unsalted butter. The small preload of food with salt should function as an appetizer that increases people's need to eat (Herman, 1996; Schulkin, 1991). In contrast, the large amount of bread, combined with the fat in the butter, should have a sating effect that decreases people's need to eat.

We were particularly interested in differences in patterns of ratings between the groups with a high and low need to eat as a function of the time of day that the study was performed. In particular, we were curious about where we would find valuation effects. One possibility is that they occur at the level of foods in general (so that preference ratings for all foods would be greater for people with a high need to eat than for people with a low need to eat). A second possibility is that the valuation effects occur only for contextually relevant foods (e.g., for breakfast foods in the morning).

A study by Gilbert, Gill, and Wilson (2002) suggests that laypeople expect that the need to eat influences their preference at the level of foods in general. Participants who were hungry during the experiment predicted that they would like eating spaghetti with meatballs equally the next morning or the next afternoon. In contrast, participants who were not hungry predicted that they would like eating the spaghetti the next day more in the afternoon than in the morning. Spaghetti, of course, is a food typically consumed in the afternoon. Our study differs from that of Gilbert et al. because it was actually performed either in the morning or in the afternoon. Thus, it is possible that people mispredict the influence of the time of day on their preferences.

In our study, we did find valuation effects, but in contrast to lay intuitions, valuation was obtained only for the foods contextually appropriate to the time of day when the study was run. Thus, need to eat increased preference for breakfast foods, but only in the morning, and it increased preference for dinner foods, but only in the afternoon. Preference ratings for foods that were not contextually appropriate for the time of day were not influenced in a statistically reliable fashion by need to eat. This finding may explain the puzzling observation that some previous studies have found weak valuation effects. The set of items for which valuation was observed in this study is narrower than we might have expected. Thus, it is possible that many goals lead to narrower valuation effects than intuition might suggest.

To be clear, the issue is not that in the morning we consume breakfast rather than dinner foods. That observation alone might have led to an interaction between type of food and time of day such that overall preference for breakfast foods would be greater in the morning than in the evening and preference for dinner foods would be greater in the evening than in the morning. Nonetheless, we might have observed valuation for foods in general. That is, a high need to eat could have increased people's preferences relative to a low need for all foods, but it did not.

Furthermore, we are not claiming that those needs that drive preferences are always specific. What we are claiming is that even if the need activated is quite abstract, the level of abstraction at which this need translates into a preference for items and hence influences action can be much more specific. Knowing that level of abstraction at which a need is translated into a preference is a crucial boundary condition for observing valuation effects. For instance, it is possible that in our initial smoking study, we did not find a valuation effect for cigarettes because respondents were stuck in a classroom where it was highly inappropriate for them to smoke. Just as food goals may involve an appropriate time, smoking goals may involve a place. Future research should investigate when this level of abstraction is high and when it is low.

In a second set of studies, we found boundary conditions on the observation that goal-conflicting items are devalued by goal activation. Devaluing goal-conflicting items may occur only as part of a particular behavioral strategy, such as a strategy of avoiding distractions or temptations. Because this strategy involves at least some avoidance, activating avoidance motivation in a person may render devaluation of goal-conflicting items more likely. From the perspective of satisfying the need to smoke, thinking about lung cancer would be a conflicting activity. Based on this reasoning, we investigated smokers' concern for items that might block goal satisfaction (Markman et al., 2007). Most important for the current discussion, we also manipulated smokers' general level of avoidance motivation (versus approach motivation). And finally, we manipulated their need to smoke.

To heighten people's general motivation to avoid losses, we used a manipulation derived from research on regulatory focus theory (Higgins, 1987, 1997). The logic of the manipulation is that when people are avoiding a particular loss in the environment, they are also vigilant to other potential losses in the environment. Thus, participants in our study were told that at some point during the experiment they would be doing a mathematics test, and then they would be doing a very boring task (e.g., alphabetizing a list). They were told that if they did well on the math test, they would not have to do the boring task. The other half of our participants were motivated toward approach goals by telling them that they would perform an interesting task (e.g., playing a game) if they performed well on the math test (for a similar manipulation, see Crowe & Higgins, 1997).[1]

After instantiating both the approach/avoidance manipulation and the manipulation of need to smoke, participants rated their degree of concern with a variety of potential problems. Some of these were health problems that other smokers stated are highly related to smoking (e.g., lung cancer and emphysema). From the perspective of satisfying a need to smoke, these are goal-conflicting items. Other concerns were health problems that are also severe but not related to smoking (e.g., AIDS). These are intermediately related items but not conflicting ones. Finally, there was a group of problems that are unrelated to smoking and also unrelated to health (e.g., financial troubles). These are unrelated items.

Let us take a look at the avoidance motivated smokers first. For the smoking-related health problems, they showed reliably less concern when they had a high need to smoke than when they had a low need to smoke. That is, the need to smoke actually drove down people's overall concern with potential problems that might prevent goal satisfaction. This is a devaluation effect that is consistent with lay theory. It is a devaluation effect because the negative evaluation of a disease got diminished. In contrast, the ratings done by participants with approach motivation were not affected by their level of need to smoke.

There are two possible explanations for this effect. One explanation is that any

goal-conflicting item will show devaluation only when participants are avoidance motivated. A second possibility is that the items in our study showed devaluation only when participants were avoidance motivated because the items themselves were negative items that participants wanted to avoid. Future research will have to address these possibilities. Nevertheless, these data show that we need to qualify the general notion that focal goals automatically devalue conflicting items.

Next, we qualify the generality of the notion that items with a moderate degree of relatedness to a focal goal are unaffected by goal activation and thus show neither valuation nor devaluation. This finding is sensible from the perspective that action should be driven toward highly goal-related items rather than intermediately related items while maintaining intermediately related items as potential substitutes. This logic may indeed hold when a person is in a general mode of approach motivation. On the other hand, what would change if a person were in the motivational mode of avoiding goal-conflicting items?

To suggest an answer, we can borrow from perception, which must solve the conceptually similar problem of detecting a signal when there are similar signals nearby that it could be confused with. For example, in perception, the problem of identifying an edge is made easier by enhancing the contrast between bright and dark illumination on the surface. This is often implemented through a neural mechanism called lateral inhibition between preceptors that code level of illumination in terms of level of neural activation (e.g., Hartline, Wagner, & Ratcliff, 1956; Marr, 1982). In lateral inhibition all receptors inhibit the ones around them. As a result, the dark side of the edge appears darker because the bright-side receptors inhibit the dark-side receptors. At the same time, because the dark-side receptors are inhibited, their inhibition of the bright-side receptors is attenuated, making the bright side "brighter." The bright-side receptors are disinhibited. Thus, the physical bright–dark difference at the edge is exaggerated by the corresponding receptors. Lateral inhibition always results in one side of a contrast being inhibited and the other being disinhibited.

Likewise, the border between items within a goal and outside a goal may show a similar contrast enhancement. So, for example, there is a conceptual "edge" between diseases related to smoking (e.g., lung cancer) and diseases unrelated to smoking (e.g., diabetes). If the need to smoke inhibits diseases related to smoking, then there will be a contrast enhancement at the edge between the smoking-related and the smoking-unrelated diseases. The need to smoke would inhibit smoking-related diseases, and therefore people's concern with diseases like lung cancer would decrease. However, we would observe relative disinhibition of smoking-unrelated diseases. Thus, the need to smoke might paradoxically *increase* people's concern with smoking-unrelated diseases.

Our study did indeed find such a lateral inhibition pattern of concern. Smokers were reliably more concerned with smoking-unrelated health problems (e.g., diabetes) when they had a high need to smoke than when they had a low need to smoke. This valuation effect (i.e., increased negativity) was evident only for avoidance-oriented smokers. This is consistent with the lateral inhibition assumption because valuation of intermediately related items should occur as a result of devaluation of conflicting items. The data show that we need to qualify the generality of the notion that intermediately related items are not affected by goals. We found valuation of intermediately related items when respondents avoided goal-conflicting items.

Finally, we qualify the generality of the notion that goal-unrelated items are devalued. For goals to influence action, some mechanism must delineate the boundary of the goal. In other words, there need to be a set of items beyond which items less similar to the goal will not be pursued. Items that get devalued by a focal goal presumably fall outside that boundary. A motivational strategy of approaching a focal goal may devalue goal-unrelated items because these items could not serve as substitutes and could hence only detract from goal pursuit. The situation may be different for motivational strategies of avoiding distractions or competing items. We have seen that such avoidance may be implemented by a mechanism of lateral inhibition, which would draw a sharp boundary closely around a goal. Lateral inhibition mechanisms draw boundaries by deactivating concepts close to a center, activating concepts a little bit further removed from the center, and leaving more distant concepts untouched. So if indeed lateral inhibition drew the boundary around the smoking goal in our prevention-oriented respondents, we would expect that, for them, completely unrelated goals would not be devalued. Indeed, our prevention-oriented respondents exhibited neither devaluation nor valuation of unrelated items (i.e., smoking-unrelated nonhealth problems). Recall that they did exhibit devaluation of conflicting items. Hence, the notion that goal-unrelated items are generally devalued requires qualification too. Goal-unrelated items were not devalued when respondents devalued goal-conflicting items.

We can now draw a more differentiated picture of how goals influence preferences in order to guide action. Rather than looking only at items that are directly relevant to a goal, be it because they are directly supportive or hindering, we have taken the perspective of looking at the pattern by which a goal changes preferences for items ranging from highly relevant to completely irrelevant. This allowed us to identify two patterns of preferences that goals impose on their environment. It turns out that the initially depicted simple picture of the influence of goals on preferences is a mix between these two patterns.

The first pattern of valuation and devaluation is illustrated in the top panel of Figure 16.1. In this case, an active goal leads to valuation of goal-related items, devaluation of goal-unrelated items, and intermediately related items falling in the middle. This data pattern we found in the smoking consumption study with smoking-related and smoking-unrelated consumption products. What we have not mentioned before is that if we manipulate approach and avoidance motivation, we obtain this pattern for approach-motivated respondents but

not for avoidance-motivated respondents. The current data, then, suggest that this pattern may be prototypical for approach motivation.

The second pattern is illustrated in the bottom panel of Figure 16.1. In this case, an active goal leads to devaluation of goal-related items, valuation of conflicting items, and valuation of intermediately related items. Goal-unrelated items are neither valued nor devalued. We obtained this pattern for various concerns as items. Thus, the data suggest that this pattern may be prototypical for avoidance motivation.

To summarize, then, we began this section with a straightforward picture of the relationship between goals and action. In particular, items related to an active goal should be valued, and items that conflict with an active goal should be devalued. The data in this section extend this view in four ways. First, valuation occurs only for items within the scope of an active goal, and this scope may not always concur with intuition. For example, we found that a moderate need to eat led to valuation for only a narrow range of items contextually relevant to the time of day that the study was run. Likewise, Ferguson and Bargh found evaluative priming only for items (e.g., water and juice) that would directly satisfy the active need.

Second, devaluation occurs in two situations. Positive items that are unrelated to an active approach goal are devalued. Thus, people with a strong need to smoke devalue consumer products. In addition, negative items that conflict with an active approach goal are devalued. Thus, we find that habitual smokers with a strong need to smoke also reduce their concern for smoking-related health concerns relative to smokers with a low need to smoke.

Third, when positive items are related to an approach goal only to an intermediate degree, they show neither valuation nor devaluation. Thus, the strength of valuation

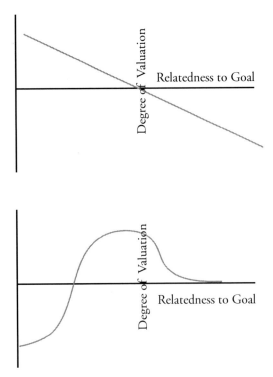

Fig. 16.1 Two patterns of valuation and devaluation. The top pattern was obtained with consumption products as items. The bottom panel was obtained with concerns as items. More positive values on the y-axis correspond to greater preference for products and to greater concerns.

and devaluation of positive items appears to be monotonically related to the relatedness of the item to the active goal.

Fourth, the pattern of valuation and devaluation for negative items exhibits a pattern reminiscent of an active inhibition. Negative items that conflict with an active goal directly are devalued (i.e., become less negative). Negative items with a moderate relationship to the active goal actually increase in their valuation (i.e., become more negative). Thus, habitual smokers reliably increase their concern with smoking-unrelated health problems like AIDS when their need to smoke increases. Finally, negative items with a distant relationship to the active goal are neither valued nor devalued. In the next section, we explore the degree to which goal activation also affects the accessibility of goal-related and goal-unrelated concepts.

Valuation, Devaluation, and Accessibility

Research on goals suggests that the activation of a particular goal may influence the accessibility of concepts related to that goal. This work also suggests that this change in goal activation may be related to changes in preferences that occur with goal activation. For example, mounting evidence supports the intuition that goal activation increases the accessibility of items that promote goal satisfaction (e.g., Aarts & Dijksterhuis, 2000; Bargh, Gollwitzer, Lee-Chai, Barndollar, & Trötschel, 2001; Forster, Liberman, & Higgins, 2005; Shah & Kruglanski, 2002; Shah, Kruglanski, & Friedman, 2003; see Chapters 17 and 29). There is also some evidence that devalued items are attenuated in their accessibility in order to render them less distracting or tempting. For example, we described Fishbach et al.'s study of successful self-regulators who exhibited devaluation of goal-conflicting items (e.g., tempting foods) when primed with words relating to

a goal (Fishbach et al., 2003). The same individuals also exhibited attenuation of the accessibility of conflicting items. When successful dieters who have a need to eat exhibit attenuated accessibility of tempting foods, they have presumably found a way to actively yet automatically inhibit the accessibility of goal-conflicting items.

The same logic does not necessarily apply to goal-unrelated items. As we have seen previously, lateral inhibition (hence active inhibition) does not seem to be the mechanism driving the devaluation of goal-unrelated items. Rather, we hypothesize that these items are devalued because the motivational system has a limited amount of activation (or energy). Focusing this activation on an active goal draws activation away from items that are unrelated to the goal. Whether such a drop in motivational energy translates into a drop in accessibility is an empirical question that we addressed with a Stroop task (Stroop, 1935) on the same items for which people also judged preferences. In the original Stroop task, color words (e.g., "RED" or "GREEN") were written in a font that was either the same color or a different color. People were then asked to name the color of the font. The classic finding is that people are slower to name the color of the font when the word names a different color than when it names the same color. More recently, this paradigm has been used to measure the accessibility of concepts (e.g., Bargh & Pratto, 1986; W. M. Cox, Fadardi, & Pothos, 2006; Jacoby, Lindsay, & Hessels, 2003). In this case, other concepts are printed in fonts of different colors. The idea is that the more accessible the concept named by a word, the slower individuals will be to identify the color of the font.

We used this task to assess the relationship between accessibility and preference. The participants were those in the study described previously in which they rated the preference of five types of consumption products that differed in the strength of their relationship to smoking. As discussed, the items most closely related to smoking exhibited valuation, and the items least related to smoking exhibited devaluation. All these items were presented to a computer screen in one of three font colors. Participants pressed a button to identify the font color.

Of particular interest was the relative speed to identify items depending on whether the participant had a high need to smoke or a low need to smoke. For cigarettes and items that are instrumentally related to smoking, people were faster to identify the font color when they had a low need to smoke than when they had a high need to smoke. This finding suggests that cigarette brand names and items instrumentally related to smoking were more accessible when people had a high need to smoke than when they had a low need to smoke. In contrast, for the items that were unrelated to smoking, they were faster to identify the font when they had a high need to smoke than when they had a low need to smoke. This finding suggests that these items that were unrelated to smoking were reliably less accessible when people had a high need to smoke than when they had a low need to smoke. In sum, the pattern of accessibility mirrors that of valuation and devaluation. In this way, our findings diverge from those of Ferguson and Bargh (2004), who found an inconsistent relationship between accessibility (as measured by evaluating priming) and explicit ratings and who observed the equivalent of valuation but not devaluation on their evaluative priming measure.

Our findings are consistent with Kruglanski et al.'s (2002) proposal that goals are represented in a semantic network that spreads activation from goals to means. From this perspective, the motivational system influences both preferences for items

and their accessibility. In the next section, we explore how motivation may influence action and preference through these mechanisms of accessibility.

Motivational Influences on Attitudes and Action

An individual's evaluation of some object is influenced by both semantic and motivational factors. This distinction between semantic and motivational factors maps onto the distinction between "cool" and "hot" psychological systems (Loewenstein, 1996; Metcalfe & Mischel, 1999; see Chapter 5). Semantic factors are those aspects of evaluations that have become part of an individual's consciously accessible representation of a particular concept. For example, a woman who is a habitual smoker may see herself as liking cigarettes. A teenage boy may think of a Corvette as car that is cool. A lifelong Democrat may have an explicit negative attitude toward Republican candidates.

In addition to this semantic component of evaluation, there is also a strong motivational aspect to evaluations. These motivational influences can change as a result of moment-by-moment changes in the strength of someone's motivation to pursue a particular goal. Thus, for example, a smoker may have a generally positive evaluation of cigarettes, but this preference for cigarettes may change when she has a high need to smoke relative to when she has a low need to smoke.

An important aspect of these motivational influences is that they are largely inaccessible to consciousness. That is, people have relatively little explicit awareness of the activation of their motivational system. Indeed, though people will often give detailed reasons for their actions, these reasons are typically drawn from available information in the environment rather than from privileged access to the representational content of the motivational system (Kruglanski et al., 2002; Markman & Brendl, 2005).

To be clear, we are arguing that (at least some) sources of people's evaluations are inaccessible to consciousness but not that their evaluations themselves are unconscious. Thus, our discussion is orthogonal to the extended debate over "implicit attitudes," defined as evaluations of items about which people do not have explicit access (Greenwald et al., 2002; Wilson, Lindsey, & Schooler, 2000).

Consider the following example. People prefer their name initials to other letters of the alphabet (Nuttin, 1985). Pelham and colleagues have found that real-world decisions (e.g., cities to live in or careers to engage in) correlate with the similarity of these decision objects to the decision makers' names (Jones, Pelham, Carvallo, & Mirenberg, 2004; Pelham, Mirenberg, & Jones, 2002). Presumably, people are unaware that these preferences may be influenced by name similarities. Most persons named Dennis would reject the idea that they chose to become a dentist because of the name similarity, even though they are aware of their liking of dentistry. To explore this phenomenon experimentally, Brendl, Chattopadhyay, Pelham, and Carvallo (2005) investigated conditions when a person named, for example, Herbert is more likely to prefer chocolate as a result of branding it Hershey's rather than Snickers. Such name-letter-branding effects occurred only when a person had an active need that related to the product under evaluation (e.g., the need to eat but not the need to drink). The data suggest that hungry respondents were aware that they felt better about one object than about the other because when they ignored their feelings, they were not influenced by name letters. Yet the data also suggest that respondents were unaware that the origin of their feeling was the relationship between the brand name and the letters in their name. At the same time, they had no difficulty coming up with evidently false but acceptable reasons for their preference, such as taste. Thus, they exhibited a "false" valuation effect. Need to eat led to a conscious valuation of an object (candy bar) based on an unconscious source (name letters).

Motivational Mechanisms

How does motivation influence accessibility? To begin with, our results are in line with the view that items that support goal satisfaction will increase in their accessibility and that items that may block goal satisfaction will decrease in their accessibility (Bruner, 1957; Ferguson & Bargh, 2004). Beyond that, our most novel finding concerning accessibility is that items that are unrelated to the goal (i.e., those that neither support nor block the goal) may also be lowered in accessibility by an active goal. Thus, goal-related items will be available for planning actions that will allow goals to be achieved. Furthermore, this accessibility will help people recognize the presence of goal-related items in the environment, which will help them recognize opportunities for goal satisfaction (Lewin, 1926; Ovsiankina, 1928; Patalano & Seifert, 1997).

Our results are also consistent with the observation that people are often unaware of the motivational influences on their behavior (Bargh & Chartrand, 1999; Bargh et al., 2001). On this view, motivation has a subtle influence of changing the overall accessibility of some concepts. In addition, in semantic memory, people are not aware of the factors that affect the accessibility of concepts. Furthermore, they cannot determine what the "baseline" level of accessibility for concepts should be. Thus, they have no way to determine what the influence of a particular motivational state is on current experiences elicited by accessibility, nor can they correct accurately for the influence of these motivational states (Loewenstein, 1996).

This view also suggests why habits are so pernicious. Motivational states influence the activation of concepts. Thus, even when someone wants to change a habit (e.g., to stop smoking), the motivational system will serve to activate concepts that support goal satisfaction (e.g., ashtrays) and to inhibit concepts that block goal satisfaction (e.g., lung cancer). Even the accessibility of goal-unrelated concepts may be attenuated, this way reducing chances that a completely unrelated behavior and usefully distracting behavior would be triggered (e.g., listening to a song instead of taking a smoke). Overcoming these effects would require significant changes in the structure of an individual's semantic network.

The difficulty of changing habits is exacerbated by the affective states that accompany motivation. So far, we have talked about manipulations of people's motivation (e.g., manipulating the need to smoke). Commonly, people talk about "craving a cigarette," "desperately wanting to buy a car," or "being hungry." When people say they "crave," "want," and "feel hunger," they refer to conscious affective states. Lay theory assumes these are the conscious markers of physiological states. However, ratings of cravings and hunger are only moderately correlated with other physiological and behavioral measures of the strength of a need (Kassel & Shiffman, 1992; Tiffany, 1990; Tiffany & Conklin, 2000). This observation suggests that these conscious experiences are not driven by physiological states in a one-to-one fashion. Instead, it appears that cravings are experienced most strongly when individuals have a strong motivation to pursue a goal yet are blocked from pursuing the goal by their habitual means.

This view of cravings suggests that they may be emotional states that are based

on appraisals (Smith, Haynes, Lazarus, & Pope, 1993). On this view, experiencing a particular emotion requires more than just the raw affective force of a situation. Individuals must also appraise the situation as relevant to a particular schema to experience that emotion (though this appraisal may be implicit; Berkowitz & Harmon-Jones, 2004). So the experience of a need state may require both the physiological signals associated with an active need and an appraisal consistent with the emotion. In the case of cravings, failing to satisfy an active goal leads to an aversive state. The latter was anticipated by Lewin's (1926) proposal that unsatisfied goals elicit a state of tension, a quasi need.

The influence of goals on the accessibility of concepts may be an important part of experiences such as cravings. Items that support goal satisfaction are increased in their accessibility and create a "cognitive obsession" with these items. Items that hinder goal satisfaction (by conflicting with it) or that are simply irrelevant to the active goal are decreased in their accessibility, making it hard for actors to think of them. As a result, individuals focus on items that will permit the active goal to be achieved.

There is one more critical issue to be addressed, however. Not all the motivational effects on action described so far are specific to the active goal. In particular, whether we see valuation or devaluation depends both on the specific active goal and on the individual's general motivational state. Positive items only show valuation or devaluation when the individual is approach motivated. Negative items only show valuation or devaluation when the individual is avoidance motivated. This finding implies that there are broad motivational states that may have a profound influence on the accessibility of particular kinds of concepts that may ultimately have a large impact on action.

We explore this issue in the next section by focusing on motivational states that may cause some observed cultural differences in cognitive performance.

Motivation and Individual Differences

There has been much interest in cultural differences in cognitive performance. There are many sources of this interest. One is the recognition that research in psychology has overrepresented data from college-educated Western-born participants. Another is that there are significant differences on average in performance on a variety of cognitive tasks by members of different cultures (Masuda & Nisbett, 2001; Nisbett, Peng, Choi, & Norenzayan, 2001; Peng & Nisbett, 1999). Finally, there is a growing appreciation of the practical benefits of understanding the reasoning processes of members of different cultures.

The source of cultural differences in cognitive performance is less clear than the existence of these differences. There are a number of significant differences between cultures that could lead to differences. For example, Nisbett and his colleagues point out that Eastern and Western cultures have a quite different intellectual heritage that may influence the thought processes of members of the culture (Nisbett et al., 2001). Obviously, there are language differences across cultures that could potentially influence cognitive performance (Gentner & Goldin-Meadow, 2003). Furthermore, members of Eastern and Western cultures differ along a number of other variables. For example, Eastern cultures tend to be relatively collectivist cultures, but Western cultures tend to be more individualist (e.g., Markus & Kitayama, 1991; Oyserman, Coon, & Kemmelmeier, 2002). Thus, there are many potential sources for any observed difference in cognitive performance across cultures.

One recent trend in research has been to explore whether cross-cultural differences in cognitive performance can be explained by individual difference variables that also explain variation in performance within members of a culture (Hong & Chiu, 2001). That is, there may be factors that lead members of a culture to differ along a variable, but this variable is the one that actually affects cognitive performance. We believe that this potential explanation is made more plausible by the findings reviewed in the previous section. That is, if the motivational system affects the information to which people are sensitive, then fairly small changes in motivational state can have significant effects on cognitive performance.

We are particularly interested in this possibility because it suggests avenues by which the motivational system can influence cognitive processing broadly. These motivational mechanisms go beyond the influence of specific goals described in the first half of this chapter. In this section, we start by identifying some individual difference characteristics that are potential candidates as variables that might lead to the observed cross-cultural differences. Then we present some evidence for the role of these variables in cognitive performance.

Motivational Variables That Affect Cognitive Performance

How can motivational variables influence cognitive performance in ways that might explain observed cross-cultural differences? An instructive case comes from research on the effects of *self-construal* on cognitive performance (Lee, Aaker, & Gardner, 2000; Markus & Kitayama, 1991). Self-construal is an aspect of a person's self-representation that refers to the degree to which people consider themselves to be connected to others in their social world. Those with a relatively *independent* self-construal tend to describe themselves using terms that do not refer to others (e.g., smart, funny, or happy). Those with a relatively *interdependent* self-construal tend to describe themselves using terms that relate the self to others (e.g., mother or wife).

Self-construal is interesting for two reasons. First, it does vary across cultures. Members of Western cultures tend to use more independent descriptors of themselves, while members of Eastern cultures tend to use more interdependent descriptors of themselves (Markus & Kitayama, 1991). Second, self-construal differences within cultures affect social judgment in ways that are consistent with observed cultural differences. For example, Gardner, Gabriel, and Lee (1999) primed independent or interdependent self-construals in members of Eastern and Western cultures and asked them to judge the importance of a group of values that reflect either individualism (e.g., freedom) or collectivist values (e.g., friendship). Typically, members of Eastern cultures find collectivist values more important than individualist values, and members of Western cultures find individualist values more important than individualist values. Gardner et al. found that people primed to have a relatively independent self-construal (regardless of what culture they came from) endorsed individualist values more strongly than collectivist values. In contrast, people primed to have a relatively interdependent self-construal endorsed collectivist values more strongly than individualist values (see also Kuhnen & Oyserman, 2002).

If self-construal were the only variable that both varied between cultures and affected judgment, we could begin to weave a story about the influence of self-construal on information processing. This story might make specific reference to aspects of the way that self relates to others. However, there are other variables that appear quite similar in the literature.

One variable of interest is fear of isolation, which is the degree to which a person is sensitive to the prospect of being socially isolated from other members of the culture (Baumeister & Leary, 1995; Noelle-Neumann, 1984). This characteristic is called "fear of isolation," though it is more a representational state than an active anxiety state. Individuals with high levels of fear of isolation are chronically sensitive to the potential that they will be negatively evaluated by members of their peer group. Indeed, the scale used to measure an individual's chronic fear of isolation examines people's sensitivity to negative evaluations (Watson & Friend, 1969).

Like self-construal, fear of isolation varies across cultures. For example, Kim and Markman (2006) gave the Fear of Negative Evaluation Scale to members of Eastern and Western cultures and found that members of Eastern cultures had higher chronic levels of fear of isolation than did members of Western cultures. On the surface, it is not clear that self-construal and fear of isolation ought to differ across cultures in the same way, nor is it clear whether they should have a common influence on information processing.

There is also evidence that people may differ in the degree to which they view the social environment as relatively fixed or relatively malleable (Hong et al., 2003). People who view their social position as fixed must attend to social relations in order to understand and maintain their appropriate place in society. In contrast, those who view their social position as malleable can focus on their own attributes and attempt to use them to alter the world around them. While there are individual differences in the degree to which people view their social position as fixed or malleable, there is also a tendency for members of Eastern cultures to see social roles as more fixed than do members of Western cultures.

We bring these lines of research together by suggesting that motivational variables like self-construal and fear of isolation influence attention to relationships in the environment in a manner similar to that observed for the malleability of social relations. Thus, individuals with a high fear of isolation or an interdependent self-construal should be more likely than those with low fear of isolation or an independent self-construal to attend to social and contextual relationships in cognitive tasks. In the next section, we discuss some preliminary evidence that bears on this point.

Explorations of Fear of Isolation and Self-Construal

We have explored the possibility that motivational factors influence people's attention to relations in the environment in three types of studies: dialectical reasoning, recognition memory, and causal induction. The first two of these were designed to replicate findings from cross-cultural research. The study of causal induction demonstrated a new phenomenon not explored in previous research.

The study of dialectical reasoning was based on previous research by Peng and Nisbett (1999), who found that East Asians had a greater relative preference for dialectical proverbs (i.e., those that embody contradictions, such as "Sorrow is born of excessive joy") than do members of Western cultures. In contrast, members of Western cultures tend to prefer nondialectical proverbs (i.e., those do not embody contradictions, such as "Half a loaf is better than none"). We believe that the ability to comprehend and appreciate the wisdom of dialectical proverbs requires more relational processing than does the ability to comprehend nondialectical proverbs. Dialectical proverbs require understanding that people, objects, and emotional states differ in their relationships to each other in ways that permit them to satisfy multiple roles in the environment.

To demonstrate that individual difference variables can have an influence on cognitive performance that is similar to observed cultural differences, we manipulated fear of isolation in a sample of American undergraduates (Kim & Markman, 2006). Fear of isolation was manipulated by asking some participants (in the high fear of isolation group) to write about at least three experiences in which they were anxious or afraid because they were isolated from a group and asking other participants (in the low fear of isolation group) to write about at least three experiences in which they were anxious or afraid because they caused someone else to be isolated from a group. This manipulation causes the two experimental groups to differ in their scores on the Fear of Negative Evaluation Scale that we described previously, though it does not lead to significant differences in emotional state or state anxiety.

After this manipulation of fear of isolation, people rated their preference for a variety of proverbs. The proverbs were taken from Peng and Nisbett's (1999) research and were selected from American, Chinese, and Yiddish sources. Consistent with our predictions, the high fear of isolation group showed a relatively greater preference for the dialectical proverbs than did the low fear of isolation group. To relate this work to cultural differences, we also ran a group of Korean participants without a manipulation of fear of isolation. This group had higher scores on the Fear of Negative Evaluation Scale than either of the two groups of Americans and also exhibited a greater preference for dialectical proverbs than did either of the two groups of American participants. Thus, participants' scores on the Fear of Negative Evaluation Scale predicted variability in preference for dialectical proverbs both within and between cultures.

Recognition memory is another way to explore the influence of context on cognitive processing. Masuda and Nisbett (2001) showed members of East Asian and Western cultures a series of pictures of animals against a background. For example, among the pictures in the study phase might be a cow in a field. Later, these participants were shown pictures and asked whether they had seen the animal before regardless of the context against which it was presented. That is, participants should respond that they saw an animal before if it was presented in the same context (e.g., a cow in a field) or a different context (e.g., a cow in a meadow) but not if they saw a different animal even if it appeared in one of the contexts seen during study (e.g., a sheep in a field). Members of East Asian cultures were more likely than members of Western cultures to erroneously respond that an animal they had seen before was new if it was presented in a new background than if it was presented in the same background.

If this observed cultural difference reflects sensitivity to contextual factors in processing, then we should be able to induce this difference in memory performance by manipulating fear of isolation in a sample of Americans. We used a similar procedure to the one in the study described in the previous paragraph to create groups that differed in their average level of fear of isolation (Kim & Markman, 2006). We then repeated the procedure from Masuda and Nisbett (2001). We found that the high fear of isolation group was more likely than the low fear of isolation group to erroneously say that animals they had seen before were new when they appeared with a new background. Thus, higher levels of fear of isolation were associated with relatively greater sensitivity to contextual information.

Contextual processing is also central to causal induction from observations. Research on causal induction often has individuals observe trials in which one or more potential causal factors may lead (probabilistically) to an effect (Spellman, 1996; White, 1988). Of interest is the kind of information that people use to determine that a potential cause either promotes or inhibits an effect. Much research suggests that people can use information about the *unconditional contingency* between a cause and an effect to assess the causal status of a potential cause (Cheng, 1997; Cheng & Novick, 1992). An unconditional contingency compares the conditional probability of an effect in the presence of a potential cause to the conditional probability of that effect in the absence of the potential cause. If the effect is more likely in the presence of the cause than in its absence, then the cause is a good candidate to promote the effect. If the effect is less likely in the presence of the cause than in its absence, the cause is a good candidate to be an inhibitor of the effect. If the effect is about equally likely in the presence of the cause as in its absence, then the factor is unlikely to be causally related to the effect.

Of course, there are many potential causal factors in the world, and often they are correlated with each other. Thus, truly assessing the causal status of a potential cause requires attending both to that cause and to other potential causal factors in the environment. Indeed, some researchers have explored the degree to which people can attend to *conditional contingencies,* which are contingencies computed assuming the presence or absence of some other (set of) candidate causes (Spellman, 1996; Tangen & Allan, 2004). Of interest for the present discussion is that being sensitive to conditional contingencies requires greater attention to contextual information in the environment than does being sensitive to unconditional contingencies because conditional contingencies must control for the presence of other potential causal factors.

We explored whether self-construal influenced people's attention to contextual information in a causal induction task (Kim, Narvaez, & Markman, 2007). First, we primed a relatively greater independent or interdependent self-construal by having participants circle the pronouns *I* and *me* (for an independent self-construal) or *we* and *our* (for an interdependent self-construal) in a set of sentences. Then participants were exposed to a series of events in which two liquids that might serve as fertilizers for plant growth were applied to plants in different combinations. After seeing which fertilizers were applied, participants were told whether the plant bloomed. The trials were constructed so that participants would reach different conclusions about the causal efficacy of the liquids depending on whether they attended to the unconditional contingency of the individual causes with the effect or the conditional contingency of the causes taking into account the presence of the alternative cause.

Consistent with the results of the studies already described, participants given a relatively interdependent self-construal showed greater sensitivity to conditional contingencies than did participants given a relatively independent self-construal. This result suggests that self-construal is another factor that affects the degree to which people attend to causal information in the environment.

To summarize, individual differences in the general motivational variables of self-construal and fear of isolation affect people's attention to contextual information in the environment. People with relatively higher level of fear of isolation and relatively more interdependent self-construals are more sensitive to context than are those with a relatively lower level of fear of isolation and relatively more independent self-construal. These variables suggest that there are core motivational factors that influence the way people encode and use information. These variables may also be at the root of observed cultural differences in cognitive processing.

Motivation, Cognition, and Action

The purpose of this chapter was to describe two levels at which the motivational system affects action. First, we focused on the level of specific goals. It is uncontroversial that people pursue a wide range of different goals and that the motivation to pursue particular goals changes over time. What is less well understood is the influence that these dynamic changes in motivational strength have on preference and action.

Our research fits with other recent studies demonstrating that motivation influences the accessibility of concepts that are related to active goals (e.g., Ferguson & Bargh, 2004; Gollwitzer, 1993; Kruglanski et al., 2002; Payne, Jacoby, & Lambert, 2005). We argue that people's expressed evaluations reflect a combination of their stored information about preferences adjusted with motivational factors that affect the accessibility of goal-related concepts. Furthermore, the motivational system affects action both by making goal-related concepts more accessible and by making information that would hinder goal pursuit less accessible (see also Fishbach et al., 2003). Hindering information is not only information that poses a conflict with goal pursuit but also information that would detract from goal pursuit because it draws attention to completely unrelated concepts.

Second, there are broad motivational influences on behavior that tune the reliance of the cognitive system on individual objects or on the relationships between objects and their environment. The causal that factors create high levels of fear of isolation and relatively interdependent self-construals (and likely other factors, such as high mortality salience; e.g., Greenberg et al., 1990; Rosenblatt, Greenberg, Solomon, Pyszczynski, & Lyon, 1989) influence individuals to attend to the relationship between objects and their context. Thus, these motivational factors have a significant influence on cognitive processing by affecting the kinds of information people process. Furthermore, because there are cultural factors that lead to chronic differences along these variables between cultures, these motivational factors also lead to cross-cultural differences in cognitive performance. Future research must explore more deeply the relationships among these motivational factors.

Acknowledgments

This research was supported by NIDA grant #1 R21 DA015211-01A1, AFOSR grant FA9550-06-1-0204, and a fellowship at the IC^2 institute to the first author. The authors thank Serge Blok, John Dennis, Micah Goldwater, Levi Larkey, Claude Messner, Lisa Narvaez, Leora Orent, and Jon Rein for helpful comments on this project.

Note

1. Higgins and his colleagues use these manipulations to induce a promotion or prevention focus. We are using the terms *approach* and *avoidance* motivation in this chapter because our results do not allow us to determine whether participants are focused on approaching positive items and avoiding negative ones or whether they are developing a sensitivity to gains and losses in a manner consistent with regulatory focus theory. Nonetheless, we do view our results as compatible with the predictions of regulatory focus theory.

References

Aarts, H., & Dijksterhuis, A. (2000). Habits as knowledge structures: Automaticity in goal-directed behavior. *Journal of Personality and Social Psychology, 78,* 53–63.

Bargh, J. A., & Chartrand, T. L. (1999). The unbearable automaticity of being. *American Psychologist, 54,* 462–479.

Bargh, J. A., Gollwitzer, P. M., Lee-Chai, A., Barndollar, K., & Trötschel, R. (2001). The automated will: Nonconscious activation and pursuit of behavioral goals. *Journal of Personality and Social Psychology, 81*(6), 1014–1027.

Bargh, J. A., & Pratto, F. (1986). Individual construct accessibility and perceptual selection. *Journal of Experimental Social Psychology, 22,* 293–311.

Baumeister, R. F., & Leary, M. R. (1995). The need to belong: Desire for interpersonal attachments as a fundamental human motivation. *Psychological Bulletin, 117,* 497–529.

Berkowitz, L., & Harmon-Jones, E. (2004). Toward an understanding of the determinants of anger. *Emotion, 4,* 107–130.

Brendl, C. M., Chattopadhyay, A., Pelham, B. W., & Carvallo, M. (2005). Name letter branding: Valence transfers when product specific needs are active. *Journal of Consumer Research, 32,* 405–415.

Brendl, C. M., & Higgins, E. T. (1996). Principles of judging valence: What makes events positive or negative. *Advances in Experimental Social Psychology, 28,* 95–160.

Brendl, C. M., Markman, A. B., & Messner, C. (2003). Devaluation of goal-unrelated choice options. *Journal of Consumer Research, 29,* 463–473.

Bruner, J. S. (1957). On perceptual readiness. *Psychological Review, 64,* 123–152.

Cabanac, M. (1971). Physiological role of pleasure. *Science, 173,* 1103–1107.

Cheng, P. W. (1997). From covariation to causation: A causal power theory. *Psychological Review, 104,* 367–405.

Cheng, P. W., & Novick, L. R. (1992). Covariation in natural causal induction. *Psychological Review, 99,* 365–382.

Cox, L. S., Tiffany, S. T., & Christin, A. G. (2001). Evaluation of the brief questionnaire of smoking urges (QSU-Brief) in laboratory and clinical settings. *Nicotine and Tobacco Research, 3,* 7–16.

Cox, W. M., Fadardi, J. S., & Pothos, E. M. (2006). The addiction-Stroop test: Theoretical considerations and procedural recommendations. *Psychological Bulletin, 132,* 443–476.

Crowe, E., & Higgins, E. T. (1997). Regulatory focus and strategic inclinations: Promotion and prevention in decision-making. *Organizational Behavior and Human Decision Processes, 69,* 117–132.

Ferguson, M. J., & Bargh, J. A. (2004). Liking is for doing: The effects of goal pursuit on automatic evaluation. *Journal of Personality and Social Psychology, 87,* 557–572.

Fikes, R. E., & Nilsson, N. J. (1971). STRIPS: A new approach to the application of theorem-proving to problem-solving. *Artificial Intelligence, 2,* 189–208.

Fishbach, A., Friedman, R. S., & Kruglanski, A. W. (2003). Leading us not into temptation: Momentary allurements elicit overriding goal activation. *Journal of Personality and Social Psychology, 84,* 296–309.

Forster, J., Liberman, N., & Higgins, E. T. (2005). Accessibility from active and fulfilled goals. *Journal of Experimental Social Psychology, 41,* 220–239.

Gardner, W. L., Gabriel, S., & Lee, A. Y. (1999). "I" value freedom, but "we" value relationships: Self-construal priming mirrors cultural differences in judgment. *Psychological Science, 10,* 321–326.

Gentner, D., & Goldin-Meadow, S. (Eds.). (2003). *Language in mind.* Cambridge, MA: MIT Press.

Gilbert, D. T., Gill, M. J., & Wilson, T. D. (2002). The future is now: Temporal correction in affective forecasting. *Organizational Behavior and Human Decision Processing, 88,* 430–444.

Gollwitzer, P. M. (1993). Goal achievement: The role of intentions. *European Review of Social Psychology, 4,* 141–185.

Greenberg, J., Pyszczynski, T., Solomon, S., Rosenblatt, A., Veeder, M., Kirkland, S., et al. (1990). Evidence for terror management theory II: The effects of mortality salience on reactions to those who threaten or bolster the cultural world view. *Journal of Personality and Social Psychology, 58,* 308–318.

Greenwald, A. G., Banaji, M. R., Rudman, L. A., Farnham, S. D., Nosek, B. A., & Mellott, D. S. (2002). A unified theory of implicit attitudes, stereotypes, self-esteem, and self-concept. *Psychological Review, 109,* 3–25.

Hartline, H. D., Wagner, H. G., & Ratcliff, F. (1956). Inhibition in the eye of the Limulus. *Journal of General Physiology, 39,* 651–673.

Herman, C. P. (1996). Human eating: Diagnosis and prognosis. *Neuroscience and Biobehavioral Reviews, 20,* 107–111.

Higgins, E. T. (1987). Self-discrepancy: A theory relating self and affect. *Psychological Review, 94,* 319–340.

Higgins, E. T. (1997). Beyond pleasure and pain. *American Psychologist, 52,* 1280–1300.

Hong, Y. Y., Chan, G., Chiu, C. Y., Wong, R. Y. M., Hansen, I. G., Lee, S. L., et al. (2003). How are social identities linked to self-conception and intergroup orientation? The moderating effect of implicit theories. *Journal of Personality and Social Psychology, 85,* 1147–1160.

Hong, Y. Y., & Chiu, C. Y. (2001). Toward a paradigm shift: From cross-cultural differences in social cognition to social-cognitive mediation of cultural differences. *Social Cognition, 19,* 181–196.

Jacoby, L. L., Lindsay, D. S., & Hessels, S. (2003). Item-specific control of automatic processes: Stroop process dissociations. *Psychonomic Bulletin and Review, 10,* 638–644.

Jones, J. T., Pelham, B. W., Carvallo, M., & Mirenberg, M. C. (2004). How do I love thee? Let me count the Js: Implicit egotism and interpersonal attraction. *Journal of Personality and Social Psychology, 87,* 665–683.

Kassel, J. D., & Shiffman, S. (1992). What can hunger teach us about drug craving? A comparative analysis of the two constructs. *Advances in Behavioural Research and Therapy, 14,* 141–167.

Kim, K., & Markman, A. B. (2006). Differences in fear of isolation as an explanation of cultural differences: Evidence from memory and reasoning. *Journal of Experimental Social Psychology, 42,* 350–364.

Kim, K., Narvaez, L. R., & Markman, A. B. (2007). Self-construal and the processing of covariation information in causal reasoning. *Memory and Cognition, 35,* 1337–1343.

Kruglanski, A. W., Shah, J. Y., Fishbach, A., Friedman, R., Chun, W. Y., & Sleeth-Keppler, D. (2002). A theory of goal systems. *Advances in Experimental Social Psychology, 34,* 331–378.

Kuhnen, U., & Oyserman, D. (2002). Thinking about the self influences thinking in general: Cognitive consequences of salient self-concept. *Journal of Experimental Social Psychology, 38,* 492–499.

Lee, A. Y., Aaker, J. L., & Gardner, W. (2000). The pleasures and pains of distinct self-construals: The role of interdependence in regulatory focus. *Journal of Personality and Social Psychology, 78,* 1122–1134.

Lewin, K. (1926). Vorsatz, Wille und Bedürfnis [Intention, will, and need]. *Psychologische Forschung, 7,* 330–385.

Loewenstein, G. (1996). Out of control: Visceral influences on behavior. *Organizational Behavior and Human Decision Processes, 65,* 272–292.

Markman, A. B., & Brendl, C. M. (2005). Goals, policies, preferences, and actions. In F. R. Kardes, P. M. Herr, & J. Nantel (Eds.), *Applying social* cognition to consumer-focused strategy (pp. 183–200). Mahwah, NJ: Lawrence Erlbaum Associates.

Markman, A. B., Brendl, C. M., & Kim, K. (2007). Preference and the specificity of goals. *Emotion, 7*(3), 680–684.

Markus, H. R., & Kitayama, S. (1991). Culture and the self: Implications for cognition, emotion, and motivation. *Psychological Review, 98,* 224–253.

Marr, D. (1982). *Vision.* New York: Freeman.

Masuda, T., & Nisbett, R. E. (2001). Attending holistically versus analytically: Comparing the context sensitivity of Japanese and Americans. *Journal of Personality and Social Psychology, 81,* 922–934.

Metcalfe, J., & Mischel, W. (1999). A hot/cool-system analysis of delay of gratification: Dynamics of willpower. *Psychological Review, 106,* 3–19.

Miller, G. A., Galanter, E., & Pribram, K. H. (1960). *Plans and the structure of behavior.* New York: Holt, Rinehart and Winston.

Nisbett, R. E., & Kanouse, D. E. (1969). Obesity, food deprivation, and supermarket shopping behavior. *Journal of Personality and Social Psychology, 12,* 289–294.

Nisbett, R. E., Peng, K., Choi, I., & Norenzayan, A. (2001). Culture and systems of thought: Holistic versus analytic cognition. *Psychological Review, 108,* 291–310.

Noelle-Neumann, E. (1984). *The spiral of silence: Public opinion, our social skin.* Chicago: University of Chicago Press.

Nuttin, J. M. (1985). Narcissism beyond Gestalt and awareness: The name letter effect. *European Journal of Social Psychology, 15,* 353–361.

Ovsiankina, M. (1928). Die Wiederaufnahme unterbrochener Handlungen [The resumption of interrupted tasks]. *Psychologische Forschung, 11,* 302–379.

Oyserman, D., Coon, H. M., & Kemmelmeier, M. (2002). Rethinking individualism and collectivism: Evaluation of theoretical assumptions and meta-analyses. *Psychological Bulletin, 128,* 3–72.

Patalano, A. L., & Seifert, C. M. (1997). Opportunistic planning: Being reminded of pending goals. *Cognitive Psychology, 34,* 1–36.

Payne, B. K., Jacoby, L. L., & Lambert, A. J. (2005). Attitudes as accessibility bias: Dissociating automatic and controlled processes. In R. R. Hassin, J. S. Uleman, & J. A. Bargh (Eds.), *The new unconscious* (pp. 393–420). New York: Oxford University Press.

Pelham, B. W., Mirenberg, M. C., & Jones, J. T. (2002). Why Susie sells seashells by the seashore: Implicit egotism and major life decisions. *Journal of Personality and Social Psychology, 82,* 469–487.

Peng, K. P., & Nisbett, R. E. (1999). Culture, dialectics, and reasoning about contradiction. *American Psychologist, 54,* 741–754.

Read, D., & van Leeuwen, B. (1998). Predicting hunger: The effects of appetite and delay on choice. *Organizational Behavior and Human Decision Processes, 76,* 189–205.

Rosenblatt, A., Greenberg, J., Solomon, S., Pyszczynski, T., & Lyon, D. (1989). Evidence for terror management theory: I. The effects of mortality salience on reactions to those who violate or uphold cultural values. *Journal of Personality and Social Psychology, 57,* 681–690.

Schulkin, J. (1991). The allure of salt. *Psychobiology, 19,* 116–121.

Shah, J. Y., & Kruglanski, A. W. (2002). Priming against your will: How accessible alternatives affect goal pursuit. *Journal of Experimental Social Psychology, 38,* 368–383.

Shah, J. Y., Kruglanski, A. W., & Friedman, R. (2003). Goal systems theory: Integrating the cognitive and motivational aspects of self-regulation. In S. J. Spencer, S. Fein, M. P. Zanna, & J. M. Olson (Eds.), *Motivated social perception: The Ontario Symposium* (Vol. 9, pp. 247–275). Mahwah, NJ: Lawrence Erlbaum Associates.

Sherman, S. J., Rose, J. S., Koch, K., Presson, C. C., & Chassin, L. (2003). Implicit and explicit attitudes toward cigarette smoking: The effects of context and motivation. *Journal of Social and Clinical Psychology, 22,* 13–39.

Smith, C. A., Haynes, K. N., Lazarus, R. S., & Pope, L. K. (1993). In search of the "hot" cognitions: Attributions, appraisals, and their relation to emotion. *Journal of Personality and Social Psychology, 65,* 916–929.

Spellman, B. A. (1996). Acting as intuitive scientists: Contingency judgments are made while controlling for alternative potential causes. *Psychological Science, 7,* 337–342.

Stroop, J. R. (1935). Studies of interference in serial verbal reactions. *Journal of Experimental Psychology, 18,* 643–662.

Tangen, J. M., & Allan, L. G. (2004). Cue interaction and judgments of causality: Contributions of causal and associative processes. *Memory and Cognition, 32,* 107–124.

Tiffany, S. T. (1990). A cognitive model of drug urges and drug-use behavior: Role of automatic and nonautomatic processes. *Psychological Review, 97,* 147–168.

Tiffany, S. T., & Conklin, C. A. (2000). A cognitive processing model of alcohol craving and compulsive alcohol use. *Addiction, 95,* S145–S154.

Watson, D., & Friend, R. (1969). Measurement of social-evaluative anxiety. *Journal of Consulting and Clinical Psychology, 33,* 448–457.

White, P. A. (1988). Causal processing: Origins and development. *Psychological Bulletin, 104,* 36–52.

Wilson, T. D., Lindsey, S., & Schooler, T. Y. (2000). A model of dual attitudes. *Psychological Review, 107,* 101–126.

The Role of Goal Systems in Self-Regulation

Arie W. Kruglanski *and* Catalina Kopetz

Abstract

This chapter discusses some of the recent goal-relevant research inspired by the social-cognitive approach. It begins by locating the contemporary goal research in the broader historical context of social-psychological theorizing about motivation and cognition. It then highlights the phenomena of goal activation, intra(goal) systemic effects, and, inter(goal) systemic effects.

Keywords: social-cognitive approach, goal activation, motivation, intrasystemic effects, intersystemic effects

Over the past 15 years, much research in social cognition has addressed goals and goal-related phenomena. The novel cognitive focus on goals as cognitive structures afforded conceptual and methodological advantages enabling new insights into classical issues. In the pages that follow, we attempt to describe and systematically discuss some of the recent goal-relevant research inspired by the social-cognitive approach.

We start by assuming a phase sequence that seems to unfold as people go about their everyday affairs. First, a goal needs to be activated by aspects of the external environment or by people's innermost associations. Typically, the goal does not come alone. It comes with an entourage of associates, including its subgoals and means of attainment. In other words, a goal system is activated, and it gives rise to goal-relevant action and its attendant outcomes. But time does not just stand still until every currently engaged objective has

been accomplished. Sooner or later, various alternative goals are likely to be activated, potentially pulling the individuals' resources away from the original activity. In accordance with the foregoing sequence of events, our discussion highlights the phenomena of goal activation, intra(goal) systemic effects, and, finally inter(goal) systemic effects. But first, by way of an introduction, we locate the contemporary goal research in the broader historical context of social-psychological theorizing about motivation and cognition.

Social Psychology and Motivational Theorizing

Despite the obvious importance of goals and goal-related phenomena for human action, until recently explicit social psychological theorizing about goals has been rather scarce (but see Ach's analysis of determination and Lewin's need theory of goal striving cited in Gollwitzer & Moskowitz,

1996). By contrast, goal concepts have been present often in cognitive models of human action. Newell, Shaw, and Simon's (1958) general problem solver model discussed means–ends relationships and a hierarchy of goals and subgoals, and G. A. Miller, Galanter, and Pribram (1960) discussed the relation between goals and plans. Nonetheless, the various cognitive models had little to say about what kinds of goals people have, how goals and goal systems develop, and how they are integrated with other aspects of human behavior. In many analyses, the organism was portrayed as a spectator rather than as a participant, as if "people only collect maps, but never go on trips" (Pervin, 1989).

Unlike the attention that cognitive psychology accorded to goal constructs, in social psychology, motivation was often contrasted with cognition. This was manifest in several major formulations and debates in social psychology. Thus, for example, the dissonance versus self-perception debate (Bem, 1972) pitted motivational (i.e., dissonance) versus cognitive (i.e., self-perception) explanations of attitude change phenomena. A similar subsequent controversy pertained to the question of whether a motivational explanation of biased causal attributions in terms of ego-defensive tendencies (cf. Kelly, 1987) is valid, given the alternative possibility of a purely cognitive explanation in terms of expectancies (D. T. Miller & Ross, 1975).

In major social psychological models of persuasion (Chen & Chaiken, 1999; Petty & Cacioppo, 1986), judgment, or impression formation (Brewer, 1988; Fiske & Neuberg, 1990; Kruglanski & Webster, 1996), distinct functions were assigned to motivational and cognitive variables. Beyond its separation from cognition, motivation has been often treated statically in social-psychological research. Specifically, individuals were classified as if in a fixed motivational state with identifiable properties. Thus, they were considered to have either a high or a low need for closure (Kruglanski & Webster, 1996; Webster & Kruglanski, 1998) or a high or a low need for cognition (Cacioppo & Petty, 1982) or to posses "learning" or "performance" goals (Dweck, 1999) assumed to systematically impact various relevant phenomena.

Yet our wishes, interests, and desires are rarely so steady or constant. Often they fluctuate from one moment to the next as we succumb to a variety of distractions, temptations, and digressions. Rather than relentlessly keeping to the task at hand, we often daydream, ruminate, or get otherwise distracted, and our shifting moods and emotional states often track our changing motivational conditions. Recently, social psychologists realized that an insight into such motivational dynamics may be gained if we abandon the separateness assumption of the "motivation" versus "cognition" program.

About 15 years ago, dating back to John Bargh's (1990) chapter on auto-motives, a fresh movement in this direction began brewing in social cognition, and it has been gathering steam ever since. It ushered in a "new look in motivation," mirroring the "new look in perception" of the late 1940s and the 1950s. The new look in perception was about how cognition is colored by motivation (Bruner, 1951). The new look in motivation is about how motivation is colored by cognition or, better yet, about motivation as (a kind of) cognition.

Although not inconsistent with the traditional approach, the new look perspective highlights very different aspects of motivational phenomena. The traditional approach targeted specific motives, neatly classified in Susan Fiske's (2003) BUCET (belonging, understanding, controlling, enhancing, and trusting) model. It paid little attention to general motivational processes.

In contrast, the new look approach pays little attention to specific motives, and it pays a great deal of attention to general processes. Furthermore, whereas the traditional approach stressed the differences between motivation and cognition, the new look stresses the commonalities. And finally, whereas the traditional approach addressed stable motivational effects (e.g., those characterizing the needs for consistency, esteem, cognition, or closure), the new look highlights motivational dynamism and flux as persons move through environments and react to them. Over the past 15 years, motivational researchers of the new look have attempted to isolate in the lab aspects of this dynamic flux that characterizes everyday living. Essentially, such flux can be discussed in terms of the following three categories: (a) goal system activation, (b) intrasystemic phenomena, and (c) intersystemic phenomena. We address each in turn.

Goal System Activation
The Allure of the Unconscious

By far, the lion's share of the new look research explored the phenomenon of goal activation. Why was this phenomenon of such an overriding interest to investigators? One possible reason was that it concerned the "when" question regarding the environmental conditions under which a given motivation will arise. A second, not mutually exclusive possibility is that its appeal derived from the mystique of the unconscious. The idea that we act without quite knowing why has fascinated psychologists since the time of Sigmund Freud to the present (e.g., Nisbett & Wilson, 1977). In this vein, recent research has indicated that people can behave, interact, and pursue their goals without knowing precisely why they are doing so or what process has put various objectives in their mind.

For instance, in research by Chartrand and Bargh (1996), participants were primed

with either an impression-formation goal (through words like "opinion," "personality," "evaluate," and "impression") or a memory goal (through words like "absorb," "retain," "remember," and "memory"). In an allegedly unrelated second experiment, they were presented a series of predicates describing behaviors suggestive of different personality traits (social, athletic, intelligent, and religious). Participants were then given a surprise recall test. Those primed with the impression-formation goal clustered their recall more than did participants primed with the goal of memorization, just as did participants in the Hamilton, Katz, and Leirer (1980) study, where corresponding goals were induced via explicit instructions.

More interestingly yet, unconscious goal activation may lead to goal-related behavior. Bargh, Gollwitzer, Lee-Chai, Barndollar, and Trötschel (2001) primed participants (via a word-search task) with achievement-related words ("succeed," "strive," "attain," and "achieve") or with cooperation words ("helpful," "support," "honest," "cooperative," and "friendly"). Both types of priming led to goal-relevant behaviors (greater achievement and greater cooperation) on a subsequent task without the participants' exhibiting awareness of the relation between the priming and the performance tasks. Other studies have been obtaining the same results: Unconscious goal activation leads to goal pursuit and to appropriate emotional reactions if the pursuit goes well or poorly (e.g., Shah, Friedman, & Kruglanski, 2002; Shah & Kruglanski, 2002, 2003).

As Bargh (2005) aptly noted, one reason why these effects seem so magical is our fundamental belief in our free will. Typically, people have the subjective experience of making a choice or forming an intention and then enacting the decision via behavior. They often take this as evidence of the causal relationship between their intention and the behavior. However, even though freedom of will may be thought of as acting in accordance with one's intentions, formation of these intentions may often be under external stimulus control.

In short, there are reasons to believe then the current fascination with the new look approach has to do with the unconscious nature of many of the observed effects. This fits well with the general Zeitgeist in social psychology these days that focuses on the unconscious (for a comprehensive review, see Hassin, Uleman, & Bargh, 2005). Beyond mere Zeitgeist, the unconscious has a great deal of cachet and mystique of its own. It evokes Freud's theorizing that had such a profound impact on our culture. However, although visionary, Freud's work rested on a questionable empirical basis. By contrast, the current new look approach is rigorously empirical. It thus provides a strong scientific antidote to the rationalism still popular in the social sciences (rational choice theory) in which conscious deliberation and intelligent choice have been a mainstay.

Diverse Sources of Goal Activation

What kinds of stimuli can activate a goal? A better question is, What kinds of stimuli cannot? Indeed, research has uncovered a wide diversity of activation sources. Semantic associates may activate a goal (Bargh et al., 2001; Chartrand & Bargh, 1996), as noted earlier. Specific person concepts (e.g., mother, father, and friend) who have a given goal for an individual may also activate it (Fitzsimons & Bargh, 2003; Shah, 2003a, 2003b). Priming by specific persons who have a given goal for themselves may activate it in others, thus producing a goal contagion (Aarts, Gollwitzer, & Hassin, 2004; see Chapter 22).

A means may activate the corresponding goal in a bottom-up fashion (Berkowitz &

LePage, 1967; Shah & Kruglanski, 2003). An opportunity to pursue a goal may activate it. In this vein, Shah and Kruglanski (2003) found that priming an opportunity to show one's capacity for "functional thinking"[1] substantially interfered with participants' pursuit of a current task of anagram solution.

Idiosyncrasy

In principle, any construct linked in an individual's mind to a goal will tend to activate it. Many such linkages are common to most individuals sharing the same culture and are based on general notions concerning norms of goal attainment (e.g., most Americans would associate the attainment of food with shopping at a grocery store). To some extent, however, the history of prior linkages may differ for different individuals. For instance, Chen, Lee-Chai, and Bargh (2001) argued that people with an exchange orientation associate power with self-oriented goals, whereas people with a communal orientation[2] associate power with goals of responsiveness to others' needs. Accordingly, priming the concept of power led "exchange-oriented" participants to allow more time for themselves in solving exercises, whereas "communal" participants under the same circumstances allowed less time for themselves.

In summary, goal activation research suggests that (a) goals can operate without individuals' awareness of their source of activation, (b) diverse stimuli previously associated with a goal can activate it, and (c) these associations are idiosyncratic. Thus, very different stimuli can activate the same goal for different persons, and the same stimulus can activate different goals for different persons. In principle, any concept could activate a goal for some people under some circumstances. Whereas the word "table" may sound neutral enough, it could activate an achievement goal for an aspiring carpenter hoping to make wonderful tables or for a gambler hoping to make a fortune at a baccarat table.

Intrasystemic Phenomena

Evidence reviewed previously in this chapter suggests that once they have been automatically activated, goals are automatically pursued. This is presumably possible because goals are cognitively associated with their corresponding means of attainment. Consequently, the activation of goals is transmitted to their corresponding behavioral plans (Aarts & Dijksterhuis, 2000; Bargh, 1990; Kruglanski et al., 2002), propelling one to action. In the following sections, we consider such intrasystemic effects pertaining to goal–means relations and their implications for goal-directed behavior and affect.

Mimicry or Means Suggestion?

An intriguing intrasystemic phenomenon is behavioral mimicry represented by the finding that under some conditions people may unwittingly (and unconsciously) adopt a way of doing things activated by an unrelated concept or event. We are referring here to what Dijksterhuis and Bargh (2001) described as "the perception-behavior expressway." Their idea was that a "mere" perception of a behavior leads to a predisposition or a tendency toward imitation (Chartrand, Maddux, & Lakin, 2005; Dijksterhuis & Bargh, 2001). Thus, in research by Bargh, Chen, and Burrows (1996), participants primed with words related to rudeness ("rude," "impolite," and "obnoxious") were more likely to interrupt a conversation than those primed with neutral words, whereas participants primed with politeness words showed the least tendency to interrupt the conversation. Similarly, participants primed with words related to the elderly stereotype walked more slowly when provided the opportunity to do so.

In related work, people behaved with greater hostility after being primed with the African American stereotype versus the White stereotype (Chen & Bargh, 1997) and performed significantly better on a Trivial Pursuit task when primed with the "professor" versus the "hooligan" stereotype (Dijksterhuis & van Knippenberg, 1998). Such a tendency to mimic the behaviors of others has been viewed as a consequence of the way humans are constituted, reflecting perhaps an evolutionary-based propensity toward a herd mentality. Like the chameleon that changes its colors to blend or fit in with its physical environment, people unwittingly change their mannerism and behaviors to blend in with their social environments (Chartrand et al., 2005).

Chartrand et al. (2005) hypothesized that mimicry may constitute an "unidentified strategy in the repertoire of behaviors that help people get along with others." In this vein, Chartrand and Bargh (1999, study 2) showed that when a confederate mimicked the posture and mannerism of the participant during an interaction, participants liked the confederate better and perceived the interaction as unfolding more smoothly than when the confederate did not mimic the participants.

Behavioral mimicry has been showed to have other benefits as well. Van Baaren, Holland, and Steenaert (2003) have showed that waitresses who mimicked their customers either verbally or physically received larger tips than waitresses who did not use mimicry. Moreover, participants mimicked by the experimenter in an alleged marketing study were more likely to engage in a prosocial behavior (picking up pens that were accidentally dropped by the experimenter) than participants who had not been so mimicked (van Baaren, Holland, Kawakami, & van Knippenberg, 2004).

These results speak to the instrumentality of unconscious imitation, suggesting that mimicry constitutes a means to a better social fit. However, it is possible that mimicry represents a broader sense of means suggestion. Priming an event or perceiving others may suggest that a way of doing things—that is, a "means" that, when coupled with an appropriate goal, such as expressing oneself in a conversation or walking—is mindlessly adopted. Consistent with this way of reasoning, Dijksterhuis and van Knippenberg (1998) suggested that the prime must trigger behaviors beneficial to performance on the subsequent task (more effort and smarter solving strategies). When the suggested behavior is incompatible with the current behavioral goals and hence is noninstrumental to their pursuit, mimicry is significantly reduced. For instance, Macrae and Johnston (1998) showed that priming participants with "helpfulness" increased their tendency to help a confederate who dropped a number of objects. But when they were told that they were running late and had to hurry to the next experimental session, the goal of "hurry" overruled the priming effect.

It also seems plausible that individuals would be less likely to adopt a suggested means, that is, to engage in mimicry to the extent that they already possessed in their repertoire a highly accessible means to the objective in question. If so, one could "immunize" individuals against means suggestion by equipping them in advance with a strongly accessible alternative means. One could also explore whether goal importance matters and whether a mindless adoption of suggested means is not restricted to relatively trivial goals about whose manner of pursuit one "does not" care much. Alternatively, one could investigate whether individuals under high need for closure, known to "snap at" or "seize and freeze" on whatever happens to be activated, show an augmented chameleon effect. These possibilities could be fruitfully explored in subsequent research.

Emotional Transfer

Linkages between goals and means can vary in strength. Such strength can be inferred from the speed of activating the means by the corresponding goal prime. Fishbach, Shah, and Kruglanski (2004) recently explored whether such association strength moderates the transfer from the goal to the means of various motivational properties, such as degree of commitment and the magnitude and quality of affect.

In one study (Fishbach et al., 2004, study 1), the degree of correspondence was measured between emotional commitment to the goal and to the means as a function of their association strength. Participants listed two attribute goals that they were striving to attain (e.g., being intelligent, happy, or beautiful) and listed one activity that they believed could help them attain each attribute (e.g., study, party, or diet, respectively). To assess association strength, participants were subliminally primed with the goals (or control words) and performed a lexical decision task with the activities (i.e., the means) as lexical targets. Then they rated the emotions they felt when thinking about possessing the attribute and the emotions they felt when engaging in the activity. Fishbach et al. found that the correlation between the magnitude of affect associated with participants' goals (e.g., a goal of becoming educated) and the magnitude of affect associated with a corresponding means (e.g., a means of studying) depended on the strength of the goal–means association as assessed by the priming task.

The notion of transfer suggests that the very same activity or means can be experienced differently depending on the goal with which it happens to be associated. Participants in one study (Fishbach et al., 2004, study 2) were primed either with the goal of weight watching or of food enjoyment or with no goal at all (control condition). They then rated the extent to which they experienced positive and negative emotions when they ate (a) vegetables, (b) fruits, (c) chocolate, (d) cake, (e) fries, and (f) hamburgers. The low-calorie food was experienced equally positively in the weight-watching, control, and food enjoyment conditions. But the high-calorie food was associated with less positive emotions in the weight-watching compared to the control condition and with the most positive emotions in the food enjoyment condition.

DYNAMIC TRANSFER OR SCHEMA-TRIGGERED AFFECT

The foregoing analysis assumes that an affective investment in the goal is transferred to one's own means of attainment. But it could also be that the previously described results attest to a semantic phenomenon of a schema-triggered affect. In other words, the goal category may be affectively charged, and this affect may spread to all the constructs with which this category happens to be associated. To tease apart the semantic and motivational interpretations of transfer, the degree of transfer occurring between one's goals and one's personal means of attainment was compared to the degree of transfer from the same goals to equally strongly associated other people's means. Participants rated their commitment to three common goals (keeping in shape, traveling, and studying) and listed either an activity that they typically pursue or an activity that other people typically pursue to attain that particular goal. The results showed, first, that personal and general means were equally strongly associated with the goals. Second, consistent with the transfer hypothesis, greater positive affect to the personal means was manifested by participants with greater (versus lesser) commitment to the corresponding goal. However, no significant relation was obtained between commitment to the goal and affect toward other people's means. These findings are consistent with the portrayal of goal systems as dynamic (rather than merely semantic) configurations.

TRANSFER OF AFFECTIVE QUALITY

Not only the magnitude but also the quality of affect may be capable of transfer from goals to means. In one study (Fishbach et al., 2004, study 3), participants listed either an "ought" goal or an "ideal" goal. Higgins's (1987, 1997) research suggests that attainment of ought goals gives rise to such emotions as relief, calm, and relaxation. By contrast, attainment of ideal goals gives rise to the emotions of happiness, pride, or enjoyment.

Participants then listed three acquaintances believed instrumental to attainment of either an ideal or an ought goal (i.e., to constitute "social means" to the goal in question). Following Higgins, King, and Mavin (1982), we assumed that the order in which the acquaintances are listed reflects the strength of their association to the goal. Participants then rated their expected emotions following goal attainment using three items related to ideal-type affect (i.e., happy, proud, and enjoy) and three items related to ought-type affect (i.e., relieved, calm, and relaxed). It was found that the affective qualities associated with ideal or ought goals were transferred to individuals related to these goals' attainment and that the degree of transfer was proportionate to the order in which these persons were listed. Thus, for an ideal-type goal, ideal-type affect and not an ought-type affect felt with respect to the first person listed was more pronounced than ideal-type affect felt with regard to the second person listed, which in turn was more pronounced than the ideal-type affect felt with respect to the third person listed. Similarly, for the ought-type goal, the corresponding (ought-type) affect and not the ideal-type affect was stronger with respect to the first two persons listed than with respect to the third person listed.

Equifinality Phenomena

Intriguing psychological phenomena are posed by the equifinality configuration in which several different means are linked to the same goal. We consider these in turn.

CHOICE

One such phenomenon concerns choice between the different means. How is such choice effected, particularly if the means are truly equifinal, that is, equally instrumental with regard to goal attainment? Chun, Kruglanski, Sleeth-Keppler, and Friedman (2005) recently explored the possibility that the choice of means would be guided by the principle of multifinality whereby, in addition to the focal goal, the chosen means would also appear to serve other active goals, increasing one's bang for the buck as it were. For instance, the means of terrorism, in addition to appearing to serve an organization's political goals, may also serve the members' emotional goals of wreaking vengeance on an enemy (Kruglanski & Fishman, 2006; see also Chapter 16).

Whereas the bang-for-the-buck principle makes a lot of sense and seems quite rational, some multifinality-driven choices appear to occur without the chooser's awareness of the goal he or she is pursuing. For instance, in Wilson and Nisbett's (1978) classic research, passersby at a department store chose among four different nightgowns of similar quality or among four identical pairs of nylon stockings. A strong position effect was found such that the two rightmost objects in the array were heavily overchosen. Yet participants seemed entirely unconscious of their bias. Instead, they justified their choices exclusively in terms of the quality of the choice objects (the nightgowns or the stockings). Chun et al. (2005) hypothesized that the choice of

the rightmost object was multifinal, satisfying not only the focal goal of choosing the best-quality items, a goal that would have been gratified equally well by any object in the array, but also a background goal of reaching quick closure after inspecting the entire array from left to right.

To explore this possibility, Chun et al. (2005) conceptually replicated Wilson and Nisbett's (1978) study with one modification. Participants' focal goal was kept constant while manipulating the presumptive background goal of closure. Participants were given the (focal) goal of choosing among four pairs of (actually) identical athletic socks, the pair that was of the best quality. To manipulate the background goal of closure, participants in one condition were placed under time pressure (Kruglanski, 2004; Kruglanski, Pierro, Mannetti, & DeGrada, 2006; Kruglanski & Webster, 1996; Webster & Kruglanski, 1998). In another condition, participants were not placed under pressure, and they were given accuracy instructions intended to reduce their need for closure (Kruglanski & Webster, 1996). If the multifinality analysis is correct, the rightward bias should replicate in the time-pressure condition and be reduced or eliminated in the accuracy condition. This is precisely what happened: 81% of participants in the time-pressure (need for closure) condition chose the two rightmost choices, replicating Wilson and Nisbett (1978). By contrast, only 33% of participants in the accuracy condition made these rightmost choices.

In both the Wilson and Nisbett (1978) and the Chun et al. (2005) study, the various means presented (the stockings and the socks) were equally instrumental to the focal goal, hence truly equifinal. In a following study by Chun et al. (2005), these authors showed that *if* the means differed in their instrumentality, the power of the background goals would be overridden. In other words, if one of the means choices was more instrumental to the focal goal than to the background goal, whereas another was more instrumental to the background than to the focal goal, a "focal override" would take place, and the means more instrumental to the focal goal would be selected, sacrificing the background goal.

The hypothesis that unconscious goal states may influence one's choices in different circumstances based on the principle of multifinality was further explored in a study conducted by Sleeth-Keppler (2005). In the study designed to test these notions, Winthrop University students were asked to make a choice between two identical sheets of construction paper, one dyed in the primary school color (garnet) and one dyed in blue (control color). Prior to making the choice, they were subliminally primed with either a school identification or a disidentification goal. Next, the goal of self-affirmation was manipulated following the procedure employed by Cohen, Aronson, and Steele (2000). Assuming that the act of identifying or disidentifying with a group subserves the higher-order goal of self-affirmation, one could argue that fulfilling that goal in a manner unrelated to group identification should decrease participants' need to identify/disidentify with their group via a goal-consistent product choice.

In line with the predictions, 80% of participants in the Winthrop identification condition chose the garnet-colored paper when no alternative means to affirm the self was provided to them (i.e., in the no-affirmation control condition). This pattern of results was perfectly reversed when the Winthrop disidentification goal was primed and no alternative self-affirmation opportunity was provided. Quite a different pattern of results emerged in the affirmation condition. Only 30.8% of the participants chose the garnet-colored sheet in the identification condition, whereas in the disidentification condition, 41.7% of participants chose the garnet-colored sheet after affirming the self.

Again, without exception, participants justified their choices in terms of the focal goal of choosing the highest-quality paper: "the red piece of paper felt sturdier and looked much less grainy than the blue one," "the paper looked smoother and of higher quality," and so on.

MULTIFINALITY AND NEED FOR CLOSURE

Beyond the bang for the buck it affords, multifinality could be appealing for another reason as well, specifically because it eliminates the unnerving ambiguity of having one's alternative goal pursuits suspended while pursuing a current focal goal. Persons who are high on the need for closure should be particularly unnerved by such an ambiguity. Hence, such individuals should exhibit a particularly pronounced preference for multifinal means. Chun and Kruglanski (2005) obtained consistent support for this hypothesis in a series of studies. Participants high (versus low) on need for closure reported that they (a) expected to attain more goals through the use of computers, (b) exhibited a stronger preference for a multifinal over a unifinal camera even though the unifinal one was of a higher quality, (c) exhibited a stronger preference for a multifinal over a unifinal cell phone even though the multifinal one was much more expensive, and (d) reported greater use of a multifinal soap (for both the face and the body) versus two separate soaps, one for the face and the other for the body. These findings were echoed by the results of Sleeth-Keppler (2005) that (e) high- versus low-need-for-closure individuals prefer multifinal friends (i.e., "friends for all seasons" who gratify multiple needs over unifinal friends relevant to one type of need only).

SUBSTITUTION

A particularly interesting feature of equifinality is the possibility of substituting one means for another in the case of failure or thwarting of goal pursuit via the initial means. The problem of substitution is fundamental to social and personality psychology, as witnessed by the attention it received from Freud (1961), who introduced the notion of symptom substitution, and from Lewin (1935), who discussed the notion of substitute tasks. But there has been little work on the mechanism of substitution as such (but see Tesser, Martin, & Cornell, 1996).

Equifinality Set Size and Commitment to Goals and Means

The possibility of substitution should increase people's tendency to commit to a given goal by increasing the expectancy of goal attainment (if not one way, then another). In other words, the larger the equifinality set size, the more subjectively likely should be goal attainment and hence the stronger should be the tendency to adopt the goal and commit to it. Pierro (2005) recently carried out a series of studies designed to address this problem. In one of the studies, participants—investment consultants in a large financial company in Rome—were asked to list two work goals they would be trying to attain in the next 6 months (they listed goals such as the acquisition of new clients and increasing the value of one's portfolio) and either a single means (e.g., use a mailing list or teamwork) or three separate means for attaining these goals. Pierro found that in the three- versus the one-means condition, participants exhibited weaker commitment to the first means but a stronger commitment to the goal. As expected, this effect was mediated by the greater likelihood of goal attainment in the three- versus the one-means condition.

Framing Linkages

Recent evidence suggests that equifinality configurations do not necessitate an extensive history of associations; instead, they may be established momentarily by framing. Shah and Kruglanski (2002) framed two instances of anagram solution as relating either to the same (promotion or prevention) goal or to different goals in which one instance of the activity was linked to a prevention goal and the other to a promotion goal. Participants then completed two different anagram tasks (each with its own promotion or prevention contingency).

It was found that failure at the first task increased performance on the second task if both had the same regulatory focus framing but not when they had different regulatory focus framing. Assuming that increased performance reflects investment of efforts in an activity, these results suggest that when two tasks are framed as connected to the same goal, failure on one increases efforts invested in the other—attesting to substitution. These investigators also found that success at the first task decreased performance on the second when it had the same (versus the different) regulatory focus framing, attesting that substitution was no longer pertinent when the objective was attained via the first means.

The "False-Proxy" Effect

As Pierro's (2005) results demonstrate, one psychological downside of equifinality is a decreased commitment to a particular means as a function of the number of means. A different intriguing downside can be labeled the "false-proxy" effect. It arises when an irrelevant activity is mistakenly substituted for a primary means with adverse consequences for subsequent goal pursuit. Along these lines, Pfeffer and Sutton (2000) discussed an organizational phenomenon wherein meetings, presentations, or committee reports are mistaken for actual action or goal progress. Pfeffer and Sutton (2000) called this "substituting talk for action."

A fascinating social-psychological phenomenon where a similar thing may be occurring concerns the psychology of promises. Consider the familiar "promises-of-the-moment" phenomenon. A friend promises one to do something or other yet fails to deliver on one's promise. This usually evokes a disappointed reaction, and one might begin to question the sincerity of the promise, the friend's moral fiber, or his or her commitment to oneself. But it is possible that the promise was not followed through precisely because it was sincere, which allowed it to be mistaken for actual goal pursuit. It could be, in other words, that for some of the people, some of the time, promises actually reduce the likelihood of action. Obviously, this could not be so universally. Some promises, after all, increase one's commitment to the promised activity. Thus, the challenge is to identify the moderators of the promises-of-the-moment effect. For instance, under cognitive load or need for closure, individuals might mistake promises for action simply because of inadequate processing resources. Similarly, high locomotors may want to believe that they have locomoted and hence be more likely to misidentify promises for actions and so on. A systematic pursuit of these issues could be profitably undertaken in future research.

Inference of Goal Progress

The false-proxy effect assumes that the experience of goal progress is an inference that occasionally could be erroneous. Intriguing evidence for this assumption has been furnished recently by Fishbach and Dhar (2005). While recognizing that the progress one is making toward a goal provides useful regulatory feedback regarding one's discrepancy from the ideal goal state (Carver, Scheier, Higgins, & Sorrentino, 1990), the investigators showed that sometimes this regulatory feedback may also justify disengagement with a goal. Fishbach and Dhar manipulated participants' inferred progress toward various goals and measured their subsequent tendency to pursue those goals versus turning to alternative objectives. Thus, in one study, progress toward the goal of a svelte figure was manipulated by asking dieters how far off they were from their ideal weight on a scale with either 5 pounds or 25 pounds as end points. The latter scale was assumed to lead dieters to believe that they had made sufficient progress since the same discrepancy from an ideal weight (e.g., of 4 pounds) would appear smaller with the wider, 25-pound scale than with the narrower, 5-pound scale. The tendency to pursue the dieting goal versus the food enjoyment goal was assessed by having participants choose a chocolate bar versus an apple as a parting gift. Consistent with the inferred progress hypothesis, 85% of participants in the wide-scale condition chose a chocolate bar over an apple, whereas only 58% did so in the narrow-scale condition.

In another study, university students were asked how much time they spent on their course work during the past day. They completed their answers on a survey form that was previously completed by a fictitious participant whose responses, while erased, were still quite visible. This fictitious respondent listed either 30 minutes—evincing a low standard, suggesting that the amount of time participants invested (e.g., 2 hours) represented considerable progress—or 5 hours—representing a high standard and suggesting that participants' time investment did not represent much progress. Indeed, participants in the low-standard condition reported greater interest in nonacademic activities (i.e., alternative goals) than those in the high-standard condition. This difference was mediated by perceived academic progress that was greater in the low- versus the high-standard condition. As a whole, then, the results of various studies indicate that substitution depends on the inference of goal progress. If such inference is low, substitution to other equifinal means will take place. If it is high, there will be a tendency to move on to alternative objectives.

To summarize, the research described in this section demonstrates the psychological importance of various intrasystemic goal phenomena. People may mimic others as a way of adopting other people's way of doing things, perceived as instrumental to various goals. The strength of associations between goals and means facilitates the transfer of various motivational properties related to the goal (such as magnitude and quality of affect) to the means in question. Finally, the number of means attached to a goal determines the amount of available choice between means and the range of substitutability of one means for possible others.

Intersystemic Phenomena
Goal Pull and Goal Shielding

The tendency to switch to alternative goals on an inference of goal progress (Fishbach & Dhar, 2005) invites the third and final section of this chapter: the realm of intersystemic phenomena. We rarely have the luxury of pursuing a single goal in isolation. More typically, various alternative goals are activated by our incessant stream of associations and by the various social and physical environments through which we locomote. Such alternative goals can pull resources away from the focal goal, and individuals may learn to shield the focal goals from unwanted interference by these rival alternatives.

Along these lines, it has been found in several studies (e.g., Shah & Kruglanski, 2002) that introducing an alternative goal undermined participants' commitment to the focal goal, hampered progress toward that goal, hindered the development of effective means

for goal pursuit, and dampened participants' emotional responses to positive and negative feedback about goal progress. In one of Shah and Kruglanski's (2002) studies, participants expected to perform two consecutive tasks, the first of which consisted of anagram solution. While working toward this focal goal, participants were subliminally primed with the second task they expected to perform later (operationally defined as the alternative goal) or with a control phrase. Commitment to the focal goal was assessed through persistence on the first task, performance success, and extent of affective reactivity to success and failure feedback. These measures of commitment showed substantial decline in the alternative goal-priming (versus control) condition. In other words, the activation of alternative goals may pull away attentional resources from the focal goal, in turn undermining commitment to such goal.

In another series of studies, Shah et al. (2002) found that activation of a given focal goal results in an inhibition of alternative goals reflected in the slowing down of lexical decision times to such goals. For instance, when a goal (versus a control word) served as a prime, this increased the lexical decision times to the alternative goals (versus control words), attesting to their inhibition, the magnitude of such inhibition being positively related to participants' commitment to the focal goal they were currently pursuing.

Overcoming Temptations
ACTIVATION PATTERNS

As the Shah et al. (2002) studies demonstrate, commitment to the focal, currently pursued goal matters, but what about commitment to alternative goals whose pursuit may be undermined by pursuit of the focal goal? In fact, successful self-regulators may have learned to spontaneously activate rather than inhibit high-commitment alternative goals undermined by pursuit of a current focal goal. We are referring here to a strategy of overcoming temptations (i.e., currently active low-commitment goals) by immediately activating the high-commitment goals with which they are in conflict.

In one of the studies by Fishbach, Friedman, and Kruglanski (2003), University of Maryland undergraduates who, by their own admission, were either successful or unsuccessful academically performed a lexical decision task after first being exposed to a subliminal prime. On some trials, the primes related to temptations to avoid studying, such as "television," "procrastinate," "phone," and "Internet," and target words related to the goal of studying, such as "study," "grades," "homework," and "graduate." On other trials, the study words were the primes and the temptation words the lexical targets. The results showed that, for successful students, temptation words activated study words to a significantly greater extent than vice versa. By contrast, for the unsuccessful students, study words activated temptation words to a greater extent than vice versa.

EVALUATION PATTERNS

Beyond such goal-activation patterns, the dynamics of overcoming temptations may include automatic shifts in evaluation. Along these lines, Fishbach et al. (2003) has shown that committed (versus less committed) self-regulators may have learned to place more positive evaluations on their high-importance goals and more negative evaluations on the temptation goals. In one of Fishbach et al.'s (2003) studies, participants listed high-importance goals ("an activity you feel it is your duty or obligation to work on") and temptations (defined as "an enjoyable activity that you ought not to do if you want to fulfill your duties and obligations"). Self-regulatory success was assessed in an allegedly unrelated study where participants reported their tendency to engage in each of their specific temptations. Then participants completed an affective priming procedure with their high-importance goals and temptations as subliminal primes and various positive and negative concepts as lexical targets. Successful self-regulators categorized more quickly positive targets following goal primes than following temptation primes and more slowly negative targets following goal primes than following temptation primes. No similar Prime × Target interaction was obtained for the less successful self-regulators.

Crowding Out Effects and Equifinality Set Size

Often the presence of alternative goals implies the need to exercise goal choice. Indeed, all the intersystemic effects discussed so far entailed a choice reflected in an inhibition of one of the goals. However, choice might not be necessary if multifinal means could be found that afforded the attainment of both (or more) of the activated goals. Such a solution should be generally preferable to individuals because it affords "eating one's cake and having it too," representing the "best of possible worlds" as it were.

But how can such quest for multifinal means be observed? Kopetz, Fishbach, and Kruglanski (2005) made two assumptions. Our first assumption states that the presence (versus absence) of alternative goals should reduce the equifinality set size (number of means perceived as appropriate) to the focal goal because the alternative goals should constrain the means to the focal goal and restrict them to a subset of means multifinal to both goals. We refer to a possible multifinality-driven restriction in the means set size (to the focal goal) as the "crowding-out" effect. Our second assumption states that the greater the commitment to the focal goal, the more the alternative goals are inhibited (Shah et al., 2002). This should remove (or relax) the multifinality constraints imposed by the alternative goal such that no reduction in the number of means should be observed anymore.

In an initial study testing these notions, participants at the food court at the University of Maryland Student Union were approached during lunch hour. Not surprisingly, they all stated that their goal was to have lunch. In one condition, we asked them to list three other goals that they had for that day. This represented the alternative-goals condition. In the no-alternatives condition, we asked them to list three goals that they had already accomplished that day. Such accomplished goals were assumed to have lost their constraining potential or, in Lewinian terms, to have their "tension system" drained. Participants then rated the extent to which they were interested in each of seven types of food available at the food court. Compared to participants in the control (no-alternatives) condition, those for whom actual (rather than accomplished) goal alternatives were activated listed significantly fewer foods in which they were interested.

These findings, although consistent with the crowding-out hypothesis, do not explore its more specific implications. To get at these, in the next study we manipulated the degree of multifinality constraints imposed by the alternative goals by varying the degree to which the two goals were perceived as related to each other. The reasoning behind this study was that if the focal goal and the alternative goal were perceived as related, the multifinality constraint imposed by the alternative goal would be weaker or easier to gratify. Consequently, the prediction was that the reduction in the number of means generated would be less extensive when the alternative goal was related versus unrelated to the focal goal. Indeed, the results revealed that participants expecting to work on two unrelated tasks (versus two

related tasks or one single task) generated significantly fewer means to the focal task. Moreover, participants in the related-task condition also generated a greater number of multifinal means. Finally, participants in the unrelated-task condition found the generation of means more difficult, and perceived difficulty mediated the number of generated means across conditions.

Whereas in the first two studies in this series the focal goal was kept constant (hunger) and what varied was the presence (or kind) of the alternative goals, in the third study the alternative goal was kept constant, and commitment to the focal goal was varied. The alternative goal common to all participants was keeping a healthy diet. The focal goal was eating, and commitment to eating was manipulated by priming participants during midday hours with eating-related words (such as "lunch," "food," and "eat") or neutral words. Participants made hungrier through the priming manipulation expressed interest in a greater variety of foods (as means to the focal goal of eating) and in a lesser proportion of multifinal foods. Finally, participants in the hungrier condition evinced slower reaction times, indicative of inhibition, to diet-related words.

The intersystemic phenomena considered previously refer to one of the fundamental challenges of everyday life: that of coordinating our significant and often conflicting pursuits. Such a challenge comes from the fact that goal pursuit is resource dependent and that attentional and energetic resources are limited. Thus, the greater the investment of resources in pursuit of a given goal, the less resources should be available for alternative goals. As a consequence, currently active goals may pull resources away from each other. It follows that the ability to inhibit alternative goals, especially those of lesser importance, confers clear self-regulatory advantages allowing one to concentrate resources on current pursuits. Indeed, our findings indicate people are capable of shielding their focal goal from alternative goals and to resist temptations by activating higher-priority goals threatened by such temptations. As Emmons (1996) noted, however, creative integration of one's strivings may be possible that would remove the detrimental effects of goal conflict on goal commitment, task performance, and affective experience. In the same vein, Cantor and Fleeson (1991, 1994) argued that people "tune" their goal pursuits in an attempt to find the most suitable solutions under their personal circumstances. Consistent with these ideas, we have seen that the conflict introduced by the simultaneous presence of multiple goals may be avoided via multifinal means affording the joint pursuit of the conflicting goals. Indeed, we have seen that people may react to constraints from multiple goals by initiating a search for multifinal means.

Concluding Comments

In this chapter, we attempted a selective overview of a novel research movement in social cognition, adopting a cognitive approach to motivational phenomena. This approach explores the mental representation of motivational constructs focusing specifically on notions of goals and means. Because of space limitations, our review was partial by necessity. Numerous further studies on these topics have been conducted, and excitement about the new "goal psychology" is far from waning. In a large measure, such excitement stems from the realization that our activities are driven often by factors outside of informed deliberation and conscious choice. Our actions originate in our goals. These, in turn, are activated by our internal stream of associations or by external stimuli with which we happen to come into contact. Furthermore, even after a given goal has been adopted,

our choice of means might be dictated by multifinality considerations operating outside of conscious awareness.

Despite the considerable amount of research that has been already carried out on goal-systemic phenomena, much of this conceptual territory remains uncharted. For instance, further work is needed to elucidate the phenomena of substitution (their conditions of occurrence and their implications), multifinality, relations between focal and background goals, and so on. Of particular interest are the processes underlying goal-systemic effects. How is goal value monitored? How are goal–means associations formed? How are processing resources managed? How is means activation translated into implementation intentions (Gollwitzer, 1999)? Answers to these questions would contribute much to our understanding of the dynamics of actions as people carry on their daily behaviors and react to the environments through which they move.

On the conceptual front, the recent developments in goal psychology usher in a new era in our understanding of the relations between motivation and cognition. Early on in the history of the cognitive revolution, motivation, if not ignored or denied, was at best tolerated as a poor relative, an "ugly duckling" among the "swans," of *encoding, inference, memory, priming,* or *categorization.* It is not as if the cognitively oriented researchers did not realize at some level that motivation matters. Rather, motivation was neglected because motivational constructs were alien to the cognitive idiom and did not fit the cognitive paradigm. Consequently, they were difficult to reconcile with the cognitive models. Rather, one had to tack them as the external appendages whose working derived from different premises, foreign to the principles of human cognition. The new goal psychology removes these paradigmatic obstacles, affording a true cognitive/motivational integration. It allows motivation to emerge as a full-fledged (social cognitive) swan rather than the ugly duckling of yesteryear.

Notes

1. An object-use task that required participants to generate as many different uses as possible for common objects was described as diagnostic of functional thinking.

2. A communal relationship is one in which the parties are concerned about each other's needs, whereas an exchange relationship is based on a tit-for-tat reciprocity.

References

Aarts, H., & Dijksterhuis, A. (2000). Habits as knowledge structures: Automaticity in goal-directed behavior. *Journal of Personality and Social Psychology, 78*,(1), 53–63.

Aarts, H., Gollwitzer, P. M., & Hassin, R. R. (2004). Goal contagion: Perceiving is for pursuing. *Journal of Personality and Social Psychology, 87*(1), 23–37.

Bargh, J. A. (1990). Auto-motives: Preconscious determinants of social interaction. In E. T. Higgins, & R. M. Sorrentino (Eds.), *Handbook of motivation and cognition: Foundations of social behavior* (Vol. 2, pp. 93–130). New York: Guilford Press.

Bargh, J. A. (2005). Bypassing the will: Toward demystifying the nonconscious control of social behavior. In R. R. Hassin, J. S. Uleman, & J. A. Bargh (Eds.), *The new unconscious* (pp. 37–58). New York: Oxford University Press.

Bargh, J. A., Chen, M., & Burrows, L. (1996). Automaticity of social behavior: Direct effects of trait construct and stereotype activation on action. *Journal of Personality and Social Psychology, 71*(2), 230–244.

Bargh, J. A., Gollwitzer, P. M., Lee-Chai, A., Barndollar, K., & Trötschel, R. (2001). The automated will: Nonconscious activation and pursuit of behavioral goals. *Journal of Personality and Social Psychology, 81*(6), 1014–1027.

Bem, D. J. (1972). Self-perception theory. In L. Berkowitz (Ed.), *Advances in experimental social psychology* (Vol. 6, pp. 1–62). New York: Academic Press.

Berkowitz, L., & LePage, A. (1967). Weapons as aggression-eliciting stimuli. *Journal of Personality and Social Psychology, 7*, 202–207.

Brewer, M. B. (1988). A dual process model of impression formation. In T. K. Srull & R. S. Wyer (Eds.), *Advances in social cognition* (Vol. 1, pp. 1–36). Hillsdale, NJ: Lawrence Erlbaum Associates.

Bruner, J. S. (1951). Personality dynamics and the process of perceiving. In R. R. Blake, & G. V. Ramsey (Eds.), *Perception: An approach to personality* (pp. 121–147). Oxford: Ronald Press.

Cacioppo, J. T., & Petty, R. E. (1982). The need for cognition. *Journal of Personality and Social Psychology, 42*, 116–132.

Cantor, N., & Fleeson, W. (1991). Life-tasks and self-regulatory processes. In M. Maehr & P. Pintrich (Eds.), *Advances in motivation and achievement* (Vol. 7, pp. 327–369). Greenwich, CT: JAI Press.

Cantor, N., & Fleeson, W. (1994). Social intelligence and intelligent goal pursuit: A cognitive slice of motivation. In V. Spaulding (Ed.), *Nebraska Symposium on Motivation* (Vol. 41, pp. 125–180). Lincoln: University of Nebraska Press.

Carver, C. S., Scheier, M., Higgins, E. T., & Sorrentino, R. M. (1990). Principles of self-regulation: Action and emotion. In *Handbook of motivation and cognition: Foundations of social behavior* (Vol. 2, pp. 3–52). New York: Guilford Press.

Chartrand, T. L., & Bargh, J. A. (1996). Automatic activation of impression formation and memorization goals: Nonconscious goal priming reproduces effects of explicit task instructions. *Journal of Personality and Social Psychology, 71*(3), 464–478.

Chartrand, T. L., & Bargh, J. A. (1999). The chameleon effect: The perception-behavior link and social interaction. *Journal of Personality and Social Psychology, 76*(6), 893–910.

Chartrand, T. L., Maddux, W. W., & Lakin, J. L. (2005). Beyond the perception-behavior link: The ubiquitous utility and motivational moderators of nonconscious mimicry. In R. R. Hassin, J. S. Uleman, & J. A. Bargh (Eds.), *The new unconscious* (pp. 334–361). New York: Oxford University Press.

Chen, M., & Bargh, J. A. (1997). Nonconscious behavioral confirmation processes: The self-fulfilling consequences of automatic stereotype activation. *Journal of Experimental Social Psychology, 33*(5), 541–560.

Chen, S., & Chaiken, S. (1999). The heuristic-systematic model in its broader context. In S. Chaiken & Y. Trope (Eds.), *Dual-process theories in social psychology* (pp. 72–96). New York: Guilford Press.

Chen, S., Lee-Chai, A. Y., & Bargh, J. A. (2001). Relationship orientation as a moderator of the effects of social power. *Journal of Personality and Social Psychology, 80*(2), 173–187.

Chun, W. Y., & Kruglanski, A. W. (2005). Consumption as a multiple goal pursuit without awareness. In F. R. Kardes, P. M. Herr, & J. Nantel (Eds.),

Applying social cognition to consumer-focused strategy (pp. 25–43). Mahwah, NJ: Lawrence Erlbaum Associates.

Chun, W., Kruglanski, A. W., Sleeth-Keppler, D., & Friedman, R. (2005). *On the psychology of quasi-rational decisions: The multifinality principle in choice without awareness.* Manuscript submitted for publication.

Cohen, G. L., Aronson, J., & Steele, C. M. (2000). When beliefs yield to evidence: Reducing biased evaluation by affirming the self. *Personality and Social Psychology Bulletin, 26*(9), 1151–1164.

Dijksterhuis, A., & Bargh, J. A. (2001). The perception-behavior expressway: Automatic effects of social perception on social behavior. In M. P. Zanna (Ed.), *Advances in experimental social psychology* (Vol. 33, pp. 1–40). San Diego, CA: Academic Press.

Dijksterhuis, A., & van Knippenberg, A. (1998). The relation between perception and behavior, or how to win a game of Trivial Pursuit. *Journal of Personality and Social Psychology, 74*(4), 865–877.

Dweck, C. S. (1999). *Self-theories: Their role in motivation, personality, and development.* Philadelphia: Psychology Press.

Emmons, R. A. (1996). Striving and feeling: Personal goals and subjective well-being. In P. M. Gollwitzer & J. A. Bargh (Eds.), *The psychology of action* (pp. 313–337). New York: Guilford Press.

Fishbach, A., & Dhar, R. (2005). Goals as excuses or guides: The liberating effect of perceived goal progress on choice. *Journal of Consumer Research, 32*(3), 370–377.

Fishbach, A., Friedman, R., & Kruglanski, A. W. (2003). Leading us not into temptation: Momentary allurements elicit overriding goal activation. *Journal of Personality and Social Psychology, 84*(2), 296–309.

Fishbach, A., Shah, J. Y., & Kruglanski, A. W. (2004). Emotional transfer in goal systems. *Journal of Experimental Social Psychology, 40*(6), 723–738.

Fiske, S. T. (2003). Five core social motives, plus or minus five. In S. J. Spencer, F. Steven, M. P. Zanna, & J. M. Olson (Eds.), *Motivated social perception: The Ontario Symposium* (Vol. 9, pp. 233–246). Mahwah, NJ: Lawrence Erlbaum Associates.

Fiske, S. T., & Neuberg, S. L. (1990). A continuum model of impression formation, from category-based to individuating processes: Influences of information and motivation on attention and interpretation. In M. P. Zanna (Ed.), *Advances in experimental social psychology* (Vol. 23, pp. 1–74). New York: Academic Press.

Fitzsimons, G. M., & Bargh, J. A. (2003). Thinking of you: Nonconscious pursuit of interpersonal goals associated with relationship partners. *Journal of Personality and Social Psychology, 84*(1), 148–163.

Freud, S. (1961). *The ego and the id.* New York: W. W. Norton. & Co, Inc.

Gollwitzer, P. M. (1999). Implementation intentions: Strong effects of simple plans. *American Psychologist, 54*(7), 493–503.

Gollwitzer, P. M., & Moskowitz, G. B. (1996). Goal effects on action and cognition. In E. T. Higgins & A. W. Kruglanski (Eds.), *Social psychology: Handbook of basic principles* (pp. 361–399). New York: Guilford Press.

Hamilton, D. L., Katz, L. B., & Leirer, V. O. (1980). Cognitive representations of personality impressions: Organizational processes in first impression formation. *Journal of Personality and Social Psychology, 39,* 1050–1063.

Hassin, R. R., Uleman, J. S., & Bargh, J. A. (Eds.). (2005). *The new unconscious.* New York: Oxford University Press.

Higgins, E. T. (1987). Self-discrepancy: A theory relating self and affect. *Psychological Review, 94*(3), 319–340.

Higgins, E. T. (1997). Beyond pleasure and pain. *American Psychologist, 52*(12), 1280–1300.

Higgins, E. T., King, G. A., & Mavin, G. H. (1982). Individual construct accessibility and subjective impressions and recall. *Journal of Personality and Social Psychology, 43*(1), 35–47.

Kelly, H. H. (1987). Causal schemata and attribution process. In E. E. Jones, D. E. Kanouse, H. H. Kelly, R. E. Nisbett, & S. Valins (Eds.), *Attribution: Perceiving the causes of behavior* (pp. 151–174). Hillsdale, NJ, England: Lawrence Erlbaum Associates.

Kopetz, C. E., Fishbach, A., & Kruglanski, A. W. (2005). *Having one's cake and eating it too: The quest for multifinal means in goal pursuit.* Unpublished manuscript, University of Maryland, College Park.

Kruglanski, A. W. (2004). *The psychology of closed mindedness.* New York: Psychology Press.

Kruglanski, A. W., & Fishman, S. (2006). The psychology of terrorism: Syndrome versus tool perspectives. *Journal of Terrorism and Political Violence, 15*(1), 45–48.

Kruglanski, A. W., Pierro, A., Mannetti, L., & DeGrada, E. (2006). Groups as epistemic providers: Need for closure and the unfolding of group centrism. *Psychological Review, 113*(1), 84–100.

Kruglanski, A. W., Shah, Y. J., Fishbach, A., Friedman, R., Chun, W. Y., & Sleeth-Keppler, D. (2002). A theory of goal-systems. In M. P. Zanna

(Ed.), *Advances in experimental social psychology* (pp. 331–376). San Diego, CA: Academic Press.

Kruglanski, A. W., & Webster, D. M. (1996). Motivated closing of the mind: "Seizing" and "freezing." *Psychological Review, 103*(2), 263–283.

Lewin, K. (1935). *A dynamic theory of personality: Selected papers* (D. E. Adams & K. E. Zener, Trans.). New York: McGraw- Hill.

Macrae, C. N., & Johnston, L. (1998). Help, I need somebody: Automatic action and inaction. *Social Cognition, 16*(4), 400–417.

Miller, D. T., & Ross, M. (1975). Self-serving biases in the attribution of causality: Fact or fiction? *Psychological Bulletin, 82*(2), 213–225.

Miller, G. A., Galanter, E., & Pribram, K. H. (1960). *Plans and the structure of behavior.* New York: Henry Holt. and Co, Inc.

Newell, A., Shaw, J. C., & Simon, H. A. (1958). Elements of a theory of human problem solving. *Psychological Review, 65,* 151–166.

Nisbett, R. E., & Wilson, T. D. (1977). Telling more than we can know: Verbal reports on mental processes. *Psychological Review, 87,* 231–259.

Pervin, L. A. (1989). Goal concepts in personality and social psychology: A historical introduction. In L. A. Pervin (Ed.), *Goal concepts in personality and social psychology* (pp. 1–17). Hillsdale, NJ: Lawrence Erlbaum Associates.

Petty, R. E., & Cacioppo, J. T. (1986). The elaboration likelihood model of persuasion. In L. Berkowitz (Ed.), *Advances in experimental social psychology* (Vol. 19, pp. 1123–1205). New York: Academic Press.

Pfeffer, J., & Sutton, R. (2000). *The knowing-doing gap: How smart firms turn knowledge into action.* Cambridge, MA: Harvard Business School Press.

Pierro, A. (2005). [The possibility for means substitution increases people's commitment to a given goal.] Unpublished raw data. University of Rome.

Shah, J. (2003a). Automatic for the people: How representations of significant others implicitly affect goal pursuit. *Journal of Personality and Social Psychology, 84*(4), 661–681.

Shah, J. (2003b). The motivational looking glass: How significant others implicitly affect goal appraisals. *Journal of Personality and Social Psychology, 85*(3), 424–439.

Shah, J. Y., Friedman, R., & Kruglanski, A. W. (2002). Forgetting all else: On the antecedence and consequences of goal shielding. *Journal of Personality and Social Psychology, 83,* 1261–1280.

Shah, J. Y., & Kruglanski, A. W. (2002). Priming against your will: How accessible alternatives affect goal pursuit. *Journal of Experimental Social Psychology, 38,* 368–383.

Shah, J. Y., & Kruglanski, A. W. (2003). When opportunity knocks: Bottom-up priming of goals by means and its effects on self-regulation. *Journal of Personality and Social Psychology, 84*(6), 1109–1122.

Sleeth-Keppler, D. P. (2005). *The multifinality principle in choice without awareness.* Unpublished manuscript, Winthrop University, Rock Hill, SC.

Tesser, A., Martin, L. L., & Cornell, D. P. (1996). On the substitutability of self-protective mechanisms. In P. M. Gollwitzer, & J. A. Bargh, (Eds.), *The psychology of action: Linking cognition and motivation to behavior* (pp. 48–68). New York: Guilford Press.

van Baaren, R. B., Holland, R. W., Kawakami, K., & van Knippenberg, A. (2004). Mimicry and prosocial behavior. *Psychological Science, 15*(1), 71–74.

van Baaren, R. B., Holland, R. W., & Steenaert, B. (2003). Mimicry for money: Behavioral consequences of imitation. *Journal of Experimental Social Psychology, 39*(4), 393–398.

Webster, D. M., & Kruglanski, A. W. (1998). Cognitive and social consequences of the motivation for closure. *The European Review of Psychology, 8,* 133–173.

Wilson, T. D., & Nisbett, R. E. (1978). The accuracy of verbal reports about the effects of stimuli on evaluations and behavior. *Social Psychology, 41*(2), 118–131.

PART 5

The Origins and Sources of Action

Acquisition, Representation, and Control of Action

Bernhard Hommel *and* Birgit Elsner

Abstract

This chapter traces the gradual emergence of action control from the experience of action-produced events. It begins by reviewing and integrating findings on the acquisition of action effects, that is, on the learning of associations between movements and perceivable outcomes in infants, children, and adults. Second, it discusses what is actually acquired by these learning processes, that is, how actions and action plans are cognitively represented. Third, it outlines how the acquired knowledge is employed in action control, that is, in the planning and production of goal-directed movement.

Keywords: action control, action-produced vents, learning, movement, acquired knowledge

"If, in voluntary action properly so-called, the act must be foreseen, it follows that no creature not endowed with divinatory power can perform an act voluntarily for the first time" (James, 1890, p. 487). There is quite a bit of information that William James wanted to communicate to the reader with this sentence. First, he incidentally introduces probably the most common definition of voluntary action by equating it with goal-directed movement. Second, he emphasizes the role of anticipation in action control, that is, the selective and directing function of predictions of action outcomes. Third, he points out that action control relies on knowledge about relationships between movements and outcomes, which, fourth, implies and presupposes the previous experience of movement–outcome relationships.

In this chapter, we trace the gradual emergence of action control from the experience of action-produced events that is suggested by this theoretical view. We do so in three steps. First, we review and integrate findings on the acquisition of action effects, that is, on the learning of associations between movements and perceivable outcomes in infants, children, and adults. Second, we discuss what is actually acquired by these learning processes, that is, how actions and action plans are cognitively represented. Third, we outline how the acquired knowledge is employed in action control, that is, in the planning and production of goal-directed movement.

Knowing What We Could Do: Acquiring Action

Although newborns are already equipped with some motor and sensory capabilities, it is widely accepted that they lack the ability to perform goal-directed actions. Nevertheless, young infants can move their bodies, and motor control develops substantially during the first 2 years. They can also perceive sensory events, including feedback from self-performed movements: Both distal (visual or auditory) and proximal (tactile or proprioceptive) action consequences can be registered from birth (for a general overview, see Kellman & Arterberry, 1998). But how do we develop from a moving and perceiving infant to an intentional agent?

By performing actions, agents try to realize goals that they have in mind, and they do so in a variety of situational contexts and by a variety of bodily movements. Accordingly, it seems unlikely that intentional action is innate. Rather, action control has to be acquired through experience in terms of both motor execution and specifying the motor patterns suited to produce the desired effects. As mentioned already, controlling an action requires the anticipation of its intended outcome (Hommel, Müsseler, Aschersleben, & Prinz, 2001; see Chapters 2 and 6). Before producing a goal-directed action, the agent has thus to build up or activate a representation of the desired effect in mind and has to use this representation to select a movement pattern that is suitable to bring about this effect—James's (1890) "ideomotor principle." This ability to anticipate the consequences of one's own actions emerges around 9 months of age (Piaget, 1952; Tomasello, 1999; Willats, 1999).

In the preceding first 8 months of life, maturation leads to a differentiation of innate behavioral patterns to increasingly coordinated and controlled movements (e.g., von Hofsten, 2004). Additionally, young infants are equipped with learning mechanisms that allow them to detect and encode contingencies between self-performed movements and environmental events, or action effects (Gergely & Watson, 1999; Piaget, 1952; Rochat, 1998; Rovee-Collier, 1987). These mechanisms

are so efficient that newborns are able to vary their sucking frequency in order to obtain a certain sensory input (e.g., hearing their mother's voice, getting a sweet liquid, or seeing certain pictures; e.g., DeCasper & Fifer, 1980; Rochat & Striano, 1999). More evidence that young infants learn action–effect contingencies comes from studies on instrumental learning: Two- to 5-month-olds are able to pick up contingencies between their own leg movements and the movements of a mobile connected to the leg (Rovee & Rovee, 1969; Watson & Ramey, 1972) or the sounds of a rattle (Rochat & Morgan, 1998), and they learn to turn their heads to obtain a milk reward (Papousek, 1967). These examples demonstrate a transition from stimulus control of behavior to action control through acquired representations of action effects (for a review, see Rovee-Collier, 1987).

Learning contingencies between self-performed movements and their to-be-expected effects increasingly enables infants to exert control over their environment. They keep practicing this control ability by reproducing pleasant effects through repeating the movement over and over again, which they typically start doing by 4 months (Piaget, 1952) or even earlier (Rovee-Collier, 1987). By 4 months, infants are also able to expect a particular outcome after having performed a well-known movement, as they smile and coo when the typical effect occurs (Lewis, Sullivan, & Brooks-Gunn, 1985; Papousek, 1969) but show distress when it does not (Watson, 1972). Around 9 months of age, infants start to act in a truly goal-oriented fashion. For example, they pull a towel to obtain an object that is out of their reach, or they remove an obstacle preventing their reach to the object (Piaget, 1952; Willats, 1999). According to Tomasello (1999), these behaviors may indicate a new level of intentional functioning, inasmuch as infants now differentiate the goal they are pursuing from the behavioral means they employ to pursue it. Most probably, infants' exploration of the contingencies between self-performed movements and their effects helps the emergence of goal-directed actions at the end of their first year (Elsner & Aschersleben, 2003).

Action–effect learning can thus be seen as a prerequisite for goal-directed action, which led Elsner and Hommel (2001) to propose a two-stage model for the acquisition of voluntary action control. Stage 1 of the model is concerned with the acquisition of contingencies between movements and effects. If a given movement and a given sensory event co-occur repeatedly in temporal proximity, their representations are connected by a bidirectional association (Elsner & Hommel, 2004). Accordingly, activating one representation on later occasions will tend to activate the other one too so that the codes of an action effect become effective retrieval cues or primes of the associated movement pattern. Stage 2 of the model refers to the use of such cues for action control, that is, to the selection of goal-directed movements by anticipating their effects (Hommel et al., 2001). Establishing a goal is assumed to activate codes of related action effects, hence to effect anticipation. Via the acquired movement–effect association, activation of effect codes will spread to the related movement pattern, which is then carried out and actually produces the expected effect. Although this model was developed to explain empirical evidence obtained in adults, its implications are meant to be valid for the emergence of intentional action control in infants as well.

Studies with adults provide strong support for the Elsner and Hommel model in general and the claim that acquired action effects play a central role in action control in particular. Indeed, novel, arbitrary action effects are spontaneously acquired and become associated with the action they ac-company, as demonstrated by the observation that the effects become effective primes of the action: Such priming effects have been observed with auditory stimuli (Elsner & Hommel, 2001, 2004), visually presented letters (Ziessler, Nattkemper, & Frensch, 2004), and words (Hommel, Alonso, & Fuentes, 2003) and even demonstrated for the affective value of visual (Caessens, Hommel, Lammertyn, & Van der Goten, 2008) and electrocutaneous feedback (Beckers, De Houwer, & Eelen, 2002). Contingencies between actions and their effects are picked up in a variety of tasks and conditions, such as in studies of choice reactions (Hommel, 1996; Stock & Hoffmann, 2002) or of the acquisition of stimulus–response sequences (Hazeltine, 2002; Hoffmann, Sebald, & Stoecker, 2001; Ziessler & Nattkemper, 2001). Further evidence that the perception of previously acquired action effects primes the associated response comes from both reaction-time experiments (Elsner & Hommel, 2001, 2004; Flach, Osman, Dickinson, & Heyes, 2006; Hommel, 1996; Kunde, 2004; Ziessler et al., 2004) and a recent brain-imaging study (Elsner et al., 2002). In this latter study using positron emission tomography, the mere presentation of previously acquired, auditory action effects was found to activate premotor brain structures (i.e., the caudal part of the rostral supplementary motor area) that are known to be involved in voluntary action planning.

Recently, action–effect learning and the priming of movements by the perception of previously acquired action effects has also been reported for 4- to 7-year-old children (Eenshuistra, Weidema, & Hommel, 2004). In this study, the younger children had greater problems in suppressing the response that was primed by the perception of a just-acquired action effect than the older ones, a finding that is consistent with the notion that action control develops substantially during childhood (e.g.,

Dowsett & Livesey, 2000; Levy, 1980). This development is commonly attributed to the maturation of the prefrontal cortex and the frontal circuits of the corpus callosum, such as changes in synaptic density and the myelinization of neural connections (e.g., Fuster, 1989; Thompson et al., 2000). Younger children's deficits in action control suggest that associative action–effect learning and the priming of movements by action effects may be important prerequisites for voluntary action but that further cognitive processes are required to adjust the behavior to situational constraints or to actual action goals, hence to make effective use of action–effect knowledge. We now turn to the question of how such knowledge is represented and how it is used to control one's action.

Bits and Pieces: Representing Action

Now that we have an idea how novel actions are acquired, let us turn to the question of what is actually acquired. Actions are often referred to as single units. This certainly applies to the behavioristic conceptualization of action as a response defined in terms of measurable characteristics, but it also applies to modern cognitive psychology. In fact, most psychological textbooks treat action as a mere indicator of the more interesting perceptual, memory, and thought processes, an output function that allows measuring the duration and accuracy of cognitive processes. Early systematic attempts to investigate and theorize about action in its own right acknowledged that actions can be complex and hierarchical (i.e., simple actions can be organized into larger action sequences; see Lashley, 1951; Miller, Galanter, & Pribram, 1960), but how a given action is cognitively represented, what its internal structure looks like, and how people identify a contextually appropriate action still was anathema.

Sensorimotor Units

Our discussion of how agents acquire knowledge about what they are doing and what they achieve by doing so suggests that people associate their actions with representations of action effects. In other words, people are storing not just the output signals (efferences) of their cognitive system to the motor units responsible for bringing about a movement but, rather, they store integrated sensorimotor units (efferences and reafferences). In modern cognitive psychology, a more detailed theoretical treatment of how action is represented emerged no earlier than in the late 1960s in the field of motor learning. Adams (1968, 1971) picked up the control-theoretical approach of Miller et al. (1960) and considered that learning an action must comprise of at least two components. On the one hand, there must be some representation of the actual perceptual outcome of an action, which can be matched against a representation of the goal—otherwise an unsupervised learner would have no idea whether a given action was accurate. On the other hand, there must be some motor function producing the actual outcome, and this function must be modifiable.

This distinction between a perceptual and a motor component echoes the similar distinction in the introspective analysis of Lotze (1852) and Harless (1861)—better known from James's (1890) summary of their basic ideas. These authors were concerned with the question of how we can select an appropriate motor pattern to reach a given goal. Only if one has information about the likely perceptual outcome of actions, so they argued, can one determine which motor pattern is likely to realize the intended effect. Indeed, models of decision making and action planning are typically well equipped with respect to the way in which action alternatives are weighted against each other, but they are commonly silent with regard to the question of how people identify the possible alternatives in the first place (e.g., Kahneman & Tversky, 2000; Morris & Ward, 2005). One reason for this theoretical neglect is that, in studies of decision making and planning, the to-be-considered set of action alternatives is presented to the subject. In real life, however, selection is often rather unconstrained—just think of the different ways you can grasp a cup of coffee. Having one's action alternatives associated with the to-be-expected consequences of these actions strongly facilitates the decision: One need only specify relevant goals (e.g., holding the cup, optimizing speed, saving energy, or avoiding heat), which then will prime the alternatives to the degree that their expected consequences are matching those goals (Hommel et al., 2001; Rosenbaum, Meulenbroek, Vaughan, & Jansen, 2001). Thus, representing actions through sensorimotor units allows for a rather smooth and automatic transition from goal specification to decision making and the ultimate selection of an action, at least in principle.

Distributed Representation

After having (re)introduced the distinction between motor (efferent) and perceptual (reafferent) components of action representations, action theorists have analyzed the motor component somewhat further. Keele's (1968) initial definition of motor programs as feedback-independent structures of muscle-specific commands, obviously reflecting the increasing impact of computer logic on psychological theorizing, soon turned out to be unrealistically inflexible. In particular, the idea that actions may be represented in terms of muscle-specific codes faces at least two serious problems: the storage problem and the novelty problem (Schmidt, 1975). The former results from the fact that each single change in a movement, be it the pressure exerted with one finger or its end position, would require the creation of a new program, which would imply the need to store an almost infinite and therefore unrealistically large number of programs. The latter refers to the inability of the muscle-specific account to explain (in a realistic fashion) how existing skills can be modified and extended to accommodate varying situations, such as changing winds in a tennis match. According to Schmidt (1975), the storage problem and the novelty problem can be solved by assuming that action is represented in terms of schemas that contain information about the fixed features of an action but leave open slots for variable parameters, such as the width of a reaching movement. This idea was revived only recently by Glover (2004).

The concept of action representations as assemblies of codes that refer to the different features of the action is fully consistent with what we know about action representations in the primate brain. Indeed, primate brains have a preference for the distributed, feature-based coding of events, and planned actions are no exception. For instance, separate networks have been found to code the direction (Bonnet & MacKay, 1989; Georgopoulos, 1990), force (Kalaska & Hyde, 1985; Kutas & Donchin, 1980), and distance (Riehle & Requin, 1989; Vidal, Bonnet, & Macar, 1991) of arm movements. This suggests that action plans are composites of codes of separately specified action features. Such a conclusion receives further support from behavioral studies. For instance, numerous studies (e.g., Lépine, Glencross, & Requin, 1989; Rosenbaum, 1980) have shown that different parameters of pointing movements can be precued through separate stimuli, with the eventual reaction time decreasing as a function of the number of precues.

If we combine the evidence that action representations are cortically represented in a distributed fashion with the assumption that the basic functional units[1] of action representations are actually sensorimotor components, it is interesting to consider whether evidence for distributed, action-specific sensorimotor units can be found in the human brain. Indeed, recent functional magnetic resonance imaging studies of Schubotz and colleagues provide evidence of such units (Schubotz, Friederici, & von Cramon, 2000; Schubotz & von Cramon, 2001, 2002). For instance, monitoring a visual series of events for a timing, color/shape, or location oddball has been found to recruit neural circuits in the premotor cortex that are also involved in the control of actions that are specifically related to these stimulus dimensions (i.e., tapping/articulation, grasping, and reaching, respectively). Likewise, having people prepare for a grasping or reaching movement increases their perceptual sensitivity toward size- or location-defined stimuli, respectively (Fagioli, Hommel, & Schubotz, 2007). Hence, processing particular features of stimuli apparently involves neural systems that control those actions that typically make use of these features. This provides clear evidence of the existence of action-specific sensorimotor units and points to an important integrative role of the human premotor cortex in the anticipation of action effects and the control of the corresponding actions. Indeed, damage to the premotor cortex has been found to hamper stimulus prediction (Schubotz, Sakreida, Tittgemeyer, & von Cramon, 2004). As suggested by Schubotz and von Cramon (2001, 2003), the premotor cortex may integrate actions and their expected consequences into a kind of habitual pragmatic body map, a representational system for the "common coding" of perceptual events and action plans (Hommel et al., 2001; Prinz, 1990).

To summarize, there is evidence that action representations are both integrated (with respect to perceptual and motor components) and distributed (with respect to the different features of an action). However, until now we have considered only the most obvious ingredients of action representations, namely, simple movements and their rather immediate sensory consequences. Let us now turn to perhaps somewhat less obvious ingredients and associates.

Affordances

Acquiring associations between actions and their effects tells the actor/perceiver something about his or her own action and, in some sense, something about his or her effector and the way it is functioning. In fact, acquiring action effects can be considered as the first step of individuation, that is, of distinguishing one's own body (which creates predictable effects) from one's environment (which creates unpredictable effects) (see Piaget, 1952; Prinz, 1992; Rochat, 1998). But actions are often directed at and dependent on the existence of objects. As Goodale et al. (1994) have demonstrated, people are able to make grasping movements to both present and remembered objects, but the kinematics of these movements look different: Whereas grasps to a present object show the typical profile of a narrow grip aperture in the beginning, a wide opening when approaching the object, and the final closing of the hand around the object, grasps to a remembered object are stereotyped with a wide and relatively invariant opening from the beginning to the end (see Chapter 11).

This example not only shows that movements are not fully prespecified before they start (as the motor program view would have suggested) but also reveals that some parameters of actions are left to be specified by the environment, the object in this case. Indeed, given the lawful relationships between some object characteristics and movement parameters (*affordances* in the sense of Gibson, 1979), it makes much more sense to exploit such relationships and outsource the control of the respective parameters of the action rather than to rely on fallible internal predictions. As discussed by Glover (2004), quite a number of such action-parameter–specific object affordances have been identified so far, such as object orientation (controlling hand orientation: Jeannerod, 1981), object position and velocity (controlling hand trajectory: Brenner, Smeets, & de Lussanet, 1998; Jeannerod, 1981), object shape (controlling hand shape: Klatzky, Fikes, & Pellegrino, 1995), and object size (controlling grasping aperture: Jeannerod, 1984).

Making use of action-related information delivered by objects makes it unnecessary to specify the respective parameters in advance, but it does require planning about which information should specify which parameter. For instance, the size of an object has rather different implications for a movement, depending on whether the actor intends to point at the object, to grasp it, or to use it to hit another object. This means that action representations need to include pointers to particular types of environmental information so that preparing oneself, say, for a grasp makes one more sensitive to size information (Fagioli et al., 2007). This action-induced facilitation of action-related stimulus information (i.e., information that can be used to specify movement parameters) can be seen as a sort of proactive attentional selection that effectively turns the cognitive system into a prepared-reflex machinery (Hommel, 2000). How beneficially this processing strategy works can be seen from observations of Prablanc and Pélisson (1990). These authors had subjects move their hands to a goal position indicated by a light that was sometimes shifted by a few centimeters after the movement had begun. Even though subjects were prevented from noticing the shift (by carrying it out during

an eye movement), they moved their hand straight to the new goal location without any signs of corrections. That is, once the location of an object has been linked to an action plan, any change in the location leads to an automatic update of the movement's parameters even if the change occurs outside the actor's awareness.

But there are also downsides to this form of self-automatization. Once a system has turned itself into a prepared-reflex machinery, it becomes vulnerable against misleading information from the "correct channels." A well-known example for this vulnerability is the Stroop effect (for an overview, see MacLeod, 1991), which is observed if people respond to the ink of color words: If the task-irrelevant meaning of the word happens to match the relevant ink color (e.g., the word RED in red ink), performance is much better than if meaning and ink do not match (e.g., the word GREEN in red ink). This obvious inability to fully ignore the meaning of the words has been taken to indicate that reading is a fully automatized skill, at least in Western cultures. However, the Stroop effect is much more pronounced if people respond verbally than by key pressing (see MacLeod, 1991). Even though one may argue that this reflects the greater experience we have in calling out words than in responding to them manually, it is a first indication that preparing for a task (pronouncing words in this case) makes the cognitive system more sensitive to stimuli that afford performing this task (i.e., words). Indeed, if subjects are not prepared to utter words but make a judgment whether a particular color is present or absent in a word, the Stroop effect disappears (Bauer & Besner, 1997).

More evidence in support of this possibility comes from the Simon effect, a variant of the Stroop effect (for an overview, see Lu & Proctor, 1995). This effect occurs if people respond to a nonspatial stimulus feature by carrying out a spatially defined response, such as a left-versus-right key press in response to the letters X and O. Stimulus location is irrelevant in this task but varies nevertheless. And it does have an effect: Performance is better if the stimulus happens to appear in a location that spatially corresponds with the proper response, hence, if in our example the X appears on the left and the O appears on the right.

Again, an automaticity account may argue that people are used to carrying out responses to spatially corresponding objects, but there is increasing evidence that this kind of automaticity is induced or at least enabled by the task. For instance, it has been shown that stimuli in the Simon task activate spatially corresponding responses up to the level of lateralized readiness potentials (LRPs; Sommer, Leuthold, & Hermanutz, 1993), an apparently strong indication of automaticity. Valle-Inclán and Redondo (1998) have looked into the conditions under which LRPs occur in a Simon task. In their study, the relevant S-R mapping was not fixed but varied randomly from trial to trial so that participants were presented not only with a stimulus but also with a display showing how the stimuli were mapped onto responses. The temporal order in which the mapping display and the stimulus were presented varied as well so that sometimes the mapping preceded the stimulus (i.e., participants knew and could have implemented the mapping before encountering the stimulus) and sometimes the stimulus preceded the mapping. When the mapping preceded the stimulus, stimulus-induced LRPs were observed; that is, the stimulus activated the spatially corresponding response regardless of which response was correct. However, when the stimulus preceded the S-R mapping, stimulus-induced LRPs were no longer observed. It thus appears that the spatial affordance of a stimulus depends on the currently implemented task set, which seems to enable the automatic processing of stimuli varying on task-relevant dimensions.

The same conclusion can be drawn from priming studies. For instance, presenting a task-irrelevant arrow prime while people are waiting for a spatial target stimulus has been shown to yield an arrow-related LRP (Eimer, 1995) even if the arrow appears subliminally (Eimer & Schlaghecken, 1998). However, arrow primes ceased to have an effect if the relevant stimuli were nonspatial (e.g., letters; Eimer & Schlaghecken, 1998). This suggests that the prime-induced activation of responses was automatic only if (and, presumably, because) the perceiver/actor intended to respond to prime-related information, which implies that "automatic" translation depends on intentions.

Taken altogether, these observations suggest that representations of actions contain pointers to environmental information that is suited to specify the concrete parameters of an upcoming or ongoing action (see Fagioli et al., 2007; Neumann & Klotz, 1994). By restricting the storage of action plans to fully predictable aspects of the action and using pointers to environmental information to fill in the aspects that cannot be predicted in advance, action plans can be tailored to context conditions of almost any degree of (in)stability. Note that this enormous benefit relies on the fact that action plans are both distributed composites and sensorimotor in nature. The reason is that environmental information specifies actions only on the level of action effects but does not provide muscle-specific information: The location of an object specifies the end point of a reaching action but not which muscles to activate for how long, and a word specifies the phonological codes to utter (which again presupposes some grapheme–phoneme translation) but not the movements of the vocal tract. If the units of action plans were not sensorimotor (and thus provide the translation rules necessary to derive muscle parameters from effect representations) and distributed (so that different stimuli or stimulus aspects can be taken to specify different parameters of the action), human action planning would be much less flexible.

A by-product of integrating actions with pointers to stimulus information that can fill in action parameters online is that object-directed actions can be carried out even in the absence of objects. As already discussed, such actions look unnatural and pantomimed (Goodale et al., 1994), but they are easy to carry out by imagining the respective object. Apparently, the pointers contained in action plans can also pick up internally generated information about an object, information that is necessarily less specific and up to date than that provided by a real object but is nevertheless sufficient to specify the open parameters. This possibility allows people to play through alternative actions (e.g., to make a difficult decision) and to carry out mental practice.

Given the rich evidence that actions are coded in a sensorimotor fashion, it makes sense to suspect that stimulus events are also coded in such a way. Indeed, several authors have suggested that representations of stimulus events may include information about the actions afforded by these stimuli (e.g., Barsalou, 1999; Gibson, 1979; Hommel et al., 2001). Action-related information seems to be integrated continuously and rather automatically, as a number of recent observations suggest. For instance, Richardson and Spivey (2000) presented subjects with short video clips that appeared in various locations, each clip showing a speaker talking about a particular topic (e.g., plays of Shakespeare). When the subjects were later asked about facts related to these topics, they tended to look spontaneously at the location where the respective clip had been presented. Apparently, the representation

of the audiovisual events also contained information about where they had been seen so that retrieving information about the clip reactivated location information, which had a direct effect on eye-movement control. Along the same lines, Hommel and Knuf (2000) had subjects perform choice responses to cued houses on a visual map-like array. After having acquired the correct house-response mappings, participants evaluated statements about the spatial relationships between pairs of houses. Pairs were judged faster if the two houses had shared the same response in the acquisition phase, even when the map was no longer visible. This suggests that response-related information became associated with the houses' representations so that accessing one member of a pair for comparison spread activation to the other via the shared response code. Hence, the principle of sensorimotor representation may apply not only to action plans but to object and event codes as well (Hommel et al., 2001).

Verbal Labels

If action representations are associated with all sorts of stimulus codes and contextual information, it is easy to see how action plans can become activated in the presence of an action-related stimulus. But humans can plan actions even in the absence of related stimuli and even outside the situational context the action is planned for—just think of the preparation for a job talk. This raises the question of how action representations are retrieved and activated under such circumstances. We have briefly touched one possibility: One may imagine the stimuli that trigger the sought-for action. In fact, this is the original solution proposed by Lotze (1852), who suggested that voluntary action control is acquired by learning to mentally simulate the trigger conditions for actions.

Another important means to control one's actions has been promoted by Vygotsky (1962). He claimed that, in the course of ontogenetic development, the increasing ability to control one's action goes hand in hand with and is strongly supported by the increasing ability to employ internal speech (see Zelazo, 1999). Infants and young children often describe the outcomes of their actions verbally only after having produced them, but very soon they begin to talk while acting, and at some point, children verbally describe the intended outcome before beginning to act. Vygotsky assumes that at this stage speech has become a self-regulatory function in specifying the goal of an action and organizing the means to achieve it. Translated into our present terminology, verbalizing action outcomes associates action effect codes with verbal labels. This provides an additional retrieval cue allowing to activate the effect codes—and thereby the whole action representation they are part of—by overt or inner speech.

There is indeed evidence of a strong relationship between (overt and covert) speech and the ability to control one's action. Luria (1959, 1961) showed that children are much better in controlling stimulus-dependent responses and in avoiding unnecessary perseverance if they verbalize their action goal and the stimulus–response mapping. For instance, asking young children to respond to a stimulus often triggered immediate responding long before the stimulus actually appeared (Luria, 1961). But once the children learned to insert a verbal self-instruction ("Go!") into the sequence of stimuli and responses (stimulus–"go"–response), they could master the task perfectly.

In adults, verbalization has been demonstrated to reduce the mental costs associated with switching from one task to another (Baddeley, Chincotta, & Adlam, 2001; Emerson & Miyake, 2003; Goschke, 2000;

Kray, Eber, & Lindenberger, 2004). Even the acquisition of new action effects can be facilitated by verbalizing the action–effect relationship (Kray, Eenshuistra, Kerstner, Weidema, & Hommel, 2006). These behavioral observations are consistent with recent neurophysiological findings on the representation of words. As pointed out by Pulvermüller (2003; Pulvermüller, Hauk, Nikulin, & Ilmoniemi, 2005), words are likely to be represented by widely distributed cell assemblies with strong links to the perceptual and motor codes of their referents. In particular, assemblies representing words that signify visual events include neurons in visual cortices, and assemblies representing words that signify actions include neurons in motor cortices.

Thus, there is evidence that action representations entertain associative links to verbal labels describing the effects produced by the action and, hence, signifying the action's pragmatic meaning. These links provide the actor with retrieval cues that can be used to activate and maintain the elements of action plans by inner and outer speech. Using them allows for setting up action plans long ahead of action execution, and it provides the opportunity to acquire, communicate, and exchange action plans quite easily.

Affective Values

In addressing the role of action effects and their representations for action control, we until now have focused on physical effects and their perceptual representations. However, actions also have affective consequences. Learning theory has emphasized the function of affective consequences for the selection of actions: Actions followed by positive affective consequences will be more likely to be carried out in the future, whereas actions followed by negative consequences will be less likely (Thorndike, 1927). Affect in that case provides the glue that binds actions to situations (Walker, 1969), but it does not become a part of the eventual binding. In other words, affect provides online criteria for associative learning, but it is no longer represented in the emerging associative structure.

Recent theories have considered a more representational role of affect, however. Rolls (1999) has suggested that, in the process of learning, animals acquire stimulus–reinforcement associations that can be used to evaluate the to be expected reinforcement properties of stimulus–response pairs. By using them, animals can "play through" if–then rules when making a decision and thus pick the behavior that maximizes the expected reinforcement. A very similar suggestion has been made by Damasio (1994). He assumes that actions become associated with so-called somatic markers, that is, representations of the bodily sensations resulting from an action. When making a decision, people can thus quickly simulate how it would feel to carry out a particular action and then go for the action that makes them feel best. Indeed, there is evidence that people show autonomic affective reactions (increased sweat production) before making risky decisions (Bechara, Damasio, Tranel, & Damasio, 1997), suggesting that they anticipate the possibly negative outcome.

Another argument supporting the assumption that representations of affect may become integrated into action representations has to do with the already discussed principle of sensorimotor representation. Affective bodily reactions can only impact decision making and action planning to the degree that they are (consciously or unconsciously) perceptually registered, which was the main point of James's (1884) theory of emotion. But once such reactions are perceptually coded, they should not be treated any differently than other, external consequences of the action (Hommel et al., 2001). That is, integration processes should treat the perception that carrying out a given action makes one tremble, sweat, and feel terrible not any different from the perception that carrying out this action, say, produces a particular auditory signal or reduces one's income by 50%. If so, the codes underlying these perceptions should be bound to their respective actions in just the same way.

Indeed, recent evidence suggests that perceptions of affective consequences are integrated with the producing action just like perceptions of nonaffective consequences. Beckers et al. (2002) used the same paradigm as Elsner and Hommel (2001). In the acquisition phase, subjects performed binary-choice responses to the grammatical category of neutral words, with one response producing a mild electroshock. In the following test phase, subjects performed the same task but now to stimulus words with positive or negative affective valence. As expected, subjects performed better when the word valence matched the valence of the response: Negative words were responded to more quickly with the response followed by a shock, whereas the opposite was true for positive words. This suggests that the actions acquired the affective valence of their effects. Findings of Caessens et al. (2008) point in the same direction. These authors had subjects perform two overlapping key-pressing tasks where the two response alternatives in the secondary task triggered the presentation of a smiley and a grumpy, respectively. The results indicated that preparing the smiley-producing response facilitated the processing of words with positive valence in the primary task, while preparing the grumpy-producing responses primed words with a negative valence. Apparently, the actions were integrated with and thus affectively marked by the affective valence of their effects.

Summary

Representations of actions are not unitary codes but rather composites of several elements. Minimally, a representation includes sensorimotor associations between the perceptual codes of particular action features and the motor program realizing them. At least in humans, action representations are also likely to comprise of pointers to action-relevant stimuli and stimulus dimensions, that is, to environmental events that specify free action parameters. Links to verbal labels make action representations easily accessible and controllable by means of inner speech and external instruction. By integrating representations of the to-be-expected affective consequences, action representations can be quickly evaluated and compared.

Picking, Weighting, and Binding: Controlling Action

When cognitive psychologists talk about action control, they often refer to processes that take place between the occurrence of an action-triggering stimulus event and the execution of the triggered action. This perspective derives from the theoretical approach of Donders (1868), who developed the first stage model of information processing. Donders assumed that human will impacts information processing by selectively translating some but not other stimuli into overt movement. To measure how long what he called the "organ of the will" needs for decision making, he manipulated stimulus and response uncertainty in choice reaction-time tasks. First, he found that informing subjects about the upcoming stimulus sped up reaction time, and he considered the amount of facilitation as a measure of the combined effect of stimulus discrimination and the "determination of the will"—assuming that with preinformation, both could be achieved before the stimulus. Then, to isolate the stimulus-related component, he employed a go/no-go task, which pairs stimulus uncertainty with response certainty. The difference between the reaction time in this task and in a choice task without preinformation, so he reasoned, should reflect the time demands of will determination. Applying this logic left Donders with an estimate of 36 milliseconds for making up one's mind. Even though some details of Donders's theoretical claims have been criticized, modified (Sternberg, 1969), and extended (Pashler & Johnston, 1989), his basic approach is still popular and heavily used to theorize about action control, such as in the study of dual-task performance (Pashler, 1994).

Donders's emphasis on online control (i.e., processes after stimulus presentation and before response execution) was not shared by everyone. Exner (1879), for instance, gained a fundamentally different impression of how action control works. Based on his introspections, he considered it difficult to believe that control intervenes between stimulus and response. Instead, he claimed that the actual control takes place long before the stimulus comes up. As a consequence, he considered the preparation for responding a truly voluntary act but the eventual action in a certain sense involuntary. The main job of voluntary processes, so he reasoned, would be to automatize the cognitive system and turn it into a "prepared reflex" (Woodworth, 1938; see Bargh & Gollwitzer, 1994; Hommel, 2000).

In view of Exner's considerations, it seems important to distinguish between the point in time at which action control is exerted (i.e., when "control processes" determining what and how will be done) and the point in time at which these control decisions become effective (i.e., when the action is carried out). With this distinction in mind, it may well turn out that what Donders had measured is not the time needed to make a decision but merely the online reflection of a (perhaps much more time demanding) decision that had been made much earlier (i.e., off-line). It is fair to say that the distinction between exertion and impact of control is widely neglected, often with severe theoretical consequences.

A prominent example is the theorizing about response inhibition. Following the spirit of Freud (1914), numerous authors have taken it for granted that unwanted response tendencies can be prevented from taking over action control only if they are actively suppressed (Logan & Cowan, 1984; Ridderinkhof, 2002). Accordingly, response inhibition has been granted the status of an executive process (e.g., Barkley, 1997; Logan, 1985) worthy and in need of further investigation. However, considering Exner's account of action control this reasoning is less straightforward than it might seem. The first flaw in this reasoning stems from the assumption that, if a particular response tendency is activated (e.g., as indicated in reaction-time patterns or LRPs) but the corresponding behavior is not shown, the tendency must have been suppressed. This is possible but by no means necessary. If response tendencies are evaluated with regard to their activation level, choosing the correct response will become more difficult (thus increasing choice reaction time) the more activated other tendencies are, but there is no need to assume that making the decision requires the suppression of these other tendencies. For example, it takes more time to determine the outcome of a (democratic) presidential election if there is more than one popular candidate, but reaching the eventual decision does not require the suppression or elimination of any votes or candidate.

The second flaw in the reasoning underlying many inhibition accounts is the strong belief that inhibition is necessarily

"active"—which is commonly meant to imply intentional online control. Again, this is a possibility, but it is neither necessary nor self-evident, nor is it parsimonious. Consider how action alternatives are typically modeled in neural networks (e.g., Cohen, Dunbar, & McClelland, 1990; Gilbert & Shallice, 2002). If R1 and R2 were alternative responses, their representations would be assumed to be linked by inhibitory connections so that activating R1 would inhibit R2 and vice versa. Now assume that R1 would be the correct response and R2 would be an incorrect alternative that is primed by some misleading stimulus. Obviously, the activation of R2 would inhibit R1, which would explain why R1 would take longer to reach the threshold for response execution. However, if R1 does reach the threshold, it must have been activated more strongly than R2 (otherwise the incorrect response R2 would be performed), which again means that R2 is inhibited. Hence, any competitive system with a built-in winner-takes-all mechanism (which is common in contemporary network models) produces inhibition of non-selected alternatives, without any particular "active" inhibition system. From this perspective, it makes sense to assume that the inhibition process is an automatic consequence of the way the cognitive system is configured and prepared rather than an achievement of online executive processes.

Considering examples of this sort, we doubt whether the seemingly clear-cut distinctions between executive and task processes or between intentional and automatic processes make sense. In fact, there is hardly any evidence that processes more complex than a knee-jerk reflex can be completely independent of the goals of an actor/perceiver and the way these goals have configured the cognitive system (see von Hofsten, 2004). That is, most or all processes are reflecting the actor/perceiver's intentions but are automatic at the same time—conditionally automatic in the sense of Bargh (1989). In the following, we therefore do not attempt to track the time points at which control is implemented (because, as pointed out, we think that the implementation precedes its impact on processing) but, rather, consider when and how control is reflected in processing and behavior. In other words, we focus more on the effects than on the causes of control. To do so, we follow the schema of Heckhausen and Gollwitzer (1987) and distinguish between the phase of action planning proper (what Heckhausen and Gollwitzer call the preactional phase), the actional phase, and the postactional phase. We thus restrict our discussion to the short-term effects of creating and executing action plans and neglect long-term effects, such as stimulus–response learning or prospective memory.

Planning Phase

As James has pointed out in our introductory reference, intentional action must be based on some anticipation of the action's outcome almost by definition. What these anticipations look like, whether they necessarily include sensory expectations (as ideomotor approaches suggest) or whether they can also be abstract, is largely unknown. However, we do have evidence that anticipations play a role in action planning. First, choice reaction times have been observed to increase if the spatial relationship between the location of a response and its visual effect is incompatible as compared to when this relation is compatible (Hommel, 1993; Kunde, 2001). Likewise, the reaction time for vocal color-word responses increase if responses are followed by the presentation of a response-incompatible color (Koch & Kunde, 2002). This means that selecting an action is accompanied by activating the codes of the expected action effects, suggesting that such codes

are mediating selection. Second, Kunde, Hoffmann, and Zellmann (2002) had subjects perform a four-alternative choice-reaction-time task in which each response produced one of two auditory effects. In some trials, the subjects were cued to prepare one response but were then required to carry out another. If this other response was expected to produce the same auditory effect as the prepared response, reaction times were faster than if the other response was expected to produce a different effect. Again, this provides evidence that codes of the expected sensory consequences of actions are involved in action planning.

Considering that actions are represented in terms of their effects and that effect codes are indeed involved in action planning, the first step in the planning process can be conceived of similarly as the biased-competition scenario that Duncan and colleagues (Desimone & Duncan, 1995; Duncan & Humphreys, 1989) have suggested for the selection of perceptual events. The scenario assumes that, to find a target stimulus among distractors, a search template is created that contains a description of the sought-for target. Representations of registered events that are assumed to compete for selection are compared with this template and receive top-down support to the degree that they match. The best-matching event thus receives the strongest support so that it outperforms its competitors and is eventually selected for further processing. Along the same lines, the action goal may be thought of as a description of the intended action in terms of the to-be-achieved perceptual effects. This action template will then prime stored sensorimotor (i.e., action–effect) links to the degree that their effects are matching the goal, which eventually will activate the best-fitting links the most. Given that action representations are not unitary but composites, several sensorimotor links are likely to be selected, each representing a relevant feature of the intended action.

In view of the evidence we have discussed so far, it seems likely that goals can refer to visual and auditory action effects, but other formats are possible as well. We have pointed out that inner speech seems to play an important role in action control and considered that action representations entertain links to verbal labels describing them. If so, it makes sense to assume that goal descriptions can also be of a verbal format so that sensorimotor structures are primed to the degree that their verbal labels match the verbal goal description. We speculate that verbal mediation of action planning is particularly important with respect to self-imposed or contextually primed strategies, such as the intention to perform particularly fast or accurately (Förster, Higgins, & Taylor Bianco, 2003). Goals may also refer to affective consequences of actions, bringing representations of affective action effects into play. Affect-related criteria may be particularly useful in cases where many action alternatives are active and competing for selection. Hence, if there are many ways to reach a particular goal, people may go for the alternative that is giving them the best "gut feeling" (i.e., the alternative that is associated with the most positive affective expectations). Finally, environmental information about the context and about action-related objects is likely to provide further biases toward particular action alternatives. Taken altogether, the selection of an action may thus represent the best compromise between functional, affective, and practical requirements and biases.

Specifying the relevant features of an action and activating the best-fitting sensorimotor links is an important first step in the action planning process, but it is presumably not yet sufficient to make a plan complete. The reason is that we commonly carry out more than one action at the same time and that we certainly entertain multiple action plans concurrently—just think of the multiple items on your daily agenda. Given that action plans are composites, this means that chances are high that multiple features belonging to more than one action plan are active at the same time—which again is likely to create confusion about which feature belongs to which plan. In other words, distributed planning creates binding problems as they exist in the processing of stimulus events (Treisman, 1996). To solve this problem and to avoid confusion and cross talk with other plans, the elements of an action plan need presumably to be integrated or bound before the plan can be executed (Stoet & Hommel, 1999). Support for this assumption comes from studies on the side effects of action planning. Müsseler and Hommel (1997) observed that creating and maintaining an action plan, such as preparing to press the left of two keys, strongly impairs the perception of visual events that share the same spatial feature, such as a left-pointing arrow. As Müsseler and Hommel argue, preparing a left action may have required or at least involved the binding of a <LEFT> feature to the action plan so that this feature was unavailable for the concurrent coding of feature-overlapping events. Consistent with this code-occupation hypothesis, Stoet and Hommel (1999) found that preparing an action with the left or right hand or foot interfered with planning another action with the same effector or on the same side. Along the same lines, Stoet and Hommel (2002) showed that holding a left or right stimulus event in short-term memory impaired the planning of a spatially corresponding manual action. Recent findings have demonstrated similar code-occupation effects in drawing movements (Schubö, Prinz, & Aschersleben, 2004) and weight judgments (Hamilton, Wolpert, & Frith, 2004).

Many researchers assume that human behavior is as flexible as it is because people can develop and apply clever strategies. Logan (1985), for instance, distinguishes between four functions of executive action control: the choice among strategies, the construction of a chosen strategy, the execution and maintenance of a strategy, and the inhibition of strategies if the goal changes. Unfortunately, however, the term "strategy" is commonly used without any definition. If we look it up in our *Collins Concise Dictionary,* we find two suggestions, "a particular long-term plan for success" and "a plan," which imply that executive control (and, thus, the handling of strategies) can be equated with the management of action plans (e.g., Norman & Shallice, 1986). Given that this management seems to be a more or less (conditionally) automatic function of activating a goal representation, which again may often be imposed by the social and physical environment (see the following discussion), we easily end up with a semantic paradox: What researchers call "strategy" may be the necessary consequence of contextual constraints and influences rather than reflecting conscious and willful decision making (as the everyday use of the term would imply). Indeed, recent findings strongly point in this direction. For instance, Bargh, Gollwitzer, Lee-Chai, Barndollar, and Trötschel (2001) found that people were doing substantially better in a word puzzle task if they had been nonconsciously primed with achievement-related words. Further experiments showed that behavior guided by these induced achievement strategies exhibits the same characteristics as behavior guided by self-set strategic goals: persistence at a task and task resumption after interruption (Bargh et al., 2001). Additionally, success and failure at nonconsciously induced strategic goals affect people's moods just like they do at conscious goals (Chartrand & Kay, 2008).

And yet, even if "strategies" may not be the most fortunate term to describe choices in the way an action is carried out, it is true that such choices can be induced and are being made: People instructed to act fast are commonly faster than people instructed to act accurately, people are more cautious (i.e., slower and more accurate) after having made a mistake, and asking someone to prioritize one of two concurrent tasks will improve his or her performance on this task. Hence, choices are being made, and they impact behavior, raising the question of how they do so. With regard to general "strategic" goals, however they may be induced, the answer is relatively easy. We have pointed out that adding a wanted feature to the goal description leads to changes in the top-down support for alternative actions competing for selection. Accordingly, adding the feature <FAST> to the goal description (e.g., as a consequence of instructing a subject accordingly) will favor action representations that also include this feature, again increasing the probability that a fast action (or a fast version of the action) will win the competition and be selected for execution. To be more precise: Given that action representations are composites, it is likely that there is only one <FAST> feature, which, if activated and bound to whatever other action components are selected, will speed up the execution.

An interesting implication of this assumption is that "strategies" may be misapplied, that is, extended to actions they were not "devised for." For instance, if instructing someone to carry out action X quickly leads to the activation of the <FAST> feature, carrying out another action Y should also be sped up. Even though we do not know of an experiment that has looked at this particular issue, there are two recent observations suggesting that our prediction may be correct. One stems from a study of Meiran, Hommel, Bibi, and Lev (2002), who had participants switch between randomly ordered tasks. People were cued in advance which task to perform next and instructed to prepare as much as possible before indicating their readiness for the upcoming task. Assuming that preparing for a task should take time (e.g., Rogers & Monsell, 1995), we expected a *negative* correlation between readiness time (the time people took to prepare) and reaction time (the time to carry out the actual task). Hence, responses should be faster the better prepared the task was. Paradoxically, however, the correlation was *positive,* indicating that long preparation went along with slow responding. Apparently, random trial-to-trial fluctuations in concentration or set for speed versus accuracy affected both readiness time and reaction time (and the underlying processes) to the same degree. This suggests that carryover effects of "strategic" parameters are possible: If one goes for speed or accuracy in preparing a task, one automatically takes over this "strategic preference" in subsequent responding.

Another carryover effect was demonstrated by Memelink and Hommel (2006), whose subjects performed a two-dimensional S-R compatibility task (i.e., a task in which the horizontal and vertical stimulus–response compatibility varied independently). This task was alternated with or was embedded in a logically unrelated "priming task" in which subjects were to discover particular stimulus–response rules. Making the horizontal dimension relevant in the priming task increased the horizontal compatibility effect, and making the vertical dimension relevant increased the vertical compatibility effect, suggesting that the attentional set induced by the priming task carried over to the compatibility task.

Preparing for an action often involves not only the specification and binding of the relevant action features but also the specification of the conditions under which the action should be carried out. Several authors have emphasized the importance of creating linkages between action plans and environmental trigger conditions for self-automatization (Bargh & Gollwitzer, 1994; Ellis, 1996; Mayr & Bryck, 2007). Hence, action planning will often involve the implementation of stimulus–response links, especially if the temporal delay between planning and execution is long. More important for our purposes (given our focus on short-term effects) is that planning an action involves the activation of the stimulus pointers that we have argued to be associated with plan elements. More needs to be known about which actions are associated with pointers to which stimulus dimensions, but a couple of connections have been revealed already, such as between grasping and shape (including size and orientation), pointing and location, tapping or speaking and rhythm, and velocity and position (Brenner et al., 1998; Fagioli et al., 2007; Jeannerod, 1981; Klatzky et al., 1995; Schubotz & von Cramon, 2003). The purpose of activating these pointers is to allow low-level action parameters to be filled in online during the actional phase (see previous section).

Actional Phase

The actional phase is entered as soon as the planned action begins. This will often be the case when the planning phase is completed or, with prospective planning, when the defined trigger event occurs. Interestingly, however, there is evidence that the execution of a plan does not need to await the plan's completion. First, action planning and action initiation can be dissociated empirically, as evident from the observation that the two processes can create different and independent dual-task bottlenecks in information processing (De Jong, 1993; Ivry, Franz, Kingstone, & Johnston, 1998; Logan & Burkell, 1986). For instance, Ivry et al. tested a split-brain patient in a dual-task experiment requiring speeded responses to lateralized stimuli. In contrast to healthy subjects who were strongly impaired if the stimulus–response mappings for two tasks were mutually incompatible (e.g., if stimuli appearing at the top and bottom of a display required top and bottom responses in one task but bottom and top responses in the other), the lack of callosal communication between the two cortical hemispheres allowed the patient to hold and apply the incompatible mappings concurrently without substantial drop in performance. And yet, the patient did show dual-task costs, suggesting that some late, postselection bottleneck was still operative.

Second, if the time available for planning is varied by means of a strict deadline technique, the kinematics of the action reflect a continuous transition from a default parameter (the average of all possible goal parameters) to the actual goal parameter (Ghez, Hening, & Favilla, 1990; van Sonderen & Denier van der Gon, 1991). This suggests that plans can be executed at any stage of (under)specification. These observations support Bullock and Grossberg's (1988) model of action-plan implementation (see also Rosenbaum, 1987). According to that model, a plan is executed whenever a respective go signal is given (which is considered to work much like James's "fiat"; James, 1890). This go signal is claimed to be nonspecific (i.e., blind to the action it launches) and temporally independent of action planning proper so that it can trigger the execution of a plan at any planning stage.

Even though we assume that actions are running more or less under "automatic pilot," this pilot is only conditionally automatic (Bargh, 1989) and thus reflects the current action goal. In particular, environmental information will get fast and automatic access to action control but only to the degree that it is rendered "legitimate"

and salient by an action-related pointer. That is, novel shape information about the target of a grasp will have direct impact on hand control, and changes in the location of a pointing target will immediately affect arm control. An excellent example for this mechanism are so-called double-step experiments in which the location of a visual goal is moved after the subject has started a reaching movement toward it. Under such circumstances, people move their hand to the new goal location without showing any signs of hesitation or correction in the speed or acceleration profiles. This is true even for conditions under which the change in location is carried out during an eye movement, thus preventing subjects from consciously perceiving the change (e.g., Prablanc & Pélisson, 1990; see also Bridgeman, Lewis, Heit, & Nagle, 1979; Goodale, Pélisson, & Prablanc, 1986). This suggests that the molar, goal-relevant parameters of the action (i.e., moving the hand to the visual target) were specified in the action plan, while the more incidental parameters (i.e., the exact movement path) were not. However, pointers were established to determine from which informational source the missing (incidental) parameters should be derived, thereby allowing information from this source to be picked up automatically (even unconsciously) and exploited to fine-tune the ongoing action.

To account for observations of this sort, a number of dual- or multiple-route models have been suggested. Milner and Goodale (1995) have attributed the off-line business of action planning to the ventral cortical pathway of visual information processing (which they somewhat unfortunately call the "perceptual" pathway) and the online specification of actions to the dorsal pathway (which they call the "action" pathway). The model has been widely discussed, and a number of theoretical flaws (Glover, 2004; Hommel et al., 2001) and empirical inconsistencies (e.g., Bruno, 2001; Franz, 2001; Jackson, 2000; Rossetti & Pisella, 2002) have been pointed out, but the basic distinction between the off-line planning process and the online specification of open parameters has found wide acceptance (e.g., Bridgeman, 2002; Glover, 2004; Hommel et al., 2001; Neumann & Klotz, 1994). Interestingly, not only can the online phase of action planning (or, perhaps better, parameter specification: Neumann & Klotz, 1994) operate independently of conscious awareness, as the findings of Bridgeman et al. (1979), Prablanc and Pélisson (1990), and others indicate, but the operations and computational products of this phase may even be inaccessible for conscious awareness in principle (Bridgeman, 2002; Glover, 2004; Keele, Ivry, Mayr, Hazeltine, & Heuer, 2003; Milner & Goodale, 1995). Even though more research on this issue is necessary, this assumption matches the observations of Münsterberg (1889) and Marbe (1901), who were perplexed to find nothing of theoretical interest in the introspective reports of their subjects about the time between a stimulus and the completion of the corresponding action. Among other things, it was this observation that was leading the members of the then-evolving Würzburg school to claim that task instructions are transformed into a cognitive task set before but not as a result of stimulus presentation.

Postactional Phase

Even though the way that actions are represented in the human cognitive system allows for the simulation of various alternatives and for the prediction of the most likely outcome of a given action, actually performing an action is the only way to find out whether one has made an appropriate choice. Accordingly, the postactional phase is important for evaluating actions, strengthening successful actions, and preventing or improving unsuccessful actions. A number of postactional activities are relevant for long-term learning, an important issue that, however, we do not focus on in this chapter. Also important are short-term adaptations that feed back into behavioral control immediately. Here we will discuss two of such adaptations: strategy adjustment and episodic binding. We introduce and discuss them separately because they are commonly investigated in different areas and with different theoretical goals in mind, but we conclude by considering how these two functions may work together.

Strategy adjustment refers to the fact that people learn from experience: We commonly do not repeat an action if it was unsuccessful, and we make active attempts to improve our actions all the time. This means that we must have had expectations about action outcomes, and/or representations of the ideal action that we compare with what we have actually achieved (Adams, 1968). Depending on the outcome of this comparison, we must be able to modify available action plans in such a way that the next execution of a given plan is likely to be more successful, thus minimizing the discrepancy between ideal and actual action. Such modifications may refer to any feature of an action, be it the smoothness of a golf swing, the affective tone of a musical piece, or the speed of a 100-meter sprint. That people can adjust all sorts of features of their action plans is obvious from many findings, such as the typical slowing down of responses after an error trial (Rabbitt, 1966), but there is not much we know about *how* the adjustment is done.

A number of recent observations suggest a possibly central role of conflict and conflict monitoring in error correction. Botvinick, Braver, Barch, Carter, and Cohen (2001) have suggested that the cognitive system may be comprised of a mechanism that is sensitive to conflict anywhere in the system, be it created by the activation of multiple stimulus representations or of multiple responses. If so, the presence or absence of conflict could be used to stimulate the adaptation of parameters and processes in perception and action control. A number of recent studies have been taken to provide support for the conflict-monitoring account. For instance, it has been observed that the impact of irrelevant, response-compatible or response-incompatible flankers on behavior increases after trials with compatible flankers and decreases after trials with incompatible flankers (Gratton, Coles, & Donchin, 1992). This may be explained by assuming that the detection of conflict leads to the (increased) inhibition of flanker processing, whereas the absence of conflict leads to either no change or a decrease of flanker inhibition (Botvinick et al., 2001; see Chapter 3). Likewise, it has been observed that stimulus–response compatibility effects become larger after compatible trials and smaller after incompatible trials (Stürmer, Leuthold, Schröter, Soetens, & Sommer, 2002), which may also be explained by conflict-induced adaptation of stimulus–response pathways.

However, the control-monitoring approach suffers from two problems, one theoretical and one empirical problem, and both of them point to a role of episodic binding. The empirical problem results from the fact that transitions between stimulus-compatible and/or response-compatible trials are often fully confounded with the sequential relationships between stimuli and responses. Assume, for instance, that a right response to a left stimulus is followed by a left response to a left stimulus. In the context of a study on control monitoring, this would count as the transition from a stimulus–response-incompatible to a stimulus–response-compatible trial. Finding that reaction time in the latter is higher than after a compatible trial (say, a right response to a right stimulus)

would be taken to mean that the conflict in the incompatible trial must have inhibited the impact of stimulus–response compatibility (e.g., Stürmer et al., 2002). Unfortunately, however, alternative interpretations are possible and, given independent evidence supporting it, in some cases even more plausible. It is known that performance is negatively affected by mismatches of stimulus–stimulus or stimulus–response conjunctions (Hommel, 1998), most likely because repeating one element leads to an automatic retrieval of the previously related elements (i.e., episodic bindings; Hommel, 2004). Accordingly, at least with two alternative tasks, it is impossible to tell whether worse performance in a compatible trial has resulted from the fact that the previous trial was incompatible or from the fact that the stimulus (or the response) is repeated while the response (or the stimulus) is not—and a clear-cut interpretation of better performance in an incompatible after a compatible trial is equally impossible (Hommel, Proctor, & Vu, 2004; Mayr, Awh, & Laurey, 2003). More recent studies have attempted to test the predictions from the conflict-monitoring approach under conditions in which episodic retrieval is unlikely to account for the findings (Ullsperger, Bylsma, & Botvinick, 2005; Wühr & Ansorge, 2005), and it seems that measurable effects remain. However, given that we still know very little about the structure of episodic traces and the conditions under which they are created, more research is clearly necessary on this issue.

The theoretical problem with the conflict-monitoring approach is that it can predict *when* adjustments are being made (i.e., whenever conflict is detected), but, as Botvinick et al. (2001) admit, it fails to explain *which* adjustments are made and *how* they are accomplished. Once this problem is solved, it may turn out that conflict monitoring and episodic retrieval do not represent mutually exclusive explanations of trial-to-trial variability but, rather, components of an adaptive network. Registering conflict in a given trial may increase the degree to which the current goal is activated. According to our present considerations, this should increase the impact of top-down processes on the competition between and eventual selection among stimulus events and, more important for present purposes, action alternatives. In particular, refreshing the goal representation should strengthen the impact of action-related pointers to the relevant stimulus and response dimensions, thereby increasing the relative impact of action-related information. As a consequence, the system would behave exactly as Botvinick et al. (2001) suggested: The detection of conflict would lead to a decreased impact of (task-irrelevant) flankers in a flanker task and of (task-irrelevant) stimulus–response compatibility in a compatibility task. Moreover, emphasizing the task-relevant feature dimensions will affect episodic retrieval in such a way that task-relevant stimulus and response features will contribute more strongly to the retrieval process; that is, repeating a task-relevant feature will be more likely to trigger the retrieval of a previous episode including that feature than repeating a task-irrelevant feature. And that task relevance affects the retrieval of episodic bindings has been demonstrated only recently (Hommel, Memelink, Zmigrod, & Colzato, 2008).

Summary

The control of human action comprises at least three different phases with distinct functions. The first, planning phase consists of specifying the relevant features of an action, activating the codes representing and controlling them, and integrating these codes into a coherent action plan. The second, actional phase consists of an interaction between the controlling action plan and sensorimotor streams that provide online information to concretize the action and to specify the parameters left open in the plan. The third, postactional phase consists of the evaluation of the action's success, the thereby informed and controlled storage of information that links the action to the current context (i.e., the creation of episodic bindings), and the adaptive modification of the action plan and the general strategy if necessary.

Conclusions

In this chapter, we have painted a picture of voluntary action as gradually emerging from sensorimotor experience, just as envisioned by James (1890). Infants, children, and adult novices in some sense observe themselves moving and extract from that experience systematic relationships between movement patterns and their sensory consequences. Representations of these consequences are then increasingly used to anticipate wanted action effects, and this at the same time primes the action producing these effects. That is, self-prediction and self-control go hand in hand. The distributed representation of action plans provides the backbone for human flexibility and adaptivity: Inappropriate plans can be quickly adapted by modifying only a few parameters, new plans can be derived from overlearned plans through extrapolation and generalization, and forgetting or cell loss can be compensated rather easily. Actions are thus at the core of larger representational networks that can include codes of the sensory and affective by-products of the action, codes of the most appropriate context, verbal descriptions of the action and its function in a particular context, and more. The representations of actions and the broader cognitive structures of which action plans are a part are not fixed or invariant, as the metaphor of a motor or action "program" may imply. Rather, action plans should be thought of as networks of feature codes that are continuously updated and tailored to the current situation and the task at hand. Once implemented, such networks in some sense automatize the actor in taking care of the intended action outcome and channeling up-to-date, online environmental information to the appropriate motor systems. Hence, somewhat paradoxically, we control our actions long before we actually carry them out.

Acknowledgments

Support from a grant of the German Research Community (DFG, Priority Program on Executive Functions, HO 1430/8-3) to BH is gratefully acknowledged. BH is member of the EPOS research school.

Note

1. We consider it reasonable to distinguish between functional units and anatomical units. Two or more elements are thus considered a functional unit if they tend to "go together," that is, if activating/involving one element will almost always lead to the activation/involvement of the other. This does not necessarily exclude the possibility that the elements of a functional unit are anatomically separable, for instance, by lesioning one component of a neural network but not the other.

References

Adams, J. A. (1968). Response feedback and learning. *Psychological Bulletin, 70,* 486–504.

Adams, J. A. (1971). A closed-loop theory of motor learning. *Journal of Motor Behavior, 3,* 111–150.

Baddeley, A., Chincotta, D., & Adlam, A. (2001). Working memory and the control of action: Evidence from task switching. *Journal of Experimental Psychology: General, 130,* 641–657.

Bargh, J. A. (1989). Conditional automaticity: Varieties of automatic influence in social perception and cognition. In J. S. Uleman & J. A. Bargh (Eds.), *Unintended thought* (pp. 3–51). London: Guilford Press.

Bargh, J. A., & Gollwitzer, P. M. (1994). Environmental control over goal-directed action. *Nebraska Symposium on Motivation, 41,* 71–124.

Bargh, J. A., Gollwitzer, P. M., Lee-Chai, A. Y., Barndollar, K., & Trötschel, R. (2001). The automated will: Nonconscious activation and pursuit of behavioral goals. *Journal of Personality and Social Psychology, 81,* 1014–1027.

Barkley, R. A. (1997). Behavioral inhibitory control, sustained attention, and executive functions: Constructing a unifying theory of ADHD. *Psychological Bulletin, 121,* 65–94.

Barsalou, L. W. (1999). Perceptual symbol systems. *Behavioral and Brain Sciences, 22,* 577–609.

Bauer, B., & Besner, D. (1997). Processing in the Stroop task: Mental set as a determinant of performance. *Canadian Journal of Experimental Psychology, 51,* 61–68.

Bechara, A., Damasio, H., Tranel, D., & Damasio, A. R. (1997). Deciding advantageously before knowing the advantageous strategy. *Science, 275,* 1293–1295.

Beckers, T., De Houwer, J., & Eelen, P. (2002). Automatic integration of non-perceptual action effect features: The case of the associative affective Simon effect. *Psychological Research, 66,* 166–173.

Bonnet, M., & MacKay, W. A. (1989). Changes in contingent-negative variation and reaction time related to precueing of direction and force of a forearm movement. *Brain, Behavior and Evolution, 33,* 147–152.

Botvinick, M., Braver, T., Barch, D., Carter, C., & Cohen, J. (2001). Conflict and cognitive control. *Psychological Review, 108,* 625–652.

Brenner, E., Smeets, J., & de Lussanet, M. (1998). Hitting moving targets: Continuous control of the acceleration of the hand on the basis of the target's velocity. *Experimental Brain Research, 122,* 467–474.

Bridgeman, B. (2002). Attention and visually guided behavior in distinct systems. In W. Prinz & B. Hommel (Eds.), *Common mechanisms in perception and action: Attention and performance XIX* (pp. 120–135). Oxford: Oxford University Press.

Bridgeman, B., Lewis, S., Heit, G., & Nagle, M. (1979). Relation between cognitive and motor-oriented systems of visual position perception. *Journal of Experimental Psychology: Human Perception and Performance, 5,* 692–700.

Bruno, N. (2001). When does action resist visual illusions? *Trends in Cognitive Sciences, 5,* 379–382.

Bullock, D., & Grossberg, S. (1988). Neural dynamics of planned arm movements: Emergent invariants and speed-accuracy properties during trajectory formation. *Psychological Review, 95,* 49–90.

Caessens, B., Hommel, B., Lammertyn, J., & Van der Goten, K. (2008). *The functional basis of backward-compatibility effects: Selecting emotional actions primes the perception of emotional words.* Manuscript submitted for publication.

Chartrand, T. L., & Kay, A. (2008). *Mystery moods and perplexing performance: Consequences of succeeding and failing at a nonconscious goal.* Manuscript submitted for publication.

Cohen, J. D., Dunbar, K., & McClelland, J. L. (1990). On the control of automatic processes: A parallel distributed processing account of the Stroop effect. *Psychological Review, 97,* 332–361.

Damasio, A. (1994). *Descartes' error.* New York: G. P. Putnam's Sons.

DeCasper, A. J., & Fifer, W. P. (1980). Of human bonding: Newborns prefer their mothers' voices. *Science, 208,* 1174–1176.

De Jong, R. (1993). Multiple bottlenecks in overlapping task performance. *Journal of Experimental Psychology: Human Perception and Performance, 19,* 965–980.

Desimone, R., & Duncan, J. (1995). Neural mechanisms of selective visual attention. *Annual Review of Neuroscience, 18,* 193–222.

Donders, F. C. (1868). *Over de snelheid van psychische processen.* Onderzoekingen, gedan in het physiologisch laboratorium der Utrechtsche hoogeschool, 2. reeks, 92–120.

Dowsett, S. M., & Livesey, D. J. (2000). The development of inhibitory control in preschool children: Effects of "executive skills" training. *Developmental Psychobiology, 36,* 161–174.

Duncan, J., & Humphreys, G. W. (1989). Visual search and stimulus similarity. *Psychological Review, 96,* 433–458.

Eenshuistra, R. M., Weidema, M. A., & Hommel, B. (2004). Development of the acquisition and control of action-effect associations. *Acta Psychologica, 115,* 185–209.

Eimer, M. (1995). Stimulus-response compatibility and automatic response activation: Evidence from psychophysiological studies. *Journal of Experimental Psychology: Human Perception and Performance, 21,* 837–854.

Eimer, M., & Schlaghecken, F. (1998). Effects of masked stimuli on motor activation: Behavioral and electrophysiological evidence. *Journal of Experimental Psychology: Human Perception and Performance, 24,* 1737–1747.

Ellis, J. (1996). Prospective memory or the realization of delayed intentions: A conceptual framework for research. In M. Brandimonte, G. O. Einstein, & M. A. McDaniel (Eds.), *Prospective memory: Theory and applications* (pp. 371–376). Hillsdale, NJ: Lawrence Erlbaum Associates.

Elsner, B., & Aschersleben, G. (2003). Do I get what you get? Learning about the effects of self-performed and observed actions in infancy. *Consciousness and Cognition, 12,* 732–751.

Elsner, B., & Hommel, B. (2001). Effect anticipation and action control. *Journal of Experimental Psychology: Human Perception and Performance, 27,* 229–240.

Elsner, B., & Hommel, B. (2004). Contiguity and contingency in action-effect learning. *Psychological Research, 68,* 138–154.

Elsner, B., Hommel, B., Mentschel, C., Drzezga, A., Prinz, W., Conrad, B., et al. (2002). Linking actions and their perceivable consequences in the human brain. *Neuroimage, 17,* 364–372.

Emerson, M. J., & Miyake, A. (2003). The role of inner speech in task switching: A dual-task investigation. *Journal of Memory and Language, 48,* 148–168.

Exner, S. (1879). Physiologie der Grosshirnrinde. In L. Hermann (Ed.), *Handbuch der Physiologie* (Vol. 2, Pt. 2, pp. 189–350). Leipzig: Vogel.

Fagioli, S., Hommel, B., & Schubotz, R. I. (2007). Intentional control of attention: Action planning primes action-related stimulus dimensions. *Psychological Research, 71,* 22–29.

Flach, R., Osman, M., Dickinson, A., & Heyes, C. M. (2006). The interaction of response effects in response effect priming. *Acta Psychologica, 122,* 11–26.

Förster, J., Higgins, E. T., & Taylor Bianco, A. (2003). Speed/accuracy in performance: Trade-off in decision making or separate strategic concerns? *Organizational Behavior and Human Decision Processes, 90,* 148–164.

Franz, V. H. (2001). Action does not resist visual illusions. *Trends in Cognitive Sciences, 5,* 457–459.

Freud, S. (1914). *Psychopathology of everyday life.* London: T. Fisher Unwin.

Fuster, J. M. (1989). *The prefrontal cortex.* New York: Raven Press.

Georgopoulos, A. P. (1990). Neurophysiology of reaching. In M. Jeannerod (Ed.), *Attention and performance XIII: Motor representation and control* (pp. 227–263). Hillsdale, NJ: Lawrence Erlbaum Associates.

Gergely, G., & Watson, J. S. (1999). Early social-emotional development: Contingency perception and the social biofeedback model. In P. Rochat (Ed.), *Early social cognition* (pp. 101–136). Hillsdale, NJ: Lawrence Erlbaum Associates.

Ghez, C., Hening, W., & Favilla, M. (1990). Parallel interacting channels in the initiation and specification of motor response features. In M. Jeannerod (Ed.), *Attention and performance XIII: Motor representation and control* (pp. 265–293). Hillsdale, NJ: Lawrence Erlbaum Associates.

Gibson, J. J. (1979). *The ecological approach to visual perception.* Boston: Houghton Mifflin.

Gilbert, S. J., & Shallice, T. (2002). Task switching: A PDP model. *Cognitive Psychology, 44,* 297–337.

Glover, S. (2004). Separate visual representations in the planning and control of action. *Behavioral and Brain Sciences, 27,* 3–24.

Goodale, M. A., Jakobson, L., Milner, A., Perrett, D., Benson, P., & Hietanen, J. (1994). The nature and limits of orientation and pattern processing supporting visuomotor control in a visual form agnosic. *Journal of Cognitive Neuroscience, 6,* 46–56.

Goodale, M. A., Pélisson, D., & Prablanc, C. (1986). Large adjustments in visually guided reaching do not depend on vision of the hand or perception of target displacement. *Nature, 320,* 748–750.

Goschke, T. (2000). Intentional reconfiguration and involuntary persistence in task-set switching. In S. Monsell & J. Driver (Eds.), *Control of cognitive processes: Attention and performance XVIII* (pp. 331–355). Cambridge, MA: MIT Press.

Gratton, G., Coles, M. G. H., & Donchin, E. (1992). Optimizing the use of information: Strategic control of activation of responses. *Journal of Experimental Psychology: General, 121,* 480–506.

Hamilton, A., Wolpert, D. M., & Frith, U. (2004). Your own action influences how you perceive another person's action. *Current Biology, 14,* 493–498.

Harless, E. (1861). Der Apparat des Willens. *Zeitschrift für Philosophie und philosophische Kritik, 38,* 50–73.

Hazeltine, E. (2002). The representational nature of sequence learning: Evidence for goal-based codes. In W. Prinz & B. Hommel (Eds.), *Common mechanisms in perception and action: Attention and performance XIX* (pp. 673–689). Oxford: Oxford University Press.

Heckhausen, H., & Gollwitzer, P. M. (1987). Thought contents and cognitive functioning in motivational vs. volitional states of mind. *Motivation and Emotion, 11,* 101–120.

Hoffmann, J., Sebald, A., & Stoecker, C. (2001). Irrelevant response effects improve serial learning in serial reaction time tasks. *Journal of Experimental Psychology: Learning, Memory, and Cognition, 27,* 470–482.

Hommel, B. (1993). Inverting the Simon effect by intention: Determinants of direction and extent of effects of irrelevant spatial information. *Psychological Research, 55,* 270–279.

Hommel, B. (1996). The cognitive representation of action: Automatic integration of perceived action effects. *Psychological Research, 59,* 176–186.

Hommel, B. (1998). Event files: Evidence for automatic integration of stimulus-response episodes. *Visual Cognition, 5,* 183–216.

Hommel, B. (2000). The prepared reflex: Automaticity and control in stimulus-response translation. In S. Monsell & J. Driver (Eds.), *Control of cognitive processes: Attention and performance XVIII* (pp. 247–273). Cambridge, MA: MIT Press.

Hommel, B. (2004). Event files: Feature binding in and across perception and action. *Trends in Cognitive Sciences, 8,* 494–500.

Hommel, B., Alonso, D., & Fuentes, L. J. (2003). Acquisition and generalization of action effects. *Visual Cognition, 10,* 965–986.

Hommel, B., & Knuf, L. (2000). Action related determinants of spatial coding in perception and memory. In C. Freksa, W. Brauer, C. Habel, & K. F. Wender (Eds.), *Spatial cognition II: Integrating abstract theories, empirical studies, formal methods, and practical applications* (pp. 387–398). Berlin: Springer.

Hommel, B., Memelink, J., Zmigrod, S., & Colzato, L. S. (2008). *How information of relevant dimension control the creation and retrieval of feature-response binding.* Manuscript submitted for publication.

Hommel, B., Müsseler, J., Aschersleben, G., & Prinz, W. (2001). The theory of event coding: A framework for perception and action planning. *Behavioral and Brain Sciences, 24,* 849–937.

Hommel, B., Proctor, R. W., & Vu, K.-P. L. (2004). A feature-integration account of sequential effects in the Simon task. *Psychological Research, 68,* 1–17.

Ivry, R. B., Franz, E. A., Kingstone, A., & Johnston, J. C. (1998). The psychological refractory period effect following callosotomy: Uncoupling of lateralized response codes. *Journal of Experimental Psychology: Human Perception and Performance, 24,* 463–480.

Jackson, S. R. (2000). Perception, awareness and action. In Y. Rossetti & A. Revonsuo (Eds.), *Interaction between dissociable conscious and nonconscious processes* (pp. 73–98). Amsterdam: John Benjamins.

James, W. (1884). What is an emotion? *Mind, 9,* 188–205.

James, W. (1890). *The principles of psychology.* New York: Dover.

Jeannerod, M. (1981). Intersegmental coordination during reaching at natural objects. In J. Long &

A. Baddeley (Eds.), *Attention and performance IX* (pp. 153–169). Hillsdale, NJ: Lawrence Erlbaum Associates.

Jeannerod, M. (1984). The contribution of open-loop and closed-loop control modes in prehension movements. In S. Kornblum & J. Requin (Eds.), *Preparatory states and processes* (pp. 323–337). Hillsdale, NJ: Lawrence Erlbaum Associates.

Kahneman, D., & Tversky, A. (Eds.). (2000). *Choices, values, and frames.* New York: Cambridge University Press.

Kalaska, J. F., & Hyde, M. L. (1985). Area 4 and area 5: Differences between the load direction-dependent discharge variability of cells during active postural fixation. *Experimental Brain Research, 59,* 197–202.

Keele, S. W. (1968). Movement control in skilled motor performance. *Psychological Bulletin, 70,* 387–403.

Keele, S., Ivry, R., Mayr, U., Hazeltine, E., & Heuer, H. (2003). The cognitive and neural architecture of sequence representation. *Psychological Review, 110,* 316–339.

Kellman, P. J., & Arterberry, M. E. (1998). *The cradle of knowledge: Development of perception in infancy.* Cambridge, MA: MIT Press.

Klatzky, R. L., Fikes, T. G., & Pellegrino, J. W. (1995). Planning for hand shape and arm transport when reaching for objects. *Acta Psychologica, 88,* 209–232.

Koch, I., & Kunde, W. (2002). Verbal response-effect compatibility. *Memory and Cognition, 30,* 1297–1303.

Kray, J., Eber, J., & Lindenberger, U. (2004). Age differences in executive functioning across the lifespan: The role of verbalization in task preparation. *Acta Psychologica, 115,* 143–165.

Kray, J., Eenshuistra, R., Kerstner, H., Weidema, M., & Hommel, B. (2006). Language and action control: The acquisition of action goals in early childhood. *Psychological Science, 17,* 737–774.

Kunde, W. (2001). Response-effect compatibility in manual choice reaction tasks. *Journal of Experimental Psychology: Human Perception and Performance, 27,* 387–394.

Kunde, W. (2004). Response priming by supraliminal and subliminal action effects. *Psychological Research, 68,* 91–96.

Kunde, W., Hoffmann, J., & Zellmann, P. (2002). The impact of anticipated action effects on action planning. *Acta Psychologica, 109,* 137–155.

Kutas, M., & Donchin, E. (1980). Preparation to respond as manifested by movement-related brain potentials. *Brain Research, 202,* 95–115.

Lashley, K. S. (1951). The problem of serial order in behavior. In L. A. Jeffress (Ed.), *Cerebral mechanisms in behavior* (pp. 112–146). New York: Wiley.

Lépine, D., Glencross, D., & Requin, J. (1989). Some experimental evidence for and against a parametric conception of movement programming. *Journal of Experimental Psychology: Human Perception and Performance, 15,* 347–362.

Levy, F. (1980). The development of sustained attention (vigilance) and inhibition in children: Some normative data. *Journal of Child Psychiatry, 21,* 77–84.

Lewis, M., Sullivan, M. W., & Brooks-Gunn, J. (1985). Emotional behaviour during the learning of a contingency in early infancy. *British Journal of Developmental Psychology, 3,* 307–316.

Logan, G. D. (1985). Executive control of thought and action. *Acta Psychologica, 60,* 193–210.

Logan, G. D., & Burkell, J. (1986). Dependence and independence in responding to double stimulation: A comparison of stop, change, and dual-task paradigms. *Journal of Experimental Psychology: Human Perception and Performance, 12,* 549–563.

Logan, G. D., & Cowan, W. B. (1984). On the ability to inhibit thought and action: A theory of an act of control. *Psychological Review, 91,* 295–327.

Lotze, R. H. (1852). *Medicinische Psychologie oder die Physiologie der Seele.* Leipzig: Weidmann'sche Buchhandlung.

Lu, C.-H., & Proctor, R. W. (1995). The influence of irrelevant location information on performance: A review of the Simon and spatial Stroop effects. *Psychonomic Bulletin and Review, 2,* 174–207.

Luria, A. R. (1959). The directive function of speech in development and dissolution. *Word, 15,* 341–352.

Luria, A. R. (1961). The development of the regulatory role of speech. In J. Tizard (Ed.), *The role of speech in the regulation of normal and abnormal behavior* (pp. 50–96). New York: Liverlight.

MacLeod, C. M. (1991). Half a century of research on the Stroop effect: An integrative review. *Psychological Bulletin, 109,* 163–203.

Marbe, K. (1901). *Experimentell-psychologische Untersuchungen über das Urteil.* Leipzig: Engelmann.

Mayr, U., Awh, E., & Laurey, P. (2003). Conflict adaptation effects in the absence of executive control. *Nature Neuroscience, 6,* 450–452.

Mayr, U., & Bryck, R. L. (2007). Low-level constraints on high-level selection: Switching tasks with and without switching stimulus/response objects. *Psychological Research, 71*, 107–116.

Meiran, N., Hommel, B., Bibi, U., & Lev, I. (2002). Consciousness and control in task switching. *Consciousness and Cognition, 11*, 10–33.

Memelink, J., & Hommel, B. (2006). Tailoring perception and action to the task at hand. *European Journal of Cognitive Psychology, 18*, 579–592.

Miller, G. A., Galanter, E., & Pribram, K. H. (1960). *Plans and the structure of behavior.* New York: Holt, Rinehart and Winston.

Milner, A. D., & Goodale, M. A. (1995). *The visual brain in action.* Oxford: Oxford University Press.

Morris, R., & Ward, G. (2005). (Eds.). *The cognitive psychology of planning.* Hove: Psychology Press.

Münsterberg, H. (1889). *Beiträge zur experimentellen Psychologie* (Heft 1). Freiburg: Mohr.

Müsseler, J., & Hommel, B. (1997). Blindness to response-compatible stimuli. *Journal of Experimental Psychology: Human Perception and Performance, 23*, 861–872.

Neumann, O., & Klotz, W. (1994). Motor responses to nonreportable, masked stimuli: Where is the limit of direct parameter specification? In C. Umiltà & M. Moscovitch (Eds.), *Attention and performance XV: Conscious and nonconscious information processing* (pp. 123–150). Cambridge, MA: MIT Press.

Norman, D. A., & Shallice, T. (1986). Attention to action: Willed and automatic control of behavior. In R. J. Davidson, G. E. Schwartz, & D. Shapiro (Eds.), *Consciousness and self-regulation* (Vol. 4, pp. 1–17). New York: Plenum Press.

Papousek, H. (1967). Experimental studies of appetitional behavior in human newborns and infants. In H. W. Stevenson, E. H. Hess, & H. L. Rheingold (Eds.), *Early behavior* (pp. 249–277). New York: Wiley.

Papousek, H. (1969). Individual variability in learned responses in human infants. In R. J. Robinson (Ed.), *Brain and early behavior* (pp. 251–266). New York: Academic Press.

Pashler, H. (1994). Dual-task interference in simple tasks: Data and theory. *Psychological Bulletin, 116*, 220–244.

Pashler, H., & Johnston, J. C. (1989). Chronometric evidence for central postponement in temporally overlapping tasks. *Quarterly Journal of Experimental Psychology, 41A*, 19–45.

Piaget, J. (1952). *The origins of intelligence in children.* New York: International Universities Press.

Prablanc, C., & Pélisson, D. (1990). Gaze saccade orienting and hand pointing are locked to their goal by quick internal loops. In M. Jeannerod (Ed.), *Attention and performance XIII* (pp. 653–676). Hillsdale, NJ: Lawrence Erlbaum Associates.

Prinz, W. (1990). A common coding approach to perception and action. In O. Neumann & W. Prinz (Eds.), *Relationships between perception and action* (pp. 167–201). Berlin: Springer-Verlag.

Prinz, W. (1992). Why don't we perceive our brain states? *European Journal of Cognitive Psychology, 4*, 1–20.

Pulvermüller, F. (2003). *The neuroscience of language.* Cambridge: Cambridge University Press.

Pulvermüller, F., Hauk, O., Nikulin, V. V., & Ilmoniemi, R. J. (2005). Functional links between motor and language systems. *European Journal of Neuroscience, 21*, 793–797.

Rabbitt, P. M. (1966). Errors and error correction in choice-response tasks. *Journal of Experimental Psychology, 71*, 264–272.

Richardson, D. C., & Spivey, M. J. (2000). Representation, space and Hollywood Squares: Looking at things that aren't there anymore. *Cognition, 76*, 269–295.

Ridderinkhof, K. R. (2002). Activation and suppression in conflict tasks: Empirical clarification through distributional analyses. In W. Prinz & B. Hommel (Eds.), *Attention and performance XIX: Common mechanisms in perception and action* (pp. 494–519). Oxford: Oxford University Press.

Riehle, A., & Requin, J. (1989). Monkey primary motor and premotor cortex: Single-cell activity related to prior information about direction and extent of an intended movement. *Journal of Neurophysiology, 61*, 534–549.

Rochat, P. (1998). Self-perception and action in infancy. *Experimental Brain Research, 132*, 102–109.

Rochat, P., & Morgan, R. (1998). Two functional orientations of self-exploration in infancy. *British Journal of Developmental Psychology, 16*, 139–154.

Rochat, P., & Striano, T. (1999). Emerging self-exploration by 2-month-old infants. *Developmental Science, 2*, 206–218.

Rogers, R. D., & Monsell, S. (1995). Cost of a predictable switch between simple cognitive tasks. *Journal of Experimental Psychology: Human Perception and Performance, 124*, 207–231.

Rolls, E. T. (1999). *The brain and emotion.* Oxford: Oxford University Press.

Rosenbaum, D. A. (1980). Human movement initiation: Specification of arm, direction and extent. *Journal of Experimental Psychology: General, 109,* 444–474.

Rosenbaum, D. A. (1987). Successive approximations to a model of human motor programming. *Psychology of Learning and Motivation, 21,* 153–182.

Rosenbaum, D. A., Meulenbroek, R. J., Vaughan, J., & Jansen, C. (2001). Posture-based motion planning: Applications to grasping. *Psychological Review, 108,* 709–734.

Rossetti, Y., & Pisella, L. (2002). Several "vision for action" systems: A guide to dissociating and integrating dorsal and ventral functions. In W. Prinz & B. Hommel (Eds.), *Attention and performance XIX: Common mechanisms in perception and action* (pp. 62–119). Oxford: Oxford University Press.

Rovee, C. K., & Rovee, D. T. (1969). Conjugate reinforcement of infants' exploratory behavior. *Journal of Experimental Child Psychology, 8,* 33–39.

Rovee-Collier, C. (1987). Learning and memory in infancy. In J. D. Osofsky (Ed.), *Handbook of infant development* (2nd ed., pp. 98–148). New York: Wiley.

Schmidt, R. A. (1975). A schema theory of discrete motor skill learning. *Psychological Review, 82,* 225–260.

Schubö, A., Prinz, W., & Aschersleben, G. (2004). Perceiving while acting: Action affects perception. *Psychological Research, 68,* 208–215.

Schubotz, R. I., Friederici, A., D., & von Cramon, D. Y. (2000). Time perception and motor timing: A common cortical and subcortical basis revealed by fMRI. *Neuroimage, 11,* 1–12.

Schubotz, R. I., Sakreida, K., Tittgemeyer, M., & von Cramon, D. Y. (2004). Motor areas beyond motor performance: Deficits in sensory prediction following ventrolateral premotor lesions. *Neuropsychology, 18,* 638–645.

Schubotz, R. I., & von Cramon, D. Y. (2001). Functional organization of the lateral premotor cortex: fMRI reveals different regions activated by anticipation of object properties, location and speed. *Cognitive Brain Research, 11,* 97–112.

Schubotz, R. I., & von Cramon, D. Y. (2002). Predicting perceptual events activates corresponding motor schemes in lateral premotor cortex: An fMRI study. *Neuroimage, 15,* 787–796.

Schubotz, R. I., & von Cramon, D. Y. (2003). Functional-anatomical concepts of human premotor cortex: Evidence from fMRI and PET studies. *Neuroimage, 20,* S120–S131.

Sommer, W., Leuthold, H., & Hermanutz, M. (1993). Covert effects of alcohol revealed by event-related potentials. *Perception and Psychophysics, 54,* 127–135.

Sternberg, S. (1969). The discovery of processing stages: Extensions of Donders' method. *Acta Psychologica, 30,* 276–315.

Stock, A., & Hoffmann, J. (2002). Intentional fixation of behavioural learning, or how R-O learning blocks S-R learning. *European Journal of Cognitive Psychology, 14,* 127–153.

Stoet, G., & Hommel, B. (1999). Action planning and the temporal binding of response codes. *Journal of Experimental Psychology: Human Perception and Performance, 25,* 1625–1640.

Stoet, G., & Hommel, B. (2002). Interaction between feature binding in perception and action. In W. Prinz & B. Hommel (Eds.), *Common mechanisms in perception and action: Attention and Performance XIX* (pp. 538–552). Oxford: Oxford University Press.

Stürmer, B., Leuthold, H., Schröter, H., Soetens, E., & Sommer, W. (2002). Control over location-based response activation in the Simon task: Behavioral and electrophysiological evidence. *Journal of Experimental Psychology: Human Perception and Performance, 28,* 1345–1363.

Thompson, P., Gied, J. N., Woods, R. P., MacDonald, D., Evans, A. C., & Toga, A. W. (2000). Growth patterns in the developing brain detected by using continuum mechanical tensor maps. *Nature, 404,* 191–193.

Thorndike, E. L. (1927). The law of effect. *American Journal of Psychology, 39,* 212–222.

Tomasello, M. (1999). *The cultural origins of human cognition.* Cambridge, MA: Harvard University Press.

Treisman, A. (1996). The binding problem. *Current Opinion in Neurobiology, 6,* 171–178.

Ullsperger, M., Bylsma, L. M., & Botvinick, M. (2005). The conflict-adaptation effect: It's not just priming. *Cognitive, Affective, and Behavioral Neuroscience, 5,* 467–472.

Valle-Inclán, F., & Redondo, M. (1998). On the automaticity of ipsilateral response activation in the Simon effect. *Psychophysiology, 35,* 366–371.

van Sonderen, J. F., & Denier van der Gon, J. J. (1991). Reaction-time-dependent differences in the initial movement direction of fast goal-directed arm movements. *Human Movement Science, 10,* 713–726.

Vidal, F., Bonnet, M., & Macar, F. (1991). Programming response duration in a precueing reaction time paradigm. *Journal of Motor Behavior, 23,* 226–234.

von Hofsten, C. (2004). An action perspective on motor development. *Trends in Cognitive Sciences, 8,* 266–272.

Vygotsky, L. S. (1962). *Thought and language.* Cambridge, MA: MIT Press. (Original work published 1934)

Walker, E. L. (1969). Reinforcement—"The one ring." In J. T. Tapp (Ed.), *Reinforcement and behavior* (pp. 47–62). New York: Academic Press.

Watson, J. S. (1972). Smiling, cooing, and "the game." *Merrill-Palmer Quarterly, 18,* 323–339.

Watson, J. S., & Ramey, C. T. (1972). Reactions to response-contingent stimulation in early infancy. *Merrill-Palmer Quarterly, 18,* 219–227.

Willats, P. (1999). Development of means-end behavior in young infants: Pulling a support to retrieve a distant object. *Developmental Psychology, 35,* 651–666.

Woodworth, R. S. (1938). *Experimental psychology.* New York: Holt, Rinehart and Winston.

Wühr, P., & Ansorge, U. (2005). Exploring trial-by-trial modulations of the Simon effect. *Quarterly Journal of Experimental Psychology, 58A,* 705–731.

Zelazo, P. D. (1999). Self-reflection and the development of consciously controlled processing. In P. Mitchell & K. J. Riggs (Eds.), *Children's reasoning and the mind.* Hove: Psychology Press.

Ziessler, M., & Nattkemper, D. (2001). Learning of event sequences is based on response-effect learning: Further evidence from a serial reaction task. *Journal of Experimental Psychology: Learning, Memory, and Cognition, 27,* 595–613.

Ziessler, M., Nattkemper, D., & Frensch, P. (2004). The role of anticipation and intention in the learning of effects of self-performed actions. *Psychological Research, 68,* 163–175.

19

Flexibility in the Development of Action

Karen E. Adolph, Amy S. Joh, John M. Franchak, Shaziela Ishak, *and* Simone V. Gill

Abstract

This chapter has two major aims. The first is to describe flexibility in motor action. Balance and locomotion in infants are used as a test case for understanding three aspects of behavioral flexibility—adaptive motor decisions, modification of ongoing activity, and new means to achieve a goal. The second aim is to illuminate the links between flexibility and development. In particular, it demonstrates that flexibility is acquired during development and that developmental changes both facilitate and impede its acquisition. It is shown that flexibility does not automatically appear when infants acquire new forms of balance and locomotion. Instead, flexibility is learned over many weeks of everyday locomotor experience in a newly acquired posture. Infants learn how to learn as they acquire the appropriate exploratory behaviors for generating information about the current constraints on action and potential alternatives for achieving their goals. Two kinds of limits on flexibility are described—one created by developmental transitions to new postural control systems and the other created by the nature of the perceptual information for friction and rigidity.

Keywords: flexibility, learning, motor action, infants, balance, locomotion

Behavioral flexibility is the essence of goal-directed action. Flexibility is the wherewithal to cope with variable and novel circumstances: selecting adaptive responses to novel instances of a problem, modifying ongoing behaviors in accordance with changes in local conditions, and finding new means to achieve a desired outcome (Adolph, 2005; Adolph & Berger, 2006). Motor actions are movements of the eyes, head, limbs, and body that are geared to getting information about or interacting with the world. Flexibility is essential for motor action because variability and novelty are endemic in everyday activities. Local conditions are continually changing. Constraints on movement are always in flux. For actions to be adaptive and functional, movements must be selected and modified to suit the demands of the current situation (Bernstein, 1996; E. J. Gibson & Pick, 2000). Motor actions must reflect the here and now while simultaneously anticipating the immediate future (von Hofsten, 2003, 2004). Motor decisions must match the actual possibilities for action.

Learning to Learn

Flexibility refers to the creative and improvisatory nature of action. Motor actions require a variety of means, not the same movements over and over. To take current conditions into account while guiding action toward the intended goal, each movement must be performed a little bit differently. Even highly practiced actions such as walking cannot be a series of rote repetitions with each step exactly like the last because the everyday environment is not like a big gymnasium with uniform, open ground. In real life, paths are cluttered and ground surfaces are infinitely variable. Walking cannot be choreographed or prescribed by a preexisting plan because the everyday environment is not like a fixed obstacle course with all the challenges known ahead of time. Instead, the precise nature of each challenge is always new. Walking speed and step length increase and decrease in preparation for navigating obstacles; legs rise to different heights to clear impediments or to lower the body; the torso twists or bends to slide through narrow passages or under barriers; arms swing freely, raise to the sides for balance, or grasp supports; double steps, back steps, cross steps, and side steps correct missteps; and new routes or alternative modes of locomotion are chosen if the path is impassable.

Flexibility, with its emphasis on discovery in the present moment, is akin to Harlow's (1949) notion of "learning to learn" (Adolph, 2002, 2005). As Stevenson (1972) put it, "The ultimate goal in any type of learning cannot be the retention of large amounts of specific information. For the most part, this information will be forgotten. What can be retained are techniques for acquiring new information, learning how to attend to relevant cues and ignore irrelevant cues, how to apply hypotheses and strategies and relinquish them when they are unsuccessful" (p. 307). In other words, rather than learning particular solutions for familiar problems, learners learn how to discover new solutions for new problems.

Perceptual information is the key to behavioral flexibility. Online exploratory behaviors generate the information needed to assess the current constraints on action and find an appropriate resolution. As J. J. Gibson (1979) pointed out, perceptual information provides the basis for adaptive motor decisions. Movements are embedded in a continuous cycle of perception and action in which what we are doing now provides feedback for deciding what to do next. Exploration and performance are fluid and interchangeable; every movement can serve both information gathering and performatory functions.

Optimally, perceptual feedback allows movements to be controlled prospectively ahead of time rather than reactively in response to an unexpected disruption (E. J. Gibson & Pick, 2000; Lee, 1993; von Hofsten, 1993). Reactive responses are often too late to prevent a mishap because the rate of neural conduction is relatively slow. Movements are prospective when modifications are anticipatory, that is, lifting a leg to clear the curb rather than attempting to recover balance after tripping on the obstacle. Prospective control requires anticipating a shift in the body's center of mass before lifting the arms rather than compensating after the fact for disrupted balance. Because movements are ongoing, prospective adjustments and reactive compensations often occur in concert (Adolph, Eppler, Marin, Weise, & Clearfield, 2000). A slight misjudgment in planning requires reactive adjustments; reactive adjustments, in turn, provide new information for planning the next step prospectively.

Chapter Overview

This chapter has two major aims. The first aim is to describe flexibility in motor action. We use balance and locomotion in infants as a test case for understanding three aspects of behavioral flexibility—adaptive motor decisions, modification of ongoing activity, and new means to achieve a goal.

Thus, we begin by describing why infant balance and locomotion make an apt model system for investigating flexibility in action. Next, we report evidence that infants do in fact exhibit behavioral flexibility and that adaptive motor decisions are related to infants' real-time exploratory behaviors that obtain the relevant perceptual information.

Our second aim is to illuminate the links between flexibility and development. In particular, we demonstrate that flexibility is acquired during development and that developmental changes both facilitate and impede its acquisition. In subsequent sections, we show that flexibility does not automatically appear when infants acquire new forms of balance and locomotion. Instead, flexibility is learned over many weeks of everyday locomotor experience in a newly acquired posture. Infants learn how to learn as they acquire the appropriate exploratory behaviors for generating information about the current constraints on action and potential alternatives for achieving their goals. Finally, we describe two kinds of limits on flexibility, one created by developmental transitions to new postural control systems and the other created by the nature of the perceptual information for friction and rigidity. We conclude with a final discussion of flexibility in development.

Infants in Balance

For adults, keeping balance is integrated into the body's movements so seamlessly and effortlessly that, like breathing, we do not appreciate its importance until something goes wrong. We do not appreciate its difficulty until we attempt to perform a new postural skill. A lower back muscle spasm is a rude reminder that posture underlies all bodily movements. Attempting to ski or roller blade for the first time is an embarrassing lesson that illustrates that the art of maintaining balance is acquired one step at a time. For infants, achieving a stable posture

is a tremendous struggle. The developmental status of infants' postural control is the primary impediment and facilitator of their ability to explore and act on the world.

Balance Is Basic

A primary reason to focus on balance and locomotion for the study of flexibility is that these behaviors are fundamental for motor action. Balance is the foundation on which all movements of the head, limbs, and torso are built (Adolph & Berger, 2006; Reed, 1982). Stationary postures are not like frozen stone statues. The term "stationary" is really a misnomer because the body is continually in motion. Unless infants are lying flat on the ground, their bodies are always fighting the pull of gravity. Even sitting and standing postures that look stationary to casual observation are actually postures in motion. High-resolution motion recordings show that the body is gently swaying inside its base of support. Electromyographic recordings show that the muscles are actively engaged in balance control. As the body sways in one direction, a compensatory sway pulls it back in the opposite direction.

Moreover, when infants move their various body parts while sitting or standing, balance becomes more complicated. As the head turns or an arm lifts, the torso must tighten to stabilize the body. A forward lean necessitates compensatory torques by opposing body parts. Like the old song says, the toe bone is connected to the foot bone, and the foot, leg, knee, hip, back, neck, and head bones are connected all the way up. Failure to generate the appropriate compensatory sway or to stabilize the body against movements of the extremities can result in loss of balance, and the baby will fall down.

Balance is also integral to locomotor postures. During locomotion, balance is dynamic because the base of support is moving rather than stationary. To achieve dynamic balance, infants must deliberately induce disequilibrium to shift the body weight outside the current base of support and to produce the propulsive forces necessary to move the body. To prevent falling, the base of support moves to 'catch' the body. In crawling and walking, for example, the base of support shifts forward in anticipation of catching the body as the moving limb swings forward from step to step. Thus, locomotion is a series of controlled near falls.

A second reason to focus on balance and locomotion is that these activities are so common. A typical walking infant, for example, is on the floor engaged in balance and locomotion for 6 hours each day. Based on naturalistic observations of infants in an indoor play room, we estimate that the average 14-month-old toddler takes nearly 15,000 steps each day, traveling the distance of 45 football fields and incurring over 100 (fortunately, inconsequential) falls (Adolph, Badaly, Garciaguirre, & Sotsky, 2008). A typical crawling infant is on the floor for 5 hours per day, taking over 3,000 crawling steps, and covering the distance of two football fields (Adolph, 2002).

A third reason for focusing on balance and locomotion is the intense demand for flexibility in everyday activities. Every movement of the body—reaching for a cup of coffee, nodding the head, even drawing a deep breath—changes the location of the center of mass and the destabilizing torques acting on the body. Every variation in the ground surface (e.g., slant, elevation, traction, rigidity), in the body's functional dimensions (growth, clothing, loads), in physical ability (strength, reaction time, coordination), in task demands (running the 50-yard-dash versus running a marathon), in the goal (being fast versus being accurate, making a beeline to the destination), and in the available perceptual information (visual cues from a distance, overhead lighting conditions, the feel of the ground underfoot)

affects the biomechanical and psychological constraints on balance and locomotion.

Developmental Constraints on Balance

We study flexibility in infants rather than adults because variability and novelty are dramatically heightened during the infancy period. The demand for flexibility is especially high. Over the first 2 years of life, infants' environments enlarge with a wealth of new surfaces and goals, their bodies undergo radical changes in size and proportions, and their motor skill levels rapidly improve. Most unique to the infancy period is the acquisition of new ways of stabilizing the body and of moving the body from place to place: Infants acquire new postural control systems in development.

For infants, environmental features can be truly novel. Frequently, infants who visit our laboratory in New York City have yet to walk over a sidewalk, play on grass, stand on sand, step onto ice, or encounter a flight of stairs. More generally, for most infants everywhere, sloping ground, deformable and slippery surfaces, loose traction, abrupt drop-offs, narrow apertures, overhead barriers, and underfoot obstacles may be novel.

Moreover, changes in infants' bodies and skills introduce them to new aspects of the environment. With the advent of independent locomotion, infants can go to see what is around the corner or in the next room. Crawlers' eyes are pointed toward the ground, and with their hands in front, tactile information inadvertently reveals the substantial properties of the ground surface. In upright postures, infants can peer over the top of the coffee table and see what is happening above their parents' knees. Their eyes are pointed farther ahead, and tactile exploration is performed primarily with the feet.

Infants' body growth is traditionally depicted as a continuous increase in size (height, weight, head circumference, and so on) with a corresponding decrease in overall chubbiness and top-heavy proportions (Kuczmarski, 2000). In actuality, growth is episodic. Infants' height, for example, stays the same for 2 to 28 consecutive days and then, in the course of a single day, suddenly increases by 0.5 to 1.65 centimeters (Lampl, Veldhuis, & Johnson, 1992). Episodic development is also characteristic of changes in infants' weight, head circumference, and leg bone growth. The long bones grow faster than the skull and muscle mass accumulates faster than fat so that infants become leaner and stronger as they grow longer, and their bodies become less light-bulb shaped and more cylindrical (Adolph & Berger, 2005). All the while, the center of mass lowers relative to the height of the body. Body growth, of course, changes the biomechanical constraints on balance and propulsion. The episodic nature of infants' body growth makes the demand for flexibility even greater.

Concurrent with changes in infants' bodies are rapid changes in their skill levels. When infants first begin crawling and walking, for example, their steps are small, shaky, and slow. New walkers splay their legs so far apart that their step widths are larger than their step lengths. Short periods with the limbs in the air are punctuated by long periods with the limbs on the floor. Step length and velocity increase exponentially over the first few months of crawling and walking, showing the negatively accelerated performance functions characteristic of improvements in motor skill acquisition (Adolph, Vereijken, & Denny, 1998; Adolph, Vereijken, & Shrout, 2003; Bril & Ledebt, 1998). As a consequence, a poorly skilled infant last week may become highly proficient next week, and a speedy, sturdy crawler will soon become a slow, unsteady walker. Infants must take these rapid changes in their abilities into account when making decisions about motor action.

Quantitative improvements in balance and locomotion are only part of the story. Changes are qualitative as well. At birth, when infants lie prone, their necks are so weak that they can barely pull their faces from the mattress to turn their heads from side to side. When held in a sitting position, their heads loll forward until their chests rest on their knees. When held upright, they cannot support any of their body weight.

Over the ensuing months, infants acquire the means to conquer gravity with a series of qualitatively different postural control systems: sitting, crawling, cruising, and walking (Figure 19.1). In a sitting posture, infants keep balance with their legs outstretched in a "V" shape or bent backward at the knees, beneath their bottoms, in a "W." Some locomote by "bum shuffling" using their arms to move their body forward or hitching using one leg to do the work of propulsion. In a crawling posture, infants keep balance only momentarily while using their bellies for support, or they keep balance on hands and knees or hands and feet with their abdomens suspended in the air. In a cruising posture, infants move upright, in a sideways position, holding onto furniture for support. Their arms do most of the work of balance and propulsion and support some of their body's weight. In a walking posture, infants face forward with their arms free, and they support all of their body weight on one leg while the other swings forward. The postures are qualitatively different because they involve different body parts for balance and propulsion, muscle actions to perform the movements, key pivots about which the body rotates, regions within which the body can sway without falling, vantage points for viewing the ground ahead, sources of perceptual information for controlling balance and locomotion, and so on.

On average, infants achieve sitting at around 6 months of age, crawling on hands

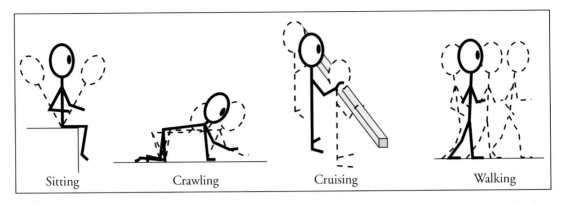

Fig. 19.1 Four postural control systems—sitting, crawling, cruising, and walking—depicted in their typical order of emergence in development. Each posture requires different strategies for maintaining balance, obtaining relevant perceptual information, and moving the body from place to place during locomotion. The dashed lines represent the body's swaying motions during static and dynamic balance. Adapted with permission from Adolph, K. E., & Eppler, M. A. (1998). Development of visually guided locomotion. *Ecological Psychology, 10,* 303–321. Lawrence Erlbaum Associates.

and knees at 8 months, cruising sideways along furniture at 9 months, and walking at 12 months (Capute, Shapiro, Palmer, Ross, & Wachtel, 1985; Frankenburg, Fandal, Sciarillo, & Burgess, 1981). However, the ages and order of acquisition vary wildly between infants. For example, some babies walk at 7 months and others at 17 months; some infants crawl before sitting or after walking, and some infants never crawl at all. The most important point is that qualitatively different forms of postural control appear staggered over many months of development so that at the same point in time, infants are experts in an earlier developing posture and novices in a later developing one.

Flexibility in Infant Action

Given the tremendous variability and novelty in infants' environments, bodies, and skills, flexible responding is an impressive feat. Here, we describe three examples of flexibility in infants' balance and locomotion. In the first example, infants faced novel variations in the surface layout: They were challenged to walk over a walkway with variable slant. In the second example, they adapted to novel variations in their bodies and skills: They walked while carrying heavy loads. In the third example, they used a tool as a means for achieving their goals: They crossed bridges of variable widths with and without a handrail available to augment their balance, and in some cases the material properties of the handrail varied.

In each task, infants demonstrated flexibility in several ways. Most important, their responses were adaptive: Their decisions about whether to walk matched the actual possibilities for walking. Moreover, they modified their ongoing exploratory activity and walking patterns in accordance with the constraints imposed by the novel manipulations, and they devised new means for dealing with the novel challenges.

Walking Over Slopes

At 14 months of age, most infants have several weeks of walking experience, but few have encountered a steep slope on their own. Although young toddlers have ample opportunity to climb up onto furniture and other elevated surfaces, few have mastered descent of furniture, stairs or drop-offs. Thus, slopes are novel, especially for descent. To assess infants' ability to cope with the challenge of going up and down slopes, 14-month-old walking infants were observed on a large, mechanized walkway (Adolph, 1995). As shown in Figure 19.2, two flat platforms flanked a middle sloping platform. Slant could be adjusted in 2-degree increments from 0 to 36 degrees by pumping a car jack that raised and lowered the bottom platform. Caregivers stood at the far side of the walkway and encouraged infants to come up or down, using toys and dry cereal as incentives. An experimenter followed alongside infants to ensure their safety if they began to fall.

Each infant was observed on the full range of slopes over dozens of trials. Because infants' body dimensions and walking skill vary widely at the same chronological age, the identical degree of slant could be perfectly safe for one infant but impossibly risky for another. Thus, risk level was determined on an individual basis using a psychophysical procedure to identify the steepest slope that each infant could walk up and walk down on at least 67% of trials—their "motor thresholds." Then infants were tested at various slopes incurring the same relative degree of risk across participants. Slopes shallower than the threshold increment were increasingly safe, meaning that the probability of walking successfully increased. Slopes steeper than the threshold increment were increasingly risky, meaning that attempts to walk were likely to result in falling.

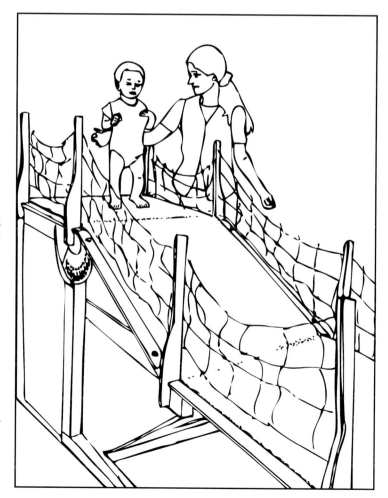

Fig. 19.2 Adjustable sloping walkway. Infants began at one end of the walkway, and caregivers (not shown) stood at the far end of the walkway offering encouragement. An experimenter (shown) walked alongside infants to ensure their safety. In addition, safety nets lined the sides of the walkway, and a plush carpet provided cushioning against falls. Adapted with permission from Adolph, K. E., & Avolio, A. M. (2000). Walking infants adapt locomotion to changing body dimensions. *Journal of Experimental Psychology: Human Perception and Performance, 26,* 1148–1166. American Psychological Association.

Motor thresholds showed large individual differences (8 to 24 degrees for uphill and 6 to 28 degrees for downhill), confirming the need for the normalization procedure. The primary question regarding flexibility was whether infants' motor decisions were adapted to their own level of walking skill and to the variations in the degree of slant from trial to trial. Would infants detect the different possibilities for walking over safe and risky slopes and adjust their behavior accordingly?

As shown in Figure 19.3A, infants' motor decisions were scaled to their own abilities. Infants attempted to walk up and down safe slopes on nearly every trial and refused to walk over increasingly risky slopes. For ascent, the average attempt rate decreased from 0.99 at the threshold increment to 0.23 on slopes ≥18 degrees steeper than the threshold increment. For descent, the attempt rate decreased from 0.94 to 0.11. The difference in attempt rates between uphill and downhill trials reflected the different consequences of falling in each condition. While walking uphill, infants' hands are in front of their bodies, and they can safely catch themselves if they fall. Walking downhill is more treacherous because infants' hands are poorly positioned to break a fall, the distance to fall is farther, and infants' bodies are moving faster as they build up forward momentum. In line with these different consequences, on uphill trials, infants appeared unruffled when they fell, but on downhill trials, they fussed as if the sensation of falling downward were aversive.

Infants also displayed flexibility by modifying their walking patterns in accordance with the degree of slant and the different demands of going uphill or down (Figures 19.3B and 19.3C). On safe slopes shallower than the threshold increment, they walked straight up or down after only a brief glance at the obstacle. Similarly,

on risky uphill slopes, latency and touching increased only slightly. But on risky downhill slopes, latency and touching increased sharply. Latency provided a crude measure of visual exploration because infants looked toward the landing platform nearly all of the time that they hesitated at the brink. Touching provided a measure of tactile exploration. Touches were typically brief (only a few seconds) but occurred on 23% of risky slopes. As they slowed down and stopped at the edge of the slope peering downward, infants touched the surface with a foot. They stood at the brink of the slope and rocked back and forth around their ankles, they took tiny steps with their feet straddling the brink, and they poked out one foot to pat or rub the sloping surface while grasping a support post with their hands to keep balance.

Additional evidence for flexibility was infants' variety of means for coping with slopes. Risky slopes required avoidance or an alternative means of descent. On risky uphill trials, infants never avoided ascent. Instead, they quickly shifted from their upright posture to all fours and clambered up the slope on hands and feet (dashed curve in Figure 19.3D). As they felt their bodies slide, they turned their toes under to get a better grip. On risky downhill trials, infants explored alternative means of descent by testing what different positions felt like before committing themselves to traversal (solid curve in Figure 19.3D). They executed multiple shifts in position (≥2 shifts) on 43% of the 225 risky downhill trials, and the number of shifts ranged up to 10. For example, in a typical long sequence, one infant shifted from standing upright to a backing position with his legs dangling down the slope, perched on hands and knees, sat down facing the bottom platform, stood back up, returned to a backing position, and finally spun around to a sitting position and slid down.

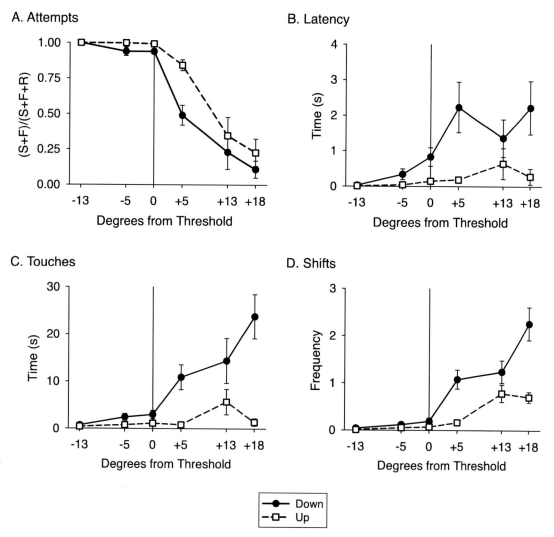

Fig. 19.3 Fourteen-month-old infants' motor decisions and exploratory behaviors on uphill (dashed curves) and downhill slopes (solid curves). Mean values of (A) attempts to walk, (B) latency, (C) accumulated duration of touching, and (D) number of position shifts. Data are shown normalized to each infant's motor threshold (denoted by solid, vertical lines at 0). On the x-axis, negative numbers to the left of the threshold represent safe slopes, and positive numbers to the right of the threshold represent risky slopes. Error bars indicate mean standard errors. Reproduced with permission from Adolph, K. E. (1995). Psychophysical assessment of toddlers' ability to cope with slopes. *Journal of Experimental Psychology: Human Perception and Performance, 21,* 734–750. American Psychological Association.

Exploratory shifts in position paid off because infants discovered varied means for descending risky slopes. They avoided descent on only 18% of downhill trials. For the remaining 82% of trials, they discovered alternative methods of locomotion (Figure 19.4). They crawled down, slid headfirst prone with their arms outstretched like Superman, slid down in a sitting position, and backed down feet first with their faces turned away from the bottom platform. Although sitting and backing were the most common descent methods, most infants used multiple means, averaging 2.23 different methods for descending risky slopes (Siegler, Adolph, & Lemaire, 1996). On trials in which infants shifted multiple times, they nearly always refused to walk and nearly always selected an appropriate alternative, providing further evidence that their shifts on the starting platform reflected a search for alternative means.

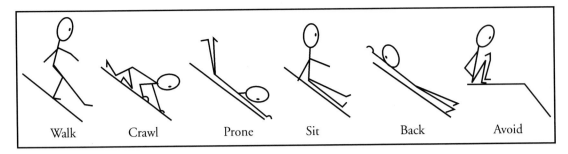

| Walk | Crawl | Prone | Sit | Back | Avoid |

Fig. 19.4 Strategies for descending slopes: walking, crawling on hands and knees, sliding head first prone, sitting, backing feet first, and avoiding descent. Adapted with permission from Adolph, K. E. (1997). Learning in the development of infant locomotion. *Monographs of the Society for Research in Child Development, 62*(3, Serial No. 251). Wiley-Blackwell Publishing Ltd.

Walking With Loads

The second example provides an even more impressive demonstration of flexibility: Fourteen-month-old walking infants adapted to experimental manipulation of their body dimensions while simultaneously gauging possibilities for walking down slopes (Adolph & Avolio, 2000). Infants were tested on an adjustable sloping walkway, but this time slant varied from 0 to 90 degrees in 4-degree increments via a push-button remote that operated an electric motor. In addition, infants wore a fitted vest with removable shoulder packs that altered their body dimensions (Figure 19.5). On some trials, the shoulder packs were filled with lead weights distributed symmetrically around their chests and backs (25% of each infant's body weight; $M = 2.59$ kg); on other trials, the packs were filled with feather weight, Polyfil stuffing. The lead-loaded packs increased infants' overall mass and raised their center of mass, making their bodies more top heavy and their balance more precarious, especially while walking down slopes. The feather-weight packs increased the circumference of infants' torsos by the same amount as the lead-weight packs but did not affect infants' ability to keep balance. As in the previous study, a psychophysical procedure was used to normalize the degree of risk to each infant's ability in each of the load conditions. But now, two psychophysical protocols were interleaved so that infants had to discover at the start of each trial whether

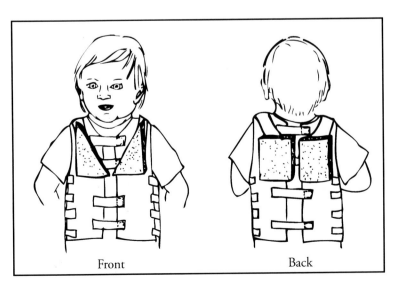

| Front | Back |

Fig. 19.5 Front and back views of adjustable vest loaded with lead weight or feather weight shoulder packs. Velcro tabs allowed quick fastening and removal of packs on infants' chests and backs. Reproduced with permission from Garciaguirre, J. S., Adolph, K. E., & Shrout, P. E. (2007). Baby carriage: Infants walking with loads. *Child Development, 78*, 664–680. Wiley-Blackwell Publishing Ltd.

the shoulder packs were loaded with the lead weights or the feather weights—that is, whether their walking skill was altered.

The lead-weight packs impaired infants' ability to walk down slopes, indicating that more top-heavy body dimensions had a detrimental effect on walking skill. Infants executed more modifications in their walking patterns (e.g., took shorter, slower steps) while descending slopes wearing feather-weight packs compared with lead-weight packs. Without the ability to modify step length and velocity with lead weights, gravity and momentum took over, pulling infants down the slope. As a consequence, infants' motor thresholds decreased while walking down slopes wearing the lead-weight packs, (M threshold for feather weights = 12.00 degrees; M threshold for lead weights = 7.60 degrees).

As in the previous study, infants scaled their motor decisions to the relative degree of risk. In both conditions, attempts to walk were high, near 1.0, on safe slopes, and decreased sharply over risky slopes to 0.32 at slopes 18 degrees steeper than the threshold increment and to 0.20 at slopes 40 degrees steeper than the threshold. In the current study, infants also showed flexible adaptation to their altered bodies and skills. They detected the added body mass induced by the lead weights and anticipated how the load would affect their walking abilities when deciding whether to walk down slopes. The same absolute degrees of slant between their feather- and lead-weight thresholds were safe while they were wearing their feather-weight packs and risky while wearing their lead-weight packs. Accordingly, infants correctly showed higher attempt rates on the same absolute degrees of slant in the feather-weight condition than in the lead-weight condition.

Infants also modified their exploratory movements in line with the degree of slant and the load condition. Latency increased with relative risk in both load conditions, meaning that infants slowed down while approaching risky slopes and hesitated longer before stepping over the brink. However, infants had to keep their bodies stiffly upright to prevent themselves from being pulled over by the lead weight packs, and this interfered with their ability to execute exploratory postural sway at the edge of the starting platform and to rock back and forth over their ankles at the brink. Thus, exploratory touching was slightly depressed in the lead-weight condition. The lead weights, however, did not interfere with infants' use of alternative means for descent. In both load conditions, they avoided descent on less than 20% of trials in which they refused to walk. They descended risky slopes by sliding down in various positions: primarily sitting and backing feet first but also crawling, headfirst prone, and clinging onto the safety nets for support while standing upright.

To determine the extent of infants' ability to modify their walking patterns in response to loads, another group of 14-month-olds were observed while carrying loads over flat ground (Garciaguirre, Adolph, & Shrout, 2007). Infants wore the same vest used in the previous study. This time, the lead weights were lighter (15% of infants' body weight), and the load was distributed symmetrically (divided evenly on the front, back, and sides of the vest as in the previous study) and asymmetrically over infants' bodies (all load carried on infants' front, back, left side, or right side). Although infants carry loads in their arms nearly as soon as they can walk, few infants carry loads on their backs in baby backpacks or over one shoulder in a baby purse or satchel, and loads are not placed on the shoulders above infants' center of mass. Thus, the manipulation of infants' body dimensions was relatively novel.

A mechanized carpet covering the flat testing surface recorded modifications in infants' footfall patterns (step length, velocity, and the period of time that their feet were on the ground and in the air). Video recordings revealed modifications in infants' posture (leaning forward, backward, and to the right and left sides) and disruptions in their walking patterns (tripping, falling, double steps with the same foot, zigzagging cross steps, and back steps).

Here, evidence for flexibility was primarily reactive because the load distribution varied from trial to trial, requiring infants to respond as they felt their bodies pulled in one direction or another as they began to walk. As in the previous study, infants kept their bodies stiffly upright in the symmetrical condition. However, in the asymmetrical conditions, infants modified their body posture by leaning. To our surprise, infants leaned with the load rather than in the opposite direction (e.g., they leaned forward like ski jumpers while carrying the front load and backward like walking into a wind tunnel while carrying the back load). In contrast, older children and adults compensate for asymmetrical loads by leaning in the direction opposite to the load (e.g., leaning forward while wearing a heavy backpack and leaning to the right while carrying a suitcase in the left hand). The adults' strategy keeps the center of mass inside the base of support. The infants' strategy allows the loads to pull the center of mass outside the base of support.

Infants' gait modifications were in response to their altered body posture. To offset the shift in their center of mass induced by leaning with the loads, they modified their footfall patterns so as to maintain dynamic balance. They shortened their step length, decreased their step velocity, planted their moving foot on the floor as quickly as possible, and increased the period of time when both feet were on the floor. In the side-load condition, infants limped, spending less time swinging their leg through the air on the side carrying the load. The back-load condition—the most novel—was most difficult, causing the highest number of gait disruptions and the greatest magnitude of gait modifications. Infants with more walking experience showed fewer gait disruptions and subtler gait modifications, indicating that they were more adept at keeping balance.

Crossing Bridges

In the third example of flexibility, infants were challenged with novel variations in the surface layout, but also provided with the opportunity to incorporate a tool into their

A) No Handrail

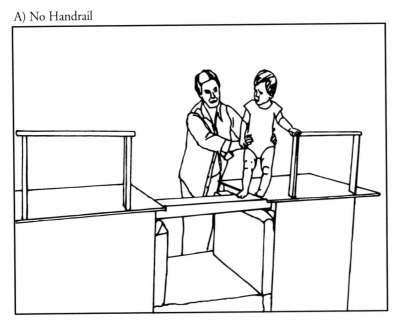

Fig. 19.6 Adjustable bridge apparatus. Two platforms were connected by bridges varying in width. A removable handrail could be placed on permanent support posts. Depending on the condition, infants were encouraged to cross bridges (A) without a handrail to augment their balance;

B) Sturdy Handrail

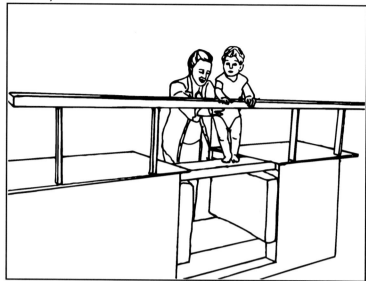

Fig. 19.6 (*continued*)
(B) with a sturdy, wooden handrail; or (C) with a wobbly handrail that deformed beneath their weight. Caregivers (not shown) encouraged infants to cross from the far side of the finishing platform. An experimenter (shown) walked alongside infants to ensure their safety. As an additional precaution, the area under the bridge was lined with foam cushions. Figures 19.6A and 19.6B reproduced with permission from Berger, S. E., & Adolph, K. E. (2003). Infants use handrails as tools in a locomotor task. *Developmental Psychology, 39*, 594–605. American Psychological Association. Figure 19.6C reproduced with permission from Berger, S. E., Adolph, K. E., & Lobo, S. A. (2005). Out of the toolbox: Toddlers differentiate wobbly and wooden handrails. *Child Development, 76*, 1294–1307. Wiley-Blackwell Publishing Ltd.

C) Wobbly Handrail
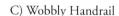

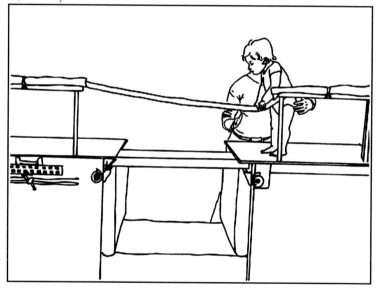

motor plan. As shown in Figure 19.6, 16-month-old walking infants were encouraged to cross bridges of variable widths (12–72 cm) spanning a deep, foam-filled precipice (Berger & Adolph, 2003). On half the trials, a solid wooden handrail spanned the walkway, and on half the trials, the handrail was removed. Caregivers coaxed infants to cross from the far side of the precipice, using toys and snacks as incentives, while an experimenter followed alongside infants to ensure

their safety. The adults did not point out the handrail or encourage infants to use it.

Infants' motor decisions depended on both bridge width and handrail presence, indicating that they detected the changing possibilities for walking and the utility of the handrail for augmenting their balance. They fell on only 6% of trials, indicating that their responses were highly adaptive. Infants ran straight across the wider bridges regardless of whether the handrail was present, and they rarely touched the handrail as they whizzed past. For example, infants walked over the 72-centimeter-wide bridge on 100% of trials regardless of handrail presence and used the handrail for crossing on only 7% of trials. However, on the narrowest bridges, attempt rates were low in both handrail conditions, and when infants crossed, they clung onto the handrail with both arms. On the 24-centimeter bridge, they walked on only 48% of trials when the handrail was absent. In contrast, infants walked on 90% of trials when the handrail was available and used it to cross on nearly every trial. On the 12-centimeter bridge, they walked on only 14% of trials when the handrail was absent. They walked on 39% of trials when it was available and used the handrail on 93% of those trials.

Infants modified their ongoing activity before stepping onto the bridge. Latency, touching the bridge and handrail, and exploratory shifts in position increased as bridge width decreased. Infants explored the bridge by rubbing it with their hands or feet. They explored the handrail by gripping and patting it. Sometimes, they explored the handrail and the bridge simultaneously by holding onto the handrail and rubbing one foot over the edge of the bridge. Infants shifted from upright to squatting, crawling, sitting, and backing positions, suggesting that they were searching for alternative means to cross. Exploratory looking, touching, and position shifts were associated with higher rates of successful crossing.

Infants also modified their walking patterns after stepping onto the bridge. They crossed the widest bridges in an average of 1.30 seconds with only a handful of large steps ($M = 5.25$). In contrast, they crossed the narrowest bridges in 31.23 seconds and 21.56 tiny steps. While crossing upright, infants implemented varied strategies, sometimes facing frontward, sometimes turning sideways to face the handrail, and sometimes turning their back to the handrail

and holding onto it with their hands behind their back.

A follow-up study showed that infants also take the material properties of the handrail into account when assessing its use a tool to augment their balance (Berger, Adolph, & Lobo, 2005). Another group of 16-month-olds were tested on the same apparatus with 10- to 40-centimeter bridges. This time, a handrail was available on all trials, but the material property of the handrail varied from trial to trial. On some trials, the handrail was made of sturdy wood and could easily support infants' full body weight. On other trials, the handrails were made of flexible foam or latex, and they drooped below infants' knees when they leaned their full weight on them.

As in the previous study, infants' motor decisions were highly adaptive: They fell on only 7% of trials. On wide bridges, infants ignored the handrail and ran straight across. On narrower bridges, attempts to walk decreased and handrail use increased. Infants hesitated longer before stepping onto the bridges, and exploratory touches of the bridge and handrail increased, especially on trials with the wobbly handrails. Exploratory touching was tailored to the material composition of the handrails. Infants tapped the wooden handrail more than the wobbly ones and squeezed, pushed, or rubbed the wobbly handrails more than the wooden one. They also explored the wobbly handrails by mouthing them.

To our surprise, infants preferred a wobbly handrail to no rail at all even though the wobbly handrails were flimsy and could not support their full weight. They crossed narrow bridges more often with the wobbly handrail than infants facing the same bridge widths with no handrail in the previous study, and their attempts were largely successful. How did infants manage to outwit three seasoned experimenters' best-laid plans? Infants devised clever, new solutions for crossing the narrow bridges by exploit-

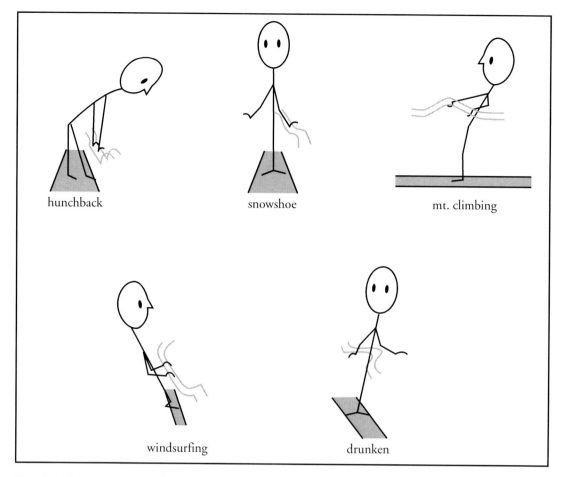

Fig. 19.7 Alternative strategies for crossing bridges with wobbly handrails. Hunchback: facing the handrail, walking sideways, stooped over, pressing down on the handrail. Snowshoe: facing forward, distributing body weight over the entire arm while gliding it over the handrail. Mountain climbing: facing forward, leaning backward, pulling up on the handrail like a rope. Windsurfing: facing the handrail, walking sideways, leaning backward and pulling up on the handrail with both hands. Drunken: facing forward, leaning against the handrail as their torsos slid along it. Reproduced with permission from Berger, S. E., Adolph, K. E., & Lobo, S. A. (2005). Out of the toolbox: Toddlers differentiate wobbly and wooden handrails. *Child Development, 76,* 1294–1307. Wiley-Blackwell Publishing Ltd.

ing the wobbly, deformable properties of the handrails (Figure 19.7). For example, 10 infants used a "hunchback" strategy in which they walked sideways (facing the handrail), stooped over like a hunchback, and pressing down on the handrail. Six children used a "mountain-climbing" strategy in which they faced forward (toward the goal), leaned back, and used the handrail like a rope to pull themselves hand over hand across the bridge. Three children used a "windsurfing" strategy in which they faced the handrail and leaned far back while pulling up on the handrail with both hands.

Acquiring Flexibility

In the previous section, we showed that infants demonstrate flexibility in response to novel variations in the surface layout and to changes in their body dimensions and skill levels. We reported evidence that infants' motor decisions were geared to the actual possibilities for action. Infants modified ongoing exploratory and loco-motor behaviors both prospectively and reactively. They gathered perceptual information to support their motor decisions and they adapted their walking patterns to the current conditions. And infants devised new means to cope with the novel challenges.

In this section, we provide evidence that flexibility is learned. When infants first begin sitting, crawling, cruising, and walking, they do not behave like the expert toddlers who dealt with slopes, loads, and bridges so competently. Their new skills, of course, are clumsy and disfluent, but novice infants do not appear to recognize the limits of their abilities. Their motor decisions are not matched to the actual possibilities for action, they do not modify their ongoing behaviors in accordance with changing constraints on balance and locomotion, and they do not search for alternative means to achieve their goal. The acquisition of flexibility requires a long, protracted period of everyday experience with balance and locomotion for infants to learn to recognize potential threats to balance, gather the relevant perceptual information, and use the information to respond adaptively—that is, for them to learn how to learn.

We illustrate the role of experience in flexibility with a longitudinal study of infants crawling and walking down slopes (Adolph, 1997). Outside the laboratory, parents agreed to keep their infants off playground slides and sloping ground surfaces for the duration of the study so that the slope task would be novel. Inside the lab, infants were observed on an adjustable sloping walkway (slant varied from 0 to 36 degrees in 2-degree increments). As in the previous slope studies, a psychophysical procedure was used to normalize risk level to each infant's ability at each test session. Infants were tested once every 3 weeks, from their first week of crawling until 13 weeks or so after they began walking. Most infants participated for more than 10 months. In addition, infants in a control group were tested at three matched session times (in their first and 10th weeks of crawling and in their first week of walking) to ensure that the results

from the test group were not due to repeated practice effects on slopes. Both groups of infants showed three types of improvements over weeks of crawling and walking experience: Their motor thresholds improved as they learned to modify ongoing crawling and walking patterns, their motor decisions became more accurate and adaptive as they learned to detect the current constraints on action, and they discovered alternative means for descending slopes.

Gait Modifications

Everyday locomotor experience was related to improvements in infants' ability to crawl and walk over flat ground and in their ability to crawl and walk down slopes (Adolph, 1997). On flat ground, infants' crawling and walking movements became larger, faster, straighter, and less variable as their bodies became stronger and more coordinated. On slopes, infants' average motor threshold increased from 17.43 degrees in their first week of crawling to 24.79 degrees in their 10th week of crawling and from 5.47 degrees in their first week of walking to 14.97 degrees in their 10th week of walking.

Part of the improvement in motor thresholds over weeks of crawling and walking resulted from infants' increasing ability to modify their steps during descent. Infants curbed forward momentum by decreasing their step length and velocity and by braking between steps. They minimized destabilizing torques by keeping their bodies vertical to ensure that their center of mass remained inside their base of support. After weeks of crawling experience, for example, infants crawled down steep slopes with their arms stiffly extended, slowly moving their hands an inch at a time, their legs nearly immobilized, flexed tightly beneath their torsos. Similarly, after weeks of walking experience, infants used a braking strategy to inch their way down steep slopes (see also Adolph, Gill, Lucero, & Fadl, 1996; Gill-Alvarez &

Adolph, 2005). Infants implemented these gait modifications before stepping over the brink, indicating that flexible adaptation of ongoing locomotor patterns was controlled prospectively based on perceptual information about the relative difficulty of descent.

The increase in the group averages over weeks of crawling, however, masks important individual differences. In their first week of crawling, about half the infants crawled on their bellies with their stomachs dragging along the floor, and half crawled on their hands and knees, with their stomachs in the air. The belly crawlers were at an advantage for descending slopes because they could slither down headfirst without having to support their body weight on their arms. As a consequence, belly crawlers began with steeper thresholds than the hands-and-knees crawlers. For infants in both crawling groups, thresholds increased over test sessions. However, when the belly crawlers finally switched to crawling on their hands and knees, their thresholds decreased temporarily, reflecting the more difficult task of crawling headfirst down slopes while supporting their raised bodies on their arms, before increasing again as they gained experience with hand-and-knees crawling. For all infants, the switch from crawling to walking caused a significant decrement in their motor thresholds, reflecting the switch to a new postural control system and the more stringent demands of descending upright.

Across sessions, better crawling and walking on flat ground predicted steeper thresholds on slopes, indicating that general locomotor proficiency transferred to the novel slope context. Further evidence that general everyday experience leads to flexibility comes from the infants in the control group, who were tested only three times. Compared with the infants in the experimental group who received hundreds of trials on slopes over more than a dozen sessions, slopes were relatively novel for infants

in the control group. Nonetheless, infants in the control group showed similar improvements in their motor thresholds from their first to tenth weeks of crawling (Ms = 15.83 and 20.31 degrees, respectively) and a similar decrement in thresholds in their first week of walking (M = 5.50 degrees). Even gait modifications that seem specific to descending slopes—braking forward momentum, keeping the body vertical rather than perpendicular to the slope, and so on—do not require practice locomoting over slopes. Rather, everyday experience is sufficient to facilitate flexible adaptation of ongoing movements in novel contexts (Adolph et al., 1996; Gill-Alvarez & Adolph, 2005).

Motor Decisions

Everyday locomotor experience also facilitated improvements in infants' motor decisions (Adolph, 1997). As in previous studies, infants always attempted to crawl and walk down safe slopes shallower than their threshold, where the probability of success was high (dashed curve in Figure 19.8). However, on risky slopes steeper than the threshold increment, infants' motor decisions became more adaptive with each week of locomotor experience (solid curve in Figure 19.8). In their first week of crawling, infants attempted impossibly risky slopes on repeated trials, necessitating rescue by the experimenter; the average attempt rate was 0.68. Although they could clearly see and feel the slant, novice crawlers plunged over the brink as if they did not recognize that the risky increments were beyond their ability. Over weeks of crawling, errors gradually decreased. By their 10th week of crawling, attempt rates averaged 0.56. By 20 weeks of crawling, infants were experts, and their attempt rates were 0.11. Their exploratory movements were fast and efficient, and most infants could discern within a few degrees of slant whether slopes were safe or risky for their

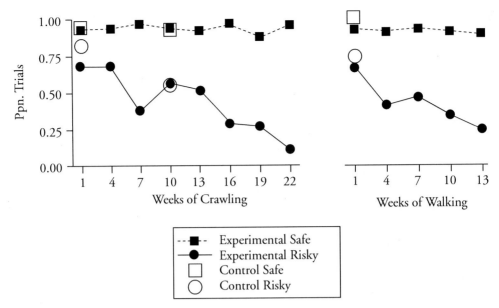

Fig. 19.8 Attempts to crawl and walk down slopes. Data were averaged over safe slopes (slopes ≤ the threshold increment, denoted by dashed lines) and risky slopes (slopes > the threshold increment, denoted by solid lines). Filled symbols represent data from the infants in the experimental group who were observed every 3 weeks, and open symbols represent data from the three sessions with infants in the control group. Reproduced with permission from Adolph, K. E. (1997). Learning in the development of infant locomotion. *Monographs of the Society for Research in Child Development, 62*(3, Serial No. 251). Wiley-Blackwell Publishing Ltd.

current level of crawling skill. Similarly, in infants' first week of walking, errors were high. They walked straight over the edge of risky slopes, and their average attempt rate was 0.66. By their 10th week of walking, attempts decreased to 0.34.

Several lines of evidence indicate that the decrease in errors over weeks of locomotor experience reflects increased flexibility. First, infants' decisions became more closely geared to their actual abilities despite weekly changes in their bodies and skills. Their motor thresholds increased over weeks of belly crawling and decreased temporarily and then increased again over weeks of hands-and-knees crawling; thresholds decreased and increased yet again after they began walking. Thus, a risky slope one week could be safe the next week when the motor threshold was steeper; a safe slope for an experienced belly crawler could be impossibly risky when the infant began crawling on hands

and knees. Second, the duration of infants' locomotor experience was a stronger predictor of their attempt rates on risky slopes than was their age at testing. Third, as shown by the open symbols on Figure 19.8, infants in the control group showed similar attempt rates at each matched session compared with the infants tested repeatedly. Finally, infants in cross-sectional studies show similar patterns of improvement when challenged with the novel slope task. For example, the 14-month-old walkers in Adolph's (1995) study showed comparable attempt rates to the infants in the longitudinal study when they were 14 months of age. Twelve-month-old crawlers, with approximately 15 weeks of crawling experience, behaved like the experienced crawlers tested longitudinally. Twelve-month-old walkers, with only 6 weeks of walking experience, behaved like the novice walkers tested longitudinally (Adolph, Tamis-LeMonda, Ishak, Karasik, & Lobo, in press; Ishak, Adolph, Lobo, Karasik, & Tamis-LeMonda, 2007). And 18-month-old walkers, with approximately 26 weeks of walking experience, behaved like the experienced walkers tested longitudinally (Lobo et al., 2007).

Alternative Means of Descent

Finally, locomotor experience was related to infants' discovery and use of varied alternatives for descending slopes (Adolph, 1997). On safe slopes, infants descended using their current locomotor methods on nearly every trial: belly crawling, crawling on hands and knees, or walking. But on risky slopes, alternative locomotor methods emerged over weeks of crawling and walking.

At first, infants dealt with recognizably risky slopes by avoiding the slope and waiting out the trial on the starting platform. After 13 weeks of crawling experience, prone descent strategies appeared. Hands-and-knees crawlers crept down on their bellies or slid spread-eagled, headfirst prone. Scooting and sliding in a sitting position appeared at about 13 weeks of crawling experience. Sometimes infants' use of sitting appeared deliberate: They sat at the edge and pushed themselves over the brink. Sometimes their use of sitting appeared serendipitous: While crawling down steep slopes, infants pushed backward so hard with their arms that they ended up in a sitting position, midslope, with their legs extended in a straddle split; eventually, they adopted the sitting position while still on the starting platform. Use of prone and sitting positions to descend slopes required infants to recognize existing strategies in their repertoires—belly crawling and sitting—as alternative means to achieve a goal.

Crawling and sliding backward feet first appeared at about 19 weeks of crawling experience. Backing was the most psychologically complex descent strategy. It required infants to execute an initial detour by turning away from the goal and then to proceed without visual guidance facing away from the goal. Most infants discovered backing in the course of trying to crawl down steep slopes. With their arms stiffly extended and legs tucked under their torsos, gravity pulled their bodies around until they were sideways or backward. Infants showed surprised at finding themselves in a backward position, sometimes exclaiming, "uh oh" and "oh no"; they crawled back up to the starting platform and peered down the slope in puzzlement. Eventually, they recognized backing as an alternative means and executed the position intentionally while still on the starting platform. Over weeks of walking, alternative descent strategies did not need to be rediscovered. Infants had only to recognize that walking was impossible on risky slopes and then draw on an existing alternative.

Limits on Flexibility

So far, we have provided evidence that infants behave flexibly in response to variable and novel conditions and that they acquire flexibility through everyday locomotor experience. In this section, we describe two kinds of limits on flexibility. Both limits involve the perceptual information that specifies possibilities for balance and locomotion. In the first case, developmental transitions in infants' posture—sitting, crawling, cruising, and walking—affect their ability to generate and use the relevant information for guiding action adaptively. During the period when infants are first mastering a new postural control system, they do not even know what the relevant information is. In the second case, limits on flexibility result from limits in the availability of perceptual information for surface substance. This limitation is critical and pervasive because the substantial properties of surfaces—friction, rigidity, mass, and so on—affect every physical encounter. In particular, novel variations in surface substance are not reliably specified by visual information from a distance, preventing infants from realizing that they are approaching a potential obstacle.

Specificity Between Developmental Transitions in Posture

Perhaps the most striking finding from the longitudinal study of infants descending slopes was that infants showed two learning curves, not one (Adolph, 1997). As illustrated in Figure 19.8, the same experienced crawlers who accurately perceived the limits of their ability to crawl down slopes attempted to walk down impossibly risky slopes when they stood up and faced the hills as novice walkers. Error rates on risky slopes were equally high in infants' first week of walking as they were in their first week of crawling (0.68 for each). They attempted to walk at the same rates as they attempted to crawl at each risky increment steeper than the motor threshold. Moreover, learning did not appear to be faster the second time around. Learning curves were parallel over weeks of crawling and walking.

Longitudinal observations provide one way to assess learning and transfer across developmental transitions in posture. An alternative approach is to keep age constant by testing infants in the same session in an earlier developing posture versus a later developing one. For example, in their first week of walking, infants were tested in six back-to-back trials on the risky 36-degree slope: two trials in their novice walking posture, two in their experienced crawling posture, and two in their novice walking posture.

Learning to learn was so specific to the earlier developing crawling posture that infants showed no evidence of transfer across consecutive trials. When started upright, infants marched straight over the edge of the 36-degree slope on two consecutive trials. Only moments later, when placed on the starting platform in their old, familiar crawling position, half the infants behaved like experienced crawlers and slid safely down. They had not forgotten or lost the alternative strategies in their repertoires; they simply did not know to use them. The other half of the infants pulled themselves up into a standing position and stepped over the brink as if they preferred to be hapless walkers rather than expert crawlers. When placed upright once again, infants attempted to walk despite the reminder that in their experienced crawling posture the slope was risky.

Specificity is not limited to the transition between crawling and walking postures or to locomotion over slopes. Infants also displayed specificity of learning when tested in an experienced sitting posture compared with a novice crawling posture at the edge of precipice (Adolph, 2000). All infants were 9.5 months of age, and all had more experience with sitting (M = 15 weeks) than with crawling (M = 6 weeks). As illustrated in Figure 19.9, the infants' goal was the same in both postures: to retrieve a toy at the far side of an adjustable gap spanning a deep precipice. An experimenter could vary the size of the gap from 0 to 90 centimeters in 2-centimeter increments by sliding a moveable landing platform along a calibrated track. Thus, infants had to decide whether they could lean forward while stretching an arm out to span the gap without falling into the precipice. Caregivers encouraged infants to cross the gap at every increment, and an experimenter spotted infants to ensure their safety if they fell over the edge.

As in the previous studies, a psychophysical procedure was used to determine relative risk levels for each infant in each posture. Motor thresholds ranged from 20 to 32 centimeters for sitting and from 2 to 18 centimeters for crawling, confirming the need for the normalization procedure. The thresholds for sitting were larger than infants' arm lengths, indicating that they leaned forward to retrieve the target.

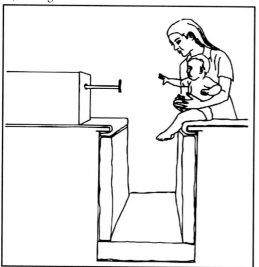
A) Sitting

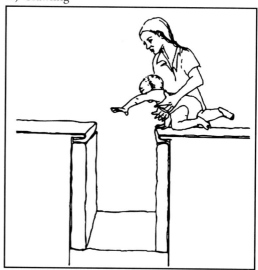
B) Crawling

Fig. 19.9 Adjustable gap apparatus. Infants were tested in (A) experienced sitting and (B) novice crawling postures. Caregivers (not shown) stood at the far side of the platform encouraging infants to cross the gap. An experimenter (shown) followed alongside infants to ensure their safety and the gap was lined with padded cushions as an additional precaution. Reproduced with permission from Adolph, K. E. (2000). Specificity of learning: Why infants fall over a veritable cliff. *Psychological Science, 11,* 290–295. Wiley-Blackwell Publishing Ltd.

Infants with the smallest thresholds for crawling placed their hand straight into the tiny gap and fell. Infants with the largest thresholds fell as they leaned forward while stretching their arms across the gap.

Infants correctly attempted to span safe gaps in both postures. But at every risky gap increment, infants responded more adaptively in the experienced sitting posture compared with the novice crawling posture. In the sitting position at the edge of risky gaps, all infants closely matched their attempts to the conditional probability of success. Attempt rates dropped from nearly 1.0 at the threshold increment to nearly 0 on gaps 18 centimeters larger than the threshold. They were so frustrated by their inability to span the risky gaps that they turned their backs to the goal so that they would not have to look at the enticing toys for the duration of each 30-second trial. In the crawling position, infants grossly overestimated their ability to span the risky gaps. They fell on 61% of risky trials and attempt rates were >.50 at gaps 18 centi-

meters larger than the threshold. Although an experimenter called infants' attention to the gap on every trial, a third of the infants plunged into the 90-centimeter gap on repeated trials—as if they thought that they could crawl into thin air.

Additionally, infants showed evidence of specificity of learning between cruising and walking. Because both cruising and walking are upright postures, traditionally, researchers have assumed that cruising is merely an early form of independent walking. However, if cruising is merely a "practice" period before infants master upright balance without support from their arms, then experience cruising should lead to more adaptive motor decisions for walking. Using a variant of the gap apparatus and a psychophysical procedure to normalize risk levels, experienced 11-month-old cruising infants were tested in two postural conditions (Adolph, 2005; Leo, Chiu, & Adolph, 2000). In the condition relevant for cruising, infants were encouraged to cruise over a solid floor with an adjustable gap (0–90 cm) in the handrail

A) Gap in Handrail

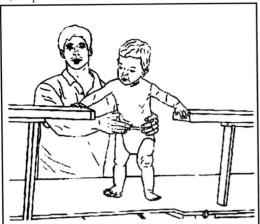

B) Gap in Floor

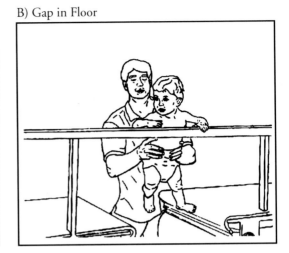

Fig. 19.10 Apparatus with adjustable gaps in handrails and floor. Infants cruised across (A) a gap in the handrail with a continuous floor and (B) a gap in the floor with a continuous handrail. Caregivers (not shown) encouraged infants from the far side of the platform, and an experimenter (shown) followed alongside infants to ensure their safety. Reprinted from Adolph, K. E., & Joh, A. S. (in press). Multiple learning mechanisms in the development of action. In A. Woodward & A. Needham (Eds.), *Learning and the infant mind.* New York: Oxford University Press.

they held for support (Figure 19.10A). In the condition relevant for walking, infants were encouraged to cruise over a solid handrail with an adjustable gap (0–90 cm) in the floor beneath their feet (Figure 19.10B). In both conditions, an experimenter showed infants the gap at the start of each trial to ensure that they saw the size of the obstacle.

As in the previous studies, infants showed more adaptive responses in the condition relevant for their experienced posture. Infants attempted to cruise over safe gaps in the handrail, and on risky gaps, they crawled to the other side or avoided traversal. But when tested with gaps in the floor, infants attempted safe and risky increments alike as if they did not realize that they needed a floor to support their bodies. A second group of 11-month-old new walkers erred in both conditions (Adolph, 2005; Leo et al., 2000). Although they could take only a few consecutive steps before falling, new walkers no longer recognized how far they could travel between gaps in the handrail, and they did not yet recognize the gap in the floor as an impediment to locomotion.

Specificity Due to Information for Surface Substance

A second cause of limitations in flexibility is not due to developmental transitions in posture. Specificity can also result from the availability of perceptual information for variations in the ground surface. Flexibility in the face of variability and novelty requires perceptual information to specify the nature of the potential challenge. Variations in the surface layout (e.g., slant, bridge width, gap size, and elevation) are signaled by a multitude of reliable depth cues (binocular disparity, convergence, motion parallax, texture gradients, and so on). Thus, as described in the previous sections, visual information from a distance can alert infants to modify their locomotor patterns and exploratory behaviors as they approach a potential obstacle. Visual and tactile exploration generate information about possibilities for action, and experienced infants—like adults—are then in a position to respond adaptively.

In contrast, novel variations in the substance of the ground surface are not reliably specified by visual information from a distance. Friction ("slipperiness" in laymen's terms) and rigidity ("hardness") are resistive forces that emerge only when the body makes contact with the surface. The size of the resistive forces depends on the two contacting surfaces and their manner of contact. For example, the probability of slipping due to inadequate frictional forces depends on the flooring material (e.g., wood, carpet, or cement), the walker's footwear (rubber-soled sneakers, nylon socks, or bare feet), the current condition of the surfaces (dust, condensation, or wear and tear), foot velocity at contact, the angle of contact (feet planted squarely or with an initial heel contact), and so on.

The widespread belief that visual cues such as shine can serve as reliable signals for emergent forces such as friction is simply incorrect because the change in resistive forces does not exist before the two surfaces come into contact (Joh, Adolph, Campbell, & Eppler, 2006). Moreover, visual cues such as shine vary with changes in the overhead lighting conditions, viewing distance and angle, and the color of the ground surface—factors that do not affect the coefficient of friction (Joh

et al., 2006). Without visual cues to prompt modifications in ongoing activity, even experienced walkers cannot detect novel changes in surface substance before they step onto the slippery or squishy surface. At that point, gait modifications become reactive rather than prospective. It is a case of too little perceptual information too late.

Several studies provide evidence for limitations on flexibility as walkers approach novel ground surfaces varying in rigidity and friction. In the most straightforward demonstrations, walkers approached a squishy or slippery obstacle on consecutive trials. On the first trial, the obstacle was novel. On subsequent trials, participants could learn from their previous encounters. For example, 15- to 39-month-old children and adults were encouraged to cross a walkway containing a large, squishy, foam pit (Joh & Adolph, 2006). The foam pit was so squishy that even the lightest infants fell if they attempted to walk over it; the foam pit was so large that infants were allowed to fall freely, landing face down in the sea of foam (Figure 19.11). An experimenter spotted the older children and adults to ensure

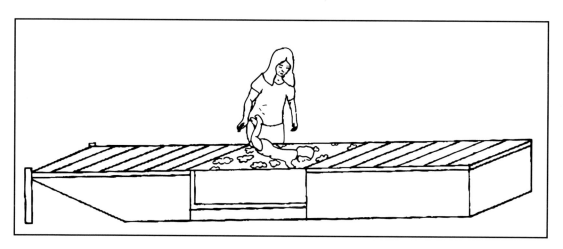

Fig. 19.11 Foam pit apparatus. Infants walked across a solid walkway containing a deformable foam pit to reach their caregivers (not shown). The foam pit was marked by changes in the color, texture, and pattern of the ground surface. The foam pit was large enough that the infants could fall into it freely without being caught. An experimenter (shown) followed the participants for safety and caught older children and adults if necessary. Reprinted from Adolph, K. E., & Joh, A. S. (in press). Multiple learning mechanisms in the development of action. In A. Woodward & A. Needham (Eds.), *Learning and the infant mind*. New York: Oxford University Press.

their safety. Most important, the foam pit was marked by salient, visual cues: It was bumpy with rounded edges, like a couch cushion, and covered with a fabric that was distinct in color, texture, and pattern from the rest of the walkway.

Even the youngest infants were expert walkers (*M* walking experience = 12.56 weeks). As described in previous sections, by 15 months, infants demonstrate flexibility to novel changes in the surface layout (e.g., Adolph, 1995). By 16 months, infants take the substance of a handrail into account but only after they explore the handrail by touching it (Berger et al., 2005). The critical question here was whether participants would recognize the deformable surface as a potential obstacle. Would they display prospective gait modifications and exploratory behaviors as they approached the foam pit and select alternative means to avoid falling?

Results were clear. Every participant in all age groups fell straight into the foam pit on their first trial. Despite the change in the appearance of the ground surface, participants did not hesitate, alter their walking patterns, or explore the foam pit by touching it. Some infants and adults gasped or screamed after falling, indicating that the deformability of the foam pit was truly unexpected. In fact, most infants fell on multiple, consecutive trials before learning to avoid the foam pit. On average, 15-month-olds fell on 7.06 consecutive trials, 21- to 39-month-olds on 2.75 to 4.83 trials, and adults on only the first trial. On the trial where participants demonstrated learning, latency to step onto the foam pit, exploratory touches with the feet and hands, and shifts in position sharply increased, providing further corroboration that without visual cues from a distance, flexible responding is impaired.

A second study with a slippery obstacle replicated the pattern of results with 15-month-olds (Adolph, Joh, & Eppler, 2008; Joh, Adolph, & DeWind, 2005). A large patch of slippery Teflon replaced the foam pit. As in the previous experiment, the Teflon was visibly different from the rest of the walkway. It was white, shiny, and smooth (like ice), whereas the beginning and ending portions of the walkway were covered with a dark blue, matte, and textured carpet. Infants wore nylon stockings to increase the likelihood of slipping on the Teflon. Because infants fell backward as they slipped, an experimenter caught them to ensure their safety. As in the previous study, infants were oblivious to the novel friction condition on their first encounter. Despite the shiny, smooth surface of the Teflon, they walked straight onto the obstacle, slipped, and fell. Again, learning over subsequent encounters required multiple trials: Infants fell repeatedly, and hesitation, tactile exploration, and means–ends exploration did not increase until the first trial where they evidenced learning.

A second line of evidence for informational limitations on flexibility comes from studies where variations in surface substance and surface layout covaried. Even when perceptual information for surface substance was provided by tactile information underfoot, infants and adults relied primarily on visual information for surface layout. For example, 14-month-old walking infants were encouraged to descend a motorized walkway with adjustable slope (0–90 degrees) under low- and high-friction conditions (Adolph, Joh, & Eppler, 2008). On some trials, the entire surface of the walkway was covered with high-friction rubber and on other trials with low-friction vinyl. Thus, underfoot information about friction was available at the beginning of each trial as infants approached the slope from the flat starting platform. As in the previous slope studies, a psychophysical procedure was used to estimate infants' motor thresholds for each friction condition to equate the relative degree of risk. On average, infants' motor thresholds were 9.12 degrees steeper on high-friction rubber (*M* = 12.25 degrees) than on low-friction vinyl (*M* = 3.12 degrees). In fact, most infants had trouble walking over the low-friction surface when the slant was set to 0 degrees. Thus, in the low-friction condition, extremely shallow slopes could be impossibly risky.

Despite continuous, underfoot information about friction as they approached the brink of the slope, infants' motor decisions were based primarily on surface slant. On safe slopes shallower than the threshold increment, infants attempted to walk on nearly every trial. However, on risky slopes, attempt rates were higher in the low-friction condition at each risky increment. Errors were especially high on slopes slightly steeper than the threshold increment. For example, on slopes 10 degrees steeper than threshold, attempt rates were 0.39 in the high-friction condition and 0.65 in the low-friction condition. As further evidence that infants responded primarily to visual information for surface slant rather than friction, they attempted to walk on the same proportion of trials in both friction conditions when data were analyzed by the absolute degree of slope. Infants did not alter ongoing walking patterns or stop at the edge of the slope to engage in tactile exploration until they saw a relatively steep slope. Thus, they stepped straight onto shallow— but impossibly risky—low-friction slopes and fell. When the visual information for surface slant prompted infants to engage in additional exploratory activity at the brink, they correctly avoided attempts to walk down risky slopes and used an alternative sliding position instead.

Reliance on visual cues for surface layout is not limited to infants. When adults were asked to gauge possibilities for descending slopes, they relied on visual information for slant rather than underfoot information for friction (Joh, Adolph, Narayanan,

& Dietz, 2007). They overestimated their abilities on low-friction vinyl by as much as 20 degrees (*M* = 9.18 degrees). Their errors had functional consequences because changes of 2 to 3 degrees were sufficient to cause adults to fall. Like the infants, however, adults showed more adaptive motor decisions when they obtained tactile information at the edge of the slope. When we allowed them to touch the low-friction slope with only half of one foot, their motor decisions matched their actual abilities (*M* difference = .09 degrees).

Conclusions: Flexibility in Development

Behavioral flexibility is so central to adaptive action that Eleanor Gibson (1994) called it a "hallmark of human behavior" (p. 71). Variability and novelty are endemic in everyday life. Happily, infants are excellent improvisers (Thelen, 1996). As we described in the previous sections, young infants display impressive flexibility in response to continually changing constraints on balance and locomotion. When faced with novel challenges such as steep slopes, narrow bridges, large gaps, and lead-weighted shoulder packs, experienced infants display adaptive motor decisions in sitting, crawling, cruising, and walking postures. Under variable conditions in the environment (variations in the degree of slant, bridge width, and so on) and in their own body dimensions and skills, infants scale their motor decisions to the actual possibilities for action. They alter their ongoing movements with subtle modifications in their locomotor patterns. They gather the requisite perceptual information with a sophisticated repertoire of exploratory movements. They discover new means to achieve their goals by intentionally testing various alternatives and by recognizing new strategies that arise in the course of trying to do something else.

For experienced infants, like adults, the only limits on flexibility appear to be informational. Novel variations in the substance of the ground surface (e.g., a deformable foam pit or a slippery slope) produce errors on the initial encounter. Flexibility may be specific to variations in the surface layout because changes in surface substance are not signaled by visual information from a distance. Infants can obtain adequate information about rigidity and friction from touching because physical contact with the obstacle creates resistive forces. However, without visual cues to prompt modifications in ongoing exploratory activity, infants do not realize the necessity of touching. The chain of exploratory behaviors is disrupted, and prospective control breaks down.

We also provided evidence in previous sections that flexibility is learned. Moreover, acquisition of flexibility requires a protracted period of experience. Infants require 10 weeks of crawling and walking experience, for example, before errors decrease below 0.50 on risky slopes and 20 weeks before errors decrease to about 0.10. What happens over those 10 to 20 weeks? Experience is not merely a euphemism for the passage of time. It is not the movement of the hands on a clock that leads to flexibility. It is the movement of infants' bodies. It is the thousands of steps, strides, turns, pauses, sways, slips, trips, and falls on the dozens of different surfaces and in the hundreds of different contexts that leads to flexibility. And during all those steps and sways and falls, infants do not amass an encyclopedia of knowledge about biomechanics and various surface properties. No list of facts or library of fixed solutions can give infants the wherewithal to cope with novelty and continual variability. Rather, infants learn how to discover the current limits and propensities of a familiar balance control system for acting in the current situation. They learn how to recognize the relevant perceptual information when it is available and how to generate the relevant perceptual information when it is not already available.

Finally, we have argued that learning to learn is nested in the larger time frame of development. The acquisition of flexibility is a tremendous developmental achievement because infants are learning about their new postural control system at the same time that the system is undergoing developmental change. That is, infants are learning about the relevant body parts for maintaining balance and propelling the body, the various muscle actions that perform compensatory swaying movements, the pivot points that their body rotates around, the sources of perceptual information that control postural and locomotor movements, and the features of the ground that support or hinder their movements—all at the same time that their bodies, skills, and environments are developing. The most extreme, qualitative developmental changes—transitions to new postural control systems—lead to specificity because the relevant body parts, muscle actions, pivot points, and so on are completely different.

Imagine building a robot that could learn to walk over various surfaces. Now imagine a robot whose body undergoes sudden growth spurts, whose strength and coordination change from week to week, and whose environment continually introduces novel surfaces. This sort of developing learning system is what developmental roboticists imagine building (Adolph, 2006). In fact, a developing learning system may be the optimal model of flexibility because the flux of developmental change may actually facilitate the task of learning to learn. If the system were static, then infants might be more inclined to learn simple facts about the environment and their bodies and skills—"this elevation is 20 centimeters high, my legs are 30 centimeters long,

I'm a terrible walker"—and to form simple associations between them—"walking over a 20-centimeter elevation will result in a fall." Such static knowledge would be maladaptive because infants' legs will grow and strengthen and their skill levels will improve. Last week's cliff can become next week's stair. Last month's barrier can become next month's chair. Ongoing developmental changes may force infants to perceive possibilities for action in relative terms: How high is this elevation relative to my current leg length and walking skill? The flux of development may push infants to acquire the information-generating behaviors that allow relative comparisons. In one's wildest fantasies, the imaginary robot could learn to display behavioral flexibility with a host of postural control systems. This robot, still far in the realm of science fiction, would begin to approximate the developmental achievement of learning to learn in sitting, crawling, cruising, and walking postures.

References

Adolph, K. E. (1995). Psychophysical assessment of toddlers' ability to cope with slopes. *Journal of Experimental Psychology: Human Perception and Performance, 21,* 734–750.

Adolph, K. E. (1997). Learning in the development of infant locomotion. *Monographs of the Society for Research in Child Development, 62*(3, Serial No. 251).

Adolph, K. E. (2000). Specificity of learning: Why infants fall over a veritable cliff. *Psychological Science, 11,* 290–295.

Adolph, K. E. (2002). Learning to keep balance. In R. Kail (Ed.), *Advances in child development and behavior* (Vol. 30, pp. 1–30). Amsterdam: Elsevier Science.

Adolph, K. E. (2005). Learning to learn in the development of action. In J. Lockman & J. Reiser (Eds.), *Action as an organizer of learning and development: The 32nd Minnesota Symposium on Child Development* (pp. 91–122). Hillsdale, NJ: Lawrence Erlbaum Associates.

Adolph, K. E. (2006, September). *Learning in the development of action.* Paper presented at the Proceedings of the Sixth International Workshop on Epigenetic Robotics: Modeling Cognitive Development in Robotic Systems, Paris.

Adolph, K. E., & Avolio, A. M. (2000). Walking infants adapt locomotion to changing body dimensions. *Journal of Experimental Psychology: Human Perception and Performance, 26,* 1148–1166.

Adolph, K. E., Badaly, D., Garciaguirre, J. S., & Sotsky, R. B. (2008). *15,000 steps: Infants' walking experience.* Manuscript in preparation.

Adolph, K. E., & Berger, S. E. (2005). Physical and motor development. In M. H. Bornstein & M. E. Lamb (Eds.), *Developmental science: An advanced textbook* (5th ed., pp. 223–281). Mahwah, NJ: Lawrence Erlbaum Associates.

Adolph, K. E., & Berger, S. E. (2006). Motor development. In D. Kuhn & R. S. Siegler (Eds.), *Handbook of child psychology: Vol. 2. Cognition, perception, and language* (6th ed., pp. 161–213). New York: Wiley.

Adolph, K. E., Eppler, M. A., Marin, L., Weise, I. B., & Clearfield, M. W. (2000). Exploration in the service of prospective control. *Infant Behavior and Development, 23,* 441–460.

Adolph, K. E., Gill, S., Lucero, A., & Fadl, Y. (1996, April). *Emergence of a stepping strategy: How infants learn to walk down hills.* Poster presented at the International Conference on Infant Studies, Providence, RI.

Adolph, K. E., & Joh, A. S. (in press). Multiple learning mechanisms in the development of action. In A. Woodward & A. Needham (Eds.), *Learning and the infant mind.* New York: Oxford University Press.

Adolph, K. E., Joh, A. S., & Eppler, M. A. (2008). *Infants' perception of affordances of slopes under high and low friction conditions.* Manuscript in preparation.

Adolph, K. E., Tamis-LeMonda, C. S., Ishak, S., Karasik, L. B., & Lobo, S. A. (in press). Locomotor experience and use of social information are posture specific. *Developmental Psychology.*

Adolph, K. E., Vereijken, B., & Denny, M. A. (1998). Learning to crawl. *Child Development, 69,* 1299–1312.

Adolph, K. E., Vereijken, B., & Shrout, P. E. (2003). What changes in infant walking and why. *Child Development, 74,* 474–497.

Berger, S. E., & Adolph, K. E. (2003). Infants use handrails as tools in a locomotor task. *Developmental Psychology, 39,* 594–605.

Berger, S. E., Adolph, K. E., & Lobo, S. A. (2005). Out of the toolbox: Toddlers differentiate wobbly and wooden handrails. *Child Development, 76,* 1294–1307.

Bernstein, N. (1996). On dexterity and its development. In M. L. Latash & M. T. Turvey (Eds.), *Dexterity and its development* (pp. 3–244). Mahwah, NJ: Lawrence Erlbaum Associates.

Bril, B., & Ledebt, A. (1998). Head coordination as a means to assist sensory integration in learning to walk. *Neuroscience and Biobehavioral Reviews, 22,* 555–563.

Capute, A. J., Shapiro, B. K., Palmer, F. B., Ross, A., & Wachtel, R. C. (1985). Normal gross motor development: The influences of race, sex and socio-economic status. *Developmental Medicine and Child Neurology, 27,* 635–643.

Frankenburg, W. K., Fandal, A. W., Sciarillo, W., & Burgess, D. (1981). The newly abbreviated and revised Denver Developmental Screening Test. *Journal of Pediatrics, 99,* 995–999.

Garciaguirre, J. S., Adolph, K. E., & Shrout, P. E. (2007). Baby carriage: Infants walking with loads. *Child Development, 78,* 664–680.

Gibson, E. J. (1994). Has psychology a future? *Psychological Science, 5,* 69–76.

Gibson, E. J., & Pick, A. D. (2000). *An ecological approach to perceptual learning and development.* New York: Oxford University Press.

Gibson, J. J. (1979). *The ecological approach to visual perception.* Boston: Houghton Mifflin.

Gill-Alvarez, S. V., & Adolph, K. E. (2005, April). *Flexibility in infant skill acquisition: How infants learn a stepping strategy.* Poster presented at the meeting of the Society for Research in Child Development, Atlanta, GA.

Harlow, H. F. (1949). The formation of learning sets. *Psychological Review, 56,* 51–65.

Ishak, S., Adolph, K. E., Lobo, S. A., Karasik, L. B., & Tamis-LeMonda, C. S. (2007, March). *Experienced crawlers and novice walkers descending slopes.* Poster presented at the meeting of the Society for Research in Child Development, Boston, MA.

Joh, A. S., & Adolph, K. E. (2006). Learning from falling. *Child Development, 77,* 89–102.

Joh, A. S., Adolph, K. E., Campbell, M. R., & Eppler, M. A. (2006). Why walkers slip: Shine is not a reliable cue for slippery ground. *Perception & Psychophysics, 68,* 339–352.

Joh, A. S., Adolph, K. E., & DeWind, N. K. (2005, November). *Learning from slipping and falling.* Poster presented at the meeting of the International Society for Developmental Psychobiology, Washington, DC.

Joh, A. S., Adolph, K. E., Narayanan, P. J., & Dietz, V. A. (2007). Gauging possibilities for action based on friction underfoot. *Journal of Experimental Psychology: Human Perception and Performance, 33,* 1145–1157.

Kuczmarski, R. J. (2000). *CDC growth charts: United States. Advance data from vital and health statistics; no. 314.* Hyattsville, MD: National Center for Health Statistics.

Lampl, M., Veldhuis, J. D., & Johnson, M. L. (1992). Saltation and stasis: A model of human growth. *Science, 258,* 801–803.

Lee, D. N. (1993). Body-environment coupling. In U. Neisser (Ed.), *The perceived self: Ecological and interpersonal sources of self-knowledge* (pp. 43–67). Cambridge: Cambridge University Press.

Leo, A. J., Chiu, J., & Adolph, K. E. (2000, July). *Temporal and functional relationships of crawling, cruising, and walking.* Poster presented at the International Conference on Infant Studies, Brighton, England.

Lobo, S. A., Koren, A., Ishak, S., Karasik, L. B., Adolph, K. E., & Tamis-LeMonda, C. S. (2007, March). *Friction underfoot affects infants' ability to cope with slopes.* Poster presented at the meeting of the Society for Research in Child Development, Boston, MA.

Reed, E. S. (1982). An outline of a theory of action systems. *Journal of Motor Behavior, 14,* 98–134.

Siegler, R. S., Adolph, K. E., & Lemaire, P. (1996). Strategy choice across the life span. In L. Reder (Ed.), *Implicit memory and metacognition* (pp. 79–121). Mahwah, NJ: Lawrence Erlbaum Associates.

Stevenson, H. W. (1972). *Children's learning.* New York: Appleton-Century-Crofts.

Thelen, E. (1996). The improvising infant: Learning about learning to move. In M. R. Merrens & G. G. Brannigan (Eds.), *The developmental psychologists: Research adventures across the lifespan* (pp. 21–36). New York: McGraw-Hill.

von Hofsten, C. (1993). Prospective control: A basic aspect of action development. *Human Development, 36,* 253–270.

von Hofsten, C. (2003). On the development of perception and action. In K. J. Connolly & J. Valsiner (Eds.), *Handbook of developmental psychology* (pp. 114–140). London: Sage.

von Hofsten, C. (2004). An action perspective on motor development. *Trends in Cognitive Sciences, 8,* 266–272.

CHAPTER

20

The Role of Memory in the Control of Action

Gordon D. Logan

Abstract

This chapter reviews studies on the role of memory in the control of action, focusing on habits, knowledge, and plans. These disparate topics are linked through a formal theory of memory and attention that points out important commonalities among them. The chapter describes the theoretical connections as well as the empirical facts, culminating with the authors' particular perspective on the role of information in the control of action.

Keywords: action control, habits, knowledge, plans, automaticity, task switching, cognitive control

The actions we perform depend not only on the stimuli available in the environment but also on what we know about the possibilities for action afforded by those stimuli. Thus, action is a joint function of perceptual information about the environment and memorial information available in various memory systems. This chapter focuses on three ways in which memorial information controls action: through habit, knowledge, and plans. Habits are common responses to familiar stimuli that can be executed with little thought and effort. In my view, habits are supported by memory retrieval. Attention to a stimulus retrieves records of past actions taken on that stimulus that serve as action plans that allow us to respond in the same way we usually respond to the stimulus. The role of memory in habits has been investigated extensively in studies of *automaticity,* particularly the ones that focus on the

acquisition and expression of automaticity in skilled performance (Logan, 1988; Logan & Etherton, 1994). Knowledge is stored information about perceptual, semantic, conceptual, and affective properties of stimuli we encounter, acquired either directly or through instruction. Knowledge can also inform the choice of action. An attended stimulus can become part of a compound retrieval cue that pulls from memory the knowledge that we require to decide how to respond to it. The role of memory in knowledge-guided action has been investigated in studies of *task switching,* in which people must choose between different ways of responding to a potentially ambiguous stimulus, like the digit 7 (Logan & Bundesen, 2003; D. W. Schneider & Logan, 2005). Plans are sets of goals to be achieved or tasks to be performed. They are often transitory, changing from one occasion to the next, so they are held in working memory to enable them to be accessed quickly when they are needed and discarded quickly when they are finished. The role of memory in implementing plans has not been investigated very extensively, but a few studies of the performance of *task sequences* offer promising insights (Logan, 2004, 2006; D. W. Schneider & Logan, 2006).

The purpose of this chapter is to review studies that my colleagues and I have conducted on the role of memory in the control of action, focusing on habits, knowledge, and plans. We have linked these disparate topics through a formal theory of memory and attention that points out important commonalities among them. The review will describe the theoretical connections as well as the empirical facts, culminating with our particular perspective on the role of information in the control of action.

What Is an Action?

For the purposes of this chapter, an action is a simple discrete response to a simple discrete stimulus, usually a key-press response to a visual stimulus. Simple actions like these form the basis of much of the literature in cognitive psychology, as evident in any issue of *Journal of Experimental Psychology: Human Perception and Performance* or *Journal of Experimental Psychology: Learning, Memory, and Cognition*. The most common measures of these simple actions are *reaction time* (RT) and error rate. Following traditions that date back to Donders (1868/1969) and Sternberg (1969), error rate is usually very low, so analyses focus on RT. Across a wide range of stimuli, responses, and tasks, mean RT ranges mostly between 200 and 2,000 milliseconds. Theories of cognition focus on events that happen in this "1.5-second" time scale on the assumption that these events represent the basic information processing operations of the cognitive system (Newell, 1990).

This restricted focus has been very fruitful. Many fascinating phenomena have been discovered and explored and many theories have been developed to explain them. The restricted focus necessarily excludes complex action sequences that extend over seconds and minutes, but researchers often assume (as I do) that these phenomena can ultimately be understood as concatenations of simple 1.5-second events. This assumption has rarely been tested; there has been enough controversy within the restricted focus to keep researchers busy for many years. Moreover, many years of cumulative progress in cognitive and information-processing psychology and the recent development of successful links to neuroscience have encouraged our belief that the focus on 1.5-second actions is important and useful even if it is not the whole story.

Habit

William James discussed habit in his classic 1890 book. Habit was an important topic in behaviorist learning theories that dominated the first half of the 20th century (e.g., Hull, 1943). It was one of several babies that were thrown out with the bathwater in the cognitive revolution of the 1950s and 1960s when researchers' interests shifted from gradual learning to single-shot apprehension and acquisition of information in studies of attention and short-term memory (e.g., Broadbent, 1958). Habit resurfaced in the 1970s in studies of automaticity, stimulated by seminal papers by Posner and Snyder (1975) and Shiffrin and Schneider (1977). The early studies in this renaissance focused on the properties of automaticity, suggesting that automatic processing was fast, effortless, obligatory, and unconscious (for reviews, see Kahneman & Treisman, 1984; Logan, 1985; Moors & De Houwer, 2006). By the 1980s, researchers became interested in factors that determined the acquisition of automaticity, proposing theories of learning that bore an uneasy resemblance to the behaviorist theories of learning that were rejected in the cognitive revolution. Anderson (1982) and W. Schneider (1985) argued that automaticity was acquired by strengthening connections between stimuli and responses, much like Hull's (1943) perspective (also see Rickard, 1997). Logan (1988) argued that automaticity was acquired by retaining memory records of each performance, much like Guthrie's (1935) perspective (see also Palmeri, 1997). The difference was that the theories of automaticity interfaced with new theories of attention and memory, going beyond behavioral definitions to describe automaticity in terms of representations and processes—the coin of the trade in cognitive theories.

Automaticity as Memory

Theories of the acquisition of automaticity suggest that automaticity is a memory phenomenon, governed by the theoretical and empirical principles that govern memory. Automatization reflects a transition from some initial strategy to memory retrieval. Shiffrin and Schneider (1977; W. Schneider, 1985) called the initial strategy "controlled processing." I prefer to call it "algorithmic processing," borrowing the computer-science definition of an algorithm as an "effective procedure" that is guaranteed to produce correct results if it is applied correctly. In my theory, subjects address a new problem domain with an algorithm they acquire through instruction or problem solving that allows them to solve the problems they are confronted with even if they have not encountered them before. Each application of the algorithm lays down an episodic memory trace—an *instance*—that represents the stimulus, the goal the subject was trying to achieve, and the response the subject executed (Logan & Etherton, 1994). Repeated exposure to

problems in the domain builds up a knowledge base of problems that can be solved by memory retrieval instead of applying the algorithm. If the domain is restricted, as is the case with many well-defined problem domains, subjects' experience may leave them with a set of instances that "covers" the domain so that they can solve any problem they encounter with memory retrieval. Problems that have been experienced before can be solved by retrieving previous solutions. Problems that have not been experienced before can be solved by retrieving solutions to similar problems that were experienced in the past (Palmeri, 1997; Ross, 1984). Eventually, subjects no longer have to think about how to solve problems; the appropriate response is retrieved directly from memory. In this way, memory controls habitual action.

A large amount of research has shown that *consistent mapping* is sufficient for the acquisition of automaticity and the expression of automaticity in skilled performance (for a review, see W. Schneider, Dumais, & Shiffrin, 1984). The idea that consistency was important was first crystallized by Shiffrin and Schneider (1977), who argued that visual search and memory search could become automatic if stimuli were mapped consistently onto responses. Other researchers generalized this idea to consistent associations between one thing and another. Logan (1990) argued that in some applications, consistent mapping of stimuli onto response categories (e.g., "yes" versus "no") was more important than consistent mapping of stimuli onto physical responses.

The reason for the importance of consistent mapping is straightforward: Subjects may associate stimuli, goals, and responses as a matter of course every time they act on the environment. But they will not get to use these associations to support performance unless the environment is consistent, that is, unless the environment requires the same responses to the same stimuli on some future occasion. Indeed, Logan (1988) showed that subjects were just as accurate at judging the frequency with which stimuli were presented with varied mapping as with consistent mapping, yet task performance improved only with consistent mapping. The information from each encounter with the stimuli was stored in memory, but it could not be expressed effectively unless the same mapping rules were used on subsequent exposures.

Automaticity in Context

Habits are often expressed in familiar environments. We work at the same desk, cook in the same kitchen, and shower in the same bathroom day after day. Our habits become associated with these contexts, making it easier to accomplish things in familiar environments. Logan and Etherton (1994) studied the effect of contextual associations in the acquisition and expression of habits. They presented two words on each trial and had subjects decide whether one of the words was a member of a target category, such as metals. The same set of targets was presented throughout practice, so stimulus-to-response mapping was always consistent. The context in which each target appeared—the *context word* that was paired with it—was either consistent throughout training (e.g., STEEL appeared with CANADA every time it was presented) or varied from one presentation to the next (e.g., STEEL appeared with CANADA and then with FRANCE). The question was whether consistent context would facilitate learning. The answer was a clear "yes." The gain in RT from the first presentation to the 16th was greater for targets paired with consistent distractors than for targets paired with varied distractors.

Logan and Etherton (1994) used a transfer test to provide converging evidence for the importance of context. At the end of training, they presented the words once more, scrambling the combinations of targets and distractors. Subjects trained with consistent pairing of targets and distractors suffered from this scrambling—their RT slowed by 99 milliseconds. However, subjects trained with varied pairing of targets and distractors showed no effect of scrambling—their RT slowed by 3 milliseconds—as if it was just one more in a long series of target–distractor re-pairings.

These context effects are important because they suggest that the stimuli that drive our habits extend beyond the intended targets of our actions to the contexts in which the targets occur. A larger portion of the environment controls our habitual actions. However, we can control the portions of the environment that control our actions by focusing attention appropriately. Logan and Etherton (1994) demonstrated this by conducting their consistent- and varied-context experiments in *focused attention conditions* in which subjects were told which of the two words could be the target (it was colored green) so they could focus attention on it and in *divided attention conditions* in which subjects were not told which word could be a target so they had to divide attention between the two words. Again, the results were clear: The effect of consistent context was greater in training and in transfer in divided attention conditions than in focused attention conditions. Focusing attention appeared to prevent retrieval of contextual associations (see also Boronat & Logan, 1997).

Knowledge

Habit only goes so far. We often find ourselves in new environments, having to act in new ways. Sometimes we have to acquire new habits. Sometimes we have to override our old habits. The flexibility required to respond to new environments in new ways is characteristic of human cognition, an essential part of the story of cognitive control of action. Memory plays an important role here, too. We seek out similarities between new situations and old ones and try to adapt our familiar habits to satisfy new goals. New situations are never completely new. There is always some commonality between past and present so that we can use our old knowledge to solve new problems.

Task Switching and Cognitive Control

Task-switching procedures have become popular methods for studying the flexibility of cognitive control. Performance is usually worse when subjects switch between tasks than when they repeat tasks—RT is longer and error rate is higher. These *switch costs* are often interpreted as measures of executive control (for reviews, see Logan, 2003; Monsell, 2003). Task switching is implemented in many different procedures, but in each one the target stimulus is ambiguous: It affords at least two different actions. Something else is required to disambiguate the stimulus and choose one action instead of the other. What that something else might be is the subject of an ongoing controversy in theories of task switching. Some attribute it to top-down cognitive control processes (Monsell & Mizon, 2006; Rogers & Monsell, 1995). Others attribute it to bottom-up memory retrieval processes (Allport, Styles, & Hsieh, 1994; Logan & Bundesen, 2003; Waszak, Hommel, & Allport, 2003). Still others attribute it to a mixture of top-down and bottom-up influences. My goal here is not to resolve this controversy. More theoretical development and empirical evidence will be required to do that. Instead, my goal is to describe one perspective on task switching that emphasizes the role of memory and prior knowledge in cognitive control.

There are empirical parallels between task switching and automaticity. Automaticity experiments involve consistent mapping of stimuli onto responses so that habits can develop and support performance. Task-switching experiments involve varied mapping of targets onto responses that past habits cannot disambiguate. Task-switching experiments are like the varied-mapping control conditions in automaticity experiments (Shiffrin & Schneider, 1977). In automaticity experiments, consistent-mapping conditions were in the foreground because they provided insights into the acquisition and expression of habits; in task-switching experiments, varied-mapping conditions are in the foreground because they provide insights into control processing.

Explicit Task Cuing

One of the more popular methods for studying task switching is the *explicit task-cuing* procedure, in which subjects are shown an ambiguous target stimulus that is preceded by an explicit cue that indicates which task to perform on the target. In many of our experiments, the target was a single digit, like 7, and the cue has been a pair of words that describe the possible responses to the digit, like Odd–Even or High–Low. When Odd–Even precedes 7, subjects must report whether 7 is odd or even; when High–Low precedes 7, subjects must report whether 7 is greater or less than 5. The advantage of this procedure is that it allows the experimental control over the time at which disambiguating information (the cue) is available to the subject, providing experimental control over the onset of cognitive control processes. The interval between the cue and the target (cue–target interval [CTI]) is manipulated to capture the time course of processing the cue (Meiran, 1996). Cues and targets are presented in random combinations, and trials are sorted post hoc into task repetitions (trials in which the task on trial $N-1$ is the same as the task on trial N) and task alternations (trials in which the task on trial $N - 1$ is different from the task on trial N). As in other task-switching procedures, RT is longer and error rate higher for task alternations than for task repetitions. These switch costs are largest when CTI = 0 and diminish smoothly as CTI increases, sometimes disappearing entirely at the longest CTI (Logan & Bundesen, 2003).

Both of these effects are important theoretically. The switch costs are interpreted as reflecting the action of cognitive control processes, which takes time and is prone to error. The reduction in switch costs with CTI is interpreted as reflecting the time course of control processing; it begins with the onset of the cue and plays out during the CTI. If the CTI is long enough, cognitive control processes will have finished their work before the target appears. My colleagues and I have presented formal models of time course functions that allow estimates of the durations of processes that encode the cue and switch between tasks (Arrington & Logan, 2004; Logan & Bundesen, 2003, 2004; D. W. Schneider & Logan, 2005).

There is an important confound in many explicit task-cuing experiments, noted independently by Logan and Bundesen (2003) and Mayr and Kliegl (2003): There is one cue for each task, so cue repetition is confounded with task repetition. Whenever the task repeats, the cue also repeats. Whenever the task alternates, the cue also alternates. The observed switch costs could reflect a benefit for processing repeated cues instead of (or as well as) the time required for executive control processing. Benefits from repetition are well known in the memory literature, having been the cornerstone of the concept of implicit memory (e.g., Logan, 1990), so the possibility that measured switch costs reflect cue-encoding benefits must be taken seriously.

One way to address this confound is to use two cues for each task. For example,

High–Low or Magnitude may cue the "greater or less than 5" task, and Odd–Even or Parity may cue the "odd–even" task. This allows three transitions between trials instead of two: *cue repetitions,* in which the cue and task both repeat (e.g., High–Low → High–Low); *task repetitions,* in which the task repeats but the cue changes (e.g., Magnitude → High–Low); and *task alternations,* in which both the cue and the task change (e.g., Odd–Even → Parity). The contrast between cue repetitions and task repetitions allows the assessment of cue-repetition benefits without a confounded task switch, and the contrast between task repetitions and task alternations allows the assessment of task switch effects without a confounded cue repetition.

Since 2003, dozens of explicit task-cuing experiments have been conducted using two cues per task. They all find substantial cue-encoding benefits. In 24 experiments conducted in our laboratory, the mean difference between cue repetitions and task repetitions (cue-encoding benefit unconfounded with task switch) was 154 milliseconds (see Logan, Schneider, & Bundesen, 2007). "True" switch costs that are unconfounded with cue-repetition effects (task alternations versus task repetitions) are generally smaller. Sometimes the differences are negligible, ranging from −2 to 14 milliseconds (Logan & Bundesen, 2003, 2004). Often, the differences are larger; the 24 experiments conducted in our laboratory yielded a mean difference of 75 milliseconds (Logan et al., 2007).

These effects are important empirically. They show that the switch costs typically measured in explicit task-cuing experiments (cue repetitions versus task alternations) reflect large cue-encoding benefits and comparatively smaller "true" switch costs. They urge caution in interpreting the effects and commend the use of two cues per task as a way of separating cue-encoding benefits from "true" switch costs (see also Arrington, Logan, & Schneider, 2007; D. W. Schneider & Logan, 2007b).

Task Switching as Compound-Cue Retrieval

The cue-repetition benefits are important theoretically. They challenge top-down interpretations of switch costs, suggesting that bottom-up cue-repetition benefits can account for large proportions of the costs. My colleagues and I have proposed a *compound retrieval cue* explanation of performance in the explicit task-cuing procedure that in principle could account for all of the effects observed with the procedure (Arrington & Logan, 2004; Logan & Bundesen, 2003, 2004; Logan & Schneider, 2006a, 2006b; D. W. Schneider & Logan, 2005). The idea is that subjects combine the cue with the target to form a compound retrieval cue and then respond with whatever the compound cue pulls from memory. The compound retrieval cue obviates the need for top-down control. While targets are ambiguous and may be mapped onto two competing responses (e.g., 7 may evoke "press left for large" and "press right for odd"), combinations of cues and targets are not ambiguous; they are mapped onto a single response (e.g., 7 and Odd–Even evoke "press right for odd," while 7 and High–Low evoke "press left for large"). Subjects can simply choose the single response associated with the compound retrieval cue without top-down intervention.

According to the compound retrieval cue theory, encoding the cue and the target are the critical operations that take time and produce errors. Cue-encoding benefits (differences between cue repetitions and task repetitions) are explained in terms of repetition priming using familiar principles from studies of implicit memory (Logan, 1990): The current cue is encoded by matching it to mental representations in long-term and short-term memory; as soon as one of the representations matches, the cue is encoded. On cue-repetition trials, the presented cue matches short-term and long-term memory, and cue-encoding time is the minimum of the two comparison processes. On task-repetition and task-alternation trials, the presented cue matches only long-term memory, so cue-encoding time is longer (Logan & Bundesen, 2003). D. W. Schneider and Logan (2005) suggested that cue encoding could benefit from semantic or associative priming as well as repetition priming, noting that two cues that indicate that the same task are necessarily related semantically and are often related associatively. Thus, a cue on trial $N - 1$ may activate a strong representation of itself and a weak representation of its associates (e.g., Magnitude activates "magnitude" strongly and "high–low" weakly). If trial N is a cue repetition, the current cue matches a strong representation in short-term memory, speeding cue encoding substantially. If trial N is a task repetition, the current cue matches a weak representation in short-term memory, speeding cue encoding to some extent. If trial N is a task alternation, the current cue does not match either representation in short-term memory, so there is no speeding of cue encoding. Thus, D. W. Schneider and Logan's (2005) priming version of the compound-cue theory can explain the (small) difference between task repetitions and task alternations as well as the (large) difference between cue repetitions and task repetitions (see also Logan & Schneider, 2006b).

The compound retrieval cue theory has not gone unchallenged (e.g., Altmann, 2006; Mayr, 2006; Monsell & Mizon, 2006; but see Logan et al., 2007). We ourselves have found evidence suggesting that cue-encoding benefits cannot account for all measured switch costs (Arrington & Logan, 2004;

Logan & Bundesen, 2004; D. W. Schneider & Logan, 2007a, 2007b). Recently, we developed a version of the explicit task-cuing procedure that separates cue encoding from target processing by requiring separate responses to the cue and the target and found true switch costs in target processing times even when all cue-encoding effects had been isolated in cue-processing times (Arrington et al., 2007). Nevertheless, the compound-cue theory suggests that a substantial part of cognitive control in the explicit task-cuing procedure may reflect knowledge-based memory retrieval.

Plans

To paraphrase Robert Burns, the "best laid plans of men," if not mice, often lead "to promised joy" because they provide focus to behavior, allowing us to direct our actions toward important goals and avoid distraction. They provide an overarching purpose to sequences of single responses, making them coherent and comprehensible. They allow us to transcend the 1.5-second universe in which our actions unfold, linking separate 1.5-second episodes together. They connect the past to the present and the present to the future. Plans are transitory, unlike habits and long-term knowledge. They are made up on the fly and changed on a whim to suit our current needs and wishes. They are held in working memory rather than long-term or procedural memory, and they fade away soon after we are done with them. Plans describe the macrostructure of action rather than the microstructure. They are one step away from action, unlike habits and algorithms for employing long-term knowledge. They are lists of intentions—goals to be achieved or tasks to be done—with no firm commitment to action. They are not task sets—states of preparation or combinations of perceptual, cognitive, and motor processes that enable performance of certain tasks. They are inputs that guide the construction of task sets and enable the execution of actions.

The idea that plans structure behavior was a central part of the cognitive revolution against behaviorism in the 1950s and 1960s (Miller, Galanter, & Pribram, 1960). Much research has addressed the processes by which people form plans to solve complex problems (e.g., Hayes-Roth & Hayes-Roth, 1988; Kotovsky, Hayes, & Simon, 1985; Thomas, 1974). My research has addressed the processes by which people implement plans after they are formed (Logan, 2004, 2006; D. W. Schneider & Logan, 2006). My goal has been to draw theoretical and empirical connections between plans, habits, and knowledge as they control simple actions that express cognitive judgments.

Plans can be cumulative or noncumulative. Cumulative plans involve steps that are all directed toward the fulfillment of an ultimate goal, such as cooking a meal or preparing a chapter. The steps in cumulative plans are related logically and conceptually; one step fulfills conditions that enable another step. You wash the vegetables before chopping them, and you chop them before you sauté them. Noncumulative plans involve steps that are unrelated and directed toward a diverse set of goals, such as a list of things to accomplish on a day at work or a list of things to do on vacation. Completion of one step need not enable another step. Meeting with a student is not a necessary precursor to checking e-mail. My research has focused on the implementation of noncumulative plans because they are simpler and easier to investigate in the laboratory. It has addressed two main issues: capacity limitations on representing plans, which follow from the idea that plans are held in working memory, and the steps involved in implementing plans, which follows from the idea that plans are not complete descriptions of task sets.

The Task Span Procedure

How many tasks can we hold in a plan without forgetting any of them? The idea that plans are held in working memory suggests that the limit should be on the order of 7 ± 2 (Miller, 1956; but see Cowan, 2001). To address this question of capacity, I developed the *task span* procedure, which is analogous to the standard memory span procedure: Subjects are given a list of N task names followed by a list of N target stimuli. They must perform each task on the list on the corresponding stimulus. If the task list was High–Low, Odd–Even, and Odd–Even and the target list was 7, 3, and 8, they would perform a magnitude judgment on 7 and a parity judgment on 3 and 8. Following tradition in the verbal memory span literature, the task span is the number of tasks subjects can perform in order without error on 50% of their attempts.

Logan (2004) measured task span by presenting subjects with lists of 1 to 10 task names followed by lists of 1 to 10 targets. Task span was 6.2 items, within the classical range of 7 ± 2 (Miller, 1956). The same subjects were tested in a memory span control condition in which they received 1 to 10 task names and recalled them in order. There, memory span was 6.9 items, which was not significantly greater than the task span. This difference is surprisingly small given that task span performance is subject to two sources of error (recalling the task names and performing the tasks), whereas memory span performance is subject to one source of error (recalling the task names). A subsequent experiment with 64 subjects showed a significant correlation between task span and memory span (r = .37), suggesting that the two procedures rely on common underlying processes.

Subjects can overcome capacity limitations on planning in two ways: chunking and practice. Analysis of serial position effects in RTs measured during task performance showed elevations in every third position, consistent with the idea that subjects organized the list in chunks of three tasks (Miller, 1956; Simon, 1980). Chunking relieves the burden on working memory by reducing the number of items to be retained (e.g., three chunks instead of nine task names). The reduced burden comes at a cost in processing time: When one chunk is finished, the next must be retrieved and unpacked, and this takes an appreciable amount of time (Anderson & Matessa, 1997). Interestingly, the extra cost in retrieval time did not increase the number of retrieval errors. Subjects took twice as long to complete a list in the task span procedure than in the memory span procedure, but their accuracy of recall was comparable (Logan, 2004).

A subsequent experiment compared task spans for lists that were presented 10 times, which would allow long-term storage, with task spans for lists that were presented only once. Performance was much better with lists that were presented 10 times. Indeed, it was not different from performance in single-task conditions, in which subjects performed the same task repeatedly. Practice allowed subjects to overcome capacity limitations, transferring control from short-term memory to long-term memory (e.g., Ericsson & Kintsch, 1995).

The Repeating Sequence Procedure

We think about our plans as well as the world around us, and that thinking takes time and produces errors just like our actions on the world. It also unfolds in the 1.5-second universe in steps that can be measured in RT and error rate. Darryl Schneider and I conducted experiments that separate these *plan-level* processes from the *task-level* processes that govern our actions on the external world. We assumed that subjects first access the plan with plan-level processing and then use the goal they retrieve to control task-level processing. The extra plan-level processing should increase RT to the first item on a list relative to subsequent items. The prediction was confirmed in task span RTs: Subjects took a long time to respond to the first item in a list and then sped through the subsequent items, just as they took longer on the first item in a chunk. The RT to the first item in the sequence increased linearly with sequence length, suggesting that subjects rehearsed the whole list before dealing with the first item (Logan, 2004).

These RT effects are suggestive of plan-level processing, but they are hard to interpret because the first item in a list is always the first item in the series of targets subjects respond to. Control conditions in which subjects perform a single task on N consecutive targets also show elevated RT for the first target (Logan, 2004). The increase in single-task conditions is smaller than the increase in task span conditions, so in principle, the effects could be separated by subtraction. However, subtraction requires strong assumptions that may not be valid (Logan, 2006). To overcome this problem, we developed the *repeating sequence* procedure, in which subjects were given a list of N tasks to perform followed by a sequence of $N \times M$ targets (e.g., High–Low, Odd–Even, Odd–Even, High–Low followed by 3, 7, 4, 6, 2, 1, 7, 8, 9, 2, 6, 1). They were told to perform each task on the list on the corresponding target and to repeat the list when they got to the end until there were no more targets (e.g., if N was 4 and M was 3, they must begin the list again on the fifth and ninth target; 2 and 9 in the previous example). We excluded the first trial in the series of $N \times M$ targets and compared RT to targets that began repetitions of the sequence with RT to targets within the

sequence. As in the task span procedure, we found elevated RT to the first targets in the sequence, indicating time-consuming plan-level processing.

To test our assumption that elevated RT to the first item in each repetition of the sequence reflected plan-level processing, we compared performance on two sequences of two tasks, characterized abstractly as AABB and ABBA. When these four-item sequences are carried out M times, they produce identical task sequences, shifted by one item. AABB repeated three times yields AABBAABBAABB, and ABBA repeated three times yields ABBAABBAABBA. Subjects could perform accurately without referring to the sequence simply by remembering the two previous trials and following the rules AB → B, BB → A, BA → A, and AA → B. If subjects followed these rules and ignored the sequence, there should be no sequence initiation effects. Performance should depend on the local transitions between tasks and not on the transitions between sequences. The B → A and A → B transitions should be slow because they reflect task switches, and A → A and B → B transitions should be fast because they reflect task repetitions.

The data suggested that subjects organized their performance in terms of sequences rather than transitions. The RT was elevated at the first position in a sequence for both ABBA and AABB sequences. Within each sequence, task alternations were slower than task repetitions, but the pattern reversed in the first position of each sequence; task repetitions (ABB<u>A</u> → <u>A</u>BBA) were reliably slower than task alternations (AAB<u>B</u> → <u>A</u>ABB). These patterns of results suggest a hierarchical relationship between plan-level processing and task-level processing: Subjects retrieve the plan or refresh it before each iteration. This retrieval or refreshment purges working memory of the traces of previous task-level processes, clearing the way for the new plan (D. W. Schneider & Logan, 2006).

Subsequent experiments showed that plans behaved (somewhat) like task sets: Sequence initiation costs were absorbed into a preparation interval, just like task-switching costs, and sequence initiation costs were greater when subjects switched between sequences than when they repeated sequences (D. W. Schneider & Logan, 2006). These modulations of sequence initiation costs suggest that it may be useful to think of executive control at the plan level as well as at the task level. The concept of task set has been difficult to define at the task level (D. W. Schneider & Logan, 2007a), but it may be more straightforward at the plan level. A task set may be a set of tasks to be performed, like the plans we examine in the task span and repeating-sequence procedures. Sets of tasks can be distinguished from each other in terms of the content of the items (e.g., ABBA is different from CDDC) and the order in which the items occur (e.g., ABBA versus AABB). Sets of tasks are essentially lists of items, so the plan-level processes that operate on sets of tasks may be understood in terms of the retrieval processes that operate in list-learning experiments (e.g., Anderson & Matessa, 1997). Models of short-term memory have proliferated recently, and it may be useful to adapt those models to task span and repeating-sequence experiments to gain insight into plan-level processing.

Toward a Theory of Memory-Based Control

An integrated theory of habits, knowledge, and plans is tantalizingly close. My colleagues and I have been working on theories that address the details of performance in experiments on automaticity, task switching, and plan implementation, and the time may be right to step back

from these detailed theories to examine the commonalities among them. The commonalities can be seen clearly from the perspective of the *instance theory of attention and memory* (ITAM), which I proposed several years ago (Logan, 2002). ITAM is a synthesis of two well-established families of theory that derive from the similarity-choice theory proposed by Luce (1959, 1963) and Shepard (1957) long ago. One family addresses attention, focusing on Bundesen's (1990) *theory of visual attention,* which, with its ancestors and progeny, provides detailed quantitative accounts of many phenomena of attention, ranging from partial report to single-cell firing rates. The other family addresses categorization, focusing on Nosofsky's (1984, 1988) *generalized context model,* which accounts quantitatively for many important details of performance in categorization tasks, ranging from perceptual identification to social judgments. ITAM is a generalization of these two families of theory that includes each theory as a special case (for details, see Logan, 2002).

The key idea in ITAM, stemming from the Shepard-Luce similarity-choice theory, is that response tendencies are governed by similarities between stimuli in the environment and representations in memory, represented as η values (η for *evidence*) and biases for particular responses or interpretations of the stimuli, represented as β values (β for *bias*). Similarities and biases combine multiplicatively to produce response tendencies (v):

$$v(c,t,i) = \eta(c,i)\eta(t,i)\beta_i \qquad (1)$$

where $\eta(t, i)$ is the similarity between a presented target and the memory representation for category i, $\eta(c, i)$ is the similarity between a presented cue or context item and the memory representation for category i, and β_i is the bias for classifying targets as members of category *i*. The response tendencies are converted to response probabilities by the Shepard-Luce choice rule:

$$P(i \mid c,t) = \frac{v(c,t,i)}{\sum_{j \in R} v(c,t,j)} \quad (2)$$

The probability of responding "category *i*" given cue or context *c* and target *t* is the ratio of the sum of the response tendencies for category *i* to the sum of the response tendencies for all categories *j* in the set of permissible responses *R*. ITAM assumes that probabilities described by Equation 2 become drift rates in random-walk evidence-accumulation processes that choose between alternative responses, yielding predictions for RT and error rate (see also Logan & Gordon, 2001; Nosofsky & Palmeri, 1997; D. W. Schneider & Logan, 2005).

Equation 1 captures the influence of habit, knowledge, and plans. Habit is represented in terms of similarities: $\eta(t, i)$ and $\eta(c, i)$. According to the instance theory of automaticity, each encounter with a target and a context cue lays down a separate trace that is represented as an η value. The ηs in Equation 1 are sums of ηs representing each of the instances encountered in the past. Repeated experience with a target increases its response tendency in a way that produces the power-function speedup that characterizes automaticity (Logan, 1988, 2002).

Equation 1 also captures the context effects described in the section on habit (Boronat & Logan, 1997; Logan & Etherton, 1994). Contexts that occur consistently with targets become associated with the categorical response given to the target; that is, each time context *c* occurs with target *t* in category *i*, $\eta(c, i)$ increases. Contexts that occur with different targets become associated with different categorical responses; that is, if

c occurs with category *i* and category *j*, then both $\eta(c, i)$ and $\eta(c, j)$ increase. Consistent contexts increase the numerator and denominator of Equation 2, increasing choice probability and speeding RT; inconsistent contexts increase only the denominator of Equation 2, reducing choice probability and slowing RT.

Knowledge is also represented in the similarities $\eta(t, i)$ and $\eta(c, i)$. Theories in the memory branch of ITAM assume that knowledge of category membership is represented in the $\eta(t, i)$ values. The compound retrieval cue theory of task-switching performance assumes that knowledge is represented in the $\eta(t, i)$ and $\eta(c, i)$ values (D. W. Schneider & Logan, 2005). The multiplication of $\eta(t, i)$ and $\eta(c, i)$ in Equation 1 explains the cue-based gating assumed by the theory. For example, let us assume that the cue Odd–Even is presented with the target 7. The target 7 evokes response tendencies $\eta(7, odd) = 1$ and $\eta(7, high) = 1$. The cue Odd–Even evokes response tendencies $\eta(Odd–Even, odd) = 1$ and $\eta(Odd–Even, high) = 0$. The combined response tendencies formed by multiplying these components are $\eta(7, odd) \times \eta(Odd–Even, odd) = 1 \times 1 = 1$ for the "odd" response and $\eta(7, high) \times \eta(Odd–Even, high) = 1 \times 0 = 0$ for the "high" response.

ITAM also captures the traditional idea of a top-down task-level task set in the response bias (β) parameters (Logan & Gordon, 2001). Top-down processes can manipulate response tendencies (Equation 1) and response probabilities (Equation 2) by varying the β values. The parameter β acts as a gain control: High values of β strengthen response tendencies, and low values of β decrease them. Thus, ITAM provides two mechanisms to account for action control in task-switching situations: top-down control through manipulations of β and bottom-up control through cue-based gating mediated by $\eta(c, i)$.

ITAM is a model of long-term memory and choice among stimuli and responses. It does not (yet) include a model of short-term memory. Thus, it accounts for habit and knowledge more directly than it accounts for planning. However, it has the machinery necessary to account for planning in the $\eta(c, i)\eta(t, i)\beta_i$ products in Equation 1. The stimulus provides $\eta(t, i)$, top-down executive control processes provide β_i, and the plan provides $\eta(c, i)$. The processes by which a task name in short-term memory gets converted to an $\eta(c, i)$ value remain to be specified, but in principle, the machinery in Equations 1 and 2 may suffice after that conversion is done.

Is Memory Everything?

Memory accounts for a lot of cognitive control of action. Habits support action in familiar environments. Cue-based gating supports action in less familiar environments and directs action toward goals when we implement plans. What else might be involved in cognitive control? One important possibility is a system that evaluates the courses of action suggested by memory, choosing the ones that are worth the most to us emotionally and motivationally. Cognitive control is useful because it gets us what we want. Thus, wants, desires, and feelings may contribute as much to cognitive control as memory does.

The memory system can be viewed as a *thought pump*—an internal process that generates ideas for possible courses of action, following the ITAM equations (Equations 1 and 2). Knowledge enters the equation through the η parameters, with cues generated by internal thoughts as well as external stimuli. Wants and desires enter the equation through the β parameters, which can be adjusted to maximize expected value (Luce, 1963). Thus, the things we think of are determined by our current knowledge and our current wants

and desires. The determinism is stochastic; the expression for response probability in Equation 2 suggests we may think different things on different occasions given the same input. However, thoughts do not compel action except in unusual cases like playing music or playing sports. In situations where more deliberation is possible, the thought pump suggests a short list of alternatives, and the evaluation system chooses the one that we commit to action. Thus, memory is part of the story but more remains to be told.

References

Allport, A., Styles, E. A., & Hsieh, S. (1994). Shifting intentional set: Exploring the dynamic control of tasks. In C. Umiltà & M. Moscovitch (Eds.), *Attention and performance XV* (pp. 421–452). Cambridge, MA: MIT Press.

Altmann, E. M. (2006). Task switching is not cue switching. *Psychonomic Bulletin and Review, 13,* 1016–1022.

Anderson, J. R. (1982). Acquisition of cognitive skill. *Psychological Review, 89,* 369–406.

Anderson, J. R., & Matessa, M. (1997). A production system theory of serial memory. *Psychological Review, 104,* 728–748.

Arrington, C. M., & Logan, G. D. (2004). Episodic and semantic components of the compound-stimulus strategy in the explicit task-cuing procedure. *Memory and Cognition, 32,* 965–978.

Arrington, C. M., Logan, G. D., & Schneider, D. W. (2007). Separating cue encoding from target processing in the explicit task-cuing procedure: Are there "true" task switch effects? *Journal of Experimental Psychology: Learning, Memory, and Cognition, 33,* 484–502.

Boronat, C. B., & Logan, G. D. (1997). The role of attention in automatization: Does attention operate at encoding, or retrieval, or both? *Memory and Cognition, 25,* 36–46.

Broadbent, D. E. (1958). *Perception and communication.* Elmsford, NY: Pergamon.

Bundesen, C. (1990). A theory of visual attention. *Psychological Review, 97,* 523–547.

Cowan, N. (2001). The magical number 4 in short-term memory: A reconsideration of mental storage capacity. *Behavioral and Brain Sciences, 24,* 87–185.

Donders, F. C. (1969). On the speed of mental processes (W. G. Koster, Trans.). In W. G. Koster (Ed.), *Attention and performance II* (pp. 412–431). Amsterdam: North-Holland. (Original work published 1868)

Ericsson, K. A., & Kintsch, W. (1995). Long-term working memory. *Psychological Review, 102,* 211–245.

Guthrie, E. R. (1935). *The psychology of learning.* New York: Harper.

Hayes-Roth, B., & Hayes-Roth, F. (1988). A cognitive model of planning. In A.M. Collins & E. E. Smith (Eds.), *Readings in cognitive science: A perspective from psychology and artificial intelligence* (pp. 496–513). San Mateo, CA: Morgan Kaufman.

Hull, C. L. (1943). *Principles of behavior.* New York: Appleton-Century-Crofts.

James, W. (1890). *Principles of psychology.* New York: Holt.

Kahneman, D., & Treisman, A. (1984). Changing views of attention and automaticity. In R. Parasuraman & D. R. Davies (Eds.), *Varieties of attention* (pp. 29–61). New York: Academic Press.

Kotovsky, K., Hayes, J. R., & Simon, H. A. (1985). Why some problems are hard—Evidence from Tower of Hanoi. *Cognitive Psychology, 17,* 248–294.

Logan, G. D. (1985). Executive control of thought and action. *Acta Psychologica, 60,* 193–210.

Logan, G. D. (1988). Toward an instance theory of automatization. *Psychological Review, 95,* 492–527.

Logan, G. D. (1990). Repetition priming and automaticity: Common underlying mechanisms? *Cognitive Psychology, 22,* 1–35.

Logan, G. D. (2002). An instance theory of attention and memory. *Psychological Review, 109,* 376–400.

Logan, G. D. (2003). Executive control of thought and action: In search of the wild homunculus. *Current Directions in Psychological Science, 12,* 45–48.

Logan, G. D. (2004). Working memory, task switching, and executive control in the task span procedure. *Journal of Experimental Psychology: General, 133,* 218–236.

Logan, G. D. (2006). Out with the old, in with the new: More valid measures of switch cost and retrieval time in the task span procedure. *Psychonomic Bulletin and Review, 13,* 139–144.

Logan, G. D., & Bundesen, C. (2003). Clever homunculus: Is there an endogenous act of control in the explicit task-cuing procedure? *Journal of Experimental Psychology: Human Perception and Performance, 29,* 575–599.

Logan, G. D., & Bundesen, C. (2004). Very clever homunculus: Compound stimulus strategies for the explicit task-cuing procedure. *Psychonomic Bulletin and Review, 11,* 832–840.

Logan, G. D., & Etherton, J. L. (1994). What is learned during automatization? The role of attention in constructing and instance. *Journal of Experimental Psychology: Learning, Memory, and Cognition, 20,* 1022–1050.

Logan, G. D., & Gordon, R. D. (2001). Executive control of visual attention in dual-task situations. *Psychological Review, 108,* 393–434.

Logan, G. D., & Schneider, D. W. (2006a). Interpreting instructional cues in task switching procedures: The role of mediator retrieval. *Journal of Experimental Psychology: Learning, Memory, and Cognition, 32,* 347–363.

Logan, G. D., & Schneider, D. W. (2006b). Priming or executive control? Associative priming of cue encoding increases "switch costs" in the explicit task-cuing procedure. *Memory and Cognition, 34,* 1250–1259.

Logan, G. D., Schneider, D. W., & Bundesen, C. (2007). Still clever after all these years: Searching for the homunculus in explicitly-cued task switching. *Journal of Experimental Psychology: Human Perception and Performance, 33,* 978–994.

Luce, R. D. (1959). *Individual choice behavior.* New York: Wiley.

Luce, R. D. (1963). Detection and recognition. In R. D. Luce, R. R. Bush, & E. Galanter (Eds.), *Handbook of mathematical psychology* (pp. 103–189). New York: Wiley.

Mayr, U. (2006). What matters in the cued task-switching paradigm: Tasks or cues? *Psychonomic Bulletin and Review, 13,* 794–799.

Mayr, U., & Kliegl, R. (2003). Differential effects of cue changes and task changes on task-set selection costs. *Journal of Experimental Psychology: Learning, Memory, and Cognition, 29,* 362–372.

Meiran, N. (1996). Reconfiguration of processing mode prior to task performance. *Journal of Experimental Psychology: Learning, Memory, and Cognition, 22,* 1423–1442.

Miller, G. A. (1956). The magical number seven, plus or minus two: Some limits on our capacity for processing information. *Psychological Review, 63,* 81–97.

Miller, G. A., Galanter, E., & Pribram, K. H. (1960). *Plans and the structure of behavior.* New York: Holt, Rinehart and Winston.

Monsell, S. (2003). Task switching. *Trends in Cognitive Sciences, 7,* 134–140.

Monsell, S., & Mizon, G. A. (2006). Can the task-cuing paradigm measure an endogenous task-set reconfiguration process? *Journal of Experimental Psychology: Human Perception and Performance, 32,* 493–516.

Moors, A., & De Houwer, J. (2006). Automaticity: A theoretical and conceptual analysis. *Psychological Bulletin, 132,* 297–326.

Newell, A. (1990). *Unified theories of cognition.* Cambridge, MA: Harvard University Press.

Nosofsky, R. M. (1984). Choice, similarity, and the context theory of classification. *Journal of Experimental Psychology: Learning, Memory, and Cognition, 10,* 104–114.

Nosofsky, R. M. (1988). Exemplar-based accounts of relations between classification, recognition, and typicality. *Journal of Experimental Psychology: Learning, Memory, and Cognition, 14,* 700–708.

Nosofsky, R. M., & Palmeri, T. J. (1997). An exemplar-based random walk model of speeded classification. *Psychological Review, 104,* 266–300.

Palmeri, T. J. (1997). Exemplar similarity and the development of automaticity. *Journal of Experimental Psychology: Learning, Memory, and Cognition, 23,* 324–354.

Posner, M. I., & Snyder, C. R. R. (1975). Attention and cognitive control. In R. L. Solso (Ed.), *Information processing and cognition: The Loyola Symposium* (pp. 55–85). Hillsdale, NJ: Lawrence Erlbaum Associates.

Rickard, T. C. (1997). Bending the power law: A CMPL theory of strategy shifts and the automatization of cognitive skills. *Journal of Experimental Psychology: General, 126,* 288–311.

Rogers, R. D., & Monsell, S. (1995). Costs of a predictable switch between simple cognitive tasks. *Journal of Experimental Psychology: General, 124,* 207–231.

Ross, B. H. (1984). Remindings and their effects in learning a cognitive skill. *Cognitive Psychology, 16,* 371–416.

Schneider, D. W., & Logan, G. D. (2005). Modeling task switching without switching tasks: A short-term priming account of explicitly cued performance. *Journal of Experimental Psychology: General, 134,* 343–367.

Schneider, D. W., & Logan, G. D. (2006). Priming cue encoding by manipulating transition frequency in explicitly cued task switching. *Psychonomic Bulletin and Review, 13,* 145–151.

Schneider, D. W., & Logan, G. D. (2007a). Defining task-set reconfiguration: The case of reference point switching. *Psychonomic Bulletin and Review, 14,* 118–125.

Schneider, D. W., & Logan, G. D. (2007b). Task switching versus cue switching: Using transition cuing to disentangle sequential effects in task-switching performance. *Journal of Experimental Psychology: Learning, Memory, and Cognition, 33,* 370–378.

Schneider, W. (1985). Toward a model of attention and the development of automatic processing. In M. I. Posner & O. S. Marin (Eds.), *Attention and performance XI* (pp. 475–493). Hillsdale, NJ: Lawrence Erlbaum Associates.

Schneider, W., Dumais, S. T., & Shiffrin, R. M. (1984). Automatic and control processing and attention. In R. Parasuraman & D. R. Davies (Eds.), *Varieties of attention* (pp. 1–27). New York: Academic Press.

Shepard, R. N. (1957). Stimulus and response generalization: A stochastic model relating generalization to distance in psychological space. *Psychometrika, 22,* 325–345.

Shiffrin, R. M., & Schneider, W. (1977). Controlled and automatic human information processing: II. Perceptual learning, automatic attending, and a general theory. *Psychological Review, 84,* 127–190.

Simon, H. A. (1980). How big is a chunk? *Science, 183,* 482–488.

Sternberg, S. (1969). The discovery of processing stages: Extensions of Donders' method. In W. G. Koster (Ed.), *Attention and performance II* (pp. 276–315). Amsterdam: North-Holland.

Thomas, J. C. (1974). An analysis of behavior in the hobbits-orcs problem. *Cognitive Psychology, 6,* 257–269.

Waszak, F., Hommel, B., & Allport, A. (2003). Task-switching and long-term priming: Role of episodic stimulus-task bindings in task-shift costs. *Cognitive Psychology, 46,* 361–413.

Automaticity In Situ and in the Lab: The Nature of Habit in Daily Life

David T. Neal *and* Wendy Wood

The marksman sees the bird, and, before he knows it, he
has aimed and shot. A gleam in his adversary's eye, a
momentary pressure from his rapier, and the fencer finds
that he has instantly made the right parry and return.
A glance at the musical hieroglyphics, and the pianist's
fingers have ripped through a cataract of notes.

—*William James* (1890, p. 114)

Abstract

This chapter examines the attributes of habits as they manifest in situ, or naturalistic environments, and
contrasts these attributes with those that have been revealed using laboratory methods. The chapter
is divided into two sections. In the first, key characteristics of habits are reviewed as they emerge in
naturalistic data, such as provided by observational studies and diary-based behavior sampling. These
approaches show that real-world habits tend to be tied to the context cues that were contiguous with
prior performance and implemented relatively independently of people's goals and intentions. In the second
section, the naturalistic profile of everyday habits is contrasted with data generated through laboratory
studies of habit. Drawing on evidence from neuroimaging studies of habit formation, it is suggested that
certain laboratory methods can inflate evidence for the goal-mediated nature of automated responding
by directing participants' conscious attention to what are typically unattended responses. In so doing, lab
procedures may yield evidence of goal mediation that does not hold in real-world, unattended habitual
responding. In contrast, naturalistic designs that use unobtrusive or post hoc assessments avoid this potential
confound because they do not necessarily alter participants' phenomenological orientation toward their
actions. The value of naturalistic methods in the study of action control mechanisms is highlighted.

Keywords: habits, naturalistic data, real-world studies, laboratory studies, diary-based behavior, goals, intentions

As the reactions of the marksman, fencer,
and pianist in James's description attest,
the world around us can serve as a powerful and automatic trigger to behavior. With
sufficient practice, the mere perception of
a contextual cue—a bird in flight, an opponent's rapier, or the notes in a melodic
sequence—can seem spontaneously to provoke the appropriate behavioral response.
Moreover, this cuing of habits is not limited
to those with special skills and talents. All of
us have followed a familiar route to work or

school guided unthinkingly by well-known
landmarks, and we have progressed mindlessly through a morning grooming ritual
while conversing with a partner or family
member.

In this chapter, we evaluate the attributes
of such habits as they manifest in situ, that
is, in the naturalistic settings in which they
spontaneously occur. Our guiding premise
is that naturalistic data can yield unique insights into the kind of automaticity underlying habitual behavior. However, we see

naturalistic data as augmenting, rather than substituting for, laboratory-based experimental paradigms designed to illuminate the basic psychological processes underlying habitual responding (e.g., Bargh & Chartrand, 1999; Hay & Jacoby, 1996; see Chapter 20). Laboratory paradigms provide powerful tools for understanding what *can* happen but provide less definitive information on what spontaneously *does* happen in everyday life. As we explain in this chapter, naturalistic data can provide this important piece of the puzzle and, in doing so, can help refine our understanding of the mechanisms underlying the habits and routines that compose much of daily life.

The chapter is divided into two sections. In the first, we review key characteristics of habits as they emerge in naturalistic data, such as provided by observational studies and diary-based behavior sampling. These approaches reveal a characteristic profile associated with habitual responding in everyday life. Specifically, real-world habits tend to be tied to the context cues that were contiguous with prior performance. Furthermore, naturalistic data show that habit performance can proceed with minimal conscious awareness and without compatible intentions guiding responding. We argue that this profile implies an underlying form of automaticity best described as context cued and non-goal-dependent[1] (Neal, Wood, & Quinn, 2006; Wood & Neal, 2007).

In the second section, we contrast the naturalistic profile of everyday habits with data generated through laboratory studies of habit. Findings from naturalistic and laboratory investigations are generally in agreement that context cues can trigger habit performance and that habit performance requires limited conscious awareness. However, a more complex picture emerges with respect to the role of goals and intentions as mediators of habitual control. Laboratory studies in animal learning, neuroscience, and cognitive psychology support the naturalistic profile in which habits are subserved by a rigid, context-cued automaticity that proceeds with minimal involvement of people's goals and intentions (Dickinson & Balleine, 2002; Hay & Jacoby, 1996; Miller & Cohen, 2001; see Chapter 26). In contrast, some work in social psychology has subsumed habits into the burgeoning literature on automatic goal pursuit (e.g., Aarts & Dijksterhuis, 2000). In this second perspective, habits involve a more flexible, goal-dependent form of automaticity in which contexts prime responses indirectly via the activation of relevant goals or intentions. Instead, habits are most accurately understood within the rigid, non-goal-dependent framing. Nonetheless, we also suggest that habits can interact with goal systems in consequential ways (Wood & Neal, 2007).

To conclude the second section of the chapter, we offer a potential explanation for the fact that some laboratory research indicates habits are rigid and context cued, whereas other laboratory research indicates habits are flexible and goal-dependent. In brief, we draw on evidence from neuroimaging studies of habit formation to suggest that certain laboratory methods can inadvertently inflate evidence for the goal-mediated nature of automated responding by directing participants' conscious attention to what are typically unattended responses. In so doing, lab procedures may yield evidence of goal mediation that does not hold during real-world, unattended habitual responding. In contrast, naturalistic designs that use unobtrusive or post hoc assessments avoid this confound because they do not necessarily alter participants' phenomenological orientation toward their actions. We conclude by highlighting the value of naturalistic methods in the study of action control mechanisms.

Habits In Situ

Naturalistic studies of habit draw from a variety of methods that seek to track people's real-world actions in minimally intrusive ways. These methods include direct observation, event- or signal-contingent sampling, and daily diaries (see Bakeman, 2000; Hektner, Schmidt, & Csikszentmihalyi, 2007). As we explain here, studies using these methods show that the habitual dimension of daily life exhibits distinct attributes within our broader behavioral repertoire. First, habits are linked to features of performance contexts, including places, and other actions, in a relatively rigid, inflexible way. Second, only limited awareness is required for habitual control. Although it might seem obvious that people pay only limited attention to habit performance, at the end of the chapter we explain that the naturalistic evidence on this issue has critical implications for interpreting experimental research on habits in laboratory contexts. Finally, we present real-world data suggesting that habits can be executed relatively independently of people's conscious goals and intentions.

Rigid Context Cuing of Performance

Barker's (1968; see also Barker & Schoggen, 1978) classic work in ecological psychology provided some of the first empirical evidence of the rigid patterns of routine actions tied to physical settings that constitute much of daily life. In these now-famous studies, trained observers directly coded the details of children's daily activities in a small Midwest U.S. town. Analyses of these records revealed a high degree of context stability in daily routines, with two individuals in the same context often exhibiting greater behavioral similarity than the same individual measured across different contexts. Accordingly, as the most proximal ecological unit to account for behavior, Barker (1968) proposed the concept of *behavior setting*, defined as "standing patterns of behavior-and-milieu" (p. 18).

Evidence that everyday responses are tied to context also emerged in our signal-contingent experience-sampling diary investigations. In these studies, college student and community participants recorded once per hour for several days what they were doing, thinking, and feeling (Quinn & Wood, 2005; Wood, Quinn, & Kashy, 2002). About 45% of the behaviors that college students listed in their diaries were deemed habitual insofar as they were consistently performed in a particular physical location almost every day. Although the community sample tended to list slightly different activities that were classified as habits, their overall profile also was one in which almost half of daily activities were repetitive and tied to particular contexts.

Additional evidence of the close link between responses and performance contexts comes from behavior prediction research in which people rated the frequency with which they performed various actions along with the stability of features of the performance context. For example, in Ji and Wood's (2007) investigation, participants who purchased fast food more frequently tended also to purchase it at the same times of day, $r(222) = .19$; participants who watched television news more frequently tended to watch it at the same locations and times of day, $rs(222) = .29$, and .32 for location and time, respectively; and participants who took the bus more frequently tended to catch a ride at the same locations and times, $rs(114) = .45$ and .40 for location and time, respectively. These data suggest that heightened frequency of performance goes hand in hand with heightened context stability, a pattern that is consistent with the context-cued nature of habitual responding.

The high degree of context stability typical of habits does not, of course, establish that those contexts play a causal role in triggering behavior. Causal arguments are difficult to test in natural environments, although suggestive evidence is available from quasi-experiments in which real-world contexts have undergone naturally occurring change. If contexts play a causal role in triggering habitual responses, then such changes should disrupt the performance of associated habits. Illustrating just this effect, Wood, Tam, and Guerrero Witt (2005) tracked disruptions to a number of students' everyday activities as they transferred enrollment from one university to another. Consistent with a causal role for contexts, students' everyday habits tended to be maintained across the transfer only if the performance context at the new university matched that at the old university. For example, students with habits to read the newspaper at the old university continued to do so at the new university only when their roommates' newspaper reading was stable across the transfer (i.e., roommates at both schools either read the paper themselves or did not). In contrast, when the reading context varied between old and new universities (i.e., when their roommates' behavior changed), students' reading habits were significantly less likely to persist at the new university. Moreover, students' intentions to read the paper were not systematically influenced by the context change, suggesting that the behavioral effects cannot be explained by reference to conscious decisions and planning. Instead, it appears that context change undermined the context–response associations underlying reading habits.

In addition to demonstrating the ways that habits can be tied to and triggered by contexts, naturalistic data provide insight into underlying cognitive and motivational processes. We turn now to consider two such process-level attributes of real-world habits: minimal awareness and insensitivity to conscious intentions. These features help to illuminate the specific form of automaticity underlying habitual control.

Conscious Awareness of Performance

The limited conscious awareness typically devoted to habit performance was demonstrated in Wood et al.'s (2002) behavior sampling study discussed in the previous section. Participants in this research recorded not only what they were doing at a particular point in time but also what they were thinking about during behavior performance. Two independent raters then judged whether participants were thinking about the behavior in which they were engaged at each recording period. Thoughts were classified as corresponding to behavior when they involved the specific actions being performed (e.g., when eating, "about how good the bread was") or implicated abstract goals and outcomes that related in some way to the actions being performed (e.g., "how I need to start eating more healthy so I can get back in the shape I was during summer"). In the case of nonhabitual behaviors, participants were thinking about what they were doing for 70% of the reports. For habitual responses, thought–action correspondence was significantly lower, and participants were thinking about what they were doing for only 40% of the reports. Thus, although some habits still attracted conscious thought during performance, such thought was significantly less common than with nonhabitual actions. Thus, consciously attending to one's habits appears to be the exception rather than the norm.

The minimal awareness required for habit performance was evident also in participants' self-report ratings of the attention and thought required to perform each behavior (Wood et al., 2002, Study 2). Compared with more novel, unfamiliar actions or those that did not typically occur in a specific context, habits were rated as requiring less attention and less thought. In addition, respondents rated the difficulty of performing each behavior listed in their diary. These ratings revealed greater ease of performing for habitual than nonhabitual actions. Thus, behaviors that people repeat in the same location almost every day possess a number of the attributes classically associated with automaticity (see Moors & De Houwer, 2006). They attract a relatively low level of thought and awareness and are experienced as easy to perform. Although perhaps not especially surprising in itself, this evidence of limited awareness of habit performance may, as we explain at the end of the chapter, be critical when interpreting the attributes of habits that have emerged in laboratory settings.

Response-Related Goals and Intentions

Naturalistic data also suggest that habit performance can proceed independently from people's current intentions. This is a significant finding because many prominent theories of behavioral control are predicated on the idea that intentions are key determinants of behavior (e.g., Ajzen & Fishbein, 2005; Austin & Vancouver, 1996; Gollwitzer & Moskowitz, 1996).

Before reviewing data on the role of intentions in habit performance, we note that real-world habits typically are *not* in conflict with intentions. This makes sense given that people's daily habits plausibly originate in purposive decision making and goal pursuit (e.g., a habit for reading a certain newspaper is likely the result of what was once a conscious, deliberative decision). Put differently, assuming that people usually repeat behaviors that serve desired outcomes, habits are likely to develop in line with intentions. Accordingly, in a meta-analytic estimate across 33 separate studies, measures of habit strength were positively correlated with the strength of intentions, $r = .43$ ($p < .01$; Ouellette & Wood, 1998). Thus, if rep-

etition initially was intentional and if intentions remained stable over time, then habit strength would correlate with intentions even when actions were repeated sufficiently to become cued by context, and hence triggered without recourse to intentions. As we discussed in detail elsewhere, a significant correlation between intentions and habit strength therefore does not, by itself, indicate that intentions are driving behavior (Wood & Neal, 2007). With respect to habits, the intention-behavior relationship is likely an epiphenomenon reflecting the fact that the habitual behavior was once an intention-driven response and thus remains consistent with intentions.[2]

Notwithstanding the overall positive relation between habits and intentions, it is obvious that habits do not always correspond with intentions. So-called bad habits reflect behaviors that are consistently out of line with what people wish they were doing. In addition, divergence between habits and intentions sometimes occurs in the form of accidental slips in everyday life. In an early example of such action slips, James (1890; see also Heckhausen & Beckmann, 1990) describes an absentminded man who enters his bedroom to change a tie for dinner and ends up getting undressed and getting into bed. While intending to change his tie, the subject of the story encountered context cues associated with a well-established habit of going to bed, and these cues co-opted or captured the stream of action in a manner that ran counter to his intentions. Using an event-sampling diary method, Reason (1990) found that such *habit capture errors* are relatively common in daily life and tend to occur when components of the intended action overlap with the habit that co-opts it (e.g., intending but failing to stop at the store on the usual drive home; see Chapters 5, 8, and 20). Thus, bad habits and action slips are exceptions to the overall tendency for habits to correspond with intentions.

Systematic evidence that well-practiced actions can be cued independently of intentions in daily life is provided in behavior prediction research. For example, Ji and Wood (2007) predicted how often college students would perform a number of everyday actions (e.g., purchase fast food) from students' earlier-reported intentions and strength of their habits (reflected in frequency of past performance and stability of performance contexts). Indicating that habitual behaviors are not guided by intentions, during the week of the study, students with stronger habits repeated their past behavior regardless of their reported intentions. Only for students with weaker habits did intentions guide actions. These findings echo those from a number of other behavior prediction studies indicating that real-world habits tend to be performed even when not aligned with current intentions and goals (e.g., Aldrich, Montgomery, & Wood, 2008; Danner, Aarts, & de Vries, 2008; Ferguson & Bibby, 2002; Ouellette & Wood, 1998; Verplanken, Aarts, van Knippenberg, & Moonen, 1998). It appears that when people have repeated actions frequently in stable contexts, context cues can activate the practiced response independently of what people intend to do. Note that these findings do not suggest that people are unable to override habitual response tendencies. When they have sufficient amounts of self-control available (Neal, Pascoe, & Wood, 2008a) and when they are using appropriate self-control strategies (Quinn, Pascoe, & Wood, 2008), people can inhibit the tendency to perform many everyday habits. However, behavior prediction research indicates that the typical pattern in everyday contexts is for people to fail to override habits that do not align with intentions.

That people perform habits in the apparent absence of a supporting intention might seem at odds with another form of real-world context-cued automaticity—implementation intentions—in which people form plans to implement a given response when they encounter a specific context (e.g., "when X occurs, I'll do Y"; Gollwitzer & Sheeran, 2006; see Chapter 29). Naturalistic data suggest that implementation intentions automate future context-cued responding and thereby increase the likelihood that people act on the relevant intentions. However, this form of automaticity differs from habits in that it depends on continued explicit endorsement of a relevant goal. Illustrating this dependence, Sheeran, Webb, and Gollwitzer (2005, study 1) had students form implementation intentions regarding the time and place at which they would study over the following week (versus control participants who did not). Participants forming these plans spent significantly more time studying only if they had a moderate or strong goal to study. Thus, although they share features of automatic cuing with habits, implementation intentions are distinct in depending on the strength of people's underlying goals and intentions.

In summary, naturalistic data arising from observational and behavior-sampling techniques suggest that real-world habitual responses are relatively rigidly tied to specific contextual cues, are implemented with limited conscious awareness, and proceed in a manner that does not depend on the presence of a supporting goal or intention. The specific pattern of habitual responses in real-world data can be distinguished from other forms of context-driven automaticity, such as implementation intentions that do require the presence of response-consistent goals or intentions. In the second half of the chapter, we contrast habits as they emerge in situ with the forms in which they appear in laboratory experiments.

Habits in the Laboratory and In Situ

Laboratory and naturalistic data converge on several points concerning the attributes of habitual automaticity. As we explain, data from the lab and from everyday life agree that habits tend to be triggered by contexts, including places, other people, and preceding actions, with only minimal conscious awareness. However, it is less clear whether the evidence of habits in the lab aligns with naturalistic data demonstrating that habits are not flexibly moderated by conflicting intentions and goals. Laboratory studies have promoted two relatively distinct views of the role of goals in habit performance (see Wood & Neal, 2007). The first perspective, associated predominantly with work in neuroscience, animal learning, and cognitive psychology, frames habits as inflexible response dispositions that are triggered directly by stimuli and thus make minimal recourse to people's goals and intentions. The second view, associated predominantly with recent work in social psychology, frames habits as a more dynamic, goal-dependent form of automaticity. After outlining these two perspectives, we propose that naturalistic habit data provide reason to favor the non-goal-dependent definition of habits. Moreover, we provide a methodological explanation for why some laboratory paradigms could produce evidence seeming to indicate that habits are dynamic and dependent on goals.

Points of Convergence: Context Cuing and Minimal Conscious Awareness

Two features of habits—context cuing and minimal conscious awareness—emerge in generally consistent ways across the full spectrum of naturalistic and laboratory paradigms. In a typical laboratory study, the context-cued nature of habitual responding might be established by having participants generate a response immediately after exposure to some context feature (e.g., a word or picture that connotes the context) that has historically covaried with that response. Con-

text cuing of the response habit is evident if response speed or accuracy is facilitated by prior exposure to the context feature (as opposed to a no-exposure control condition). The underlying logic follows our definition of habits: Responses and contexts that have historically co-occurred will become associated in memory so that activation of the context can automatically facilitate the linked response. In these studies, context features take myriad forms, including abstract experimental stimuli (e.g., auditory tones; Rah, Reber, & Hsiao, 2000; tarot cards, Neal, Pascoe, & Wood, 2008b), physical settings (e.g., a shopping mall or university; Aarts & Dijksterhuis, 2000; a sports stadium, Neal, Lally, & Wood, 2008), and prior responses in a learned sequence (see Graybiel, 1998). In each case, exposure to the habit-relevant context cue has been shown to facilitate performance of the linked response.

The second attribute of real-world habits, limited awareness, also emerges reliably in laboratory settings. This attenuated awareness is found with respect to various features of the habitual response: A person may lack awareness of the context cue that triggered performance, awareness of the response itself, or awareness of the causal relationship between the context and response (or, conceivably, any combination of these features). Whereas naturalistic paradigms have limited power to tap these subtle process-level distinctions, laboratory studies have provided fine-grained tests of people's awareness of each feature. For example, masked priming studies have shown that visual cues (e.g., everyday objects such as a key or a mallet) can prime previously associated behavioral responses (i.e., a precision grasp for a key or a power grasp for a mallet) even when presented under conditions that preclude conscious awareness of the cue during response selection and execution (e.g., Tucker & Ellis, 2004). Other studies have shown that elements of the response implementation itself also attract reduced awareness once the response has been rendered habitual. In particular, this pattern is evident in the fact that attention-demanding secondary tasks impair non-habit based responding while leaving habitual control intact (e.g., Foerde, Knowlton, & Poldrack, 2006). Neuroimaging studies of skill acquisition support a similar conclusion by showing that attention-related brain structures (e.g., dorsolateral prefrontal cortex) exhibit reduced activity during the execution of habitual compared with nonhabitual responses (e.g., Floyer-Lea & Matthews, 2004).

With respect to awareness of the causal connection between context and response, implicit learning studies have established that it is possible to attend consciously both to a cue and a response and yet to be unaware (a) that there is a pattern of historical covariation between the two and (b) that this pattern is facilitating responding (e.g., Lewicki, Hill, & Bizot, 1988; Rah et al., 2000). In illustration, Rah et al.'s (2000) participants completed a visual serial reaction time task while simultaneously performing a second, auditory tone-counting task. Participants were informed that the two tasks were unrelated. However, in reality, the visual stimuli were predicted probabilistically by the preceding auditory tone. After repeated exposure to the context–response pairings, participants showed faster reaction times in probe trials if the visual stimuli were presented after auditory cues with which they historically covaried. Thus, participants were consciously aware of the triggering cue (the auditory tone) and were consciously aware of the response (the button press), but they were unaware of the specific patterns of context–response covariation. Despite lacking this awareness, participants gave responses that were facilitated by the covariation information.

The attributes of context cuing and minimal conscious awareness that emerge in naturalistic studies of habit thus are largely mirrored in studies in the laboratory. Just as with habits in situ, laboratory-generated habits can be triggered by historically co-varying context cues in a manner that by-passes conscious awareness. Furthermore, the control inherent in lab procedures has enabled researchers to identify the extent to which people are aware of each component of habitual responding (i.e., consciousness of context cues, responses, and the covariation of cues and responses).

A Point of Divergence: Do Habits Depend on Goals and Intentions?

The naturalistic behavior sampling data and the behavior prediction work presented at the beginning of this chapter suggest that habits emerge in the form of narrowly defined context–response mappings that are implemented in a manner that is not dependent on a supporting goal or intention. This pattern was evident in the close association between habits and the contexts in which they have historically occurred and in the failure of habits to be moderated by the favorability of intentions. Anecdotal observation suggests that real-world habits often exhibit additional features suggesting they are insensitive to current goals and intentions. First, people rarely substitute habitual behaviors (e.g., a habit of daily jogging) for alternative behaviors that meet the same ostensible goal (e.g., switching from jogging to cycling). Second, real-world habit performance often persists even when the value or relevance of the ostensible goal has changed or dissipated (e.g., when one has successfully lost the 15 pounds that initially inspired the daily running). Thus, both naturalistic data and anecdotal experience suggest that real-world habits proceed in a manner that is relatively rigid and not dynamically sensitive to people's current goals and intentions.

Unlike the two attributes discussed in the previous section (context cuing and reduced awareness), laboratory data provide mixed conclusions regarding the role of goals and intentions within habitual responding. As we explain here, some laboratory paradigms provide an image of habits as context-cued responses that proceed even in the absence of facilitating intentions and goals. However, other laboratory paradigms suggest that habits reflect a more dynamic goal-dependent form of automaticity.

LABORATORY DATA SUGGESTING THAT HABITS ARE RIGID AND CONTEXT CUED

Three laboratory-based approaches have played especially prominent roles in advancing the view that habits are subserved by rigid, context-cued automaticity. These approaches encompass (a) neuroimaging studies of behavioral automation (see Kelly & Garavan, 2005), (b) animal learning studies of reinforcer devaluation effects (see Dickinson & Balleine, 2002), and (c) cognitive studies of habit control (e.g., Neal et al., 2008b; Neal, Lally, & Wood, 2008). The first line of evidence that habits are context cued and not mediated by people's current goals comes from neuroimaging studies that have tracked the role of goal-related brain systems over the course of habit development. In a typical laboratory study in this area, the neural correlates of task performance are monitored as participants repeat a motor task until it becomes habitual according to some behavioral criterion (e.g., absence of dual task interference effects). The neural patterns that emerge in such studies typically reveal that habit formation is associated with a significant redistribution of brain activity (see reviews in Jonides, 2004; Kelly & Garavan, 2005). Importantly, this redistribution characteristically features reduced activation of the prefrontal cortex (PFC; Floyer-Lea & Matthews, 2004; Raichle et al., 1994; Sakai et al., 1998). Given

that the PFC is considered critical to the selection and pursuit of goals (Miller & Cohen, 2001), the relative quiescence of this system during habit performance suggests that goals play a limited role in habit performance.

Neuroimaging studies also have provided evidence of the relative rigidity of habitual control (see Foerde et al., 2006; Reber, Knowlton, & Squire, 1996). For example, Foerde et al.'s (2006) participants practiced a probabilistic learning task under conditions that encouraged reliance on either declarative or procedural (i.e., habit) memory. Specifically, they learned to predict two weather outcomes (rain or shine) via probabilistically associated visual cues under either single-task conditions or dual-task conditions (encouraging use of declarative or procedural/habit-based memory respectively). Imaging data confirmed that these variations in learning conditions determined whether participants relied predominantly on declarative memory (i.e., medial temporal lobe) or procedural/habit memory (i.e., striatum). Participants in the declarative and procedural learning conditions acquired similar levels of proficiency at the task, but those encouraged to use procedural, habit-based memory performed significantly worse in a post test of their ability to apply their skill flexibly in a new context (see also Reber et al., 1996). Thus, consistent with naturalistic research on habits, neuroimaging studies suggest that habits rely on a relatively inflexible form of automaticity that involves associations between specific responses and context cues and is not dynamically responsive to current goals or novel contexts.

A second source of laboratory evidence comes from animal learning studies addressing the changing impact of goals as responses are practiced into habits (see Dickinson & Balleine, 2002). These studies, conducted primarily with rats, suggest that habitual responses are relatively insensitive to variations in the value of the reward-related outcomes of the responses, whereas nonhabitual responses vary dynamically with such variations. This *reinforcer devaluation insensitivity* phenomenon was established using a paradigm in which rats first underwent moderate training (e.g., 120 trials) or extended, habit training (e.g., 360 trials) in which they received reinforcement (e.g., food pellets) for performing a simple action (e.g., lever pressing). The outcome (e.g., food acquisition) was then devalued by overfeeding the rats or by pairing the food with a toxin. Such reinforcer devaluation depressed animals' subsequent performance of minimally trained responses but had little effect on habits (e.g., Balleine & Dickinson, 1998; Yin, Knowlton, & Balleine, 2004). This pattern typically is interpreted as evidence that habits involve behavioral control that has become autonomous from the specific goals and outcomes that initially motivated the response.

The third line of laboratory evidence for the non-goal-dependent view comes from behavioral studies of human habits. For example, we recently tested the effects of goal priming on habit-based automaticity through a study in which we adapted the weather prediction paradigm outlined above that is commonly used by cognitive neuroscientists studying procedural/habit based memory (Neal et al., 2008b). After learning to predict the weather using a method that fostered reliance on either declarative or procedural/habit-based memory, participants were primed with an achievement goal or no goal via a scrambled-sentence task. Activation of the achievement goal improved performance of those relying on declarative memory. However, achievement priming actually significantly impaired performance of those using habit-based procedural memory. We replicated this effect in a second study using an explicit goal priming technique (i.e., offering a cash bonus tied

to performance). These results suggest that, contrary to the pattern typically associated with goal-dependent responses, goal priming does not facilitate, and can actually impair, habit-based automaticity.

Providing further evidence that habits are not dependent on goals, in another line of work, we have focused specifically on the link between context cues and habitual responses (Neal, Lally, & Wood, 2008). The aim of the study was to test whether contexts exert their effects on habitual behaviors directly or whether they work indirectly by activating goals that then drive behavior. To address this, we used an experimental paradigm to test whether a simple behavioral response (habitual speech intensity in a given context) can be triggered by relevant contexts without changes in relevant goals. Participants were exposed to one of two contexts (*sports stadiums* or *kitchens*) as part of a "visual acuity test" similar to the *Where's Waldo* children's books. We reasoned that those who frequently attend sports stadiums may have acquired a habitual tendency to speak loudly in that environment. To assess the effect of context on goals, participants rated their desire to be represented to other participants by a loud versus quiet confederate (a pilot test confirmed that participants with the goal of speaking loudly preferred being represented by the loud confederate). Consistent with predictions, exposure to sports stadiums led to a significant increase in speech intensity, but only for participants who had a frequent and consistent behavioral history of visiting sports stadiums over the prior six months. Furthermore, path analyses confirmed that the effects of context on speech habits were not mediated by changes in participants' goals related to speech intensity (i.e., their desire to be represented by the loud confederate). Thus, these data support the view that contexts can trigger directly associated habits (in this case, simple speech intensity) without the mediating involvement of goals.

In summary, these three lines of laboratory-generated data present a relatively coherent case for the non-goal-dependent nature of habit-based automaticity. Despite varying paradigms that span multiple levels of analysis (neural, cognitive, and behavioral) and populations (human and nonhuman), habits emerge consistently as context-cued responses that are executed with minimal recourse to the goals and intentions that may initially have propelled responding. This pattern is evident in habits' reduced reliance on brain areas associated with goal pursuit, their persistence despite variations in goal relevant outcomes, and their failure to be facilitated by goal priming techniques that are known to facilitate goal-dependent responses.

LABORATORY DATA SUGGESTING THAT HABITS ARE DYNAMICALLY DEPENDENT ON GOALS

The rigid, context-cued profile outlined in the prior sections of this chapter stands in contrast with an alternative set of laboratory data in social psychology indicating that habits are a form of automatic goal pursuit. As the burgeoning literature on automatic goal pursuit has shown, goal-mediated forms of automaticity can be distinguished from more direct, context-cued automaticity along a number of dimensions (see Chartrand, Dalton, & Cheng, 2008; Moors & De Houwer, 2006). Particularly relevant for current purposes, automatic goal pursuit appears to be fluidly dependent on currently active goals (e.g., Bargh, Chen, & Burrows, 1996; Macrae & Johnston, 1998). That is, the intensity (e.g., persistence, speed, accuracy) of automatic goal pursuit appears to vary dynamically as a function of a person's currently active goal states. We have argued that habit automaticity lacks this attribute because it is implemented independently of goal states (see Neal et al., 2006; Wood & Neal, 2007).

A number of laboratory-based studies, however, have yielded data suggesting habits

possess this dynamic, goal-dependent feature (e.g., Aarts & Dijksterhuis, 2000; Sheeran, Aarts, Custers, Rivis, Webb et al., 2005). Aarts and Dijksterhuis (2000) conducted an ingenious series of studies exploring the impact of activating various travel goals (e.g., shopping at the city center mall) on the mental accessibility of people's habitual modes of travel to those destinations (e.g., bicycle, car). Specifically, participants judged as quickly as possible whether a given travel mode (e.g., bicycle) was a realistic means for getting to a previously presented location (e.g., Heuvelgalerie, a popular mall in the Netherlands city of Eindhoven). These judgments were made faster if (a) the relevant travel goal had been activated in an earlier task and (b) the bicycle was a habitual means for the participant to get to the location. The researchers interpreted this pattern as evidence that the activation of habitual associations in memory is dependent on goal activation and hence that habits are a form of automatic goal pursuit. An analogous pattern of results was reported by Sheeran, Aarts et al. (2005), who found that priming an alcohol consumption–related goal (socializing) made habitual drinkers but not nonhabitual drinkers respond more quickly to drinking-related action words and increase their likelihood of accepting a voucher for free drinks.

The pioneering laboratory studies of Aarts and Dijksterhuis (2000) and Sheeran, Aarts et al. (2005) appear to support the view that habits represent a goal-dependent form of automaticity. Although these studies offer a compelling demonstration of how goals can affect conscious, reflective decision making and behavior, in our view, their findings do not generalize to real-world habits. First, as we outlined in the first half of this chapter, naturalistic data suggest that habits are executed in a manner that pays little heed to people's currently active goals and intentions (e.g., Ji & Wood, 2007; Wood et al., 2005). Second, subsuming habits into the automatic goal pursuit literature would run counter to the many laboratory studies in neuroscience, animal learning, and cognitive psychology that support the non-goal-dependent nature of habitual control (e.g., Dickinson & Balleine, 2002; Miller & Cohen, 2001). Third, as we elaborate here, at least some laboratory paradigms used to study the role of goals within habitual responding include methodological elements that may invoke goal-dependent control over responses that would otherwise be non-goal-dependent.

Divergence Explained? Attention to Action in the Lab

Why have some laboratory paradigms indicated that habits reflect a dynamic, goal-dependent form of automaticity whereas others indicate that habits are rigid and non-goal-dependent? We speculate that this divergence can be explained in part by a methodological feature concerning the level of conscious attention that participants are asked to devote to task elements. We based this suggestion on recent neuroimaging studies demonstrating that attention to action moderates whether or not goal-related brain systems are active during the performance of habitual responses (e.g., PFC; Jueptner et al., 1997; Rowe, Friston, Frackowiak, & Passingham, 2002). If some laboratory procedures require participants to devote greater conscious awareness to their habitual responses than is typical in naturalistic settings, then this heightened awareness may induce goal-oriented control over what are typically not goal-dependent responses. In such paradigms, non-goal-dependent habits may appear to be dependent on goals.

The neuroimaging studies relevant to this potential confound have first isolated the neural correlates of normal habit acquisition and then examined changes to these neural correlates when participants were forced to direct conscious attention to their habitual responses during performance. For example, in Jueptner et al.'s (1997) study, positron emission tomography (PET) scans were taken as participants learned and then performed a habitual sequence of complex finger movements. As we mentioned in the prior section of the chapter, the established effect in the literature is that goal-related brain systems (i.e., the PFC) that were engaged while participants were first learning the task subsequently disengaged after the behavior became well learned and was executed habitually. Jueptner et al. (1997) replicated this basic effect. However, their study included an additional condition in which participants at the end of learning were asked to direct conscious attention to the performance of the habitual sequence. Specifically, they "were asked to 'think of the next movement' once they finished the previous one" (p. 1314). In this condition, the PET data showed that participants re-engaged PFC activation in a manner similar to initial learning. Thus, when consciously attending to the performance of their habitual response, brain activity consistent with goal-mediated control emerged despite this activity being absent when the response was performed without attention. These findings, along with comparable ones by Rowe et al. (2002), suggest that a habitual response that is otherwise executed with minimal attention and without recourse to goal-mediated control can appear to be goal mediated if tested under conditions in which the response is subject to conscious attention.

We believe that Jueptner et al.'s (1997) and Rowe et al.'s (2002) findings offer a potential explanation for the conflicting laboratory evidence regarding the role of goals within habitual responding. Their studies suggest that procedural manipulations that heighten conscious attention to action can lead to the recruitment of goal systems during a habitual response that would otherwise be executed without the involvement of those systems. As Wood et al.'s (2002) naturalistic data suggest, during habit performance, people's conscious thoughts are often directed to something other than their actions. In contrast, paradigms like those used by Aarts and Dijksterhuis (2000) and Sheeran, Aarts et al. (2005) appear to require that participants attend to their habitual responses by, for example, judging whether the response is an appropriate means to some end. Such instructions presumably increased participants' conscious attention to their responses during testing, and the Jueptner et al.'s (1997) neuroimaging data suggest that this heightened attention could have artificially promoted goal-oriented control, thus generating the appearance that habits depend on goals.

To test more directly whether conscious attention can heighten goal-oriented control, Neal, Lally, and Wood (2008) tested the role of goals in habitual responding using two different paradigms. The study recruited habitual and non-habitual runners and tested associations between running and the idiosyncratic goals (e.g., "fitness") and contexts (e.g., "gym") that participants had previously reported as being linked to their running. One paradigm used a subliminal priming method that prevented participants from consciously attending to the associations being measured. In contrast, the second paradigm explicitly required participants to attend to these associations in a manner similar to Aarts and Dijksterhuis' (2000) participants. The non-conscious task demonstrated context-priming effects but no goal-priming effects, such that habitual runners responded faster to the word "run" when primed with relevant contexts but not when primed with relevant goals. On the conscious, explicit judgment task however, significant goal priming effects were found. These data support the idea that experimental methods that require participants to attend consciously to habitual responses can yield evidence for goal-dependant operation despite that such

evidence is absent when using techniques that allow for unattended responding.

If attention to action is in fact a potential confound in studies assessing the role of goals in habitual responding (or other automatic responses), then it is important for researchers to select methods that do not heighten conscious attention to levels that deviate from the relevant real-world context to which generalization is sought. Control participants in Jueptner et al.'s (1997) research who were simply asked to perform a habit in the PET scanner without altered attention did not recruit goal-related brain systems during response execution. Also, neuroimaging studies demonstrating the decreased involvement of goal-related brain systems in habit development typically require that participants simply perform their responses in the magnet without any instructions about conscious monitoring (Floyer-Lea & Matthews, 2004; Sakai et al., 1998). Other studies limit conscious monitoring by, for example, having participants engage in an attention-demanding secondary task during habit formation (e.g., Foerde et al., 2006) or by using techniques such as subliminal priming (see Bargh & Chartrand, 2000). Additionally, to avoid artificially directing attention to habitual responses, naturalistic paradigms collect data retrospectively rather than concurrently with the response under examination. For example, in behavior-sampling studies, participants reported on the attention required by habit performance at the end of the day or when cued randomly by a beeper (e.g., Wood et al., 2002). By this strategy, naturalistic paradigms can avoid directing participants to attend to responding during performance and thus avoided inadvertently engaging goal-directed control over that responding.[3]

In summary, in light of the potentially confounding role of attention to action in some previous laboratory studies, we believe that the weight of current evidence supports the non-goal-dependent, context-cued definition of habitual control. This view is supported by naturalistic studies showing that habits are tied to narrowly defined contexts and implemented without compatible intentions and also by laboratory data showing that habits involve reduced reliance on goal-related brain systems and proceed despite changes in goal-related outcomes.

Summary and Implications for the Nature of Habitual Control

We have argued that naturalistic data can provide valuable insights into the nature of habits that augments knowledge emerging from more controlled paradigms in the laboratory. We highlighted the many points of convergence between naturalistic and laboratory-based studies of habit. In particular, both approaches show that features of a person's context (e.g., people, places, preceding actions) can be powerful, automatic triggers of habit performance, and that habits are executed with minimal recourse to conscious awareness.

There is less agreement with respect to the role that people's goals and intentions play in determining habit performance. Although some forms of real-world automaticity (e.g., implementation intentions) are sensitive to people's current goal states, established habits in naturalistic settings appear to be context cued and do not depend on goals and intentions. This naturalistic profile is consistent with laboratory data generated in neuroscience, animal learning, and some cognitive paradigms. However, it conflicts with some recent social psychological laboratory data indicating that habits are a form of goal-dependent automaticity. In resolution of this inconsistency, we argued that some laboratory procedures used in social psychological lab studies may inadvertently inflate evidence for the role of goals by increasing participants' conscious attention to their action. When attention

is not artificially directed toward habit performance, habits emerge as a form of non-goal-dependent automaticity involving relatively direct, rigid associations between context features and responses.

On a broader level, we hope that this discussion highlights the value of using naturalistic methods to study basic mechanisms of action control. Perhaps most important, naturalistic methods allow researchers to subject laboratory-generated models to the crucible of the real world and thereby identify patterns of convergence and divergence across the two domains. As we have tried to show here, naturalistic data also can play a role in arbitrating between competing models emerging from the laboratory and, in doing so, can refine our understanding of basic mechanisms and processes.

Notes

1. We use the term *context cued* in a manner similar to Moors and De Houwer's (2006) notion of stimulus-driven responding. That is, a context-cued response relies on direct cognitive associations between stimuli, in the form of context cues (e.g., people, places, and preceding actions), and responses. This form of automaticity can be distinguished from automatic goal pursuit, which is mediated through implicit or nonconscious goals. We have speculated elsewhere that these direct, context-cued responses, although not goal mediated, may sometimes exhibit motivational properties in the form of diffuse reward value that is not oriented toward acquiring a specific outcome (Neal, Wood, & Quinn, 2006; Wood & Neal, 2007). In this chapter, we do not address the distinction between motivated and nonmotivated context-cued responses, but, in principle, the attributes of habitual control we discuss here, should be equally applicable to both subtypes of context-cued responding.

2. We note there are additional processes that may plausibly result in intentions predicting habit performance in an epiphenomenal, or non-causal, manner. One candidate is post hoc inferences (see Bem, 1972). People might infer their intentions from their past behavior, reasoning that "I did it in the past, I must intend do it in the future." Following Bem's (1972) self-perception theory, people are especially likely to follow this reasoning process and to use behavior to infer internal states when internal dispositions are weak, ambiguous, or uninterpretable. We speculate that habits are especially suited to such inferences because people have only limited access to the associative mechanisms guiding such action. Thus, there are several factors that can explain why intentions sometimes predict, but do not actually drive, habitual behavior (see also, Wood & Neal, 2007).

3. Of course, such self-report procedures come with their own limitations; in particular, participants need to be willing and able to report on the features of automaticity under investigation.

References

Aarts, H., & Dijksterhuis, A. (2000). Habits as knowledge structures: Automaticity in goal-directed behavior. *Journal of Personality and Social Psychology, 78,* 53–63.

Ajzen, I., & Fishbein, M. (2005). The influence of attitudes on behavior. In D. Albarracín, B. T. Johnson, & M. P. Zanna (Eds.), *The handbook of attitudes* (pp. 173–221). Mahwah, NJ: Lawrence Erlbaum Associates.

Aldrich, J. A., Montgomery, J., & Wood, W. (2008). *Turn out as a habit.* Manuscript under review.

Austin, J. J., & Vancouver, J. B. (1996). Goal constructs in psychology: Structure, process, and content. *Psychological Bulletin, 120,* 338–375.

Bakeman, R. (2000). Behavioral observation and coding. In H. T. Reis & C. M. Judd (Eds.), *Handbook of research methods in social and personality psychology* (pp. 138–159). Cambridge: Cambridge University Press.

Balleine, B. W., & Dickinson, A. (1998). Goal-directed instrumental action: Contingency and incentive learning and their cortical substrates. *Neuropharmacology, 37,* 407–419.

Bargh, J. A., & Chartrand, T. L. (1999). The unbearable automaticity of being. *American Psychologist, 54,* 462–479.

Bargh, J. A., & Chartrand, T. L. (2000). The mind in the middle: A practical guide to priming and automaticity research. In H. T. Reis & C. M. Judd (Eds.), *Handbook of research methods in social and personality psychology* (pp. 253–285). New York: Cambridge University Press.

Bargh, J. A., Chen, M., & Burrows, L. (1996). Automaticity of social behavior: Direct effects of trait construct and stereotype activation on action. *Journal of Personality and Social Psychology, 71,* 230–244.

Barker, R. G. (1968). *Ecological psychology.* Stanford, CA: Stanford University Press.

Barker, R. G., & Schoggen, P. (1978). Measures of habitat and behavior output. In R. G. Barker & et al. (Eds.), *Habitats, environments, and human behavior: Studies in ecological psychology and ecobehavioral science from the Midwest Psychological Field Station, 1947–1972* (pp. 229–244). San Francisco: Jossey-Bass.

Bem, D. J. (1972). Self-perception theory. In L. Berkowitz (Ed.), *Advances in experimental social psychology* (Vol. 6, pp. 1–62). San Diego, CA: Academic Press.

Chartrand, T. L., Dalton, A., & Cheng, C. M. (2008). The antecedents and consequences of nonconscious goal pursuit. In J. Shah & W. Gardner (Eds.), *Handbook of motivation science* (pp. 342–355). New York: Guilford Press.

Danner, U. N., Aarts, H., & de Vries, N. K. (2008). Habit vs. intention in the prediction of future behaviour: The role of frequency, context stability and mental accessibility of past behaviour. *British Journal of Social Psychology, 47,* 245–265.

Dickinson, A., & Balleine, B. (2002). The role of learning in the operation of motivational systems. In H. Pashler & R. Gallistel (Eds.), *Stevens' handbook of experimental psychology: Learning, motivation, and emotion* (Vol. 3, 3rd ed., pp. 497–533). New York: Wiley.

Ferguson, E., & Bibby, P. A. (2002). Predicting future blood donor returns: Past behavior, intentions, and observer effects. *Health Psychology, 21,* 513–518.

Floyer-Lea, A., & Matthews, P. M. (2004). Changing brain networks for visuomotor control with increased movement automaticity. *Journal of Neurophysiology, 92,* 2405–2412.

Foerde, K., Knowlton, B. J., & Poldrack, R. A. (2006). Modulation of competing memory systems by distraction. *Proceedings of the National Academy of Sciences of the United States of America, 103,* 11778–11783.

Gollwitzer, P. M., & Moskowitz, G. B. (1996). Goal effects on action and cognition. In E. T. Higgins & A. W. Kruglanski (Eds.), *Social psychology: Handbook of basic principles* (pp. 361–399). New York: Guilford Press.

Gollwitzer, P. M., & Sheeran, P. (2006). Implementation intentions and goal achievement: A meta-analysis of effects and processes. *Advances in Experimental Social Psychology, 38,* 69–120.

Graybiel, A. M. (1998). The basal ganglia and chunking of action repertoires. *Neurobiology of Learning and Memory, 70,* 119–136.

Hay, J. F., & Jacoby, L. L. (1996). Separating habit and recollection: Memory slips, process dissociations, and probability matching. *Journal of Experimental Psychology: Learning, Memory, and Cognition, 22,* 1323–1335.

Heckhausen, H., & Beckmann, J. (1990). Intentional action and action slips. *Psychological Review, 97,* 36–48.

Hektner, J. M., Schmidt, J. A., & Csikszentmihalyi, M. (2007). *Experience sampling method: Measuring the quality of everyday life.* Thousand Oaks, CA: Sage.

James, W. J. (1890). *The principles of psychology.* New York: Dover.

Ji, M., & Wood, W. (2007). Habitual purchase and consumption: Not always what you intend. *Journal of Consumer Psychology 17,* 261–276.

Jonides, J. (2004). How does practice makes perfect? *Nature Neuroscience, 7,* 75–79.

Jueptner, M., Stephan, K. M., Frith, C. D., Brooks, D. J., Frackowiak, R. S., & Passingham, R. E. (1997). Anatomy of motor learning I: Frontal cortex and attention to action. *Journal of Neurophysiology, 77,* 1313–1324.

Kelly, A. M. C., & Garavan, H. (2005). Human functional neuroimaging of brain changes associated with practice. *Cerebral Cortex, 15,* 1089–1102.

Lewicki, P., Hill, T., & Bizot, E. (1988). Acquisition of procedural knowledge about a pattern of stimuli that cannot be articulated. *Cognitive Psychology, 20,* 24–37.

Macrae, C. N., & Johnston, L. (1998). Help, I need somebody: Automatic action and inaction. *Social Cognition, 16,* 400–417.

Miller, E. K., & Cohen J. D. (2001). An integrative theory of prefrontal cortex function. *Annual Review of Neuroscience, 2,* 167–202.

Moors, A., & De Houwer, J. (2006). Automaticity: A theoretical and conceptual analysis. *Psychological Bulletin, 132,* 297–326.

Neal, D. T., Lally, P., & Wood, W. (2008). *Power of context: Habits do not depend on goals.* Manuscript under review.

Neal, D. T., Pascoe, A. T., & Wood, W. (2008a). *Self control strength and habit performance: Boon and bane of goal pursuit.* Unpublished manuscript, Duke University, Durham, NC.

Neal, D. T., Pascoe, A., & Wood, W. (2008b). *Effects of goal enhancement on habit-based responding.* Manuscript under review.

Neal, D. T., Wood, W., & Quinn, J. M. (2006): Habits: A repeat performance. *Current Directions in Psychological Science, 15,* 198–202.

Ouellette, J. A., & Wood, W. (1998). Habit and intention in everyday life: The multiple processes by which past behavior predicts future behavior. *Psychological Bulletin, 124,* 54–74.

Quinn, J. M., & Wood, W. (2005). *Habits across the lifespan.* Unpublished manuscript, Duke University, Durham, NC.

Quinn, J. M., Pascoe, A. M., & Wood, W. (2008). *Strategies of self-control: Habits are not tempting.* Manuscript under editorial review.

Rah, S. K. Y., Reber, A. S., & Hsiao, A. T. (2000). Another wrinkle on the dual-task SRT experiment: It's probably not dual task. *Psychonomic Bulletin and Review, 7,* 309–313.

Raichle, M. E., Fiez, J. A., Videen, T. O., Macloed, A. M., Pardo, J. V., Fox, P. T., et al. (1994). Practice-related changes in human brain functional anatomy during non-motor learning. *Cerebral Cortex, 4,* 8–26.

Reason, J. (1990). *Human error.* Cambridge: Cambridge University Press.

Reber, P. J., Knowlton, B. J., & Squire, L. R. (1996). Dissociable properties of memory systems: Differences in the flexibility of declarative and nondeclarative knowledge. *Behavioral Neuroscience, 110,* 861–871.

Rowe, J., Friston, K., Frackowiak, R., & Passingham R. (2002). Attention to action: Specific modulation of corticocortical interactions in humans. *NeuroImage 17,* 988–998.

Sakai, K., Hikosaka, O., Miyauchi, S., Takino, R., Sasaki, Y., & Putz, B. (1998) Transition of brain activation from frontal to parietal areas in visuomotor sequence learning. *Journal of Neuroscience, 18,* 1827–1840.

Sheeran, P., Aarts, H., Custers, R., Rivis, A., Webb, T. L., & Cooke, R. (2005). The goal-dependent automaticity of drinking habits. *British Journal of Social Psychology, 44,* 47–63.

Sheeran, P., Webb, T. L., & Gollwitzer, P. (2005). The interplay between goal intentions and implementation intentions. *Personality and Social Psychology Bulletin, 31,* 87–98.

Tucker, M., & Ellis, R. (2004). Action priming by briefly presented objects. *Acta Psychologica, 116,* 185–203.

Verplanken, B., Aarts, H., van Knippenberg, A., & Moonen, A. (1998). Habit versus planned behaviour: A field experiment. *British Journal of Social Psychology, 37,* 111–128.

Wood, W., & Neal, D. T. (2007). A new look at habits and the habit-goal interface. *Psychological Review, 114,* 143–163.

Wood, W., Quinn, J. M., & Kashy, D. (2002). Habits in everyday life: Thought, emotion, and action. *Journal of Personality and Social Psychology, 83,* 1281–1297.

Wood, W., Tam, L., & Guerrero Witt, M. (2005). Changing contexts, disrupting habits. *Journal of Personality and Social Psychology, 88,* 918–933.

Yin, H. H., Knowlton, B. J., & Balleine, B. W. (2004). Lesions of dorsolateral striatum preserve outcome expectancy but disrupt habit formation in instrumental learning. *European Journal of Neuroscience, 19,* 181–189.

CHAPTER

22

Mimicry: Its Ubiquity, Importance, and Functionality

Tanya L. Chartrand *and* Amy N. Dalton

Abstract

This chapter examines the importance of mimicry in social life. It begins with a review of the various types of mimicry that researchers have uncovered. Research documenting verbal, facial, emotional, and behavioral mimicry is discussed, along with evidence for its automatic and nonconcious nature. Next, it is argued that mimicry has major social implications both within the mimicry interaction and beyond it. Evidence is reviewed linking mimicry to rapport and empathy, affiliation motives, and prosocial behavior. Mimicry also appears to impact the individuals being mimicked in nonsocial ways. It influences the cognitive processing style engaged in, the amount of regulatory resources they have, and the attitudes and preferences that they hold. Finally, four different theoretical approaches to the question of why humans mimic are discussed. These include conceptualizing mimicry as a communication tool, as a passive response based on an automatic perception-behavior link, as an adaptive behavior serving an important evolutionary function, and as a translator of neural responses into an understanding of the social environment.

Keywords: mimic, verbal mimicry, facial mimicry, emotional mimicry, behavioral mimicry, social lives

Humans are strongly inclined to notice how others are different from themselves and to draw on these differences—be they socio-economic, ethnic, or religious—as a source of tension. Indeed, one need only open a history book or turn on the evening news to get a glimpse of how our differences spark conflict in the world. Fortunately, we have another strong inclination that operates as a countervailing force, serving to unite us to others from our infancy. This force is mimicry. Humans automatically mimic other people, and this mimicry facilitates social interactions and interpersonal bonding. We create a sense of similarity by imitating each other in various ways. This mimicry has a powerful effect in facilitating rapport

and conveying feelings such as liking and empathy. Mimicry serves an important interpersonal function.

The notion that individuals mimic the behaviors of others has long been of interest to psychologists (e.g., James, 1890). The past 30 years in particular has seen a surge of research exploring the subtle and unintentional ways in which people imitate their social interaction partners, including mimicry of facial expressions, emotions, speech patterns, and physical movements. This unconscious mimicry is notably different from conscious imitation or modeling, an important part of social learning theory (Bandura, 1977). To better understand why we mimic and to articulate the functions mimicry serves, systematic investigations into mimicry's wide ranging consequences have been conducted, as have investigations into factors that facilitate and inhibit nonconscious mimicry. In light of these trends, this chapter unfolds in the following manner. First, we briefly introduce the various types of mimicry that research has explored. Our approach in this section is one of highlighting representative studies rather than exhaustively reviewing the literature (for more comprehensive reviews, see Chartrand, Maddux, & Lakin, 2005; Dijksterhuis & Bargh, 2001; Hatfield, Cacioppo, & Rapson, 1994). The second section of this chapter discusses the importance of mimicry by reviewing the consequences and moderators of it. Third, we discuss four different theoretical approaches to the question of why we mimic. In so doing, we review empirical support for each of these theoretical approaches.

What Do We Mimic?

When interacting with a person who is lively and animated, one will gesture more. When conversing with a person who has a distinct accent, one's own speech will develop traces of that accent. Even the mere observation of a person who feels sullen and somber will provoke similar feelings. Essentially, social environments are contagious, and people spontaneously imitate or mimic what they see in their social worlds. As these examples illustrate, a broad range of human experience is mimicked. Moreover, mimicry can transpire without an intention to mimic and without any awareness that mimicry is occurring (Chartrand & Bargh, 1999; Scheflen, 1964). In this section, we review evidence for mimicry of speech patterns, mimicry of facial expressions and emotions, and mimicry of nonverbal behaviors, including physical postures, gestures, and mannerisms. At the same time, we review evidence for the automatic and nonconscious nature of mimicry.

Verbal Mimicry

Research finds that a number of verbal tendencies are mimicked. Simner (1971) conducted research with infants and demonstrated that newborns as young as 2 to 4 days old will cry in response to another infant's crying. What is fascinating about Simner's research is the finding that infants do not mimic synthetic cries, suggesting that newborn infants can actually discriminate between real and artificial cries. Research on mimicry of speech patterns conducted with adult participants has shown that speakers tend to adopt each others' accents, latency to speak, speech rate, and utterance duration (e.g., Cappella & Planalp, 1981; Giles & Powesland, 1975; Matarazzo & Wiens, 1972; Webb, 1969). Speakers also use the same syntax (i.e., structure their sentences the same way) as their conversation partners, and this tendency has been shown to persist over multiple sentences (Bock, 1986).

There is evidence that at least some forms of verbal mimicry occur automatically. Levelt and Kelter (1982) demonstrated that during conversations, people use the same words and clauses that their interaction partners use. In one study, they included a condition in which participants were put under cognitive load. The results showed that mimicry occurred even when cognitive resources were highly taxed, suggesting that speakers imitate the words and clauses used by an interaction partner automatically. Another example comes from the work of Provine (1986), who put an end to years of speculation by demonstrating that yawning is indeed contagious—when we see another person yawn, we yawn automatically (see the discussion later in this chapter; see also Platek, Critton, Myers, & Gallup, 2003).

Facial Mimicry

Research has also shown spontaneous mimicry of facial expressions. O'Toole and Dubin (1968) reported that mothers tend to open their mouths in response to their infants opening their mouths to feed. They interpreted this finding as an application of George Herbert Mead's (1934–1967) notion of "taking the role of the other"—the idea that humans adopt each other's psychological standpoints. Zajonc, Adelmann, Murphy, and Niedenthal (1987) found that facial similarity in married couples increased over time and conjectured that this similarity arose as a consequence of married couples frequently mimicking each other's facial expressions. Chartrand and Bargh (1999) examined facial mimicry in a series of laboratory experiments and found that participants mimicked the facial expressions of confederates with whom they interacted, smiling more when they interacted with a confederate who smiled compared to a confederate who did not smile.

Dimberg, Thunberg, and Elmehed (2000) provided compelling evidence that mimicry of facial expressions occurs automatically. Three groups of participants were exposed either to happy, sad, or neutral faces for 30 milliseconds, followed by a neutral face for 5 seconds. This short presentation duration in combination with the backward masking technique prevented participants from consciously perceiving the target (happy or sad) stimuli. While participants viewed the stimuli, their spontaneous facial electromyographic activity was recorded. Dimberg et al. were specifically interested in the activity of the zygomatic major muscle, which elevates the lips during a smile, and the corrugator supercilii muscle, which knits the eyebrows during a frown. Past research had shown that activity in these muscles was spontaneously evoked by exposure to happy and angry faces, respectively (Dimberg & Thunberg, 1998). Dimberg

et al. reasoned that if distinct emotional responses can be automatically elicited, then unconscious exposure to happy or sad faces should differentially activate these muscles. The results showed that despite participants' lack of awareness of the happy or sad faces, their facial emotional response patterns showed that zygomatic major muscle activity was highest in response to happy faces and that corrugator supercilii muscle activity was highest in response to sad faces. This pattern of results suggested that facial mimicry occurred spontaneously and unconsciously in response to subliminally perceived stimuli.

Emotional Mimicry

Facial stimuli have been shown to elicit not only facial mimicry but also emotional responses (e.g., Lundquist & Dimberg, 1995). Research has begun to focus on mimicry of psychological states, including emotions (see Hatfield et al., 1994) and moods (Neumann & Strack, 2000). On the basis of facial feedback research suggesting that actions can automatically elicit feelings, Neumann and Strack (2000) tested the proposition that observing another person's emotional expression would elicit a congruent affective state in an observer. Participants listened to a cassette of a target reciting an affectively neutral speech in either a slightly happy or a slightly sad voice. In one study, participants subsequently reported experiencing corresponding mood states. In another study, participants who repeated back the content of the speech imitated the affective tone of the speaker's voice, suggesting that participants adopted a mood state congruent with that of the speaker.

One important moderator of emotion contagion appears to be expressiveness (Friedman & Riggio, 1981; Sullins, 1991). Friedman and Riggio (1981) found that highly expressive participants transmitted their moods to other, less expressive participants. Amazingly, this effect emerged when the group of participants sat together silently and therefore occurred strictly via nonverbal communication. Sullins (1991) found that this effect is further moderated by the type of mood that is being displayed. When the mood being displayed is a happy mood, both high- and low-expressive participants pass their moods on to others. However, when the mood is negative, high-expressive participants pass their mood to others more than their low-expressive counterparts.

Behavioral Mimicry

Perhaps the first to scientifically investigate behavioral mimicry, the psychotherapist Albert Scheflen was interested in the insights provided by postures and body positioning into the dynamics between interacting individuals. Scheflen (1964) videotaped 18 therapists conducting psychotherapy sessions and analyzed these tapes in order to determine the sorts of behavioral patterns individuals used to communicate. Scheflen argued that mimicry, which he called postural congruence, was an indicator of similarity in views or similarity in roles among interacting individuals.

Other research has looked at behavioral mimicry in more controlled settings. Bernieri (1988; Bernieri, Reznick, & Rosenthal, 1988) conducted a clever study designed to test whether naive judges rate "real" interactions as more synchronous. To do this, Bernieri videotaped several different mother–child interactions, always with the mother on the right and the child on the left. He then created various versions of videos in which mothers were sometimes paired with their own children and sometimes with other children. Participants watched these videos and rated how physically in sync the pairs were. Mothers were judged to be more in sync with their own children than with other children.

Bavelas, Black, Chovil, Lemery, and Mullett (1988) looked at left/right leaning behavior when an observer and target were facing each other. Their interest was in determining whether an observer's motions mirrored the direction of a target (mirror mimicry) or whether an observer's motion is the same as the target's if the observer is rotated into the target's position (rotational mimicry). Across three experiments, the researchers found that participants displayed mirror mimicry—they mirrored the leaning of the target they observed (see also LaFrance & Broadbent, 1976).

Chartrand and Bargh (1999) focused on mimicry of specific mannerisms and confirmed that mimicry occurs spontaneously in dyadic interactions. Participants engaged in a photo description task with two confederates one after the other. The first either moved their foot or touched their face throughout the session. The second confederate performed the behavior the first did not. Hidden videocameras recorded the participants' mannerisms, and coders blind to the hypothesis and condition later rated the amount of participants' face touching and foot moving during the two sessions. Results revealed that participants changed their behavior to match the behavior being displayed in their current environment: They moved their foot more when they were with the foot-moving confederate than the face-touching confederate, and they touched their face more when with the face toucher than the foot mover. This led Chartrand and Bargh (1999) to coin the phrase "the chameleon effect" to describe this nonconscious behavioral mimicry—individuals modulated their own behaviors to blend in with their current environment.

Why Is Mimicry Important?

Is nonconscious mimicry just a funny tendency we humans have, something we should leave to the realm of entertaining dinner conversation? Or is it justifiable as an important topic of scientific inquiry? There is now strong evidence for the latter. Mimicry serves a critical function not only in our social interactions but for us as individuals as well. There has been a recent surge of research examining the consequences that ensue from imitating others as well as the variables that moderate mimicry effects. These studies illuminate the importance of mimicry in our daily lives. For one, it serves as social glue, binding and bonding people together. Nonconscious mimicry helps us affiliate with others when we are feeling ostracized or different from others or when we are interacting with someone in power. It makes us feel closer to others and leads us to help other people more. It brings our attitudes in line with those of others, saves precious cognitive resources, and improves self-regulation. It also impacts the way we see ourselves and the cognitive processing style we engage in. Mimicry is not just an interesting phenomenon—it is a fundamental, critical process that serves many functions, many of which are currently being uncovered. In this section, we review the social and nonsocial impact of mimicry and answer the questions "is mimicry important?" and "is it worthy of scientific inquiry?" with a resounding "yes."

The Social Impact of Mimicry: Mimicry and Our Interactions With Others

Liking and Rapport

Some of the earliest work on mimicry was conducted in the domains of counseling and clinical psychology, where researchers were interested in the implications of nonverbal behaviors in interactions between psychologists and their clients (Charney, 1966; Dabbs, 1969; Scheflen, 1964). For instance, Charney (1966) examined postural congruence in the context of psychotherapy

sessions and found that mimicry increased over the course of a single session and that this increase in mimicry correlated significantly with an increase in rapport between the therapist and client.

LaFrance and Broadbent (1976) hypothesized that nonverbal behavioral mimicry would also be a good index of group rapport. They assessed this hypothesis in college seminar classrooms and indeed found that students rated rapport as higher in classrooms in which there was greater congruence between the body and arm positions of teachers and students. Other research also shows a strong link between mimicry and rapport. For example, the results of a meta-analysis conducted by Tickle-Degnen and Rosenthal (1990) showed that the three facets of rapport—mutual attention, coordination, and positivity—are associated with particular nonverbal behaviors, with the coordination element of rapport being highly linked with mimicry.

The information communicated by nonverbal behavioral mimicry can be understood even by naive, outside observers of an interaction. Grahe and Bernieri (1999) conducted an experiment in which participants were asked to judge rapport in dyadic interactions based on different types of information. Specifically, the participants were given access to the details of the dyadic interaction based on a transcript, audio playback, video playback, video with transcript, or video and audio playback. The results suggested that participants given video information who therefore had access only to nonverbal behavioral information were the most accurate judges of rapport in an interaction. It is somewhat counterintuitive to find evidence that nonverbal behavior may be more important than verbal behavior as an index of rapport.

Although LaFrance and Broadbent's (1976) correlational data did not allow for the conclusion that mimicry causes rapport to develop, experimental research does support this conclusion. In a series of studies, Chartrand and Bargh (1999) manipulated mimicry in the context of dyadic interactions to show that rapport is a consequence of mimicry. The dyad partners were complete strangers who presumably had no intention to affiliate and certainly no preexisting rapport. One member of each dyad was a research confederate who was instructed to either mimic or not mimic the postures and mannerisms of the research participants while they completed a joint task. When questioned after the interaction, participants who were mimicked liked the confederate more and perceived their interactions as having run more smoothly than participants who were not mimicked. These findings provide firm evidence that mirroring the behaviors of interaction partners facilitates social bonding.

Affiliation Goals

Given that mimicry leads to liking and rapport, it is functional that the motivation to build rapport can automatically increase nonconscious mimicry. Lakin and Chartrand (2003) found that compared to participants without a goal to affiliate, participants who either implicitly or explicitly held such a goal tended to mimic the face-touching behavior of a target while watching the target perform various clerical tasks on videotape. In a second study, they found that compared to participants who succeeded at an affiliation goal in an online interaction with a confederate, those who failed at an affiliation goal tended to mimic more the foot-moving behavior of a second confederate with whom they interacted. The researchers asked the second confederates (who were blind to participants' experimental conditions) to rate their interactions with the research participants, providing a measure of how successful participants were at affiliating. Confederates rated participants who failed at an affiliation

goal as more likable and rated the interactions as smoother. These studies suggest that behavioral mimicry is a "strategy" that people employ nonconsciously to affiliate with others. Moreover, this strategy works.

Note that in the Lakin and Chartrand (2003) studies, the affiliation goal was directly given to (or primed in) participants. What are the naturalistic triggers of an affiliation goal? Situations that activate such a goal in individuals should lead those individuals to engage in more mimicry. This idea has been tested recently.

FEELING TOO DIFFERENT FROM OTHERS

One situation that should lead to an affiliation goal (and subsequent mimicry) is feeling too dissimilar from an important in-group. According to Brewer's (1991) optimal distinctiveness theory, people are in a continual quest to balance their need for *distinctiveness* (i.e., seeing themselves as different from others) and their need for *assimilation* (i.e., seeing themselves as similar to others). This leads to the prediction that individuals who currently feel too different from an important group should want to assimilate and should therefore engage in behaviors that bring them closer to the group (i.e., mimicry). In a study testing this, Uldall, Hall, and Chartrand (2008) gave participants false feedback on a bogus "personality inventory" that suggested that they had either a relatively rare or a relatively common personality profile (compared to other undergraduate students at the same institution). After they received the false feedback, they engaged in a task with a confederate who moved her foot throughout the interaction. As expected, participants who were made to feel too distinct by being placed in the rare category mimicked the confederate more than those who were made to feel the same as everyone else by being placed in the common category. Thus, participants mimicked more when they were in a situation where they felt too different from a peer group.

OSTRACISM

The need to belong is a prominent quality of the human species, perhaps even universally shared (Baumeister & Leary, 1995; Leary & Baumeister, 2000). Because of our high need to form interpersonal bonds, social exclusion can be devastating (Leary, 2001). How do individuals cope with social exclusion? One route is through mimicry. Lakin, Chartrand, and Arkin (in press) studied the moderating role of social exclusion in the form of ostracism and how it promotes mimicry. Based on research showing that socially excluded individuals are more likely to engage in behaviors to promote inclusion, the authors reasoned that some of these behaviors might be automatic means of affiliation, including mimicry.

Ostracism was manipulated in the context of an online ball-tossing game called Cyberball (see Williams, Cheung, & Choi, 2000). Each participant played this online game with three other "participants" who were actually computer controlled to include or exclude the participant from the game. Following the game, participants completed what they believed to be an unrelated study in which they were to describe pictures to another participant (actually a confederate not associated with the Cyberball game). The results of several experiments using this procedure suggest that being ostracized does in fact increase participants' tendency to mimic another person. Mimicry was especially pronounced when participants were excluded by members of their in-group and subsequently interacted with another member of their in-group. It appears that participants tried to recover from their exclusion experience by affiliating with a new interaction partner who could help them reestablish their group identity more than one who could not (i.e., out-group members). Moreover, the participants were successful: The interaction partner for the picture description task rated interactions with excluded participants as smoother than interactions with included participants. These findings highlight once more that mimicry is automatically used to affiliate with others even though this heightened mimicry occurs without intention, awareness, or conscious control.

SELF-MONITORING

Cheng and Chartrand (2003) examined the moderating role of self-monitoring in participants' tendency to mimic in different social contexts that varied in affiliative cues. Not only did high self-monitors engage in more mimicry than low self-monitors, but compared to low self-monitors, high self-monitors automatically responded differentially to social contexts that varied in affiliative cues. In one study, the researchers hypothesized that high self-monitors would be more likely to mimic someone who they believed to be a peer than a nonpeer. High self-monitors who interacted with an alleged college student enrolled in the same introductory psychology class engaged in more mimicry (here, operationalized as foot moving) than high self-monitors who interacted with an alleged high school student or graduate student or than low self-monitors. In a second study, the researchers tested the hypothesis that compared to low self-monitors high self-monitors would respond more to social cues indicating that another is more powerful than they are by engaging in more mimicry than if that other was less powerful than they. They found that high self-monitors who were randomly assigned a "worker" role engaged in more mimicry (here, operationalized as face touching) than high self-monitors who were assigned a "leader" role. Essentially, Cheng and Chartrand (2003) found that among participants high in self-monitoring, social contextual details could trigger greater amounts of mimicry, but among participants low in self-monitoring, mimicry was less likely to occur regardless of one's social context.

Recently, researchers have proposed that mimicry's relationship with affiliation and liking might be due to a more general effect of mimicry on prosocial orientation. We now turn to research describing the link between mimicry and prosociality.

Prosocial Orientation

As previously described, mimicry leads to prosocial emotion (more feelings of liking and rapport) toward the mimicker. If mimicry leads to a general prosocial orientation, however, it should go beyond the dyad. Ashton-James, van Baaren, Chartrand, Decety and Karremaas (2007) found evidence for this. In one study, participants who were mimicked subsequently reported feeling closer to others in general than nonmimicked participants. This not only is additional evidence of prosocial orientation, but also suggests that the positive feelings engendered by mimicry extend beyond the dyad.

A second study looked at an implicit measure of feeling close to others—seating distance. Following a mimicry manipulation, participants were asked to take a seat in a hallway where several chairs were lined up. Several items were placed on one chair, intended to look like the belongings of another "participant." Ashton-James et al. (2007) were interested in how close participants sat to this ostensibly occupied seat. The results revealed that participants who had been mimicked in the first part of the experiment sat closer to the occupied seat than participants who had not been mimicked, reflecting greater implicit closeness to others. Again, the prosocial orientation fostered by mimicry appears to go beyond the mimicry interaction.

One prosocial emotion more specific than liking or feeling close to others is interpersonal trust. Do the prosocial feelings that mimicry engenders influence trust? Trust is particularly important in negotiations, and Maddux, Mullen, and Galinsky (2008) therefore studied the bargaining power of mimicry. Specifically, they investigated mimicry at the bargaining table to determine what effects it might have on negotiation agreements. Participants were business school students enrolled in a negotiations class. In one study, participants were each paired with one other student, and the pair was instructed to carry out a job employment negotiation. The researchers measured both individual gain from the negotiation (the extent to which individually preferred options were selected) and joint gain from the negotiation (which captured the extent to which mutually preferred options were selected). They found that mimicry had no effect on individual gains but did impact joint gains. Interactions in which one of the participants had been instructed to mimic their opponent yielded higher joint gain compared to interactions in which neither participant was instructed to engage in mimicry. Moreover, the more participants mimicked their opponents, the higher the resulting joint gain.

In a second study, a task was used that made it particularly difficult to come to a mutually preferred agreement. Again, participants interacted in dyads in which one member of the dyad was instructed to mimic their opponent or neither was instructed to mimic their opponent. The results showed that mimicry greatly increased the likelihood that a dyad would come to an agreement. As in the first study, the more participants actually mimicked their opponents, the more likely they were to come to an agreement. Finally, this study showed that the effect of mimicry on making a deal was mediated by overall dyad trust. Mimicry fostered trust, which in turn facilitated deal making.

Several recent studies have gone beyond prosocial emotions to explore whether mimicry also affects prosocial behaviors, such as helping others. In one study examining monetary generosity toward others as a measure of prosociality, waitresses were instructed to either recite back verbatim their customers' orders or to paraphrase the orders. The results revealed that the waitresses received larger tips from customers they mimicked than from customers they did not mimic (van Baaren, Holland, Steenaert, & van Knippenberg, 2003).

Another study found that participants who were mimicked by their experimenter not only helped that experimenter pick up more pens that "fell" to the floor but also were more helpful to people not directly involved in the mimicry situation by helping a second (nonmimicking) experimenter pick up pens and by donating more generously to a charitable cause (van Baaren, Holland, Kawakami, & van Knippenberg, 2004). These findings confirm a link between mimicry and prosociality and suggest further that mimicry has behavioral consequences (not just affective consequences). Moreover, it provides additional support for the notion that mimicry's effects extend beyond the dyad—that is, beyond the interacting (mimicking and mimicked) individuals.

Ashton-James et al. (2007) have proposed that the relationship between mimicry and prosociality is mediated by self-construal such that being mimicked causes a person to adopt a more interdependent self-construal, which in turn affects their prosocial feelings and behaviors. This prediction was derived from studies by van Baaren, Maddux, Chartrand, De Bouter, and van Knippenberg (2003), who found that an interdependent self-construal was associated with

more mimicry than an independent social construal. These results were obtained both when self-construal was primed and when it was inferred from cultural differences between Americans (independent) and Japanese (interdependent).

Ashton-James et al. (2007) conducted a study to test whether mimicry affects prosocial behavior via self-construal. In this study, participants were mimicked or not by an experimenter in an initial interaction and then completed the Twenty Statements Test (Kuhn & McPartland, 1954), a measure of working self-concept in which participants provide 20 different responses to the question "Who am I?" that are later coded to be independent (describe a personal attribute) or interdependent (describe a social role). After completing the self-concept measure, participants were asked if they would be interested in filling out an extra survey for a researcher who did not have funds to pay participants. The results revealed that participants who were mimicked described themselves in a more interdependent manner and were subsequently more likely to volunteer to complete the extra survey. Moreover, interdependence was shown to mediate the relationship between the mimicry manipulation and volunteering. The authors interpreted their findings as an important step in understanding *why* mimicry has positive social consequences.

The Nonsocial Impact of Mimicry: Mimicry and the Individual

Mimicry clearly influences our interactions with others. Is the impact of mimicry limited to the social domain, or does it influence the individual as well? That mimicry is associated with a particular type of self-construal (i.e., interdependence) and with high self-monitoring hints that mimicry may affect the individual, but it is only suggestive. Stronger evidence would demonstrate that mimicry has outcomes that are clearly nonsocial and is influenced by nonsocial states of mind. For instance, does mimicry influence one's attitudes and preferences, one's self-regulation in nonsocial tasks, or one's cognitive processing style? Is mimicry influenced by one's current emotional and mental state? The answer to all these questions is yes, and it is to this evidence that we now turn.

Persuasion

The prosocial consequences of mimicry have sparked a great deal of interest among researchers interested in its potential persuasive appeal. After all, people are more persuaded by individuals whom they like and who are similar to them (see Cialdini, 2001). Because mimicry has been shown to foster both liking (Chartrand & Bargh, 1999) and a sense of similarity (Bavelas, Black, Lemery, & Mullett, 1986; Bavelas et al., 1988), it is no surprise that researchers have started to explore the potential link between mimicry and attitude change.

Van Swol (2003) asked participants to play the role of a manager of a pharmaceutical company and make a decision as to which of three cholesterol-lowering drugs to market. The three drugs were pretested to be equally viable options. Participants were told that they would be asked to defend their choice in a discussion with two other individuals. The two individuals with whom participants interacted were research confederates. In their discussion, both confederates disagreed with the participant's choice and instead endorsed one of the other two drugs. However, one confederate mimicked the participant throughout the discussion, and the other did not. Following the group discussion, participants rated the mimicking confederate as more confident and more persuasive than the nonmimicking confederate. Interestingly, however, the participant was not more likely to adopt the mimicking confederate's viewpoint over the nonmimicking confederate's viewpoint.

In other words, though mimicry increased the perception of persuasiveness, it did not increase persuasion in this study. This finding was replicated in a similar study (van Swol & Drury, 2007a). Participants interacted with a confederate who disagreed with them on a particular issue and who either imitated their nonverbal behaviors or did not. Although participants rated the confederate as more persuasive and more knowledgeable following mimicry compared to no mimicry, the participants were no more persuaded in the mimicry condition compared to the no-mimicry condition.

However, countering this work is other research that did in fact find differences in persuasion among mimicked and nonmimicked participants. Bailenson and Yee (2005) conducted a fascinating study in which participants were mimicked not by humans but by digital avatars. These avatars were programmed either to mimic the head movements of participants who interacted with them in a virtual environment or to play back head movements from a different participant. The avatar delivered a persuasive message advocating a campus security policy that would require students to carry their student identification cards at all times. The results revealed that avatars that mimicked participants were subsequently rated to be more persuasive and were even evaluated more favorably on a series of trait measures. Moreover, mimicked participants were more in agreement with the avatar's persuasive appeal than were nonmimicked participants. Even though participants were interacting with a nonhuman mimicker, social influence occurred.

Both Scheflen (1964) and LaFrance (1982) proposed that mimicry might be a consequence of sharing viewpoints, but this proposition was first experimentally tested by van Swol (2003; van Swol & Drury, 2007b). Van Swol and Drury (2007b) examined whether the tendency to mimic another individual would be moderated by whether this person expressed opinions similar or dissimilar to their own. Participants read about two vacation destinations and chose which one they preferred. Following this, they discussed their choice with two other individuals, both of whom were confederates to the experiment. One confederate supported the participants' choices, and the other confederate disagreed with the participants' choices. The participants displayed more mimicry of the confederate who expressed agreement compared to the confederate who expressed disagreement.

Recent research in marketing has begun to examine the ways in which mimicry can affect people's preferences for consumer products. Tanner, Ferraro, Chartrand, Bettman, and van Baaren (2008) proposed two routes by which this can occur. The *mimicking consumer path* suggests that individuals automatically mimic the consumption behaviors of other people and that such mimicry then affects preferences toward the product(s) consumed. The *mimicked consumer path* suggests that being mimicked leads to increased prosociality, which affects preferences for products presented in dyadic interactions.

In a test of the mimicking consumer path, Tanner et al. (2008) had participants observe a confederate who was consuming one of two snacks while engaging in an unrelated task. Some participants had these same snacks available for their personal consumption, and others did not. The results showed that participants were more likely to consume the same snack that the confederate was consuming (if they were able to), and they subsequently reported more favorable attitudes toward the consumed snack. Moreover, they found that the mimicry mediated the effect on preferences. Importantly, participants

who merely observed the confederate and did not consume the snacks themselves were unaffected by the confederates' consumption behavior, further suggesting that the results were due to mimicry and not mere observation. This is the first research to focus on the downstream personal consequences (as opposed to social consequences) of mimicking others.

The authors also tested the mimicked consumer path. In two studies, a facilitator told participants about a new snack product that was about to be launched on the market. After the interaction, participants were asked to taste the product and rate how much they liked it, whether they would recommend it to friends, and whether they planned to purchase it themselves. The quantity that they consumed was also calculated at the end as an implicit measure of liking. In both studies, those who were mimicked had more favorable attitudes (as assessed by the measures above) toward the snacks.

In the second study, the facilitator was also either invested in the product's success (i.e., as a salesperson would be) or not. The authors made the counterintuitive prediction that the effect of mimicry would be stronger for invested facilitators than noninvested facilitators. They reasoned that the prosocial orientation induced in mimicked participants would lead to more "helping" behavior toward the invested facilitator, who presumably needed the "help" more than the uninvested facilitator. Thus, in the case where the facilitator has a clear stake in the outcome, the prosocial orientation would manifest itself as a greater tendency to like what is being presented. This prediction was supported by the study results. Overall, the studies by Tanner et al. suggest that mimicry can affect product preferences in two ways: Consumers automatically mimic the consumption of others, and this goes on to affect their preferences, and consumers are mimicked by others, and this affects preferences for products being presented (and even "sold to") by the mimicker.

Cognitive Style

Noting the apparent link between mimicry and greater environmental attunement, van Baaren, Horgan, Chartrand, and Dijkmans (2004) explored the relation between behavioral mimicry and cognitive style. Cognitive style refers to the ways that individuals tend to process information in terms of perception, organization, and response to stimuli. Van Baaren and colleagues focused on field-dependent versus field-independent processing style and proposed a link between mimicry and field-dependent processing style because field dependence is associated with a greater attunement to and reliance on contextual details. The researchers found that greater field dependence, whether chronic or situationally induced, was related to a greater tendency to mimic a target's behavior. They also found that participants processed information in a more context-dependent manner if they were mimicked than if they were not mimicked in a previous interaction. Again, this research suggests that mimicry is facilitated by factors that are associated with greater attunement to one's context. Van Baaren et al. further showed that cognitive style was a consequence of mimicry. Participants who were mimicked subsequently processed information in a more field-dependent manner compared to participants who were not mimicked.

Mood

One's mental state (cognitive processing style) therefore influences mimicry. So too does one's emotional state. Based on evidence that a positive mood leads people to rely more on automatic processes whereas a negative mood leads people to rely on more deliberate forms of action (e.g., Schwarz

& Clore, 1996), van Baaren, Fockenberg, Holland, Janssen, and van Knippenberg (2006) hypothesized that people in a positive mood would mimic more than people in a negative mood. The results of both correlational and experimental studies supported this hypothesis. In one study, a positive or a negative mood was induced by having participants watch either a funny or a sad video clip. Then participants were told that for the next part of the study they would listen to two short pieces of music. Their attention was again directed to the television screen, where they watched an experimenter start the first piece of music (this was actually a prerecorded video). The experimenter remained on the screen while the music played. A second experimenter was then depicted on the screen starting the second piece of music and also stayed on screen for the duration of the piece. The video segments were presented such that participants saw the experimenter play with a pen in one of the video segments but not in the other (the order was counterbalanced). Participants were videotaped while watching the video segments, and their behavior was later coded for the amount of pen playing participants displayed. The results revealed that participants in a positive mood played with their pens more when watching the experimenter who played with the pen than the one who did not. However, participants in a negative mood did not show more pen playing when they viewed the experimenter who played with the pen. Simply put, participants in a positive mood engaged in mimicry of the experimenter, but participants in a negative mood did not.

Self-Regulation

While most research has focused on the positive consequences of mimicry, recently attention has turned to the costs of poorly coordinated mimicry in social interactions. Drawing on recent research showing that poorly coordinated social interactions pose a self-regulatory burden on interactants (Finkel & Campbell, 2001), Dalton, Chartrand, and Finkel (2007; see also Finkel et al., 2008) explored whether there are basic self-regulatory consequences of well-coordinated or poorly coordinated behavioral mimicry. They proposed that poorly coordinated mimicry can disturb nonconscious social coordination processes, thereby increasing the effort required by a social interaction. This basic hypothesis was confirmed in a series of experiments that used a two-task paradigm: Participants interacted with a confederate who either mimicked or antimimicked (adopted different) physical postures, mannerisms, and gestures, and then participants completed a self-regulatory task on their own. Using measures ranging from fine motor skills to consumption of junk food, the authors showed that interactions involving mimicry or antimimicry differentially impacted self-regulatory performance on the second task. For example, participants who were mimicked during an interaction procrastinated less on a subsequent boring math task than those not mimicked.

Another study that included a mimicry, an antimimicry, and a control condition (in which the participant and confederate were separated by a divider) uncovered that the effect of mimicry on self-regulation is driven by antimimicry depleting regulatory resources rather than by mimicry replenishing regulatory resources (Dalton et al., 2007). But the authors argued that antimimicry per se was not depleting. Rather, antimimicry was depleting only when it was inconsistent with schemas for a given type of social interaction. To test this hypothesis, they examined moderation by participant race. Drawing on research suggesting that nonverbal behaviors tend to differ markedly between same-race

and cross-race interactions, the authors reasoned that although antimimicry was depleting in same-race interactions, the presence of mimicry would be schema inconsistent and therefore depleting during a cross-race interaction. The results confirmed that antimimicry interactions impaired self-regulation (assessed via Stroop task interference) in same-race interactions but actually produced the opposite effect in cross-race interactions. Moreover, mimicry's social consequences were dissociated from its self-regulatory consequences: Although mimicry depleted participants in cross-race interactions, they enjoyed mimicry interactions more.

In another study (Dalton et al., 2007, experiment 4), the authors demonstrated that experiencing poorly coordinated mimicry actually increases the attentional demands imposed on participants. The results of this last experiment suggest that poorly coordinated mimicry increases the monitoring and regulation required by an interaction and can thereby lead to subsequent impairments in self-regulatory functioning.

Taken together, research linking mimicry to self-regulation bolsters the notion that well-coordinated mimicry is an adaptive and automatic response. But these studies highlight that the adaptiveness of mimicry comes not only from its role in facilitating positive social interactions but also from its capability to save much-needed cognitive resources.

Thus far, we have reviewed a number of moderators and consequences of mimicry. (Mimicry has also been linked to empathy and perspective taking, which is discussed in detail later in this chapter.) To conclude, the literature documenting mimicry's moderators and consequences is extensive and continues to grow. As the mimicry literature matures, researchers can piece together more and more insights into mimicry's functionality, examining the relationships between variables and triangulating around a theory as to why we mimic others so frequently and automatically and why it has the powerful impact that it does. In the following section, we describe current and past perspectives on why mimicry occurs.

Why Do We Mimic?
Mimicry as Communication

Research has traditionally adopted a heavy focus on the link between mimicry and rapport, so it is no surprise that one of the earliest theories of mimicry highlighted this link. This theory of mimicry contends that mimicry communicates understanding and togetherness and therefore fosters an empathic bond between interactants that leads to positive social outcomes (Bavelas et al., 1988; Bernieri, 1988; Condon & Ogston, 1966; Condon & Sander, 1974; LaFrance, 1979, 1982).

This proposition stemmed from literature on the communicative function of nonverbal behavior in general (e.g., Scheflen, 1964). An example from this broader research tradition is the findings of Kraut and Johnston (1979), who were interested in the communicative function of facial expressions. In a field study, they found that people were more likely to respond to happy situations with a smile when there was another person around than when they were alone, suggesting that the smile served a communicative function. Bavelas, Black, Lemery, and Mullet (1986) used the findings of Kraut and Johnston (1979) as a starting point for a controlled laboratory study designed to address whether mimicry is communicative. Specifically, they tested whether mimicry is an interpersonal event and whether it is actually received as a nonverbal message that conveys similarity or togetherness (see also Bavelas et al., 1988).

In one study (Bavelas et al., 1986), participants were seated in an experimental testing room and watched as two experimenters moved a television into the testing room. One of the experimenters wore a finger splint to signal that he had an injured finger. The study was rigged so that the television would appear to crush the splinted finger as the experimenters positioned it in front of the participants. Two experimental conditions were included. In one condition, the injured experimenter looked at the participant while he experienced his injury, and in the other condition, the experimenter hunched forward while he experienced his injury so that the participant could see only his facial profile. The experiment showed that participants who witnessed the experimenter wince because of a (fake) injury often winced in response, and the size of the participants' winces reflected how well they could view the wince on the face of the experimenter.

The results of this first study suggested to the researchers that mimicry is in fact an interpersonal response—mimicry occurred the most when interactants could see it occurring. But they also sought to determine whether mimicry is a communicative act. To show that mimicry is communicative, they would need to show that the facial expressions displayed by the participants were meaningful to others. In a second experiment, the researchers provided precisely this evidence. They gave naive decoders videotaped excerpts of the participants watching the staged injuries and asked them to rate the facial expressions of the participants on several dimensions. The naive judges saw only the participants and not the experimenter, so they could not tell what condition participants were in. The results revealed that the facial expressions of participants who saw the face of the injured experimenter (compared to those who saw only the experimenter's facial profile) were judged to be more knowing, caring, and appropriate. The authors concluded that mimicry functions to communicate an observer's vicarious response to an interaction partner.

The conclusion that mimicry occurs because of its communicative function could not account for studies documenting mimicry among participants who were alone and watching videotaped stimuli (Bavelas, Black, Lemery, MacInnis, et al., 1986; see also Hsee, Hatfield, Carlson, & Chemtob, 1990). If mimicry only exists as a communicative response, then why would it occur when a person is alone? Chartrand and Bargh (1999) put forth a different explanation for mimicry, one that could account for these earlier findings. Rather than focusing on the function that mimicry serves, these researchers discussed it in terms of the structures that enable mimicry to occur.

Mimicry as a Passive and Automatic Response

Rather than focusing on the communicative function of mimicry, Chartrand and Bargh (1999) focused instead on the preconscious nature of mimicry, arguing that mimicry is a passive and automatic response. They conducted a series of studies that demonstrated that mimicry occurs automatically. They found that under minimal conditions, among strangers who have no goal to affiliate with each other, mimicry still occurs. They surmised that because mimicry is an automatic response, it does not depend on the operation of goals such as communication or affiliation during the interaction. To get at the automatic nature of the effect, they questioned participants following the dyadic interactions. Specifically, they asked their participants a series of questions designed to probe for awareness of the mimicry. No participants reported that they were aware that mimicry had occurred even when specifically asked about it.

The mechanism considered responsible for mimicry was a passive perception–behavior link. The notion of a perception–behavior link has its roots in the notion of ideomotor action, first proposed by Carpenter (1874) and James (1890). Ideomotor action occurs when the mere act of thinking about an action increases the likelihood of performing that action (see Chapters 2 and 18). Essentially, the regions of the brain that become active on thinking about an action are the same regions that become active when we engage in that action ourselves. Seeing another person engage in a behavior is another way to heighten activation. Thus, we are more likely to engage in a particular behavior when we perceive another person engage in that same behavior. That is, there is a direct and automatic "perception–behavior link." In the following section, we discuss evidence for this link.

BEHAVIORAL EVIDENCE FOR A PERCEPTION–BEHAVIOR LINK

Most of the evidence supporting the existence of a perception–behavior link comes from neuropsychological research on mirror neurons with nonhuman subjects (Gallese, Fadiga, Fogassi, & Rizzolatti, 1996; Rizzolatti, Fogassi, & Gallese, 2001; for a review, see Dijkersterhaus & Bargh, 2001). Using monkeys as research subjects, researchers have even begun to develop a physiological model for the perception–behavior link (Rizzolatti & Craighero, 2004; Rizzolatti et al., 2001; Rumiati & Bekkering, 2003; Williams et al., 2000).

Because the methods are generally unfeasible with human participants, researchers have developed clever techniques to demonstrate the existence of a perception–behavior link in humans. Sebanz, Knoblich, and Prinz (2003) used a spatial compatibility task called the Simon Task (Craft & Simon, 1970; Simon, 1990) to test whether perceiving action performed by another individual in fact activates a cognitive representation for that action in the self. In the task, a finger wearing either a red or a green ring was presented on a computer screen, and participants had to ignore the direction that the finger was pointing (left, right, or forward) and instead indicate its color by left or right clicking a computer mouse. The responses could be either compatible (finger points toward the correct button), incompatible (finger points toward the incorrect button), or neutral (finger points forward).

One group of participants completed this task alone, and results revealed a spatial compatibility effect—responses were faster on compatible trials and slower on incompatible trials as compared to neutral trials. A second group of participants completed a go/no-go version of the Simon Task in which they responded either to only the red rings or only the green rings and again had to ignore the direction of the pointing finger. This second group of participants completed this task under two different counterbalanced-order conditions: individually (e.g., responding only to red and ignoring green) or with a partner (if responding to red and ignoring green, the partner would respond to green and ignore red).

Sebanz et al. (2003) found that although the task instructions were the same for the participants in both go/no-go conditions (e.g., respond to red and ignore green), the fact that the task was performed either individually or next to a partner had an effect on the pattern of performance. When the task was completed individually, response times were relatively fast for all three types of trials. When the task was completed with a partner, response times were faster on compatible trials than on incompatible trials. In other words, when participants completed the go/no-go version with a partner, their pattern of performance suggested a spatial compatibility effect, mirroring the pattern shown by the first group of participants, who completed the entire task alone. Note that because participants in these go/no-go reaction-time tasks need respond to only one stimulus, spatial compatibility effects

usually do not occur. But the authors predicted and found such an effect when the task was completed with a partner.

The authors surmised that participants working with a partner mentally represented their partner's action in the same way they represented their own and that because the representations involved with perceiving the actions of the partner are the same representations that would become active when perceiving and planning one's own actions, participants performed as though they were completing the entire task alone even though they were actually completing the go/no-go version of the task. In another study, the authors ruled out a social facilitation explanation for these effects. Together, the studies provide behavioral evidence for a perception–behavior link.

NEUROPSYCHOLOGICAL EVIDENCE FOR A PERCEPTION–BEHAVIOR LINK

Recent investigations using functional magnetic resonance imaging (fMRI) and positron emission tomography also support the perception–behavior link postulated by ideomotor theory (see Chapter 13). Jeannerod and colleagues (Decety, Jeannerod, Germain, & Pastene, 1991; Jeannerod, 1994, 1997) examined activities such as weightlifting and running and showed that both mentally simulating these activities and performing these activities activated the same premotor cortex neurons in humans (see also Decety & Grezes, 1999; Iacoboni et al., 1999). Likewise, Paus, Petrides, Evans, and Meyer (1993) showed that thinking about words or gestures activated the anterior cingulated cortex in the same way as saying these words or performing these gestures (Chapter 7).

While these studies demonstrate a link between cognition and action, they do not show a link between the perception of another person's behavior and action. However, evidence for such a link does in fact exist. Several other areas, such as the posterior parietal cortex (Ruby & Decety, 2001) and the cerebellum (Grossman et al., 2000), show similar activation when one performs or imagines and when one observes another perform the same action. These neuropsychological studies provide the most direct evidence for a link between one's own and another's perception–action systems. Researchers have conceptualized this link in a variety of different ways, all of which are variants of the basic ideomotor action hypothesis.

CONCEPTUALIZING THE PERCEPTION–BEHAVIOR LINK
Shared Representations

Prinz (1990, 1997) proposed the common-coding hypothesis, a shared representational system for perception and action that extends the ideomotor action hypothesis to perception of events and actions, and to imitation. Action is presumed to be represented in terms of its perceivable effects (not in terms of the actions per se). These representations automatically give rise to actual behavior after a certain threshold level of activation is reached. This hypothesis has received empirical support with the discovery of "mirror neurons" in humans (Iacoboni et al., 1999; Koski, Iacoboni, Dubeau, Woods, & Mazziotta, 2002) and macaque monkeys (Metzinger & Gallese, 2003; Rizzolatti et al., 2001). Mirror neuron research suggests that common coding occurs in single neurons in the brain. Gallese et al. (1996) discovered premotor cortex neurons in the macaque monkey that fired both when the monkey grasped an object and when the monkey observed an experimenter grasp the object, hence the name "mirror neurons." Other evidence suggestive of common coding comes from a study conducted by Fadiga, Fogassi, Pavesi, and Rizzolatti (1995) that showed that perceiving a target grasping an object and grasping the object oneself result in similar muscular responses (see also Musseler & Hommel, 1997).

Schemas

Other arguments in favor of a perception–behavior link have been made in terms of schemas (e.g., Barresi & Moore, 1996). Unlike the shared representations account, which posits shared systems within the brain, the schema arguments are made from a purely cognitive perspective. According to this perspective, the schemas that activate when one produces an action have significant semantic overlap with the schemas that activate when one perceives and interprets the actions of others. Therefore, these two types of schemas tend to be active at the same time. Thus, not only does perception incite action, but action activates the corresponding behavioral representation and its overlapping interpretational schema (Berkowitz, 1984; Carver, Ganellen, Froming, & Chambers, 1983) and thereby influences the interpretation of one's perceptual landscape (Mussweiler, 2003).

Barresi and Moore's (1996) theory proposes that schemas structure the different sources of information, and therefore first-person and third-person information as well as imagined and perceived information cannot be confused. Because schemas are assumed to impose structure, this theory implies that when one perceives one's own action (e.g., on a videotape), the same system is involved in perception and action, but when one perceives another's action, different systems are involved in perception and action. Two hypotheses derive from Barresi and Moore's theoretical assumptions. First, individuals should be better able to recognize themselves than others, and, second, individuals should be better able to predict the future effects of their own actions than the effects of the actions of others. Self-recognition does appear superior to other recognition, whether looking at recognition of clapping (Repp, 1987), drawing style (Knoblich & Prinz, 2001), or body movement (Beardsworth & Buckner, 1981). Moreover, it appears that the effects of self-generated action are in fact more predictable than the effects of other-generated action. One study demonstrated that research participants more accurately predicted a dart's landing position on a dartboard when they were watching videos of their own throws compared to the throws of other individuals (Knoblich & Flach, 2001). This schema-based approach to the perception–behavior link is supported not only by these studies but also by neuropsychological evidence that different systems are involved in the perception of self versus others (see the discussion later in this chapter).

Theoretical explanations of the perception–behavior link are useful because they explain how it is that we humans can constantly engage in mimicry without intending to and even without being aware that it is occurring. But evidence for a perception–behavior link and explanations of the cognitive architecture supporting mimicry behavior do not shed light on why mimicry occurs in the first place. Dijksterhuis and Bargh (2001) argue that humans inherited the perception–behavior link from evolutionary ancestors, such as fish and frogs, which relied on perceptual processes to facilitate adaptive behavioral responding. Could it be that the perception–behavior link is a mere by-product of biological inheritance, or is it the case that the perception–behavior link serves an important and unique function to humankind? For these insights, we first turn to a social evolutionary theory of the origins of mimicry and then to recent research and theory in neuropsychology.

Mimicry From an Evolutionary Perspective

Ample evidence has been reviewed in this chapter suggesting that mimicry serves important social functions. For instance, mimicry communicates feelings of empathy to interaction partners and leads to prosocial feelings and behavior toward others. However, it may be erroneous to conclude that mimicry exists *because* of its consequences. These consequences might have evolved over time and actually have little to do with the origin of mimicry itself. The evolutionary perspective on mimicry accepts that the basic perception–behavior link was inherited from prehuman species for its physical survival value, then emphasizes that the prevalence of mimicry among humans today is largely because of its social survival value (Chartrand et al., 2005; Lakin, Jefferis, Cheng, & Chartrand, 2003). This approach highlights the social moderators and consequences of mimicry, which attest to its adaptive nature and social utility, while also acknowledging the cognitive structure supporting the basic perception–behavior link as the predecessor of these social functions.

According to this approach, basic survival benefits might have led to the automatization of mimicry in the evolution of humankind. Imagine, for instance, that you are a caveman (or cavewoman). You spend your day picking berries and hunting bison, all the while hoping that a large bear does not chase you down and eat you. Suppose that you are out berry picking with your fellow cavefolk, and suddenly several of them drop their berries and start running for the hills. Do you pause, assess the situation, and rationally decide whether you should follow? Or, at the sight of the others running, do you also bolt for the hills? In this situation, a caveman who thinks likely dies. A cavewoman who mindlessly follows the others likely survives. If situations of this sort occurred frequently enough in humans' evolutionary history, then the development of an automatic imitative response would be highly adaptive for survival.

Today, large bears are not hiding in most of our berry bushes. But the cognitive mechanism that enabled adaptive responses in the lives of our predecessors is still in place. In addition, there could still be some value to automatically mimicking those around us, as mimicry does have many positive consequences. So it is no surprise that humans are hardwired to automatically mimic one another. As early as 1 month after birth, infants smile in response to the smiles of other people and stick out their tongues when they observe others doing the same (Meltzoff & Moore, 1977), and by 9 months, infants begin to mimic emotional expressions (Termine & Izard, 1988).

In the next section, we turn to some very recent research from the behavioral mimicry and neuropsychology literatures that might be fruitful in refining current conceptualizations of mimicry. Recent developments demonstrate not only that the perception–behavior link is rooted in our cognitive architecture but also that social responses, such as empathy and perspective taking, are linked to our cognitive architecture. The picture that emerges in light of these findings illustrates that mimicry may be an important process mediating the relation between the perception–behavior link and social responses.

Merging Old With New: The Social Neuroscience Approach to Mimicry

Theories of mimicry started with an emphasis on its social functions and then turned to an emphasis on its cognitive roots. It appears theorizing may come full circle, with research coming to the fore that links social responses to cognitive architecture. Given the importance of mimicry,

empathy, and liking in facilitating social interactions, it might come as no surprise that these social feelings and behaviors have neural underpinnings. Knoblich and Sebanz (2006) made the provocative statement that basic perception–action links—evident at the level of single neurons—can actually facilitate positive social interactions and are in fact *crucial* for many social interactions. Another emerging line of research gives us reason to believe that at least some types of mimicry are rooted in the same neural substrates as empathy (Platek, Mohamed, & Gallup, 2005). In light of these and other findings, which are described later, we raise the possibility that mimicry mediates the link between various neural systems implicated in social interaction and their associated social responses, be they cognitive, behavioral, or affective. Granted that the evidence supporting this theory is incomplete, the proposition is exciting and worthy of consideration.

A social neuroscience approach to mimicry argues that it is through the perception–behavior link that we not only mimic others but also understand our social surroundings. From this perspective, mimicry is essential for translating neural responses into an understanding of social stimuli. Such an approach requires that links exist between neural substrates and mimicry; between neural substrates and social responses, including perspective taking and empathy; and between mimicry and social responses. Previously, evidence was reviewed regarding the neural underpinnings of mimicry. We review evidence for the other proposed links next.

MIMICRY AND EMPATHY

Early definitions of mimicry, such as that of Charles Darwin, viewed mimicry as synonymous with empathy. Evidence supporting this comes from some of the earliest research done on mimicry. The traditional theory viewed mimicry as an indicator of empathy, a vicarious cognitive or emotional experience. For instance, Maurer and Tindall (1983) examined postural congruence effects on client perception of counselor empathy. Adolescents interacted individually with a school psychologist (counselor) to discuss career plans. Counselors either mimicked or did not mimic the client's leg and arm positions throughout the meetings. Immediately following the meetings, clients were asked to rate the counselor's level of empathy via the 16-item Empathy scale of the Barrett-Lennard (1962) Relationship Inventory. As predicted, the researchers found that clients who were mimicked by their counselors perceived these counselors to be more empathic. Therefore, these findings provide evidence for a link between mimicry and empathy.

More recently, the neural mechanisms involved in empathy have received a lot of attention (e.g., Jackson, Brunt, Meltzoff, & Decety, 2005). This research has been conducted as a way of exploring the perception–action model (Jackson & Decety, 2004; Preston & de Waal, 2002), which is a variant of the more general perception–behavior link and proposes specifically that the perception of emotions activates the neural mechanisms that generate those emotions. Jackson et al. (2005) conducted a magnetic resonance imaging study in which they showed participants pictures of people with their hands and feet in painful or nonpainful situations. Participants experienced both "self" and "other" perspectives and were asked to rate the level of pain from these different perspectives. The researchers found many similarities in the neural networks involved in processing pain from "self" and "other" perspectives; however, they also found differences. These differences imply that empathic responding is not the same as self-responding; empathy

does not involve a complete adoption of the perspective of another. The authors argued this research helps identify the neural bases of empathy.

Based on this and similar research, Decety and colleagues have argued that the neural architecture involved with the coupling of perception and action plays a significant role in the experience of empathy (Decety & Jackson, 2004; Goldman & Sripada, 2005; Meltzoff & Decety, 2003; Preston & de Waal, 2002). These findings are key in supporting the idea that social behaviors that serve social functions can have neural substrates. Empathy is rooted in basic cognitive structures, as is mimicry.

Research on contagious yawning has taken a similar path. The notion that contagious yawning is a sign of empathy is not new (Lehmann, 1979). Contagious yawning has been described as a primitive reflection of the capacity to empathize with others. However, more recently, neuropsychological research has been gathered that supports the theoretical link between mimicry of yawning and empathy. Platek et al. (2003) showed that susceptibility to contagious yawning was positively correlated with a variety of indices of empathy, including performance on theory of mind tasks and a self-face recognition task. The authors stated that contagious yawning might have been occurring as a result of unconscious empathy and speculated on the basis of other research that unconscious mental simulation by mirror neurons might partially mediate the effect.

Platek et al. (2005) sought to provide fMRI data on the neural substrates involved in contagious yawning. They showed that viewing someone yawn activates brain areas involved in self-processing (e.g., self-referential processing and theory of mind) and concluded that their findings support the notion that contagious yawning is part of the neural network involved in empathy.

This line of research suggests that at least one type of mimicry (contagious yawning) has neural substrates and that these neural substrates are part of the same system involved in empathic responding, perspective taking, and self-processing more broadly.

Taken together, these findings suggest that mimicry is associated with empathy and that both empathy and mimicry are rooted in brain architecture, particularly the architecture implicated in the perception–behavior link. The existence of these links hints at the possibility that mimicry is essential for social responses such as empathy to occur. More direct evidence for the potential mediating role of mimicry in the relationship between brain and social responding will come in our discussion of mimicry and perspective taking, to which we now turn.

MIMICRY AND PERSPECTIVE TAKING

Research supports an association between mimicry and perspective taking, the cognitive component of empathy (Davis, 1983). Chartrand and Bargh (1999) demonstrated that individual differences in the propensity to take the perspective of others moderate the propensity to mimic others. Specifically, Chartrand and Bargh (1999) found greater mimicry of a target's behavior among research participants who scored high on a self-report measure of perspective taking than among those who were relatively low in perspective taking.

There is other evidence for a relationship between perspective taking and mimicry. Wallbott (1991) demonstrated that mimicry increases the propensity to take the perspective of another person in terms of understanding the meaning of their facial emotional expressions. Participants viewed pictures of strangers and were asked to judge the emotional expression conveyed on the stranger's face as happy, angry, sad, and so on. While they viewed the pictures, participants spontaneously mimicked the facial

expressions that they saw. Importantly, Wallbott found that the more participants mimicked a facial expression, the more accurate they were at their judgments. This suggests that the more we mimic another person, the more able we are to understand their perspective, thereby hinting at mimicry's mediational role.

Jackson, Meltzoff, and Decety (2006) investigated the neural circuits involved in imitation and perspective taking in an fMRI study. The researchers had participants watch videos of an actor performing simple hand or foot actions. The clips were varied such that they depicted the actions either from the first-person or third-person perspective. The researchers also varied whether participants were instructed to passively observe the videos or imitate the actions performed in the videos. They found that motor production systems were activated equally whether actions were observed or imitated, as ideomotor theories would contend. They also found more activation in the motor production system from the first-person than the third-person perspective, in line with an assumption of ideomotor theory that suggests that more sensory feedback would be available through the first-person perspective as well as differential activation in particular regions. Other research (Samson, Apperly, Kathirgamanathan, & Humphreys, 2005) has examined the regions implicated in third-person perspective and shown that lesions to this region impair perspective-taking abilities. Together, research suggests that the same neural substrates are implicated in imitative behavior and perspective taking. This fact is suggestive of a common biological system linking these various social responses.

Importantly, it appears that mimicry is crucial for perspective taking to occur. Adolphs, Damasio, Tranel, Cooper, and Damasio (2000) examined the ability of their research participants to categorize the facial expressions of others and were specifically interested in how participants with a lesion in the somatosensory cortex would perform on this task. Participants with somatosensory cortex lesions were impaired at judging emotional expressions, and according to the authors, their impairments occurred because their lesions compromised the mimicry response and resulting somatosensory feedback that facilitate the ability to understand the emotional expressions of others. These data provide compelling evidence for the idea that mimicry mediates the relationship between neural substrates and social responses.

To summarize, these findings bolster the argument that mimicry and perspective taking are supported by the same underlying neural systems. Importantly, the research of Wallbott, as well as that of Adolphs and colleagues, provide clues that mimicry might mediate the link between the neural substrates and their corresponding social responses. At the very least, this research suggests interdependence in the social responses of mimicry and perspective taking.

Humans possess a biologically based system of socially directed cognitions and behaviors, including perspective taking, mimicry, and empathic responding. We have reviewed evidence for the neural substrates of these various social responses. This evidence highlights the overlap in the neural underpinnings of these responses and provides preliminary evidence suggesting that these responses are interdependent. We believe that emerging research in social neuroscience will begin to play a more focal role in our conceptualizations of mimicry by addressing the fundamental theoretical issue of why mimicry occurs.

Conclusion

Mimicry functions as social glue; its presence is magnified when people are motivated to affiliate with others, when we experience certain moods, and when we are processing our environments in certain ways. Research is starting to reveal effects of mimicry that extend beyond the social interaction—mimicry affects how we process the world around us, our openness to persuasion, and even our ability to self-regulate. In this chapter, we described the theoretical and empirical issues that researchers of mimicry have tackled as well as those that have only begun to be understood. Converging evidence suggests that the fundamental purpose of mimicry appears to reside in its capacity to facilitate smooth and enjoyable social interactions. Emerging evidence goes one step further and suggests that mimicry's social role is fundamentally tied to the perception–behavior link that supports it.

References

Adolphs, R., Damasio, H., Tranel, D., Cooper, G., & Damasio, A. R. (2000). A role for somatosensory cortices in the visual recognition of emotion as revealed by three-dimensional lesion mapping. *Journal of Neuroscience, 20,* 2683–2690.

Ashton-James, C. E., van Baaren, R., Chartrand, T. L., Decety, J., & Karremass, J. (2007). Mimicry and me: The impact of mimicry on self-construal. *Social Cognition, 25,* 518–535.

Bailenson, J. N., & Yee, N. (2005). Digital chameleons: Automatic assimilation of nonverbal gestures in immersive virtual environments. *Psychological Science, 16,* 10, 814–819.

Bandura, A. (1977). *Social learning theory.* Englewood Cliffs, NJ: Prentice Hall.

Barresi, J., & Moore, C. (1996). Intentional relations and social understanding. *Behavioral and Brain Sciences, 19,* 107–154.

Barrett-Lennard, G. T. (1962) Dimensions of therapist responses as causal factors in therapeutic change. *Psychological Monographs, 76*(2, Whole No. 562).

Baumeister, R. F., & Leary, M. R. (1995). The need to belong: Desire for interpersonal attachments as a fundamental human motivation. *Psychological Bulletin, 117,* 97–529.

Bavelas, J. B., Black, A., Chovil, N., Lemery, C. R., & Mullett, J. (1988). Form and function in motor mimicry. Topographic evidence that the primary function is communicative. *Human Communication Research, 14,* 275–299.

Bavelas, J. B., Black, A., Lemery, C. R., MacInnis, S., & Mullett, J. (1986). Experimental methods for studying "elementary motor mimicry." *Journal of Nonverbal Behavior, 10,* 102–119.

Bavelas, J. B., Black, A., Lemery, C. R., & Mullett, J. (1986). "I *show* how you feel": Motor mimicry as a communicative act. *Journal of Personality and Social Psychology, 50,* 322–329.

Beardsworth, T., & Buckner, T. (1981). The ability to recognize oneself from a video recording of one's movements without seeing one's body. *Bulletin of the Psychonomic Society, 18,* 19–22.

Berkowitz, L. (1984). Some effects of thoughts on the anti- and prosocial influences of media events: A cognitive neoassociationistic analysis. *Psychological Bulletin, 95,* 410–427.

Bernieri, F. (1988). Coordinated movement and rapport in teacher-student interactions. *Journal of Nonverbal Behavior, 12,* 120–138.

Bernieri, F., Reznick, J. S., & Rosenthal, R. (1988). Synchrony, pseudo synchrony, and dissynchrony: Measuring the entrainment process in mother-infant interactions. *Journal of Personality and Social Psychology, 54,* 243–253.

Bock, J. K. (1986). Syntactic persistence in language production. *Cognitive Psychology, 18,* 355–387.

Bosbach, S., Cole, J., Prinz, W., & Knoblich, G. (2005). Understanding another's expectation from action: The role of peripheral sensation. *Nature Neuroscience, 8,* 1295–1297.

Brewer, M. B. (1991). The social self: On being the same and different at the same time. *Personality and Social Psychology Bulletin, 17,* 475–482.

Cappella, J. N., & Planalp, S. (1981). Talk and silence sequences in informal conversations III: Interspeaker influence. *Human Communication Research, 7,* 117–132.

Carpenter, W. B. (1874). *Principles of mental physiology.* London: John Churchill.

Carver, C. S., Ganellen, R. J., Froming, W. J., & Chambers, W. (1983). Modeling: An analysis in terms of category accessibility. *Journal of Experimental Social Psychology, 19,* 403–421.

Charney, E. J. (1966). Postural configurations in psychotherapy. *Psychosomatic Medicine, 28,* 305–315.

Chartrand, T. L., & Bargh, J. A. (1999). The chameleon effect: The perception-behavior link and social interaction. *Journal of Personality and Social Psychology, 76,* 93–910.

Chartrand, T. L., Maddux, W., & Lakin, J. (2005). Beyond the perception-behavior link: The ubiquitous utility and motivational moderators of nonconscious mimicry. In R. Hassin, J. Uleman, & J. A. Bargh (Eds.), *The new unconscious* (pp. 334–361). New York: Oxford University Press.

Cheng, C. M., & Chartrand, T. L. (2003). Self-monitoring without awareness: Using mimicry as a nonconscious affiliation strategy. *Journal of Personality and Social Psychology, 85,* 1170–1179.

Cialdini, R. (2001). *Influence: Science and practice.* Needham Heights, MA: Allyn and Bacon.

Condon, W. S., & Ogston, W. D. (1966). Sound film analysis of normal and pathological behavior patterns. *Journal of Nervous and Mental Disease, 143,* 338–347.

Condon, W. S., & Sander, L. W. (1974). Synchrony demonstrated between movements of the neonate and adult speech. *Child Development, 45,* 456–462.

Craft, J. L., & Simon J. R. (1970). Processing symbolic information from a visual display: Interference from an irrelevant directional cue. *Journal of Experimental Psychology, 83,* 415–432.

Dabbs, J. M. (1969). Similarity of gestures and interpersonal influence. *Proceedings, 77th Annual Convention of the American Psychological Association, 4,* 337–339.

Dalton, A. N., Chartrand, T. L., & Finkel, E. J. (2008). *The depleted chameleon: Self-regulatory consequences of social asynchrony.* Unpublished manuscript.

Davis, M. H. (1983). Measuring individual differences in empathy: Evidence for a multidimensional approach. *Journal of Personality and Social Psychology, 44,* 113–126.

Decety, J., & Grezes, J. (1999). Neural mechanisms subserving the perception of human actions. *Trends in Cognitive Sciences, 3,* 172–178.

Decety, J., & Jackson, P. L. (2004). The functional architecture of human empathy. *Behavioral and Cognitive Neuroscience Reviews, 3,* 71–100.

Decety, J., Jeannerod, M., Germain, M., & Pastene, J. (1991). Vegetative response during imagined movement is proportional to mental effort. *Behavioural Brain Research, 42,* 1–5.

Dijksterhuis, A., & Bargh, J. A. (2001). The perception-behavior expressway: Automatic effects of social perception and social behavior. In M. Zanna (Ed.), *Advances in experimental social psychology* (Vol. 30, pp. 1–40). New York: Academic Press.

Dimberg, U., & Thunberg, M. (1998). Rapid facial reactions to different emotionally relevant stimuli. *Scandinavian Journal of Psychology, 39,* 39–45.

Dimberg, U., Thunberg, M., & Elmehed, K. (2000). Unconscious facial reactions to emotional facial expressions. *Psychological Science, 11,* 86–89.

Fadiga, L., Fogassi, L., Pavesi, G., & Rizzolatti, G. (1995). Motor facilitation during action observation: A magnetic stimulation study. *Journal of Neurophysiology, 73,* 2608–2611.

Finkel, E. J., & Campbell, W. K. (2001). Self-control and accommodation in close relationships: An interdependence analysis. *Journal of Personality and Social Psychology, 81,* 263–277.

Finkel, E. J., Campbell, W. K., Brunell, A. B., Dalton, A. N., Chartrand, T. L., & Scarbeck, S. J. (2006). High-maintenance interaction: Inefficient social coordination impairs self-regulation. *Journal of Personality and Social Psychology, 91,* 456–475.

Friedman, H. S., & Riggio, R. (1981). The effect of individual differences in nonverbal expressiveness on transmission of emotion. *Journal of Nonverbal Behavior, 6,* 96–104.

Gallese, V., Fadiga, L., Fogassi, L., & Rizzolatti, G. (1996). Action recognition in the premotor cortex. *Brain, 119,* 593–609.

Giles, H., & Powesland, P. F. (1975). *Speech styles and social evaluation.* London: Academic Press.

Goldman, A., & Sripada, C. (2005). Simulationist models of face-based emotion recognition. *Cognition, 94,* 193–213.

Grahe, J. E., & Bernieri, F. J. (1999). The importance of nonverbal cues in judging rapport. *Journal of Nonverbal Behavior, 23,* 253–269.

Grossman, E., Donnelly, M., Price, R., Pickens, D., Morgan, V., Neighbor, G., et al. (2000). Brain areas involved in perception of biological motion. *Journal of Cognitive Neuroscience, 12,* 898–929.

Hatfield, E., Cacioppo, J., & Rapson, R. (1994). *Emotional contagion.* New York: Cambridge University Press.

Hsee, C. K., Hatfield, E., Carlson, J. G., & Chemtob, C. (1990). The effect of power on susceptibility to emotional contagion. *Cognition and Emotion, 4,* 327–340.

Iacoboni, M., Woods, R. P., Brass, M., Bekkering, H., Mazziotta, J. C., & Rizzolatti, G. (1999). Cortical mechanisms of human imitation. *Science, 286,* 2526–2528.

Jackson, P. L., Brunet, E., Meltzoff, A. N., & Decety, J. (2005). Empathy examined through the neural mechanisms involved in imagining how I feel versus how you feel pain. *Neuropsychologia, 44,* 752–761.

Jackson, P. L., & Decety, J. (2004). Motor cognition: A new paradigm to study self other interactions. *Current Opinion in Neurobiology, 14,* 259–263.

Jackson, P. L., Meltzoff, A. N., & Decety, J. (2006). Neural circuits involved in imitation and perspective-taking. *NeuroImage, 31,* 429–439.

James, W. (1890). *Principles of psychology.* New York: Holt.

Jeannerod, M. (1994). The representing brain: Neural correlates of motor intention and imagery. *Behavioral and Brain Sciences, 17,* 187–245.

Jeannerod, M. (1997). *The cognitive neuroscience of action.* Oxford: Blackwell.

Koski, L., Iacoboni, M., Dubeau, M., Woods, R. P., & Mazziotta, J. C. (2002). Modulation of cortical activity during different imitative behaviors. *Journal of Neurophysiology, 89,* 460–471.

Knoblich, G., & Flach, R. (2001). Predicting the effects of actions: Interactions of perception and action. *Psychological Science, 12,* 467–472.

Knoblich, G., & Prinz, W. (2001). Recognition of self-generated actions from kinematic displays of drawing. *Journal of Experimental Psychology: Human Perception and Performance, 27,* 456–465.

Knoblich, G., & Sebanz, N. (2006). The social nature of perception and action. *Current Directions in Psychological Science, 15,* 99–104.

Kraut, R. E., & Johnston, R. E. (1979). Social and emotional messages of smiling: An ethological approach. *Journal of Personality and Social Psychology, 37,* 1539–1553.

Kuhn, M. H., & McPartland, T. S. (1954). An empirical investigation of self-attitude. *American Sociological Review, 19,* 68–76.

LaFrance, M. (1979). Nonverbal synchrony and rapport: Analysis by the cross-lag panel technique. *Social Psychology Quarterly, 42,* 66–70.

LaFrance M. (1982). Posture mirroring and rapport. In M. Davis (Ed.), *Interaction rhythms: Periodicity in communicative behavior* (pp. 279–298). New York: Human Sciences Press.

LaFrance, M., & Broadbent, M. (1976). Group rapport: Posture sharing as a nonverbal indicator. *Group and Organization Studies, 1,* 328–333.

Lakin, J., & Chartrand, T. L. (2003). Using nonconscious behavioral mimicry to create affiliation and rapport. *Psychological Science, 14,* 334–339.

Lakin, J. L., Chartrand, T. L., & Arkin, R. M. (in press). *I am too just like you: The effects of ostracism on nonconscious mimicry.* Psychological Science.

Lakin, J. L., Jefferis, V. E., Cheng, C. M., & Chartrand, T. L. (2003). The chameleon effect as social glue: Evidence for the evolutionary significance of nonconscious mimicry. *Journal of Nonverbal Behavior, 27,* 145–162.

Leary, M. R. (Ed.). (2001). *Interpersonal rejection.* New York: Oxford University Press.

Leary, M. R., & Baumeister, R. F. (2000). The nature and function of self-esteem: Sociometer theory. In M. P. Zanna (Ed.), *Advances in experimental social psychology* (Vol. 32, pp. 1–62). San Diego, CA: Academic Press.

Lehmann, H. E. (1979). Yawning: A homeostatic reflex and its psychological significance. *Bulletin of the Menninger Clinic, 43,* 123–136.

Levelt, W. J. M., & Kelter, S. (1982). Surface form and memory in question answering. *Cognitive Psychology, 14,* 78–106.

Lundquist, L. O., & Dimberg, U. (1995). Facial expressions are contagious. *Journal of Psychophysiology, 9,* 203–211.

Maddux, W. W., Mullen, E., & Galinsky, A. (2008). Chameleons bake bigger pies: Strategic behavioral mimicry facilitates integrative negotiations outcomes. *Journal of Experimental Social Psychology, 44,* 461–468.

Matarazzo, J., & Wiens, A. (1972). *The interview: Research on its anatomy and structure.* Chicago: Aldine Atherton.

Maurer, R. E., & Tindall, J. H. (1983). Effect of postural congruence on client's perception of counselor empathy. *Journal of Counseling Psychology, 30,* 158–163.

Mead, G. H. (1967). *Mind, self, and society from the standpoint of a social behaviorist* (C. W. Morris, Ed.). Chicago: University of Chicago Press. (Original work published 1934)

Meltzoff, A. N., & Decety, J. (2003). What imitation tells us about social cognition: A rapprochement between developmental psychology and cognitive neuroscience. *Philosophical Transactions of the Royal Society of London. Series B. Biological Sciences, 358,* 491–500.

Meltzoff, A. N., & Moore, M. K. (1977). Imitation of facial and manual gestures by human neonates. *Science, 198,* 75–78.

Metzinger, T., & Gallese, V. (2003). The emergence of a shared action ontology: Building blocks for a theory. *Consciousness and Cognition, 12,* 549–571.

Musseler, J., & Hommel, B. (1997). Blindness to response-compatible stimuli. *Journal of Experimental Psychology: Human Perception and Performance, 23,* 861–872.

Mussweiler, T. (2003). Comparison processes in social judgment: Mechanisms and consequences. *Psychological Review, 110,* 472–489.

Neumann, R., & Strack, F. (2000). "Mood contagion": The automatic transfer of mood between persons. *Journal of Personality and Social Psychology, 79,* 211–223.

O'Toole, R., & Dubin, R. (1968). Baby feeding and body sway: An experiment in George Herbert Mead's "Taking the role of the other." *Journal of Personality and Social Psychology, 10,* 59–65.

Paus, T., Petrides, M., Evans, A. C., & Meyer, E. (1993). Role of human anterior cingulate cortex in the control of oculomotor, manual, and speech responses: A positron emission tomography study. *Journal of Neurophysiology, 70,* 453–469.

Platek, S. M., Critton, S. R., Myers, T. E., & Gallup, G. G., Jr. (2003). Contagious yawning: The role of self-awareness and mental state attribution. *Cognitive Brain Research, 17,* 223–227.

Platek, S. M., Mohamed, F. B., & Gallup, G. G., Jr. (2005). Contagious yawning and the brain. *Cognitive Brain Research, 23,* 448–452.

Preston, S. D., & de Waal, F. B. M. (2002). Empathy: Its ultimate and proximate bases. *Behavioral and Brain Science, 25,* 1–72.

Prinz, W. (1990). A common coding approach to perception and action. In O. Neumann & W. Prinz (Eds.), *Relationships between perception and action* (pp. 167–201). Berlin: Springer-Verlag.

Prinz, W. (1997). Perception and action planning. *European Journal of Cognitive Psychology, 9,* 129–154.

Provine, R. R. (1986). Yawning as a stereotypical action pattern and releasing stimulus. *Ethology, 71,* 109–122.

Repp, B. H. (1987). The sound of two hands clapping: An exploratory study. *Journal of the Acoustical Society of American, 81,* 1100–1109.

Rizzolatti, G., & Craighero, L. (2004). The mirror neuron system. *Annual Review of Neuroscience, 27,* 169–192.

Rizzolatti, G., Fogassi, L., & Gallese, V. (2001). Neurophysiological mechanisms underlying the understanding and imitation of action. *Nature Reviews: Neuroscience, 2,* 661–670.

Ruby, P., & Decety, J. (2001). Effect of subjective perspective taking during simulation of action: A PET investigation of agency. *Nature Neuroscience, 4,* 546–550.

Rumiati, R. I., & Bekkering, H. (2003). To imitate or not to imitate: How the brain can do it, that is the question. *Brain and Cognition, 53,* 479–482.

Samson, D., Apperly, I. A., Kathirgamanathan, U., & Humphreys, G. W. (2005). Seeing it my way:

A case of a selective deficit in inhibiting self-perspective. *Brain, 128,* 1102–1111.

Scheflen, A. E. (1964). The significance of posture in communication systems. *Psychiatry, 27,* 316–331.

Schwarz, N., & Clore, G. L. (1996). Feelings and phenomenal experiences. In E. T. Higgins & A. Kruglanski (Eds.), *Social psychology: Handbook of basic principles* (pp. 433–465). New York: Guilford Press.

Sebanz, N., Knoblich, G., & Prinz, W. (2003). Representing others' actions: Just like one's own? *Cognition, 88,* B11–B21.

Simner, M. L. (1971). Newborn's response to the cry of another infant. *Developmental Psychology, 5,* 136–150.

Simon, H. A. (1990). A mechanism for social selection and successful altruism. *Science, 250,* 1665–1668.

Sullins, E. S. (1991). Emotional contagion revisited: Effects of social comparison and expressive style on mood convergence. *Personality and Social Psychology Bulletin, 17,* 166–174.

Tanner, R., Ferraro, R., Chartrand, T. L., Bettman, J. & van Baaren, R. (2008). The convincing chameleon: The impact of mimicry on persuasion. *Journal of Consumer Research, 34,* 754–766.

Termine, N. T., & Izard, C. E. (1988). Infants' responses to their mothers' expressions of joy and sadness. *Developmental Psychology, 24,* 223–229.

Tickle-Degnen, L., & Rosenthal, R. (1990). The nature of rapport and its nonverbal correlates. *Psychological Inquiry, 1,* 285–293.

Uldall, B., Hall, C., & Chartrand, T. (2008). *Optimal distinctiveness and mimicry.* Manuscript in preparation.

van Baaren, R. B., Fockenberg, D. A., Holland, R. W., Janssen, L., & van Knippenberg, A. (2006). The moody chameleon: The effect of mood on nonconscious mimicry. *Social Cognition, 24,* 426–437.

van Baaren, R. B., Holland, R. W., Kawakami, K., & van Knippenberg, A. (2004). Mimicry and pro-social behavior. *Psychological Science, 15,* 71–74.

van Baaren, R. B., Holland, R. W., Steenaert, B., & van Knippenberg, A. (2003). Mimicry for money: Behavioral consequences of imitation. *Journal of Experimental Social Psychology, 39,* 393–398.

van Baaren, R. B., Horgan, T. G., Chartrand, T. L., & Dijkmans, M. (2004). The forest, the trees and the chameleon: Context-dependency and mimicry. *Journal of Personality and Social Psychology, 86,* 453–459.

van Baaren, R. B., Maddux, W. W., Chartrand, T. L., De Bouter, C., & van Knippenberg, A. (2003). It takes two to mimic: Behavioral consequences of self-construals. *Journal of Personality and Social Psychology, 84,* 1093–1102.

van Swol, L. M. (2003). The effects of nonverbal mirroring on perceived persuasiveness, agreement with an imitator, and reciprocity in a group discussion. *Communication Research, 30,* 461–480.

van Swol, L. M., & Drury, S. (2007a). Mimicry and persuasion. Unpublished raw data.

van Swol, L. M., & Drury, S. (2007b). Mimicry and persuasion II. Unpublished raw data.

Wallbott, H. G. (1991). Recognition of emotion from facial expression via imitation? Some indirect evidence for an old theory. *British Journal of Social Psychology, 30,* 207–219.

Webb, J. T. (1969). Subject speech rates as a function of interviewer behaviour. *Language and Speech, 12,* 54–67.

Williams, K. D., Cheung, C., & Choi, W. (2000). Cyberostracism: Effects of being ignored over the internet. *Journal of Personality and Social Psychology, 79,* 748–762.

Zajonc, R. B., Adelmann, K. A., Murphy, S. T., & Niedenthal, P. M. (1987). Convergence in the physical appearance of spouses. *Motivation and Emotion, 11,* 335–346.

PART 6

Control, Choice, and Volition

23 Free Willpower: A Limited Resource Theory of Volition, Choice, and Self-Regulation

Roy F. Baumeister, Matthew T. Gailliot, *and* Dianne M. Tice

Abstract

This chapter focuses on the conscious, controlled processes corresponding to free will. It is argued that the traditional folk notions of willpower and character strength have some legitimate basis in genuine phenomena. The very idea of free will, though controversial at some exalted levels of metaphysical debate, may be grounded in the fact that some behaviors do emerge from a difficult and costly inner process that differs from the simpler, more common way of behaving.

Keywords: free will, action control, controlled process, behavior

How does action occur? For centuries, thinkers have struggled to answer that question on the basis of shifting assumptions. The idea of free will, though now rather in disfavor, expressed the popular and philosophical view that behavior reflects the outcome of a struggle between an autonomous, relatively virtuous, possibly spiritual self and the baser forces of external demand and inner cravings. The assumption that two different processes battle it out to determine action has been fundamental in theological views, such as in beliefs about the judgment of individual souls based on whether they chose virtuous or sinful acts. Likewise, it is central to some modern legal judgments that assign punishment not just on the basis of the action and its (criminal) consequences but also on the supposed state of mind of the perpetrator—reserving lesser punishments for crimes committed in

mental states (including passionate anger, fear, intoxication, interpersonal influence, and legally defined insanity) that supposedly reduce the capacity of the nobler part of the self to restrain the wickeder impulses so as to do the right thing.

Modern psychological thought rejected many traditional ways of thinking about action control but has seen a revival of some of these. Early behaviorism embraced a style of explanation based on stimulus and response, as if that ought to be sufficient. That simple theoretical model came to be seen as inadequate to account for the complexity of (especially human) behavior, whereas a more cognitive behaviorism accepted the importance of inner processes mediating between stimulus and response, such as the recognition that how a person responds to an ambiguous remark or task failure depends on how the person interprets it. Perhaps ironically, the blossoming interest in inner processes has shifted attention away from the study of action, and most social psychology articles today simply assess ratings of thoughts, feelings, and attitudes (Baumeister, Vohs, & Funder, 2007). In a sense, the study of inner processes that was originally intended to illuminate behavior has now come to replace the study of behavior. Nonetheless, to the extent that modern psychologists do discuss behavior, they accept the distinctions between automatic and controlled processes, or conscious and nonconscious ones (e.g., Lieberman, Gaunt, Gilbert, & Trope, 2002; Smith & DeCoster, 1999, 2000). Behavior can thus result from at least two very different kinds of inner processes. Yet most of the work on that distinction focuses on automaticity. Bargh's (1994) classic paper identified "four horsemen of automaticity," and even though three of the four criteria named in the title actually referred to controlled rather than automatic processes, the emphasis there as elsewhere has been on automatic processes.

Thus, in a nutshell (i.e., to oversimplify), the major approach to explaining behavior in modern social psychology emphasizes automatic, nonconscious determinants of behavior. Conscious processes are regarded with suspicion, with the prominent exception of emotion. That is, emotion is widely regarded as an important direct cause of behavior, as indicated by the high frequency with which researchers report tests of emotion as mediator (so that conscious emotion is regarded as a likely direct cause of behavior). We think that emotion is a poor champion of the ability of conscious processes to direct action. While preparing their review article, Baumeister, Vohs, DeWall, and Zhang (2007) tallied 176 statistical tests for mediation by emotion in the *Journal of Personality and Social Psychology* from January 2002 to July 2005. Only 18% of these tests were significant at the .05 level. Moreover, the dependent variables for many of the successful mediation analyses were cognitions rather than behaviors. In other words, emotion is frequently tested but rarely confirmed as a proximal (mediating) cause of behavior. Thus, even the one conscious process that is popularly regarded as important for causing behavior turns out not to be very successful after all. The central conclusion of the review by Baumeister et al. (2007) was that the direct causation of behavior is not the main function of conscious emotion, even though it is widely assumed to be.

Emotion may be conscious, but it is not controlled, which may explain why researchers have been comfortable studying it as a possible cause of behavior (see Chapter 14). Full control of action suggests the concept of free will, which some researchers reject on theoretical grounds as hard to describe and therefore nonexistent. Others who accept the possibility of free will may think it is nonetheless not worth studying because insofar as people can freely choose to do anything, there would be no regular patterns in behavior that could be translated into significant findings, journal publications, and career advancement. In other words, even where free will might exist, many researchers assume that it is useless as a topic of scientific study.

The purpose of this chapter is to provide an overview of our research program, which has focused on the neglected sibling in action control—that is, the conscious, controlled processes. We do not mean to criticize the strong focus on automatic, nonconscious processes or the fine body of research it has yielded. We seek only to complement it with some effort to understand how the controlled, effortful form of action control operates.

Put in terms of free will, we accept that considerable evidence has shown that people's behavior is causally influenced by factors outside of their awareness and volition (e.g., Wegner, 2002; Chapter 27). Yet perhaps not all conscious volition is an illusion. Our findings suggest that the traditional folk notions of willpower and character strength have some legitimate basis in genuine phenomena. The very idea of free will, though controversial at some exalted levels of metaphysical debate, may be grounded in the fact that some behaviors do emerge from a difficult and costly inner process that differs from the simpler, more common way of behaving.

Definitions

We understand self-regulation as the self's capacity for altering the self. To regulate is to change, so self-regulation entails attempts (at least) to change some aspect of the self. The most common form of self-regulation involves overriding and restraining an impulse so as not to act on it (see Chapters 3 and 30). Baumeister, Heatherton, and Tice (1994) estimated that about 90% of self-regulation is what they called self-stopping, as in preventing oneself from overeating, from acting aggressively, from spending too much money, or from consuming alcohol or drugs (either totally or beyond some limit) and in other ways preventing an action.

The view of self-regulation as altering the self may seem different from treatments of it as goal-directed or standard-guided behavior, but the difference is mainly one of emphasis. Carver and Scheier (1981) treated self-awareness processes as central to self-regulation insofar as it involves comparing oneself to standards, and they borrowed the idea of feedback loops from cybernetic theory (e.g., Powers, 1973) to describe this process. The TOTE acronym for feedback loops characterizes the process as test, operate, test, exit, with the self-aware testing step consisting of appraising the self and comparing it to the standard.

Those authors paid less attention to how the self-changing operations are actually carried out. Our emphasis on changing the self corresponds to the "operate" phase in their scheme.

We use the terms *self-control* and *self-regulation* interchangeably, although in recent years there has been rising usage of a subtle distinction. Specifically, "self-control" is often used to refer specifically to conscious, effortful forms of self-regulation (which are in fact our focus). There can, however, be nonconscious and relatively automatic acts of self-regulation, and these, being automatic, are not called self-control. The nonconscious forms of self-regulation may follow different causal principles and do not rely on the same resources as the conscious and effortful ones. Put more simply, nonconscious self-regulation does not require willpower (or not nearly as much). We readily acknowledge its existence and value, but our work has been devoted to understanding the conscious and effortful processes, to which both terms (self-regulation and self-control) are applicable.

From their survey of the published literature, Baumeister et al. (1994) observed that self-regulation has mainly been studied in the following four large spheres. *Emotion regulation* involves the effort to initiate, prolong, or escape from a particular emotional state, with the most common being the attempt to get out of a bad mood or distressing feeling (Thayer, 1996). *Thought control* involves regulating cognitive processes, including directing attention to or away from a particular idea (most notably suppressing unwanted thoughts; Wegner, 1989), as well as guiding inference and decision processes toward particular outcomes (Baumeister & Newman, 1994). *Impulse control* involves directing behavior on the basis of desires and cravings, with the most common form being efforts to restrain oneself from acting on socially or personally unacceptable wishes, such as aggressive or sexual impulses and cravings for problematic foods or substances. Finally, *performance management* involves the attempt to bring one's task performance into line with various standards, and these efforts include persisting in the face of failure, overcoming fatigue or distractions, maintaining optimal performance despite pressures, and the like.

"Free will" is itself a contentious term and even to use it is to invite skepticism if not indignant contempt. Our use of the term is not intended to make metaphysical claims. Rather, like the term "willpower," we borrow a colloquial expression that we think calls attention to a real empirical difference. In other words, we are not arguing that people have free will in the most exalted sense of the term—only that there are at least two different ways of acting, one of which is appropriately regarded as freer than the other. Freedom entails not being the inevitable result of causes, especially causes located outside the person and previously in time. Our analysis is consistent with that of Kant (1797/1967): Unfree action is driven by external responses, whereas freedom, to the extent that it is real, involves acting on the basis of one's own moral reasoning reflected in unconstrained choosing.

Philosophical treatments of free will typically invoke two major types of phenomena (e.g., Dennett, 1984, 2003; Kane, 2002). One is self-control, as in doing the morally right thing and resisting temptation. The other is rational choice. Rational choice is a well-recognized aspect of human behavior. In fact, it is the predominant approach in several social sciences such as political science and economics. As Searle (2001) has contended, however, rationality, defined as the ability to use logical reasoning to evaluate different options and reach an objectively correct conclusion as to which is best, would be useless without

at least a modicum of free will. (Otherwise, the person could figure out what would be best to do but then not be able to do it.) Free will in the sense of being able to alter one's behavior on the basis of cognitive appraisals and inferences is thus an important contributor to human rationality.

In other words, we think that the current and sometimes hostile debates about free will arise because two sides talk past each other on the basis of very different definitions. Those most hostile to the notion of free will insist on regarding it as a random action, independent of all circumstances and external factors. Those more sympathetic to the idea (including us) emphasize rational choice and self-control. Baumeister (2008) proposed that, seemingly paradoxically, the evolution of free will probably cultivated it for the sake of improving the capacity to follow rules than for the capacity to act in random, unpredictable ways.

Benefits of Self-Regulation and Rationality

In order to argue that natural selection would have favored the emergence of free will, it is necessary to show that it confers advantages. This can be done by considering self-regulation and rationality as the two main types of free will.

In recent years, evidence has accumulated steadily for the benefits of self-regulation, though naturally these are mainly studied in the context of modern society rather than those of our evolutionary past. Still, the list is impressive. Most of the problems that afflict individuals and society these days involve failures of self-control in some sense: addiction, crime, violence, unwanted pregnancy, obesity, debt, smoking, failure to exercise, lack of savings, sexually transmitted diseases, underachievement, gambling, and the rest (e.g., Baumeister et al., 1994; Gottfredson & Hirschi, 1990). Good self-control predicts good relationships, adjustment, mental and physical health, and academic success (Mischel, Shoda, & Peake, 1988; Shoda, Mischel, & Peake, 1990; Tangney, Baumeister, & Boone, 2004). Some of these benefits are covered in greater detail later in this chapter.

As for rational choice, its benefits seem to be taken for granted without requiring empirical documentation. Perhaps researchers find that journal editors are not willing to publish articles that show people fare better when they act rationally as opposed to stupidly. In any case, intelligence has been shown to predict career success (positively) across an astonishingly broad range of professions, from scientist to waitress and janitor (Jensen, 1998). The superior ability to make rational choices is presumably linked to that success.

Given that both self-regulation and rational choice seem likely to provide substantial benefits, it would not be surprising that natural selection might have favored early humans who showed any signs of these. In particular, living in a human culture requires people to conform to social rules and offers them enough information to increase the beneficial effects of rational choice, so human evolution may in particular have promoted these forms of free will (see Baumeister, 2005, 2008). For readers who object to the usage of the term "free will," it may be more acceptable to propose that recent evolution selected in favor of individuals who could continually modify their behaviors by self-regulation and rational choice. This chapter is concerned with how that novel, difficult, but highly adaptive style of action control operates.

Self-Regulation and Limited Resource

Our own interest in willpower began with a survey of the research on self-regulation (Baumeister et al., 1994). An open-minded reading of that scattered literature led to the impression that self-control sometimes seemed to operate like a limited resource or muscle. In particular, when there were demands on that resource, self-control seemed then and afterward to lose some of its power and effectiveness. The idea of volition as using some energy ("willpower") thus gained plausibility as one possible explanation for how people control themselves.

Laboratory experiments provided further evidence that self-regulation depends on a limited resource. In these initial studies, participants engaged in initial self-control tasks, such as trying to stifle or amplify their emotional responses to films or to suppress forbidden thoughts. Afterward, these participants showed decrements in other (quite different) self-control tasks, such as persisting in the face of failure (Muraven, Tice, & Baumeister, 1998). In one vivid demonstration, hungry participants were instructed to resist the temptation to eat chocolates and cookies and to eat radishes instead. Afterward, they gave up much faster on a discouraging, frustrating task involving unsolvable geometric puzzles (Baumeister, Bratslavsky, Muraven, & Tice, 1998). Control condition participants whose initial task did not require self-control performed relatively better on the second task. The implication was that the first self-control task depleted some vital resource that was then unavailable to facilitate performance on the second task.

These initial studies pointed to two further conclusions beyond the mere validity of the idea of willpower. First, the same resource appears to be used for very different acts and forms of self-regulation. We noted earlier that Baumeister et al. (1994) identified four main spheres of self-regulation (emotion regulation, thought control, impulse control, and performance management). The laboratory studies on depletion routinely crossed these boundaries and effects carried over from one to another. For example, one study might manipulate impulse control and then measure performance management, and another might manipulate thought control and then measure emotion regulation (Baumeister et al., 1998; Muraven et al., 1998). A priori, it was possible that different forms and spheres of self-control depended on completely different processes, but these findings suggest that all draw on a common resource. That is, the same stock of willpower is used for dragging oneself out of bed in the morning, saying no to a second piece of pie, holding one's tongue when talking with an obnoxious neighbor, blocking a tiresome tune from running through one's mind, and making oneself stay at the computer until the report is done.

Second, the resource appears to be highly limited. When Muraven first proposed conducting experimental tests of the limited resource idea, based on his reading of our 1994 book, some of us had doubts as to whether a one-shot laboratory study could find significant results. We thought perhaps that willpower depletion would be evident only in hugely demanding, real-world situations, when an onslaught of overwhelming demands such as final examinations or crash diets would consume so much willpower that the effects would show up elsewhere. Obviously, we were wrong. Laboratory participants showed effects of depletion after just a few minutes of a seemingly easy self-regulation task, such as trying not to think about a white bear.

The fact that depletion effects occur so readily points to another important distinction. The subjective experience of feeling depleted may not be essential to getting its effects. To be sure, when people have exhausted themselves in acts of self-discipline or effortful exertion, they may have both the subjective experience of being depleted and the underlying physiological fact of depletion. But the underlying physiological reality apparently is sufficient to cause

behavioral effects long before it shows up in subjective feelings of being exhausted or depleted.

It is important not to overstate how limited the resource is. Depletion effects do not indicate that the resource has been fully exhausted. Rather, behavioral effects appear when the resource is just partly depleted (a point to which we return shortly). More broadly, the human capacity for self-regulation seems far greater than what has been observed in other animals but perhaps far less than what many human ideals and moral systems might require. One can justly admire the immense flexibility and discipline with which people alter their behavior to suit an astonishing array of standards—and one can with equal correctness bemoan the widespread lack of self-discipline as indicated by self-indulgence, debt, impulsivity, laziness, sin, and other failings. With willpower, in other words, the glass is both half full and half empty.

Choice Depletes Willpower

If willpower were solely used for self-regulation, it would already be an important aspect of the self because self-regulation is highly adaptive and contributes to the immense flexibility of human behavior. But recent work suggests that the same resource is used for both self-regulation and effortful choice.

An early finding linking self-regulation to choice was provided by Baumeister et al. (1998). Borrowing from research on cognitive dissonance (e.g., Linder, Cooper, & Jones, 1967), they had some participants deliberately choose to make a counterattitudinal speech in favor of a big tuition increase. Other participants were simply assigned the same topic without choice. Afterward, participants performed an ostensibly irrelevant task that measured persistence in the face of failure. Participants who had made the choice to make that speech gave up significantly faster than those in the no-choice control condition. Although there were potential alternate explanations based on dissonance processes and other possibilities, this finding at least suggested that making a deliberate choice depleted some vital resource that would otherwise have been used for self-regulation of performance.

A long series of further studies by Vohs, Baumeister, Schmeichel, Twenge, Nelson, and Tice (2008) has confirmed that choice depletes willpower. The approach was stimulated by Twenge's recollection of her bridal registry: After spending several hours making choices about what pattern and style to have on her future soup spoons, gravy boats, and countless other items, she recalled feeling exhausted and depleted.

In the various studies in this investigation, participants were first induced to make many small choices, such as between psychology course options or between consumer items. No-choice condition participants viewed the same items, thought about them, and made ratings of them, but they did not choose among them. Afterward, self-regulation was measured in a variety of ways, and it consistently showed decrements among the participants who had made choices (relative to the no-choice controls). They quit faster on the cold pressor task (i.e., holding one's hand in ice water), they ate more cookies but drank less bad-tasting beverage, they solved fewer math problems, and the like. A field study found that shoppers at a mall who had made more decisions during their shopping trip quit faster on a difficult task (multiplication problems) even after controlling for gender, socioeconomic status, amount of money spent, and amount of time already spent at the mall.

Thus, making choices affects subsequent self-regulation. It works the other direction, too: Depletion caused by self-regulation can alter decision making. Pocheptsova, Amir, Dhar, and Baumeister (in press) had participants engage in an initial self-control task, such as the Stroop task or a simple attention-control exercise, after which they were given a decision-making problem. Three main findings emerged.

First, depleted participants were more inclined to postpone or avoid making any decision as long as they had the option of not deciding. This finding supports the view that choosing is effortful because it shows that depleted participants preferred to avoid choosing.

Second, when they chose along a continuum, depleted participants were more likely to choose extremes rather than compromise. The implication is that compromise is a more effortful kind of decision because it requires integrating multiple criteria, whereas a simpler style of choosing merely attends to one dimension and selects the option that maximizes it (e.g., picking the cheapest; see Simonson, 1989).

Third, depleted participants were more susceptible to the so-called attraction or asymmetric dominance effect (Huber, Payne, & Puto, 1982). This is an irrational style of choosing in which the chooser is swayed by an unappealing "decoy" option to select another option near it. To illustrate, consider a choice between two apartments: an expensive one that is conveniently close to one's workplace and a cheaper one that entails a relatively long commute. Suppose these are sufficiently well balanced that half the people choose the one and half choose the other. Now imagine another decision that includes the same two options plus a so-called decoy. The decoy is much like the first apartment, being expensive and convenient—but it is a little bit more expensive and a bit less convenient than the first option. Clearly, it would be stupid to choose this option, and in fact no participants do. Logically, however, once they have ruled out this option, participants should be back to the same place as those who faced the original form of the dilemma, namely, choosing between the other two options. Therefore, one would expect the same breakdown of preferences (as we said, 50–50). What Huber et al. (1982) observed, however, was that participants who faced the three-way decision were affected by the decoy even though nobody selected it. They were significantly more likely to choose the first apartment than the second. Somehow having the decoy option in the mix ended up making them choose the option that "dominated" (hence the term "asymmetric dominance") the decoy.

In essence, the decision problem in these studies involves one easy decision and one hard decision, and the irrational but tempting course is to let the easy decision also guide the hard decision. Pocheptsova et al. (in press) replicated this pattern but found that it was significantly stronger among depleted than among nondepleted participants.

Taken together, the results of the Pocheptsova et al. (in press) studies show that depletion shifts decision makers toward more simplistic, less effortful ways of choosing.

To be sure, some decisions are more depleting than others. Moller, Deci, and Ryan (2006) showed that choosing to do what you clearly want to do over an unattractive alternative is not depleting. Novemsky and Baumeister (2006) measured self-regulation after participants had made one of several different hypothetical decisions. All the decisions involved trade-offs among different criteria, a type of decision that people generally find difficult and aversive (Luce, Bettman, & Payne, 1997). In some cases, however, the decision was set up such that there was an optimal choice, such as one for which a small increase in price yielded a very large increase in quality (and beyond which further price increases yielded minimal gains

in quality). These were less depleting than ones that were "true" trade-offs in the sense that there was no optimal choice point. When people can quickly find the right answer or best option, the decision process is apparently less depleting than when all options are about equally appealing.

Thus, self-regulation affects choice, and choice affects self-regulation, even when the choices and the self-regulation seemingly have nothing to do with each other. The effects occur because both deplete a common resource needed for both. These findings are important for the theory of free will. We noted earlier that philosophical discussions of free will typically involve two types of examples, namely, self-control and rational choice. Our laboratory work has shown that the two are linked. Both self-control and choice depend on and consume the same resource. (Rationality, as in intelligent reasoning, also uses the same resource, a fact to which we will return in the section on applications.)

The fact that the same resource was used for effortful choice as for self-regulation moved us to replace our initial term "regulatory depletion" with the broader "ego depletion." The allusion to ego was in homage to Freud, who was one of the last and only psychological theorists to propose that energy processes are important in the functioning of the self. For more than half a century after Freud's death, self theory was dominated by cognitive processes (e.g., self-esteem and self-concept). Cognitions are certainly important, but apparently the self also operates on the basis of a kind of limited energy resource that is expended during its most important and effortful actions.

The overarching idea behind this work is that evolution furnished the human mind with a relatively new, distinctive and possibly unique, powerful way of choosing. New findings on memory for choices provides further evidence that there are at least two different processes for choosing. These studies focused on memory for choices, and they support the conclusion that a depleted self chooses differently from a nondepleted self. The Pocheptsova et al. (in press) studies showed that the outcome of the choice is different as a function of whether the person is depleted or not. Studies by Schmeichel, Gailliot, and Baumeister (2005) have shown that the different ways of choosing leave different memory traces.

The first finding by Schmeichel et al. (2005) was that, under normal conditions, the self remembers its own choices especially well. This went beyond the self-reference effect (Rogers, Kuiper, & Kirker, 1977) and related effects because all items were chosen for the self and thus had self-reference. Even so, people remembered what they chose for themselves better than what someone else chose for them. Apparently, the process of choosing leaves a strong memory trace, consistent with the assumption that it requires a costly and effortful process.

More important, the self-choice effect did not occur when participants were depleted. The implication is that the depleted self chooses via a more casual, superficial, heuristic, or otherwise incompletely rational process that accordingly leaves a much weaker memory trace. Moreover, this did not appear to reflect the direct impact of self-regulation on memory retrieval (which had in fact been the original hypothesis for the investigation of Schmeichel et al., 2005) because when the depletion manipulation was administered after participants had made their choices, their memory for their choices was still quite good. Nor did it appear to reflect different outcomes of choices. In essence, then, participants faced the same choices and selected the same options, but when they did this after self-regulatory depletion, they remembered the outcomes less well than normally. Thus, there are different pathways to choosing, one of which leaves a much stronger memory trace than the other.

What Gets Depleted?

As mentioned earlier, we adopted the somewhat Freudian term "ego depletion" because Freud had spoken about the self (ego) in energy terms. But Freud's usage of energy terms and concepts remained the vaguest of metaphors, and he never felt it necessary to measure or document any actual, physical quantities of energy. Our initial usage of energy terms was comparably metaphoric, but we certainly anticipated wanting eventually to provide a physiological dimension to our theories.

To be sure, the cognitively oriented Zeitgeist dictated that we wondered first whether the appearance of energy depletion would eventually turn out to be a cognitive process after all. Possibly participants responded to our so-called depletion manipulations, in which they engaged in preliminary acts of self-control, by inferring that they were poor at self-control or by losing a sense of self-efficacy. Such theories were addressed directly by Wallace and Baumeister (2002). They measured self-efficacy and found it unchanged by the manipulations and unrelated to depletion effects. They also manipulated feedback about success and failure on the first self-control task so that some participants were led to regard themselves as good at self-control and others as poor, but these manipulations had no impact on the behavioral outcomes. These findings lent further support to the energy model.

None of this means that cognitions are irrelevant. Later we review evidence that intelligent performance is systematically impaired during ego depletion (Schmeichel, Vohs, & Baumeister, 2003). Moreover, fascinating work by Vohs and Schmeichel (2003) has established that depletion is marked by alterations in the subjective flow of time, creating a kind of "extended now" in which the present moment seems to last longer than usual, while past and future awareness is diminished.

Another alternative explanation was that the initial exercise depleted participants' willingness to exert themselves for the experiment. In fact, over the years, this alternative has been the most common and popular one among reviewers and other critics of the research. The gist is that signing up for an experiment entails a kind of implicit contract by which the participant consents to undergo a certain amount of exertion, unpleasantness, or other obligation. The first self-control task in our study is generally an unpleasant one, so participants might feel that by the time they complete it, they have done enough to satisfy their implicit contract. Hence, they are less willing to put forth their best effort on the second task (the dependent measure).

Several findings cast severe doubt on the implicit contract explanation. Muraven et al. (1998) still found depletion effects after eliminating the difference in the unpleasantness in the first task: Specifically, the depleting task involved writing one's thoughts while suppressing thoughts of a white bear, while the control task involved three-digit multiplication problems. If anything, the multiplication was regarded as more unpleasant than the thought suppression exercise, but only the thought suppression exercise produced a depletion effect. Another relevant finding was by Baumeister et al. (1998) in which depleted participants willingly sat longer than nondepleted ones in front of a boring movie. If the depletion manipulation had exhausted participants' goodwill or satisfied their implicit sense of obligation, then they should have left the experiment sooner rather than later. (Additional findings that are difficult to reconcile with the implicit contract explanation are

reviewed by Baumeister, Gailliot, DeWall, & Oaten, 2006.)

A direct test of the implicit contract and exhausted goodwill theory was undertaken by Gailliot, Baumeister, et al. (2007; though this particular study was deleted from the final, published version of the article). This study sought to offset depletion by allowing participants a pleasant indulgence. More precisely, the initial depletion manipulation was followed by giving some participants a tasty milkshake made with ice cream. It succeeded, and participants who ate the ice cream (which in principle ought to restore their sense of goodwill and obligation to exert themselves for the rest of the study) did in fact persist longer on the unsolvable search task than depleted participants who did not get any snack and merely spent the same interval reading magazines. Unfortunately for the implicit contract theory, however, the design included a second control in which participants consumed a neutral-tasting, joyless shake made with Half & Half rather than ice cream. Although there was no pleasure to be had in consuming that shake, it nonetheless counteracted the depletion manipulation such that participants persisted just as long on the subsequent task as participants in the delicious (ice cream) milkshake condition.

Our initial reaction to the Half & Half condition was disappointment because it clearly spoke against the hypothesis that a pleasurable indulgence would offset the effects of ego depletion. But then we began to reflect on what might have caused that surprising result. If it was not the pleasure or goodwill, could it have been the calories?

The idea that ego depletion is a matter of depleting energy from food had a certain appeal. As we said, psychologists had long since stopped using energy models to make their theories, but the resurgence of biological thinking into psychology during the 1990s had made energy models plausible in a new way. After all, the human body is undeniably an energy-consuming system, and indeed life itself is in part a process of energy transactions. All psychological processes involve some kind of brain activity, which is itself a matter of electrical energy.

In particular, glucose is fuel for the brain. In essence, the body ingests food, extracts and processes its energy so as to put glucose into the bloodstream, and then consumes this glucose wherever it requires energy, including the brain (and muscles, of course). A review of the glucose research literature by Gailliot and Baumeister (2007a) found abundant suggestive support for a link between glucose and self-control. Specifically, both acute and chronic glucose deficiencies are associated with self-control problems. For example, samples of criminals have been found to have elevated rates of glucose abnormalities, children who skip breakfast have poorer attention control and more behavior problems in school, higher (complex) cognitive processes have been shown to consume a significant amount of blood glucose and to deteriorate when glucose is lacking, diabetics tend to have poorer attention control and emotion control deficits, and manipulations of glucose tend to yield significant changes in behavior, such as when improving the diet of incarcerated convicts yields a notable reduction in violent and disciplinary incidents.

Three main sets of findings from further laboratory experiments by Gailliot, Baumeister, et al. (2007) cemented the link between glucose and ego depletion. First, exerting self-control resulted in significant reductions in blood glucose afterward. Second, the lower the blood glucose level after the first self-control task, the poorer the self-control performance on the second task. Third, manipulations of glucose level (accomplished by administering a glass of lemonade made with sugar as compared to similar-tasting but glucose-free lemonade made with a sugar substitute) repeatedly counteracted depletion manipulations.

We do not wish to claim that glucose dynamics are the only aspect of ego depletion. But they appear to be a significant part of it. Glucose in the bloodstream is a vital part of the body's (and the brain's) energy supply, and acts of self-control consume significant amounts of it. When it is low, further attempts at self-regulation are impaired.

The broader implication is that willpower is more than a metaphor. Glucose provides the power in willpower. We even have some recent data suggesting that the degraded patterns of decision making that depleted people show can be counteracted by administering a dose of glucose (Masicampo & Baumeister, 2008).

We may then begin to speculate about what the evolution of executive control processes (i.e., free will) entailed. Our animal ancestors essentially had automatic, nonconscious styles of choosing and acting. In retrofitting the primate psyche to make a cultural being, evolution found a way to use the body's energy in a new way of choosing. This second pathway may be biologically expensive, so it can only be used occasionally, but it permits a great improvement in flexibility and adaptability of individual behavior. In particular, its evolutionary emergence permitted a dramatic improvement in self-control and rational choice.

Empowering Self-Control

Self-regulation and rational choice—free will—constitute an important and very adaptive dimension of human action control. Ego depletion will reduce people's ability to make use of these, with potentially harmful or costly effects on behavior. Therefore, an important class of practical questions is concerned with how to boost free will, either as chronic improvement in willpower or at least counteracting the short-term depredations caused by ego depletion. We have identified a variety of factors that appear to help. These can be sorted into short-term interventions that counteract ego depletion and long-term effects that seek to create lasting improvement in self-control.

Short-Term Boosts

Motivation can help. Muraven (1998; see also Muraven & Slessareva, 2003) offered participants cash incentives for performing well on a second self-control task after they were depleted by the first task. (For example, in one study, after an initial manipulation of depletion versus no depletion, participants were offered 25 cents for each ounce of a bad-tasting vinegar-based beverage they consumed.) Depleted participants responded remarkably well to the incentive as indicated by very good performance. Thus, a motivational incentive can offset the effects of depletion.

Some researchers responded to the motivation findings by concluding that ego depletion is essentially a motivational deficit. We do not find that interpretation compelling (especially in light of the glucose findings noted previously). An analogy with physical, muscular strength is helpful. Muscles do become physiologically fatigued after exertion, so athletic performance tends to get worse as people get tired. A motivational incentive (such as a crucial goal-line play) can cause even tired athletes to perform at a high level again. But that does not mean that tiredness is merely a matter of reduced motivation. Muscles really do get tired. As with any resource, people may spend it freely when it is abundant, and they use it more sparingly when it is partly depleted—but even sparing use allows for a liberal expenditure when something especially important is at stake.

The view that ego depletion involves managing a limited resource rather than simply losing interest or motivation gains further credibility from studies on conservation. Muraven (1998; see also Muraven, Shmueli, & Burkley, 2006) showed that people conserve their limited resources when anticipating further demands on them. These procedures essentially involved three tasks: a first one to manipulate depletion, a second one that was the crucial measure, and a third, anticipated one that the participant was told would place demands on self-control. Depleted participants withheld effort on the second task when they anticipated needing to exert self-control on the third one. All these findings fit very well with the view of depletion as the consumption of a limited resource such as glucose.

Motivation may also account for the role of emotion. A series of studies by Tice, Baumeister, Shmueli, and Muraven (2007) included conditions in which depletion manipulations were followed by procedures aimed at inducing positive emotion (such as by having participants watch a brief comedy video). These also offset the impact of depletion. It is possible that the positive emotion has some physiological effect (such as freeing up more glucose for the bloodstream) that genuinely counteracts depletion. But it seems more likely that positive emotion merely makes people more willing to spend more of their depleted resources on the second task.

Possibly the most useful and elegant way to counteract depletion is to reduce the demands on free will. Gollwitzer and his colleagues (e.g., see Gollwitzer, 1999) have divided the action process into two phases, a "weighing," or deliberative, phase in which basic decisions are made and a "willing," or implemental, phase in which the person carries out the plans and intentions that stemmed from the deliberative phase. Implementation relies mainly on automatic processes and so should not require anywhere near as many executive resources as the deliberative phase. Accordingly, researchers have found that implementation intentions help counteract the effects of depletion, such as impaired performance on the Stroop task (Webb & Sheeran, 2003).

Long-Term Interventions

We have also devoted some effort to strengthening self-control per se (for a review, see Baumeister et al., 2006). Although results have been uneven and a variety of attempts have failed to produce discernible benefits, other studies have succeeded. Moreover, the potential importance of such interventions for therapy, occupational achievement, and general adjustment would certainly warrant multiple efforts to explore any possibility of improving self-control.

Our efforts have continued to explore the muscle analogy for self-control. That is, a muscle gets tired when it is used, just like self-control becomes weaker and less effective after an initial depleting act—but across time, regular exercise makes muscles stronger. Would regular exercises in self-control likewise improve self-control, akin to the Victorian concept of building character? Our interventions have assigned participants a variety of minor self-control tasks to perform on their own for a period of some weeks. It would hardly be surprising if these practices enable people to perform better on the same exercises subsequently. The crucial test, therefore, is whether exercising self-control in one domain leads to improvement in another domain.

Initial evidence was provided by Muraven, Baumeister, and Tice (1999). Participants underwent a laboratory study on depletion in order to assess their susceptibility to depletion. Then some of them spent 2 weeks performing self-control exercises, such as trying to improve their posture, to watch and record what they ate,

or to maintain a good mood. On returning to the laboratory, participants who had done the self-control exercises showed less susceptibility to depletion as compared to control participants. (The mood regulation exercises, incidentally, were a complete failure, but the other exercises yielded better results.)

Studies by Oaten and Cheng (2006, 2007) used longer and more targeted interventions. In one, participants received financial counseling and strove to improve their money management. In another, they adopted a physical exercise regimen. Carrying out these exercises led to significant improvements not only in the target domain but also in other, unrelated spheres. For example, the participants who performed the physical exercise or money management regimens also ended up reporting better discipline at housework; at curbing their consumption of tobacco, alcohol, and caffeine; and at eating healthier food (which would actually go against the money regimen insofar as healthy food is costlier than junk food) and studying more and watching less television. They also showed significant improvements (both in absolute terms and relative to a control group) on laboratory-based measures of attention control.

A last set of interventions was explored by Gailliot, Plant, Butz, and Baumeister (2007). Participants performed a variety of self-control exercises for 2 weeks, including using their nondominant hand for familiar tasks such as brushing their teeth, regulating their verbal behavior by speaking in complete sentences, avoiding contractions and colloquialisms, and the like. Prior to performing these exercises, some participants had been shown (in an initial laboratory session) to find it difficult to avoid using stereotypes and to be depleted after such a task, but after the 2 weeks of exercise, these same participants were able to avoid using stereotypes without adverse consequences.

Taken together, these findings do not clearly indicate that the baseline level of self-control can be improved. Rather, they show that exercise makes people less susceptible to depletion. By analogy, physical exercise can increase muscle power or stamina, and these findings would correspond to increasing stamina rather than power. Put another way, some acts of self-control demonstrably cause depletion, but after people engage in self-control exercises for some period of time, they can perform those same acts of self-control without being depleted to the same degree.

Applications to Common Behavior Patterns

Before closing, we review some of the major spheres of behavior that have been shown to be affected by ego depletion (see also Muraven & Baumeister, 2000). The breadth of this assortment can be taken as a sign of the fundamental and wide-ranging importance of self-regulation in human life and indeed as an index of how much free will people often exert.

Intelligent Performance

Intelligent thought has long been recognized as one of humanity's most important characteristics, indeed to the extent that humans named their own species *Homo sapiens* in recognition of this intelligence. Intelligence tests were developed in large part to predict school performance and have been tremendously successful at doing so. Yet self-control also predicts school performance, indeed sometimes even better than IQ scores do (Duckworth & Seligman, 2005; Tangney et al., 2004; Wolfe & Johnson, 1995). To be sure, it is possible that some of the variance on self-control scores is attributable to differences in intelligence, but then again the opposite is also possible, namely, that self-control affects IQ test scores. If the latter, then some of the

variance normally attributed to intelligence should properly be ascribed to self-control.

The contribution of self-control to intelligence is evident in the fact that people perform less intelligently when depleted. A series of studies by Schmeichel et al. (2003) showed that depleted participants scored lower on some measures of intelligent performance—though not all. The pattern was revealing. Depletion led to lower scores on logic and reasoning tests, cognitive extrapolation, and thoughtful reading comprehension, but it did not affect scores on simple tests of general knowledge or performance at rote memorization and recall. The implication is that controlled processes are impaired by depletion, whereas automatic processes are not. The most advanced and difficult acts of human thought involve taking one set of information and moving from it by following rules of inference to reach other conclusions. This is the sort of thinking that the self must supervise, and hence it appears to be most degraded when the self's energy is depleted. In contrast, putting information into memory and retrieving it, without operating on it to transform it or draw conclusions, is a straightforward matter that is not degraded by ego depletion.

Intimate Relationships

The importance of self-control to relationships has been suggested by a variety of findings. Tangney et al. (2004) noted that people who scored high on trait self-control reported better close relationships and family relationships. Finkel and Campbell (2001) found that high scores on trait self-control were positively correlated with relationship accommodation in the sense that people with good self-control claimed to adjust better to their partners and to resolve conflicts in constructive ways. Vohs, Baumeister, and Finkenauer (2006) tested several competing hypotheses about how the distribution of self-control scores in a couple would predict relationship satisfaction and duration in both romantic relationships and same-sex friendships. The researchers started by computing the difference between the trait self-control scores of the two partners. The well-supported principle that similarity fosters attraction would predict that relationships would be best off with a small difference (because that would mean partners were very similar to each other). In contrast, the idea that complementarity works best—opposites attract or at least opposites complement each other in helpful ways—would predict that larger differences would predict better outcomes. The evidence failed to support either hypothesis, and in fact the difference between partners' self-control trait scores had a negligible correlation with relationship outcomes. In contrast, the *sum* of the partners' trait self-control scores had a significant positive correlation with both relationship satisfaction and duration. The more total self-control, the better the relationship is.

Why? Studies by Vohs and Baumeister (2006) showed that a variety of relationship-enhancing behaviors deteriorated among depleted people, suggesting that self-control is important for sustaining these behaviors. First, depleted members of romantic couples spent more time than others looking at attractive photos of other members of the opposite sex. Showing interest in alternative partners on this same task has been shown to predict relationship breakup (Miller, 1997). Thus, self-control may be useful for restraining one's potential interest in people who could in principle tempt one away from one's current partner.

Second, depletion increased self-serving attributional biases at the expense of one's partner. In this study, romantic partners performed a task together and got feedback that they had either succeeded (were very creative) or failed. When asked to allocate credit or blame, nondepleted couples did so in ways that reflected well on each other, but depleted individuals blamed their partner for failure and hogged credit for success. Neither blaming problems on your partner nor hogging credit for joint success seems like a good recipe for long-term relationship success.

Third, depletion shifted people toward favoring more destructive styles of dealing with conflicts and problems. Participants were asked what they would do in response to various problematic acts by their partner (in current, past, and future or hypothetical relationships). Their responses were categorized using Rusbult's (1983; Rusbult, Zembrodt, & Gunn, 1982) typology of exit, voice, loyalty, and neglect. Depletion led to an increase in destructive (exit and neglect) and passive (neglect and loyalty) responses and a corresponding reduction in constructive and active responses (especially voice).

More research is needed, but it appears that good relationship skills depend on self-control. Depletion may be one process that causes people to treat their relationship partners in ways that can undermine the relationship. Indeed, depletion seems very plausibly a mediator of the harmful effects of work stress on relationships.

Aggression

Restraining aggression is an important key to human society, and in fact many writers have regarded human aggression as the single biggest obstacle to peaceful human coexistence in culture and civilization (e.g., Freud, 1930). Hence self-control is likely very important for restraining aggression. An interdisciplinary survey of studies on violence and evil by Baumeister (1997) concluded that breakdowns in self-control are often the main proximal cause of violence.

Recent findings suggest that depletion increases aggression. Stucke and Baumeister

(2006) found that depleted participants were more aggressive than others toward someone who had frustrated them. DeWall, Baumeister, Stillman, and Gailliot (2007) replicated and extended these findings, confirming that depletion increases aggression only if there is already a (separate) impulse to act aggressively and, furthermore, that the depletion manipulations themselves do not cause aggression. In other words, ego depletion does not give rise to aggressive impulses—rather, it releases them by weakening the normal restraints against them.

Converging evidence for the importance of self-control for restraining aggressive and antisocial behaviors was provided in developmental studies by Finkenauer, Engels, and Baumeister (2005). They replicated familiar findings that adolescent misbehavior patterns, such as delinquency, were predicted by parenting styles, but they showed that the trait self-control was an important mediator of those effects. Some styles of parenting instill strong self-control and thereby reduce problem behaviors, whereas other parenting patterns fail to promote self-control (and may even undermine it), resulting in higher rates of problems.

Helping

Prosocial behavior represents and important and remarkable evolutionary achievement. Early evolution endowed animals with increasingly powerful brains so that they could survive and reproduce better. In a sense, the brain is there to take care of the body, so psychological (brain) processes tend to be naturally selfish. Human evolution took a step forward, at least in the respect that enlightened self-interest required making oneself acceptable to one's cultural group, which often entails restraining selfish impulses. Thus, seemingly paradoxically, enlightened self-interest came to mean overcoming the natural selfishness, at least to the extent of being unselfish enough to

remain socially acceptable to one's group. Respecting the rules and norms of culture became a prerequisite to belonging to the group, and belonging to the group was the best way for humans to survive and reproduce. Hence, one likely context for the evolution of self-control and, indeed, free will is that the process enabled the natural inner beast to be transformed into a civilized being (see Baumeister, 2005). Consistent with that view, humans make altruistic and even self-sacrificing behaviors for the sake of nonrelatives, which is quite rare in the animal world.

Our laboratory research has confirmed that good self-control contributes to prosocial behavior. Most notably, helping is reduced when people are in a state of ego depletion (Gailliot, Baumeister, et al., 2007). A dose of glucose can restore the helpfulness of depleted people, however. Various other findings indicate that people are more prone to violate norms and other rules when depleted (Gailliot & Baumeister, 2007a, 2007b).

Existential Threats

Terror management theory has proposed that people are strongly motivated by fear of death (e.g., Pyszczynski, Greenberg, & Solomon, 1997). Numerous studies have shown that when people are led to think about death, they respond as if threatened, such as by derogating others who criticize their culture and worldview. Recent work indicates that ego depletion may be responsible for many terror management effects. Depletion increases people's susceptibility to disturbing thoughts of death, and thinking about death produces a depleted state in the sense that self-control is generally impaired afterward (Gailliot, Schmeichel, & Baumeister, 2006). Perhaps most surprisingly, a glass of lemonade containing glucose (sugar) is sufficient to eliminate the worldview defense effect from thinking about death (Gailliot, Baumeister, et al., 2007). Lemonade made with artificial sweetener tasted just as good but was no help against the threat of death.

Impulses and Appetites

Humans naturally desire many things that give them pleasure and satisfaction, but they often encounter problems when they get too many of these things. Overeating, addiction, drunkenness, promiscuity, and the like all reflect excessive indulgence in what could otherwise be healthy, life-sustaining or life-enhancing pleasures (see Chapter 24). Hence, much of the day-to-day functioning of the capacity for self-control involves restraining these desires and impulses. When people are depleted, however, the problematic excesses may begin.

Eating is an important sphere of self-control. Unlike with, say, drugs or alcohol, a zero-tolerance lifestyle is not possible with eating insofar as everyone must eat almost every day. Vohs and Heatherton (2000) showed that ego depletion leads to overeating of sugary, fattening foods. Actually, they found this pattern mainly among dieters. This again confirms the role of self-regulation for restraining behavior (as in our earlier comments about self-stopping). By definition, dieters try to restrain their eating, so depletion increases eating by weakening these restraints. Nondieters, meanwhile, are not holding back from eating, so they do not eat any more when depleted.

Alcohol consumption is another behavior that can range from a simple pleasure to a costly, destructive addiction. Muraven, Collins, and Nienhaus (2002) showed that problem drinkers consumed more alcohol when they were depleted by a recent thought-suppression exercise than when not depleted. This effect was found even when they were anticipating a driving test

and therefore ought to have known to try to remain sober. (No participants were actually sent out on the road in an intoxicated state.) Thus, again, depletion weakened the normal restraints and controls, this time on drinking.

Sexual behavior is likewise often subject to restraint and control, and in fact all known societies impose some controls on sex. Gailliot and Baumeister (2007b) showed that depletion led to increases in a variety of problematic sexual behaviors, ranging from using sexual words inappropriately to indicating greater willingness to have illicit, extramarital sexual relations. A behavioral study in the laboratory found that depleted couples engaged in more extensive sexual behavior than nondepleted ones—but this was found only among relatively new, uncommitted couples for whom presumably sexual desire regularly conflicted with the various restraining forces of modesty and caution. Couples with a more extensive sexual history did not change their behavior when depleted, most likely because they were not routinely restraining their physical affection. These findings parallel the effects of depletion on eating: Restrained eaters (dieters) and restrained lovers (new partners) indulged more after depletion, whereas unrestrained types (nondieters and established couples) did not.

Interracial Interactions

As America has become both more racially integrated and diverse and more focused on racial conflict, the problems of behaving properly when interacting with someone of a different race have become more prevalent. People struggle to say and do the right thing, such as by stifling any prejudiced or otherwise inappropriate responses.

Two sets of findings confirm the link between self-regulation and acting appropriately during interracial (and presumably other) interactions. First, interacting with someone from a different race is depleting, especially for people with prejudices (Richeson & Shelton, 2003; Richeson & Trawalter, 2005; Richeson, Trawalter, & Shelton, 2005). Apparently, the exertion of restraining one's inappropriate behaviors consumes self-regulatory resources, causing poorer performance on seemingly unrelated self-control tasks afterward.

Second, when people are depleted, they are more likely to express prejudicial or otherwise inappropriate views. For example, in one study, depletion increased the use of stereotypes of the elderly (Gordijn, Hindriks, Koomen, Dijksterhuis, & van Knippenberg, 2004). Depleted people are more likely to use and express stereotypes.

The importance of self-regulation for coping with prejudice and interracial contacts was confirmed in a different way by Inzlicht, McKay, and Stondon (2006). Black and female students took tests that they were told measured intellectual ability or math ability, which was presumed to activate stereotype threat for them, and afterward they performed worse on self-control tasks such as squeezing a handgrip and the Stroop task. In contrast, students from the same groups who took tests that were presented as nondiagnostic of ability or as having shown no gender differences performed fine at self-regulation afterward. Thus, the more people believe that they are encountering prejudice against them, the poorer their subsequent self-control.

Money

Finally, money is also a sphere of behavior in which self-control is important. Many people in modern societies find themselves in serious and long-standing difficulties because of failing to control their money adequately, such as by spending too much, incurring debts, and failing

to save. Vohs and Faber (2007) showed that depleted participants scored higher on a measure of impulsive spending, suggesting that depletion makes people more willing to buy things they do not need on a spontaneous, unplanned basis. Laboratory studies confirmed that pattern. In one, participants were asked to indicate the maximum price they were willing to pay for various items, and depleted participants indicated higher prices overall. In another, participants were given $10 for their participation and then, ostensibly in an unrelated event, invited to purchase items from the bookstore. The opportunity to buy was wholly unexpected, so one can reasonably assume that any purchases were purely impulsive. Control participants bought almost nothing, whereas depleted participants on average spent over half their stake for these items (Vohs & Faber, 2007). Thus, depletion weakens one's normal restraints on spending money.

Conclusion

The broad implication of this work confirms that there are at least two very different styles of action control in human life. Whereas most researchers have focused their best creative energies on illuminating the power and reach of automatic processes, our work has been aimed at illuminating the other form, for which we have perhaps recklessly borrowed the conventional term "free will." Our findings indicate that this style of conscious, controlled process requires effort and consumes a limited resource, a major part of which involves glucose in the bloodstream.

The controlled processes corresponding to free will have been studied mainly in connection with self-control and rational choice. There may be others, but these are clearly among the most important and common manifestations. They reveal a style of action control that is much less evident in other species. We think that one crucial development in the evolution of the human psyche involved cultivating the capacity to convert the body's glucose energy into complex, culturally useful actions—again, most notably, self-control and rational choice.

When the body's energy resources have been depleted, self-control and rational choice are often impaired. These effects of ego depletion do not have to wait until the resource is down to the final dregs, and many of them seem to occur quite early in the depletion process, apparently reflecting an effort to conserve the remaining resources. Depleted people reason less well, act in more impulsive and self-indulgent ways, fail to curb their antisocial and destructive tendencies, make less rational choices, and in other ways depart from the idealized model of reasonable and virtuous action that makes for the most successful members of civilized, cultural life.

References

Bargh, J. A. (1994). The four horsemen of automaticity: Awareness, intention, efficiency, and control in social cognition. In R. S. Wyer Jr. & T. K. Srull (Eds.), *Handbook of social cognition* (pp. 1–40). Hillsdale, NJ: Lawrence Erlbaum Associates.

Baumeister, R. F. (1997). *Evil: Inside human violence and cruelty.* New York: Freeman.

Baumeister, R. F. (2005). *The cultural animal: Human nature, meaning, and social life.* New York: Oxford University Press.

Baumeister, R. F. (2008). Free will in scientific psychology. *Perspectives on Psychological Science, 3,* 14–19.

Baumeister, R. F., Bratslavsky, E., Muraven, M., & Tice, D. M. (1998). Ego depletion: Is the active self a limited resource? *Journal of Personality and Social Psychology, 74,* 1252–1265.

Baumeister, R. F., Gailliot, M., DeWall, C. N., & Oaten, M. (2006). Self-regulation and personality: How interventions increase regulatory success, and how depletion moderates the effects of traits on behavior. *Journal of Personality, 74,* 1773–1801.

Baumeister, R. F., Heatherton, T. F., & Tice, D. M. (1994). *Losing control: How and why people fail at self-regulation.* San Diego, CA: Academic Press.

Baumeister, R. F., & Newman, L. S. (1994). Self-regulation of cognitive inference and decision processes. *Personality and Social Psychology Bulletin, 20,* 3–19.

Baumeister, R. F., Vohs, K. D., DeWall, C. N., & Zhang, L. (2007) How emotion shapes behavior: Feedback, anticipation, and reflection, rather than direct causation. *Personality and Social Psychology Review, 11,* 167–203.

Baumeister, R. F., Vohs, K. D., & Funder, D. C. (2007). Psychology as the science of self-reports and finger movements: Whatever happened to actual behavior? *Perspectives on Psychological Science, 2,* 396–403.

Carver, C. S., & Scheier, M. F. (1981). *Attention and self-regulation: A control theory approach to human behavior.* New York: Springer-Verlag.

Dennett, D. C. (1984). *Elbow room: The varieties of free will worth wanting.* Cambridge, MA: MIT Press.

Dennett, D. C. (2003). *Freedom evolves.* New York: Viking/Penguin.

DeWall, C. N., Baumeister, R. F., Stillman, T., & Gailliot, M. T. (2007). Violence restrained: Effects of self-regulation and its depletion on aggression. *Journal of Experimental Social Psychology, 43,* 62–76.

Duckworth, A. L., & Seligman, M. E. P. (2005). Self-discipline outdoes IQ in predicting academic performance of adolescents. *Psychological Science, 16,* 939–944.

Finkel, E. J., & Campbell, W. K. (2001). Self-control and accommodation in close relationships: An interdependence analysis. *Journal of Personality and Social Psychology, 81,* 263–277.

Finkenauer, C., Engels, R. C. M. E., & Baumeister, R. F. (2005). Parenting behavior and adolescent behavioral and emotional problems: The role of self-control. *International Journal of Behavioral Development, 29,* 58–69.

Freud, S. (1930). *Civilization and its discontents* (J. Riviere, Trans.). London: Hogarth Press.

Gailliot, M. T., & Baumeister, R. F. (2007a). The physiology of willpower: Linking blood glucose to self-control. *Personality and Social Psychology Review, 11,* 303–327.

Gailliot, M. T., & Baumeister, R. F. (2007b). Self-regulation and sexual restraint: Dispositionally and temporarily poor self-regulatory abilities contribute to failure at restraining sexual behavior. *Personality and Social Psychology Bulletin, 33,* 173–186.

Gailliot, M. T., Baumeister, R. F., DeWall, C. N., Maner, J. K., Plant, E. A., Tice, D. M., et al. (2007). Self-control relies on glucose as a limited energy source: Willpower is more than a metaphor. *Journal of Personality and Social Psychology, 92,* 325–336.

Gailliot, M. T., Plant, E. A., Butz, D. A., & Baumeister, R. F. (2007). Increasing self-regulatory strength can reduce the depleting effect of suppressing stereotypes. *Personality and Social Psychology Bulletin, 33,* 281–294.

Gailliot, M. T., Schmeichel, B. J., & Baumeister, R. F. (2006). Self-regulatory processes defend against the threat of death: Effects of mortality salience, self-control depletion, and trait self-control on thoughts and fears of dying. *Journal of Personality and Social Psychology, 91,* 49–62.

Gollwitzer, P. M. (1999). Implementation intentions: Strong effects of simple plans. *American Psychologist, 54,* 493–503.

Gordijn, E. H., Hindriks, I., Koomen, W., Dijksterhuis, A., & van Knippenberg, A. (2004). Consequences of stereotype suppression and internal suppression motivation: A self-regulation approach. *Personality and Social Psychology Bulletin, 30,* 212–224.

Gottfredson, M. R., & Hirschi, T. (1990). *A general theory of crime.* Stanford, CA: Stanford University Press.

Huber, J., Payne, J. W., & Puto, C. (1982). Adding asymmetrically dominated alternatives: Violations of regularity and the similarity hypothesis. *Journal of Consumer Research, 9,* 90–98.

Inzlicht, M., McKay, L., & Stondon, J. (2006). Stigma as ego depletion: How being the target of prejudice affects self-control. *Psychological Science, 17,* 262–269.

Jensen, A. R. (1998). *The g factor.* Westport, CT: Praeger.

Kane, R. (2002). *Oxford handbook of free will.* New York: Oxford University Press.

Kant, I. (1967). *Kritik der praktischen Vernunft* [Critique of practical reason]. Hamburg: Felix Meiner Verlag. (Original work published 1797)

Lieberman, M. D., Gaunt, R., Gilbert, D. T., & Trope, Y. (2002). Reflection and reflexion: A social cognitive neuroscience approach to attributional inference. In M. Zanna (Ed.), *Advances in experimental social psychology* (Vol. 34, pp. 199–249). New York: Elsevier.

Linder, D. E., Cooper, J., & Jones, E. E. (1967). Decision freedom as a determinant of the role of incentive magnitude in attitude change. *Journal of Personality and Social Psychology, 6,* 245–254.

Luce, M. F., Bettman, J. R., & Payne, J. W. (1997). Choice processing in emotionally difficult decisions. *Journal of Experimental Psychology: Learning, Memory, and Cognition, 23,* 384–405.

Masicampo, E. J., & Baumeister, R. F. (2008). Toward a physiology of dual-process reasoning and judgment: Does seeing one's own capability for wrongdoing predict forgiveness? *Journal of Personality and Social Psychology, 94,* 495–515.

Miller, R. S. (1997). Inattentive and contented: Relationship commitment and attention to alternatives. *Journal of Personality and Social Psychology, 73,* 758–766.

Mischel, W., Shoda, Y., & Peake, P. K. (1988). The nature of adolescent competencies predicted by preschool delay of gratification. *Journal of Personality and Social Psychology, 54,* 687–696.

Moller, A. C., Deci, E. L., & Ryan, R. M. (2006). Choice and ego-depletion: The moderating role of autonomy. *Personality and Social Psychology Bulletin, 32,* 1024–1036.

Muraven, M. (1998). *Mechanisms of self-control failure: Motivation and limited resources.* Unpublished doctoral dissertation, Case Western Reserve University, Cleveland, OH.

Muraven, M. R., & Baumeister, R. F. (2000). Self-regulation and depletion of limited resources: Does self-control resemble a muscle? *Psychological Bulletin, 126,* 247–259.

Muraven, M., Baumeister, R. F., & Tice, D. M. (1999). Longitudinal improvement of self-regulation through practice: Building self-control through repeated exercise. *Journal of Social Psychology, 139,* 446–457.

Muraven, M., Collins, R. L., & Nienhaus, K. (2002). Self-control and alcohol restraint. An initial application of the self-control strength model. *Psychology of Addictive Behaviors, 16,* 113–120.

Muraven, M., Shmueli, D., & Burkley, E. (2006). Conserving self-control strength. *Journal of Personality and Social Psychology, 91,* 524–537.

Muraven, M., & Slessareva, E. (2003). Mechanisms of self-control failure: Motivation and limited resources. *Personality and Social Psychology Bulletin, 29,* 894–906.

Muraven, M., Tice, D. M., & Baumeister, R. F. (1998). Self-control as limited resource: Regulatory depletion patterns. *Journal of Personality and Social Psychology, 74,* 774–789.

Novemsky, N., & Baumeister, R. (2006). [Ego depletion and consumer decisions]. Unpublished raw data.

Oaten, M., & Cheng, K. (2006). Longitudinal gains in self-regulation from regular physical exercise. *British Journal of Health Psychology, 11,* 717–733.

Oaten, M., & Cheng, K. (2007). Improvements in self-control from financial monitoring. *Journal of Economic Psychology, 28,* 487–501.

Pocheptsova, A., Amir, O., Dhar, R., & Baumeister, R. F. (in press). Deciding without resources: Resource depletion and choice in context. *Journal of Marketing Research.*

Powers, W. T. (1973). *Behavior: The control of perception.* Chicago: Aldine.

Pyszczynski, T., Greenberg, J., & Solomon, S. (1997). Why do we need what we need? A terror management perspective on the roots of human social motivation. *Psychological Inquiry, 8,* 1–20.

Richeson, J. A., & Shelton, J. N. (2003). When prejudice does not pay: Effects of interracial contact on executive function. *Psychological Science, 14,* 287–290.

Richeson, J. A., & Trawalter, S. (2005). Why do interracial interactions impair executive function? A resource depletion account. *Journal of Personality and Social Psychology, 88,* 934–947.

Richeson, J. A., Trawalter, S., & Shelton, J. N. (2005). African Americans' implicit racial attitudes and the depletion of executive function after interracial interactions. *Social Cognition, 23,* 336–352.

Rogers, T. B., Kuiper, N. A., & Kirker, W. S. (1977). Self-reference and the encoding of personal information. *Journal of Personality and Social Psychology, 35,* 677–688.

Rusbult, C. E. (1983). A longitudinal test of the investment model: The development (and deterioration) of satisfaction and commitment in heterosexual involvements. *Journal of Personality and Social Psychology, 45,* 101–117.

Rusbult, C. E., Zembrodt, I. M., & Gunn, L. K. (1982). Exit, voice, loyalty, and neglect: Responses to dissatisfaction in romantic involvements. *Journal of Personality and Social Psychology, 43,* 1230–1242.

Schmeichel, B. J., Gailliot, M. T., & Baumeister, R. F. (2005). *Ego depletion undermines the benefits of the active self to memory.* Manuscript submitted for publication.

Schmeichel, B. J., Vohs, K. D., & Baumeister, R. F. (2003). Intellectual performance and ego depletion: Role of the self in logical reasoning and other information processing. *Journal of Personality and Social Psychology, 85,* 33–46.

Searle, J. R. (2001). *Rationality in action.* Cambridge, MA: MIT Press.

Shoda, Y., Mischel, W., & Peake, P. K. (1990). Predicting adolescent cognitive and self-regulatory competencies from preschool delay of gratification: Identifying diagnostic conditions. *Developmental Psychology, 26,* 978–986.

Simonson, I. (1989). Choice based on reasons: The case of attraction and compromise effects. *Journal of Consumer Research, 16,* 158–174.

Smith, E. R., & DeCoster, J. (1999). Associated and rule-based processing: A connectionist interpretation of dual-process models. In S. Chaiken & Y. Trope (Eds.), *Dual-process theories in social psychology* (pp. 323–336). New York: Guilford Press.

Smith, E. R., & DeCoster, J. (2000). Dual-process models in social and cognitive psychology: Conceptual integration and links to underlying memory systems. *Personality and Social Psychology Review, 4,* 108–131.

Stucke, T. S., & Baumeister, R. F. (2006). Ego depletion and aggressive behavior: Is the inhibition of aggression a limited resource? *European Journal of Social Psychology, 36,* 1–13.

Tangney, J. P., Baumeister, R. F., & Boone, A. L. (2004). High self-control predicts good adjustment, less pathology, better grades, and interpersonal success. *Journal of Personality, 72,* 271–322.

Thayer, R. E. (1996). *The origin of everyday moods.* New York: Oxford University Press.

Tice, D. M., Baumeister, R. F., Shmueli, D., & Muraven, M. (2007). Restoring the self: Positive affect helps improve self-regulation following ego depletion. *Journal of Experimental Social Psychology, 43,* 379–384.

Vohs, K. D. & Baumeister, R. F. (2006). *Self-regulatory depletion impairs relationship-maintaining behavior patterns.* Manuscript in preparation, University of Minnesota.

Vohs, K. D., Baumeister, R. F., & Finkenauer, C. (2006). *Self-control and relationships: Similarity, complementarity, or simple sum?* Manuscript in preparation.

Vohs, K. D., Baumeister, R. F., Schmeichel, B. J., Twenge, J. M., Nelson, N. M., & Tice, D. M. (2008). Making choices impairs subsequent self-control: A limited resource account of decision making, self-regulation, and active initiative. *Journal of Personality and Social Psychology, 94,* 883–898.

Vohs, K. D., & Faber, R. J. (2007). Spent resources: Self-regulatory resource availability affects impulse buying. *Journal of Consumer Research, 33,* 537–547.

Vohs, K. D., & Heatherton, T. F. (2000). Self-regulatory failure: A resource-depletion approach. *Psychological Science, 11,* 249–254.

Vohs, K. D., & Schmeichel, B. J. (2003). Self-regulation and the extended now: Controlling the self alters the subjective experience of time. *Journal of Personality and Social Psychology, 85,* 217–230.

Wallace, H. M., & Baumeister, R. F. (2002). The effects of success versus failure feedback on further self-control. *Self and Identity, 1,* 35–41.

Webb, T. L., & Sheeran, P. (2003). Can implementation intentions help to overcome ego-depletion? *Journal of Experimental Social Psychology, 39,* 279–286.

Wegner, D. M. (1989). *White bears and other unwanted thoughts.* New York: Vintage.

Wegner, D. M. (2002). *The illusion of conscious will.* Cambridge, MA: MIT Press.

Wolfe, R. N., & Johnson, S. D. (1995). Personality as a predictor of college performance. *Educational and Psychological Measurement, 55,* 177–185.

Decision Utility, Incentive Salience, and Cue-Triggered "Wanting"

Kent C. Berridge *and* J. Wayne Aldridge

> This is good news and bad news for utilitarians: the limbic system reward pathways seem to correspond to a utility pump, but specialized brain circuitry processes experience in ways that are not necessarily consistent with relentless maximization of hedonic experience.
>
> —*Daniel McFadden, Frisch Lecture, Econometric Society World Congress, London, August 20, 2005 (McFadden, 2005)*

Abstract

This chapter examines brain mechanisms of reward utility operating at particular decision moments in life—moments such as when one encounters an image, sound, scent, or other cue associated in the past with a particular reward or perhaps just when one vividly imagines that cue. Such a cue can often trigger a sudden motivational urge to pursue its reward and sometimes a decision to do so. Drawing on a utility taxonomy that distinguishes among subtypes of reward utility—predicted utility, decision utility, experienced utility, and remembered utility—it is shown how cue-triggered cravings, such as an addict's surrender to relapse, can hang on special transformations by brain mesolimbic systems of one utility subtype, namely, decision utility. The chapter focuses on a particular form of decision utility called incentive salience, a type of "wanting" for rewards that is amplified by brain mesolimbic systems. Sudden peaks of intensity of incentive salience, caused by neurobiological mechanisms, can elevate the decision utility of a particular reward at the moment its cue occurs. An understanding of what happens at such moments leads to a better understanding of the mechanisms at work in decision making in general.

Keywords: decisions, reward utility, decision-making, mesolimbic system, predicted utility, decision utility, experienced utility, remembered utility, incentive salience

How do brain representations of the utility of a reward guide decisions about whether to pursue it? Our focus here is on brain mechanisms of reward utility operating at particular decision moments in life—moments such as when you encounter an image, sound, scent, or other cue associated in your past with a particular reward or perhaps just vividly imagine that cue. Such a cue can often trigger a sudden motivational urge to pursue its reward and sometimes a decision to do so. In drug addicts trying to quit, a cue for the addicted drug might trigger urges that rise to compulsive levels of intensity despite prior commitments to abstain, leading to the decision to relapse into taking the drug again. Normal or addicted, the urge and decision may well have been lacking immediately before the cue was encountered. The decision to pursue the cued reward might never have happened if the cue had not been encountered. Why can such cues momentarily dominate decision making?

This question has both psychological and neural answers, and it may be useful to consider them together. In particular, we think that a full psychological answer involves a particular subtype of reward utility. To help make this answer clear, we draw on a utility taxonomy that distinguishes among subtypes of reward utility: predicted utility, decision utility, experienced utility, and remembered utility (Kahneman, Wakker, & Sarin, 1997). We show how cue-triggered cravings, such as the addict's surrender to relapse, can hang on special transformations by brain mesolimbic systems of one utility subtype, namely, decision utility. The particular form of decision utility we focus on here is called incentive salience, a type of "wanting" for rewards that is amplified by brain mesolimbic systems. Sudden peaks of intensity of incentive salience, caused by neurobiological mechanisms to be described, can elevate the decision utility of a particular reward at the moment its cue occurs. An understanding of what happens at such moments will lead to a better understanding of the mechanisms at work in decision making in general.

Decisions and Reward Utility Types

When making decisions on hedonic grounds, a good decision is to choose and pursue the outcome, from among all available options, that will be liked best when it is gained. That is, a good decision maximizes reward utility. However, reward utility is not all of one type. To identify the types of reward utility involved in cue-triggered decisions, we draw here on a four-type utility framework proposed by Daniel Kahneman and colleagues: predicted utility, decision utility, experienced utility, and remembered utility (Kahneman et al., 1997).

Predicted utility is the expectation of how much a future reward will be liked. It is based on cognitive or associative prediction of the rewarding value an outcome will have when it is gained in the future.

Decision utility is the subtype of reward utility most directly connected to an actual decision (although most difficult to isolate in psychological terms from other subtypes, especially from predicted utility). As the name suggests, decision utility is the essence of an actual decision at the moment it is made, the valuation of the outcome manifest in choice and pursuit. Most typically, decision utility is revealed by what we actually decide to do.

Experienced utility is what most people think of the term "reward." It is the hedonic impact of the reward that is actually experienced when it is finally gained. It is the affective pleasure component of reward utility. For many, experienced utility is the essence of what reward is all about.

Remembered utility is the memory of how good a previous reward was in the past. It is the reconstructed representation of the hedonic impact carried by the remembered reward. Whenever we decide about outcomes we have previously experienced in our past, remembered utility is perhaps the chief factor that determines predicted utility: We generally expect future rewards to be about as good as they have been in the past.

Ordinarily in optimal decisions, all these subtypes of reward utility may be maximized together. But sometimes a decision is less than optimal, and then subtypes of utility may diverge from each other. A major contribution of Kahneman's utility taxonomy has been to identify cases where predicted or remembered utility diverges from actual experienced utility (Gilbert & Wilson, 2000; Kahneman, Fredrickson, Schreiber, & Redelmeier, 1993; Kahneman et al., 1997). Such divergence can lead to bad decisions on the basis of wrong expectations, called "miswanting" by Gilbert and Wilson (2000; Morewedge, Gilbert, &

Wilson, 2005). If one has a distorted remembered utility because of memory illusions of various sorts, one will have a distorted predicted utility. Decisions made on the basis of false predicted utility are likely to turn out to fail to maximize eventual experienced utility. Or if predicted utility is distorted for reasons other than faulty memory, such as by inappropriate cognitive theories about what rewards will be like in the future, then decisions will again turn out wrong. In either case, predicted utility will fail to match actual experienced utility, and the decision is liable to be wrong.

Thus, if decisions are guided principally by predictions about future reward (if decision utility equals predicted utility), then faulty predictions mean that wrong decisions will be made (decision utility does not equal experienced utility). We may thus choose outcomes that we turn out not to like when our predictions about them are wrong. We choose them because we wrongly expect to like them in such cases (and perhaps because we wrongly remember having liked them in the past)—but then we turn out not to like them after all.

The previously described mismatch captures much of what is discussed under the label of miswanting and decisions that fail to maximize utility. But Kahneman's taxonomy has a further use for an even more intriguing form of miswanting that we exploit here. This might be called irrational miswanting because it can lead to an outcome being wanted even when an outcome value is correctly predicted to be less than desirable. In this case, we suggest that decision utility may fail to match predicted utility (Berridge, 1999, 2003a; Robinson & Berridge, 1993). If decision utility exists as a distinct psychological variable (with a somewhat separate neurobiological mechanism), it might sometimes dissociate from predicted utility—just as decision utility (together with predicted utility) sometimes

dissociates from experienced utility (Berridge, 1999, 2003b; Robinson & Berridge, 1993). If at any time decision utility could grow above predicted utility, that could mean choosing an outcome that we actually expected not to like at the moment of decision (and that we not only expected not to like but also turned out not to like in the end).

Rational Decisions Versus Irrational Decisions

This brings us squarely to the topic of decision rationality. Decision rationality has been defined in various ways, so we wish to be clear about our own definition. First, unlike some, we do not demand consistency of preference. For psychologists and neuroscientists, there are many good reasons why individual preferences will change from time to time, so we would not call irrational any mere inconsistency of preference. Second, we would also suggest that the rationality of a decision has nothing at all to do with whether an impartial judge or the majority of other people would like the same outcome. Individual tastes are idiosyncratic (as the adage goes, *de gustibus non est disputandum:* there is no use disputing about individual differences in tastes). For the purpose of decision rationality, we simply accept individual tastes for what they are—differences in individual characteristics of experienced utility that make different things liked by different people (or even by the same person at different times).

Further, the rationality of a decision does not even depend on whether deciders themselves end up eventually liking their chosen outcome. Deciders can be mistaken about whether they will like an outcome they choose, as in mispredicted miswanting mentioned previously. People often choose an outcome they expect to like but then are disappointed to find they actually do not like it. That is not irrational—in those cases choosers may have done the best they can—they were simply wrong in their expectations of predicted utility. Reasons for being wrong about the predicted utility of an outcome can include ignorance for never-experienced outcomes, incorrect theories about the goodness of a hypothetical outcome or about one's own hedonic tastes, and mistaken memories about having liked something in the past (incorrect remembered utility) (Gilbert & Wilson, 2000; Kahneman et al., 1997). All these can make a decision mistaken, wrong, bad, and regrettable—even stupid. But by themselves, they do not make a decision irrational, however wrong the decision turns out to be.

We suggest that a decision remains rational as long as one chooses what one expects to like best, that is, as long as decision utility equals predicted utility. If predicted utility of an outcome is high, then choosing that outcome is rational by definition. If you believe that you will like an outcome, you are rational to choose it, to want it, and to pursue it actively—you should pursue it precisely to the degree that you expect to like it. If you turn out not to like the outcome after all, well, blame your theories, memories, or understanding of the world. But decision rationality cannot be held responsible for the eventual unhappy experienced utility because rationality in this sense cannot be held accountable for the accuracy of your predictions—only for the consistency with which you act on them.

An irrational decision is to choose what you expect not to like. That is, a decision is irrational when its decision utility does not equal predicted utility. When decision utility is greater than predicted utility, if that can happen, then one might be said to choose what one does not expect to like (not only what one mistakenly expects to like). To choose what one does not expect

to like is to choose in a way that is strongly irrational, as we define irrationality. For the purpose of identifying irrational decision mechanisms in the experiments here, this is the definition we will rely on: that one chooses disproportionately to expectation of liking so that decision utility is greater than predicted utility. Here we describe a mechanism that under specific conditions produces irrational decisions, even by our restrictive definition of irrationality, though we believe it evolved to motivate good decisions in normal life.

Brain Mechanisms of Reward Utility

Insights into rewards and decisions would be enhanced by an understanding of their brain mechanisms. Affective neuroscience studies of reward have shown that many brain structures are activated by reward utilities (Berridge, 2003b; Davidson, Shackman, & Maxwell, 2004; Kringelbach, 2004; Montague, Hyman, & Cohen, 2004; Schultz, 2006; Shizgal, 1999; Shizgal, Fulton, & Woodside, 2001). These include regions of the neocortex, especially the prefrontal cortex (ventromedial, orbitofrontal, and anterior cingulate areas), the insular cortex (which includes taste sensory representations), and the amygdala.

But what brain mechanisms actually cause reward utility as generator mechanisms? So far, the most potent causal demonstrations for actually causing reward utility have come chiefly from manipulations of brain structures below the cortex: subcortical limbic structures (Berridge, 2003b; Shizgal, 1999). We focus our analysis of experienced utility and decision utility generation on these subcortical structures, such as mesolimbic dopamine systems, nucleus accumbens, and ventral pallidum.

Before we focus on details, we must emphasize that neither cortical nor subcortical regions operate on their own and that massive reciprocal projections link them together. Connections from subcortical to cortical regions are undoubtedly required for translation of "liking" and other basic utilities generated in subcortical limbic structures into consciousness and cognitive representations. In return, descending projections from the cortex to subcortical limbic structures permit cognitive appraisals or voluntary intentions to modulate basic emotional reactions (Davidson, Jackson, & Kalin, 2000). Still, if one has to choose just a few brain mechanisms as causal generators of reward utility, the best candidates for utility generators come mostly from below the cortex.

Brain Mesolimbic Utility Generator

Perhaps the most famous subcortical reward generating substrate has been the mesolimbic dopamine system that sends its dopamine-containing fibers up from midbrain to the nucleus accumbens and related structures, passing through the lateral hypothalamus on the way. The nucleus accumbens in turn projects heavily downward, most densely above all to the ventral pallidum, a relatively little known but highly intriguing limbic structure that sits just in front of the lateral hypothalamus near the bottom of the forebrain. The ventral pallidum projects back upward into thalamocortical circuits that reach the orbitofrontal cortex, the cingulate cortex, and the insular cortex as well as downward to deeper brain structures. This looping mesolimbic dopamine–accumbens–pallidum–cortical system is a useful brain circuit to turn to in order to tease apart reward utility types. We take examples from studies of both humans and animals. Humans provide the most vivid insights into psychological dissociations, while animal studies give the clearest revelation of underlying mechanisms.

Do Strongly Irrational Decisions Exist? (Decision Utility Is Greater Than Predicted Utility)

The point of our subcortical focus here is to show how rational and irrational decision utility, especially as cue-triggered "wanting," might be generated by brain systems in particular circumstances. To start with, you might well wonder, are there really any cases where people irrationally want what they neither like nor expect to like? We think there may be some cases generated by subcortical manipulations, though these cases have not always been recognized for what they are. A good example might be false "pleasure electrodes," perhaps a case of neuroscientific mistaken identity.

False Pleasure Electrodes— Decision Utility Without Experienced Utility?

Pleasure electrodes have been famous since the 1950s but may generally turn out not to live up to their name. These are stimulation electrodes in the subcortical forebrain that rats and people would work to stimulate, pressing a lever or button thousands of times in a few hours to activate (Heath, 1972; Olds & Milner, 1954; Shizgal, 1999). What intense pleasure (experienced utility) and expectations of pleasure (predicted utility) must occur in order to motivate such intense wanting to activate the electrode (decision utility)—or so you might think.

But maybe most "pleasure electrodes" are not so pleasurable after all. For example, one of the most famous cases ever was "B-19," implanted with stimulation electrodes by Heath and colleagues as a young man in the 1960s (Heath, 1972). B-19 voraciously self-stimulated his electrode and protested when the stimulation button was taken away. In addition, his electrode caused "feelings of pleasure, alertness, and warmth (goodwill); he had feelings of sexual arousal and described a compulsion to masturbate" (Heath, 1972, p. 6). Still, did B-19's electrode really cause an intense pleasure sensation? The answer seems to be no. B-19 was never quoted as saying that the sensation was pleasurable in the papers and books written by Heath, not even an exclamation or anything like "Oh wow—that feels nice!"

Rather than simple pleasure, stimulation of B-19's electrode evoked the desire to stimulate again and again, along with strong sexual arousal. It never produced actual sexual orgasm or clear evidence of actual pleasure sensation. Clearly, the stimulation did not serve as a substitute for sexual acts.

Decades later, another patient showed similar findings, this time a woman with an electrode implanted in deep subcortical forebrain (Portenoy et al., 1986). She stimulated her electrode at home compulsively to the extent that "at its most frequent, the patient self-stimulated throughout the day, neglecting personal hygiene and family commitments" (Portenoy et al., 1986, p. 279). When her electrode was stimulated in the clinic, it produced a strong desire to drink liquids, some erotic feelings, and a continuing desire to stimulate again. Notably, records indicate that "though sexual arousal was prominent, no orgasm occurred" (Portenoy et al., 1986, p. 279). "She described erotic sensations often intermixed with an undercurrent of anxiety. She also noted extreme thirst, drinking copiously during the session, and alternating generalized hot and cold sensations" (Portenoy et al., 1986, p. 279). Clearly, this woman felt a mixture of subjective feelings, but the description's emphasis is on aversive thirst and anxiety. Like patient B-19, there is no evidence of distinct pleasure sensations. Although stimulation made B-19 want to perform sexual acts and the woman had erotic thoughts, neither

patient had orgasmic sensations from his or her electrode (in contrast to the failure of these forebrain-stimulating electrodes, spinal cord stimulation has been suggested to actually improve sexual function by enhancing orgasmic performance; Meloy & Southern, 2006).

What could brain stimulation be doing, if not inducing pleasure? This helps pinpoint the idea of incentive salience, a psychological process of reward "wanting" that is a form of decision utility (Berridge, 2003a; Berridge & Robinson, 1998; Robinson & Berridge, 1993). Incentive salience is different from reward "liking" or pleasurable hedonic impact that corresponds to experienced utility. We suggest that brain stimulation in these patients evoked only intense "wanting"—but not "liking." Brain stimulation may have caused incentive salience to be attributed to stimuli perceived at surrounding moments, including people (who became more interesting and appealing), the room (which became attractive and "brightened up"), and most especially the button and the act of pushing it (which became irresistible to do again). The button itself is most closely paired with electrode activation and so becomes a conditioned stimulus attributed most with incentive salience. If brain stimulation elevated "wanting" attribution to the button as a form of decision utility without a corresponding increase in experienced utility, a person might well "want" to activate their electrode again and again, even if it produced no pleasure sensation. That would be mere incentive salience "wanting"—without hedonic "liking."

Does the electrode hijack decision utility alone as we suggest? Or does it also hijack predicted utility as well as decision utility, causing false expectations of future reward? That is, the electrodes might produce a false declarative expectation that the activation will produce an intensely liked pleasure even though the last one never did. If so, then both predicted utility and decision utility would exceed the eventually experienced utility or the lack of pleasure actually received. We return to this issue in the animal affective neuroscience experiments later in this chapter.

One would like to know more about the experience, expectations, and motives of these people with brain self-stimulation. The information available from past studies of patients is frustratingly sparse and crude. It is possible that better information might be gathered in the future, now that a revival of deep brain stimulation and electrode implantation appears to be under way (e.g., as an experimental treatment for Parkinson's disease). Better information is something to be hoped for.

Animal Affective Neuroscience Experiments: Isolating Decision Utility

Some better information can be gained from affective neuroscience experiments with animals because in them one can use painless brain manipulations to better tease apart "wanting" from "liking." Our own analyses of reward utility types began over a decade ago in part with an animal equivalent of the electrode patients. In rats as well as people, "rewarding" brain electrodes typically turn on motivations to eat, drink, have sex, and so on if the electrode stimulation is given freely. Why do rats eat, say, when a reward electrode is turned on? Early hypotheses suggested that they ate more food because stimulation made them like food more (Hoebel, 1988). But an early study in our lab with Elliot Valenstein led to the different conclusion that the electrode increased the incentive salience or decision utility of food, causing rats to "want" to eat it without increasing "liking" for its hedonic impact or experienced utility (Berridge & Valenstein, 1991).

How can "wanting" and "liking" possibly be told apart in rats? We have tackled this by assessing affective reactions that are very specific to hedonic impact "liking" (Figure 24.1). They are not influenced by independent changes in "wanting." The affective reactions are "liking" facial expressions that are elicited sweet tastes, of which several expressions are homologous in human infants and many animals, including apes, monkeys, and rats (e.g., tongue protrusions). By contrast, nasty, bitter tastes elicit "disliking" expressions (e.g., gapes). Such affective "liking"/"disliking" reactions provide windows into brain systems that paint a pleasure gloss onto sweet and related taste sensations because the expressions change when brain manipulations alter the pleasant hedonic impact of those tastes.

Brain Limbic Hedonic Hot Spots Generate Experienced Utility ("Liking")

Using this approach, recent studies by Susana Peciña, Kyle Smith, Stephen Mahler, Sheila Reynolds and others in our laboratory have begun to map neural substrates that generate a basic experienced utility for sweetness hedonic impact (Mahler, Smith, & Berridge, 2007; Peciña & Berridge, 2000, 2005; Peciña, Smith, & Berridge, 2006; Reynolds & Berridge, 2002; Smith & Berridge, 2005; Tindell, Smith, Peciña, Berridge, & Aldridge, 2006). These studies have identified a number of hedonic hot spots: neuroanatomical sites where specific neurochemical signals are able to cause increases in the hedonic impact of sweetness "liking" (Figure 24.1). Such experiments use painless microinjections, delivered by previously implanted brain cannulae, to activate a brain substrate. Tiny droplets of morphine-type drugs (called opiate drugs because they activate opioid brain chemicals) are delivered to a hot spot in a brain structure such as the nucleus accumbens, where they activate

**Positive Hedonic
'liking'**

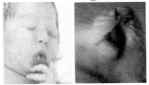

**Negative Aversive
'disliking'**

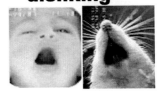

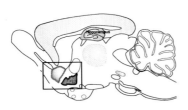

Nucleus
Accumbens

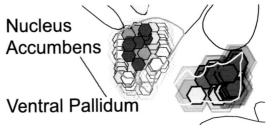

Ventral Pallidum

Opioid Hedonic Hotspots

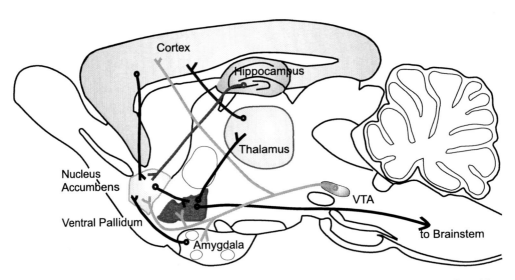

Fig. 24.1 "Liking" reactions and brain hedonic hot spots. Top: Positive hedonic "liking" reactions are elicited by sucrose taste from human infant and adult rat (e.g., rhythmic tongue protrusion). By contrast, negative aversive "disliking" reactions are elicited by bitter quinine taste. Below: Forebrain hedonic hot spots in limbic structures where mu opioid activation causes a brighter pleasure gloss to be painted on sweet sensation. Red/yellow shows hot spots in nucleus accumbens and ventral pallidum where opioid microinjections caused the biggest increases in the number of sweet-elicited "liking" reactions. Based on Peciña and Berridge (2005), Smith and Berridge (2005), and Peciña, Smith, and Berridge (2006).

the opioid circuits and cause increased hedonic "liking" reactions to the sweet taste of sugar. By moving microinjections to different locations in the structure, we can map the boundaries of the hedonic hot spot, and by varying the drug content, we can identify the neurochemical systems that paint the pleasure gloss of this basic experienced utility onto sweet sensation (Peciña et al., 2006; Tindell et al., 2006).

Hedonic hot spots, each about a cubic millimeter in size in rats (in humans, hot spots might be closer to a cubic centimeter if proportional to overall brain size), exist in subcortical limbic structures such as the nucleus accumbens and the ventral pallidum (Peciña et al., 2006; Tindell et al., 2006). In these hot spots, microinjection of the drug DAMGO activates mu opioid receptors on neurons and causes sweet tastes to elicit double or triple the number of positive hedonic "liking" reactions they normally would. In other words, DAMGO in these hot spots activates an experienced utility mechanism that magnifies the pleasure impact of sweet tastes to make them more "liked." At the same time, the microinjections that cause "liking" (experienced utility) also cause greater "wanting" (decision utility): The rats seek out food and eat three times as much as normal. Accordingly, neurons in a hedonic hot spot appear to code both "liking" and "wanting" by their firing rates (Tindell, Berridge, Zhang, Peciña, & Aldridge, 2005; Tindell et al., 2006).

Mesolimbic Dopamine Generates "Wanting" but Not "Liking"

In contrast with opioid microinjections that induce both "liking" and "wanting" for rewards, deep brain electrode stimulation that makes rats eat more nonetheless fails to increase "liking" reactions to sweetness (Berridge & Valenstein, 1991). If anything, the electrode caused more "disliking" reactions to be elicited by sugar taste (as if making it more similar to a bitter taste). In other words, the rats do not seem to eat more because they "like" food more. Instead, rats eat more despite not "liking" it more or even in some instances actually "disliking" food more. This seems to be a brain-based separation among utility types for food reward: increased decision utility ("wanting" and food consumption) without increased experienced utility ("liking" reactions to sugar).

We have observed a number of other similar brain manipulations that caused increases in motivational "wanting" but failed to increase pleasure ("liking") for the same reward (Reynolds & Berridge, 2002; Robinson & Berridge, 2003; Wyvell & Berridge, 2000, 2001). Many of these brain manipulations that dissociated decision utility from experienced utility have involved the brain's mesolimbic dopamine system, which was once thought to cause sensory pleasure. Our work, combined with other neuroscience evidence, has led to the contrary conclusion that dopamine fails to live up to its pleasure neurotransmitter label. Dopamine systems simply seem unable to cause pleasure, as assessed by "liking" reactions, unless accompanied by other neural events, even though dopamine activation can induce powerful motivation to acquire food and other rewards in animals and humans. We have tried both activating and suppressing dopamine in several ways, but it never alters pleasure reactions (Berridge, 2007; Berridge & Robinson, 1998; Tindell et al., 2005).

So if dopamine is a faux pleasure, what is its real psychological role? Our studies led us to suggest that modulating reward "wanting" rather than "liking" best captures what dopamine does. In particular, by "wanting," we mean the attribution of incentive salience to reward stimuli, which makes them be perceived as attractive incentives (Berridge, 2007; Berridge & Robinson, 1998; Tindell et al., 2005). For most of us in our everyday experience, "liking" and "wanting" usually go together for pleasant rewards, as two sides of the same psychological coin. But "wanting" may be separable in the brain from "liking," and mesolimbic dopamine systems mediate only "wanting." We and our colleagues coined the phrase incentive salience for the particular psychological form of "wanting" that we think is mediated by brain dopamine systems.

What Is "Incentive Salience"?

"Wanting" is not "liking." "Wanting" is not a sensory pleasure in any sense. And "wanting" cannot increase positive facial reactions to sweet taste or the hedonic impact of any sensory pleasure. Indeed, incentive salience is essentially *nonhedonic* in nature, even though it is important to the larger composite of processes that motivate us for reward. Faced with a number of goals (e.g., thirst versus hunger), "wanting" evolved to serve as a means to make decisions among different types of rewards (e.g., water versus food). Thus, "wanting" may provide a common neural currency or a comparison yardstick for decision utility in evaluating multiple choices (Shizgal, 1997). Usually "liking" and "wanting" for pleasant incentives do go together, but specific manipulations of dopamine-related brain mechanisms may sometimes pull them apart.

We believe that brain dopamine systems especially attribute incentive salience to reward representations at moments when a cue is encountered that has been associated with the reward in the past (or perhaps even vividly imagined). Incentive salience is attributed to Pavlovian cues following what have been called Bindra–Toates rules of learned incentive motivation (Berridge, 2001; Bindra, 1978; Toates, 1986). When a cue is attributed with incentive salience by mesolimbic brain systems, it causes both that cue and its reward to become momentarily more intensely attractive and sought. The cue actually takes on "motivational magnet" properties of its reward: It can become almost ingestible if it is a cue for food reward, drinkable if a cue for water reward, attractive in a drug-related way for cues for drug reward, and so on (and animals have been known to try to eat or drink their incentive cues in studies of what is called Pavlovian "autoshaping"). Related conditioned stimulus (CS) effects may be visible in human crack cocaine addicts who "chase ghosts" and visible CSs, scrabbling on the kitchen floor after white crumbs resembling crack crystals even if they know the crumbs are only sugar. The cue also is able to trigger increased "wanting" for its actual reward, priming the motivational desire in cue-triggered "wanting"—such as when a cue reminds you that it is lunchtime and you suddenly feel hungry.

Physiological drive states such as hunger or thirst directly modulate the incentive salience attributed to cues relevant to their particular reward. They also modulate the hedonic impact of the rewards themselves. For example, hunger makes food taste better than usual, whereas physiological sodium appetite makes salty tastes "liked" more, and these physiological states also make learned cues for those rewards instantly attractive and "wanted." Multiplicative interactions between reward cues and relevant physiological appetite states are a defining feature of incentive salience "wanting."

"Wanting" Versus Ordinary Wanting

The quotation marks around the term "wanting" serve as caveat to acknowledge that incentive salience means something different from the ordinary common language sense of the word *wanting*. For one thing, "wanting" in the incentive salience sense need not have a conscious goal or declarative target. Wanting in the ordinary sense, on the other hand, nearly always means a conscious desire for an explicitly expected outcome. In the ordinary sense, we consciously and rationally want those things we expect to like. Conscious wanting and core "wanting" differ psychologically and probably also in their brain substrates, with cognitive wanting mediated by cortical structures and incentive salience "wanting" mediated more by subcortical systems.

Reward "wanting" or incentive salience is thus just one type of decision utility. It is only decision utility—not experienced utility (which is more similar to "liking") or predicted utility (prediction or expectation of future reward). And it is not even all of decision utility—it can leave out the cognitive beliefs and resolutions that constitute more cognitive wants. If we are correct in our hypothesis, then this specificity of "wanting" means that selective activation of mesolimbic dopamine systems can produce truly irrational decisions. Activation of brain mesolimbic mechanisms for incentive salience can lead to "wanting" what is neither "liked" nor even expected to be liked sufficiently to rationally justify the decision to pursue (and thus sometimes not even wanted in a more abstract cognitive sense: irrational "wanting" impulses that occur despite not cognitively wanting).

Cue-Triggered "Wanting" as a Special Subtype of Decision Utility

Reward cues are often potent triggers for urges and decisions to pursue and consume those rewards. Why are cues so motivationally potent? The incentive salience hypothesis offers a specific answer because it posits that reward cues are attributed with dopamine-driven incentive salience by mesolimbic circuits.

These conclusions come largely from animal experiments on cue-triggered decision utility, which we describe now. Such experiments have sometimes used a procedure called Pavlovian instrumental transfer, which for our purposes can be thought of as a way of isolating incentive salience as cue-triggered "wanting." In those studies, the rats are first trained to work (press a lever) for the real rewards. Since rewards come only every so often, animals learn to persist in working to earn reward even when sparse. In a separate training session, rats are presented with rewards under conditions where they do not have to

work. Besides not having to work for the reward, the significant change here is that each reward is associated with an auditory tone cue 10 to 30 seconds long. Just as with Pavlov's dogs, the cues come to signify reward for the animals, becoming Pavlovian conditioned stimuli (CS+). With these two steps, training is complete.

Testing begins after the training is completed. A special experimental feature is employed, namely, extinction tests. Rats are tested for their willingness to work for rewards later under extinction conditions, so called because the rewards are no longer delivered at all. Since there are no real rewards any longer, the rats have only their expectations of reward to guide them. Naturally, without real rewards to sustain efforts, performance in the extinction test gradually falls. But since the rats originally learned that perseverance pays off, they persist for quite some time in working based largely on their ordinary wanting for reward. The amount of work (number of lever presses) the animals are willing to perform under these conditions of no reward delivery is the measure of "wanting." Since no actual rewards are delivered (i.e., extinction), the analysis is not confounded by consumption of rewards.

The crux of the matter to reveal cue-triggered "wanting" is to test the effects of Pavlovian cues, the tones formerly presented in association with the rewards, in various states of brain mesolimbic activation. These cues are presented once in a while as the rats continue to work—or not, as the case may be. During this extinction test, cues come and go while the rats work in order to get a reward that is never delivered. Finally, brain mesolimbic activation is manipulated by varying whether the rats receive a drug microinjection that causes increases in dopamine release.

Dopamine Magnifies Cue-Triggered "Wanting"

Cindy Wyvell used this test in our laboratory and found a form of truly irrational choice that depended on mesolimbic (dopamine) activation (Wyvell & Berridge, 2000, 2001). She used amphetamine microinjections into the brain nucleus accumbens to activate mesolimbic dopamine systems. Amphetamine causes dopamine neurons to release their dopamine into synapses so that it can reach other neurons. Wyvell found that dopamine activation caused a transient but intense form of irrational pursuit linked to incentive salience (Figure 24.2). One group of rats received amphetamine microinjections before their behavioral test, while another group received saline. During this test, their baseline performance could be guided only by their expectation of the cognitively wanted sugar because they received no real sugar rewards. And while they pursued their expected reward, the Pavlovian reward cue (light or sound for 30 seconds) was occasionally presented to them over the course of the half-hour session.

Wyvell's findings were consistent and clear. Amphetamine microinjection en-hanced "wanting" for sugar. Animals worked for the rewards, and during the presentation of the Pavlovian cue, they showed peaks of dramatically harder work; that is, their level of "wanting" increased. Amphetamine in their brains selectively raised the height of those "wanting" peaks without changing the baseline plateau on which the peaks sat or anything else. It should be noted that there are two types of wanting assessed here: (a) ordinary wanting, where the rat is guided primarily by its cognitive expectation that it will like the worked-for sugar reward, and (b) cue-triggered "wanting," or incentive salience attributed by mesolimbic systems to the representation of sugar reward that is activated by the cue. Dopamine activation selectively quadrupled cue-triggered "wanting," causing a specific elevation in this particular form of decision utility. A similar specificity, in reverse, has been found for suppressing effects of dopamine-blocking drugs on cue-triggered "wanting" (Dickinson, Smith, & Mirenowicz, 2000).

Even though the dopamine rise in Wyvell's experiments was relatively constant over the half-hour test, the elevation in "wanting"

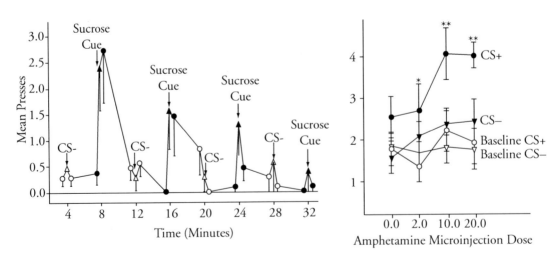

Fig. 24.2 Irrational cue-triggered "wanting." Transient irrational "wanting" comes and goes with the cue (left). Amphetamine microinjection in nucleus accumbens magnifies "wanting" for sugar reward—but only in presence of reward cue (CS+). Cognitive expectations and ordinary wanting are not altered (reflected in baseline lever pressing in absence of cue and during irrelevant cue, CS–) (right). Based on Wyvell and Berridge (2000).

was not. It required two conditions simultaneously: dopamine activation plus the presence of the cue previously associated with reward. Thus, the "wanting" peak was repeatedly reversible, even over the short span of a half-hour test session, coming and going with the 30-second cue (Wyvell & Berridge, 2000). This exaggeration of a "cue-triggered wanting" phenomenon caused by activating mesolimbic dopamine demonstrated by Wyvell was both irrational (detaching from stable expectations of reward value expressed by lever pressing for reward between cues) and transient (always decaying within a minute of the cue's end).

In a related experiment, Wyvell tested the effect of amphetamine microinjections on the experienced utility of real sugar by measuring positive hedonic "liking" reactions of rats as they received an infusion of sugar solution into their mouths. The amphetamine never increased rats' positive facial reactions elicited by the taste of real sugar, indicating once again that dopamine did not increase "liking" for the sugar reward. Thus, Wyvell found that activation of dopamine neurotransmission in the accumbens did not change ordinary wanting based on cognitive expectation of liking (measured by baseline performance on the lever), nor did it alter "liking."

In an elevated dopamine state, hyper-"wanting" is triggered by an encounter with reward cues, and at that moment it exerts its irrational effect, disproportionate to the cognitively expected hedonic value of the reward. In other words, we suggest that at the moment of a reward cue, decision utility diverges from predicted utility if the brain is dopamine stimulated by amphetamine. One moment, the dopamine-activated brain of the rat simply wants sugar in the ordinary sense, although the decision is tempered by the fact that there is no reward presented during extinction. The next moment, when the cue comes, the dopamine-activated

brain both wants sugar and "wants" sugar to an exaggerated degree, according to the incentive salience hypothesis (Figure 24.2). A few moments after the cue ends, it has returned to its rational level of wanting appropriate to its expectation of reward. Moments later still, the cue is reencountered again, and excessive and irrational "wanting" again takes control.

The irrational level of pursuit thus has two sources that determine its occurrence and duration: a physiological factor (brain mesolimbic activation) and a psychological factor (reward cue activation). It seems unlikely that mesolimbic activation altered rats' cognitive expectation of how much they would like sugar (which might have rationally increased desire even though their expectation would be mistaken). That is because amphetamine was present in the nucleus accumbens throughout the entire session, but the intense enhancement of pursuit lasted only while the cue stimulus was actually present.

Human Drug Addiction as Sensitized "Wanting"

Human drug addiction may be a special illustration of irrational "wanting" driven by mesolimbic brain systems (Robinson & Berridge, 1993, 2003). Addictive drugs not only activate brain dopamine systems when the drug is taken but also may sensitize them afterward. Neural sensitization means that the brain's mesolimbic system is hyperreactive and therefore more easily activated by drugs or related cues for a long time and maybe even permanently. The mesolimbic system reacts more strongly than normal if the drug is taken again. This state of hyperactive reactivity is gated by associative cues and contexts that predict the drug. Neural sensitization occurs to different degrees in different individuals. Some individuals are susceptible to sensitization, but others are not, depending on many factors, ranging from genes to prior experiences as well as on the drug itself, the dose, and so on (Robinson & Berridge, 1993, 2003).

Efforts to apply these insights gave rise to the incentive-sensitization theory of addiction, developed primarily by Terry Robinson, which specifies the role sensitization of incentive salience may play in driving addicts to compulsively take drugs (Robinson & Berridge, 1993, 2003). This theory suggests that if the mesolimbic system of addicts becomes sensitized after taking drugs, they may irrationally "want" to take drugs again—even if they have fully emerged from withdrawal by the time they relapse and even if they decide they don't "like" the drugs very much (or at least like them less than they like the lifestyle they will lose by taking them). This incentive-sensitization theory of addiction thus accounts for why addictive relapse is so often precipitated by encounters with drug cues that trigger excessive "wanting" for drugs. In a sensitized mesolimbic state, the reward cues trigger a momentary rise in decision utility that far outstrips any predicted or experienced utility of the drugs. Drug cues are attributed with more incentive salience than other cues because they are associatively paired with strong drugs. Drug cues could trigger irrational "wanting" in an addict whose brain was sensitized even long after withdrawal was over (because sensitization lasts longer) and regardless of expectations of "liking."

Actual evidence that sensitization does indeed cause irrational cue-triggered "wanting" was recently found by Cindy Wyvell in an affective neuroscience animal study of mesolimbic sensitization by drugs similar to the study described previously (Wyvell & Berridge, 2001). Rats that had been previously sensitized by amphetamine responded to a sugar cue with excessive "wanting" despite not having had any drug for 10 days. Even though the rats were

drug free at the time of testing, sensitization (i.e., the brain in a state of permanent mesolimbic excitability) caused excessively high cue-triggered "wanting" for their reward. For sensitized rats, irrational "wanting" for sugar came and went transiently with the Pavlovian cue associated with the sugar reward, just as if they had received a brain microinjection of drug to immediately activate the mesolimbic system—but they had not. Their persisting pattern of cue-triggered irrationality seems consistent with the incentive-sensitization theory of human drug addiction (Robinson & Berridge, 1993, 2003). Similarly, neural sensitization by drugs has been found to increase other cue and motivation effects, such as conditioned reinforcement, and the persistence of motivated performance on second-order schedules and instrumental breakpoint in animals (Vanderschuren & Everitt, 2005; Vezina, 2004).

Separating Neural Codes for Predicted Utility From Decision Utility

A crucial question about enhancements of cue-triggered "wanting" discussed previously is whether the mesolimbic increase applies to predicted utility as well or just decision utility. It is clear that decision utility was elevated in the previously mentioned experiments by prior sensitization or direct amphetamine effects. But did dopamine magnify decision utility purely and alone? Or could dopamine elevation also have raised predicted utility too? If so, a sensitized individual might hold mistakenly exaggerated expectations for future reward, expecting eventual experienced utility to be higher than it really will be. If that happened, then decision utility would also elevate and passively trail after predicted utility. After all, if one mistakenly expects a reward to be better than it will be, then one may choose to pursue it more than one otherwise would.

Contemporary Dopamine Models of Predicted Utility

A prediction error interpretation (mistakenly elevated expectation of reward) is highlighted by recent intriguing hypotheses about dopamine and predictive reward learning in computational neuroscience. These have suggested that dopamine neurons may help mediate the associations and predictions involved in reward learning, either via stamping in associations to an unconditioned stimulus (UCS) prediction error or by modulating the strength of learned predictions or learned habits elicited by a CS (Dayan & Balleine, 2002; McClure, Berns, & Montague, 2003; Montague et al., 2004; O'Doherty, Dayan, Friston, Critchley, & Dolan, 2003; Schultz, 2002, 2006; Schultz, Dayan, & Montague, 1997).

Elegant and influential studies by Wolfram Schultz and colleagues, for example, have led to suggestions that the firing of dopamine neurons may code the predicted utility of a CS cue that predicts reward (and the prediction error of a surprising UCS reward itself). For example, dopamine firing has been suggested by learning theorists to approximate the Rescorla–Wagner model of Pavlovian conditioning, that is, $\Delta V = \alpha\beta(\lambda - V)$, and the temporal difference model of gradual associative learning, that is, $V(s_t) = \langle \sum_{i=0} \gamma^i r_{t+1} \rangle$ (Montague et al., 1996; Rescorla & Wagner, 1972; Schultz, 2002). In those dopamine-learning models, firing by dopamine neurons to a CS cue that predicts reward encodes its predicted utility (V). If a UCS reward has failed to be predicted and thus is surprising, dopamine neurons may fire again, suggested by these models to encode the prediction error: $(\lambda - V)$ or $\delta(r)$.

The crucial feature of such learning models, when applied to predicted utility of reward and to mesolimbic dopamine function, is that dopamine elevation can generate new learning only by creating a UCS prediction error if the experienced utility of UCS is greater than CS expected. This feature results from the fact that previously learned values are "cached" and can be changed only incrementally and only by having further opportunities to learn a changed new relationship between CS and UCS.

Teasing Apart Predicted Utility and Decision Utility

For example, if one elevates learning parameters in the models, as a dopamine rise might produce (according to these dopamine-prediction models), the predicted utility V carried by a CS+ does not immediately change. Instead, in the next learning trial, the UCS will cause a larger prediction error or faster learning rate, which will be saved until the next trial. Evidence for new learning is postponed until it can be demonstrated in subsequent trials. The new learning is then reflected in a gradually incremented increase in predicted utility generated the next times the CS is encountered.

Thus, a startling feature of Wyvell's behavioral effects of amphetamine and sensitization on cue-triggered "wanting" described previously (and the neural recording experiment described in the next section) is that mesolimbic activation occurred after all learning trials were completed. It did not need to be relearned. It was immediate on the first cue presentations in the activated mesolimbic state. Even on the very first trial, the next time the cue was encountered, CS+ decision utility was elevated. Dopamine activation did not occur before training, so there was no possibility that learning could have enhanced subsequent prediction errors (increased predicted utility). In the Wyvell experiment, mesolimbic activation was delayed until after learning, when it was too late to be able to promote predicted utility via boosting the association between CS+ and UCS. Mesolimbic activation still increased cue-triggered "wanting," indicating that it could not have generated increased predicted utility as suggested by these temporal difference–based computational models.

But perhaps mesolimbic dopamine activation could be reinterpreted as having caused excessive general or cue-triggered predicted utility, expressed as overoptimistic expectations about the quality or quantity of upcoming rewards. In plain language, what if dopamine caused a cue to carry higher predicted utility than it ordinarily would as well as higher decision utility? If so, the elevation of predicted utility by amphetamine or sensitization would become similar to the standard types of wrong decisions or miswanting identified by Kahneman and colleagues, Gilbert and colleagues, and others (Gilbert & Wilson, 2000; Kahneman et al., 1997; Loewenstein & Schkade, 1999). Those wrong choices are based on wrong expectations. That means that they need not be irrational by the criteria we have adopted—wrong as the decisions remain—as long as the choice's decision utility matches predicted utility.

We believe we can rule out such a possibility for dopamine-based irrational "wanting" described previously. But we have to turn to inside the brain in order to do it. What happens to utility from the brain's point of view when dopamine is released?

Neuronal Coding of Predicted Utility and Decision Utility in Limbic Ventral Pallidum

A recent study of neural coding in our laboratory examined changes in predicted utility versus decision utility caused by mesolimbic dopamine activation (Tindell et al., 2005). This dissertation study was conducted primarily by Amy Tindell

in the Aldridge laboratory and focused on the ventral pallidum, a mesolimbic output structure. Tindell used recording electrodes to study the firing patterns of neurons that receive the impact of dopamine elevation and the relationship of neuronal firing to predicted utility, decision utility, and experienced utility of sugar rewards and their Pavlovian cues.

We focused on the ventral pallidum for neural coding of reward utility because it is a "limbic final common path" for reward signals in mesocorticolimbic circuits. The ventral pallidum integrates reward-related information from the nucleus accumbens (compressed as much as 29 to 1) with other structures (Kalivas & Nakamura, 1999; Oorschot, 1996; Zahm, 2000). It especially integrates dopamine influences with reward signals because the ventral pallidum receives the heaviest projections sent from the nucleus accumbens neurons that most famously get mesolimbic dopamine and also receives direct mesolimbic dopamine inputs itself. The output of the ventral pallidum is directed back to cortex through the thalamus and also onward to brain stem nuclei.

Serial Cues Uncouple Predicted Versus Decision Utilities

In order to tease apart predicted utility from decision utility, we used two different cues in series to predict the sugar reward (Tindell et al., 2005). A 10-second auditory tone cue (CS+1) was followed by a 1-second auditory click cue (CS+2), which finally was followed immediately by a sugar pellet (UCS). The two different CSs have very different ratios of predicted utility to decision utility.

The first tone cue has the most prediction utility because it predicts everything that follows: It predicts the click cue 10 seconds later and the sugar pellet 1 second after that. Once a rat learns this relationship, which usually takes only a few dozen presentations of the series, the CS+1 tone cue tells the animal everything there is to know about upcoming signals and rewards for the immediate future. By contrast, the second click cue is completely redundant as a predictor. It adds no new information. Rats can easily keep track of the 10- to 11-second interval between first tone and sugar—they do not need the second cue to tell them sugar is coming. In fact, they begin to hover around the sugar dish a few seconds before it arrives. Thus, the CS+1 tone cue carries greatest predicted utility. It sets all expectations for the future. That means that if mesolimbic activation can raise predicted utility, it should best be evident in changes in neuronal firing elicited by the CS+1 tone cue.

But the second click cue still has something the first tone cue does not: the greatest decision utility. The CS+2 click carries the greatest incentive salience. It occurs at the moment of highest incentive motivation or "wanting" for sugar, reflected in part by rat's eager hovering around the dish at that moment. If mesolimbic activation causes increases in decision utility that occur without any matching increase in predicted utility, then this should be most evident in amplification of neuronal firing elicited by the CS+2 click cue. And it should occur even if there is no change in firing to the CS+1 tone. That profile of activation would indicate that decision utility is greater than predicted utility at the moment of the CS+2 cue, setting the stage for the possibility of strongly irrational choice.

Finally, the sugar reward UCS that comes last carries the greatest experienced utility. The sweet sugary pellet is the event that is actually "liked" best. It is also the teaching signal event, the reward value that "stamps in" an association or that instructs a predictive actor in an actor–critic model that a reward event has occurred. One should expect a change in sugar-elicited neuronal firing if

mesolimbic activation causes elevations in either hedonic impact, associative stamping in, or UCS prediction errors generated as teaching signals. And just to double-check if hedonic impact "liking" is enhanced by mesolimbic activation, we also examined whether amphetamine or drug sensitization caused any elevation in "liking" reactions of rats to the taste of sugar.

Dopamine and Sensitization Specifically Elevate Coded Signal for Decision Utility

Rats were trained for 2 weeks, and then some were sensitized while others were treated with a saline placebo over another 2-week period. Sensitization leaves mesolimbic neurons structurally changed and ready to release more dopamine than normal when stimulated by drugs or certain other events (Robinson & Kolb, 2004). Then all the rats were implanted with recording electrodes in their ventral pallidum and allowed to recover for another 2 weeks. To decode reward utilities in neuronal firing patterns, we used a novel computational technique, "profile analysis," developed by our colleague Jun Zhang, that compares firing of neurons to different stimuli, asking whether the greatest firing is elicited by either the CS1, the CS+2, or the UCS to identify the maximal stimulus for each neuron. This technique allows us to identify how mesolimbic activation changes the stimulus preference "profile" of ventral pallidal (VP) neurons.

We found that individual VP neurons usually fire to all three stimuli but not equally to all (Figure 24.3). Ordinarily, predictive utility seems to dominate neuronal coding in VP in the sense that the neurons fire most to the CS+1 (next to the CS+2 and only moderately to the sugar). But decision utility was purely and specifically elevated by mesolimbic activation, including dopamine elevation, caused by either prior

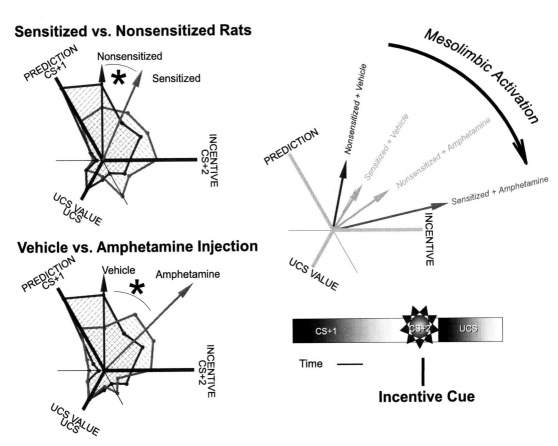

Fig. 24.3 Mesolimbic activation magnifies decision utility coding by neuron firing in ventral pallidum. Population profile vector shifts toward incentive coding with mesolimbic activation. Profile analysis shows stimulus preference coded in firing for all 524 ventral pallidum neurons. Ordinarily, neurons prefer to code predicted utility (firing maximally to CS+1 tone). Sensitization and amphetamine administration each shift neuronal coding preference toward decision utility (firing maximally to the CS+2 click) and away from predicted utility of CS+1 (without altering signal for experienced utility of the sugar UCS). Combination of sensitization with amphetamine shifts ventral pallidum coding profiles even further toward the signal for pure decision utility or incentive salience. Thus, as mesolimbic activation increases, ventral pallidum neurons increasingly carry coded signals for decision utility (relative to predicted utility and experienced utility signals). Entire populations are shown by shaded areas. Arrows shows the maximal averaged response of the population under each treatment. Based on Tindell, Berridge, Zhang, Peciña, and Aldridge (2005, pp. 2628 and 2629, figs. 6 and 7).

drug-induced neural sensitization or simply injecting the rats with amphetamine just before test (to make mesolimbic neurons release extra dopamine). Dopamine-related brain activation shifted the profiles of VP neural activation toward incentive coding of decision utility at the expense of prediction coding of predicted utility (Figure 24.3). The elevations in decision utility appeared to add together across amphetamine and sensitization treatments, combining to produce an even greater enhancement of decision utility than either treatment alone.

This may model the special vulnerability of a sensitized addict at a moment of trying to take "just one hit" again who thus maximally boosts the drug's decision utility and so precipitates a previously unintended binge of relapse and drug consumption.

It is noteworthy that the shift toward neuronal incentive coding was immediate on the first test trials and did not require any relearning (Figure 24.4). That immediate change supports the incentive-sensitization hypothesis and stands in contrast to the alternative dopamine-learning hypotheses

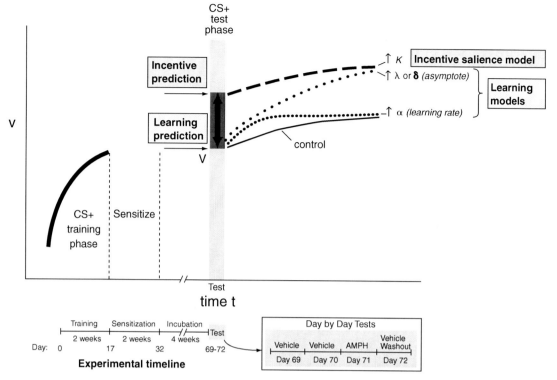

Fig. 24.4 Decision utility increment happens too fast for relearning. Time line and alternative outcomes for neuronal firing coding of reward cue after mesolimbic activation of sensitization and/or amphetamine in ventral pallidum recording experiment (Tindell, Berridge, Zhang, Peciña, & Aldridge, 2005). The incentive salience model predicts that mesolimbic activation dynamically increases the decision utility of a previously learned CS+. The increased incentive salience coding is visible the first time the already-learned cue is presented in the activated mesolimbic state. Learning models by contrast require relearning to elevate learned predicted utilities. They predict merely gradual acceleration if mesolimbic activation increases rate parameters of learning and gradual acceleration plus asymptote elevation if mesolimbic activation increases prediction errors. Actual data support the incentive salience model. Based on data from Tindell et al. (2005).

that require further training trials for the boosted prediction error of an increased reward, for example, $(\delta)t$, to magnify relearned predictions (V). It appears that in a dopamine-activated or sensitized state, incentive coding by VP neurons might mediate increased cue-triggered "wanting" and could lead to the compulsive relapse of addiction, especially for drug cues that occur close in time to their reward. And strengthening of the decision utility signal occurred at the expense of relative weakening of the predicted utility signal after drug and sensitization dopamine activations.

Finally, these shifts toward VP incentive coding were not due to enhanced UCS hedonic impact ("liking"). Behavioral hedonic

"liking" reactions to sucrose taste remained constant or even diminished slightly with sensitization and amphetamine administration. In other words, mesolimbic activation caused increases in cue-triggered "wanting" as coded by VP neurons when encountering a CS+ for sugar reward without any increase in experienced utility or "liking" for sugar itself.

In normal life, such enhancement of incentive salience might occur during normal appetite states, such as hunger. Incentive salience or cue-triggered decision utility normally depends on integrating two separate factors: (a) current physiological/neurobiological state and (b) previously learned associations about CS+ (Berridge,

2004; Toates, 1986). Integrating current physiological state with learned cues allows behavior to be guided dynamically by appetite-appropriate stimuli without need of further learning (e.g., Pavlovian cues associated with food are immediately more attractive to a hungry animal). Drug sensitization or acute amphetamine may each "short-circuit" this neurobiological system and directly increase the incentive value attributed to particular conditioned stimuli, triggering greater "wanting" and pursuit of their reward (Robinson & Berridge, 2003; Tindell et al., 2005).

Explanation for Cued Hyperbolic Temporal Discounting?

The shift toward incentive coding suggests how sensitization and addictive drugs may prime motivational behavioral responses of addicts to drug-related stimuli by amplifying the incentive impact of encountering a UCS-proximal drug CS+. Finally, it suggests a mechanism to help explain hyperbolic temporal discounting, at least in cue-triggered decisions. Temporal discounting is well recognized in addicts (Ainslie, 1992), and neuroimaging has shown that mesolimbic systems code immediate rewards (McClure, Laibson, Loewenstein, & Cohen, 2004). But temporal discounting is usually just described and accepted as a given. Although it is sometimes posited as a mechanism that drives choices, little is known about the explanatory mechanism for hyperbolic discounting itself. Part of the explanation may be that limbic activation causes circuits involving the ventral pallidum to fire more to cues for a temporally close reward and therefore selectively enhance their incentive salience, causing excessive cue-triggered "wanting" for the close reward. This also may be why "visceral states" sometimes exacerbate temporal discounting effects (Loewenstein & Schkade, 1999).

Irrational Decision Utility From Mesolimbic Activation

We suggest that both the Wyvell and Tindell experiments described previously are examples of decision utility being greater than predicted utility at the same moment. Thus, both are examples of irrational "wanting," defined as "wanting" something more than one expects to like. In the Wyvell cue-triggered "wanting" experiments, the elevated decision utility is a peak of frenzied pursuit of the sugar reward, at least for a while. The reward cue causes a momentary irrational desire, during which decision utility is greater than predicted utility (as well as decision utility being greater than experienced utility). In the Tindell neuronal firing experiments, the magnified firing bursts of VP neurons at the moment of the cue with the most incentive salience reflects a neural mechanism that may drive irrational "wanting." Irrational "wanting" happens best when a reward cue occurs simultaneously with mesolimbic activation, especially dopamine-related activation. Individuals may then "want" what they do not want cognitively. The high incentive salience type of "wanting" exerts its power independent of more cognitive wants. For example, a recovering brain-sensitized addict may sincerely want in every cognitive way to remain abstinent from drugs but may nonetheless be precipitated by a chance encounter with drug cues into intense "wanting" despite cognitive desires and thus relapse into taking drugs again. Further, they may not predict associatively in a manner that would justify their "want." The addict may accurately predict that drug pleasure will not be enough to offset the adverse consequences of taking the drug yet will still "want" to take it. The decision utility is irrational in the sense that their immediate "want" exceeds what they know cognitively they will not like (or, at least, will not "like" proportionally to their excessive "want").

Importantly, incentive salience attributions are encapsulated and modular in the sense that people may not have direct conscious access to them and find them difficult to cognitively controls (Robinson & Berridge, 1993, 2003; Winkielman & Berridge, 2004). Cue-triggered "wanting" belongs to the class of automatic reactions that operate by their own rules under the surface of direct awareness (see Chapters 5 and 23; Bargh & Ferguson, 2000; Bargh, Gollwitzer, Lee-Chai, Barndollar, & Trötschel, 2001; Dijksterhuis, Bos, Nordgren, & van Baaren, 2006; Gilbert & Wilson, 2000; Wilson, Lindsey, & Schooler, 2000; Zajonc, 2000). People are sometimes aware of incentive salience as a product but never of the underlying process. And without an extra cognitive monitoring step, they may not even be always aware of the product. Sometimes incentive salience can be triggered and can control behavior with very little awareness of what has happened. For example, subliminal exposures to happy or angry facial expressions, too brief to see consciously, can cause people later to consume more or less of a beverage—without being at all aware their "wanting" has been manipulated (Winkielman & Berridge, 2004). Additional monitoring by brain systems of conscious awareness, likely cortical structures, is required to bring a basic "want" into a subjective feeling of wanting.

Applications to Human Decision Making

Although our experiments used drugs and sensitization to manipulate brain dopamine systems in rats, people have brain dopamine systems too, which are likely to respond in similar ways. Human mesolimbic systems can be equally activated by drugs and addiction. And perhaps more relevant to everyday decisions, the same dopamine brain systems are also spontaneously activated by natural appetite states and in many emotional situations.

As a result of all this, an irrational "want" for something can occur despite cognitively not wanting it, cognitively wanting not to "want," or cognitively wanting something else. An irrational cue-triggered "want" may even surprise the person who has it by its power, suddenness, and autonomy. This may explain why some long-term drug addicts can proclaim (perhaps even truthfully) to not enjoy their drug as they once did while at the same time they may take part in criminal activity in order to acquire the drug.

Both rewarding and stressful situations activate brain mesolimbic dopamine systems. This seems to raise the possibility for decision utility elevations when reward cues occur simultaneously with brain activation at moments requiring a choice. If a person's brain dopamine system were highly activated and the person encountered a reward cue at that moment, then the person might irrationally elevate the decision utility of the cued outcome over and above both its experienced utility and its predicted utility. That person would be under the control of a decision utility peak. The person might "want" the cued reward just like the rat even if the person cognitively expected not to like it very much.

Of course, for general psychologists the primary value of issues discussed here may be a better insight into the mechanisms that underlie more normal decision making. Most decisions in ordinary life are rational, choosing and wanting what one expects to like best (Higgens, 2006). In those cases, there is no divergence between underlying brain mechanisms of incentive salience and reward prediction. Instead, these mesolimbic dopamine mechanisms of decision utility simply provide motivational oomph to help power behavioral choices that were guided by more cognitive, cortical mechanisms based on the predicted utility of potential outcomes. When choice is optimized, the multiplicity of underlying mechanisms may be seamlessly papered over, and only a psychologist would know that there are multiple mechanisms beneath the surface.

But the underlying multiplicity remains whether a given decision is rational or not. And the potential remains for irrational dissociation at future moments. Such phenomena might not be restricted to basic consumption behavior but could extend to interact with more abstract and even economic decisions too (Bernheim & Rangel, 2004; Camerer & Fehr, 2006). Whether hijacked decision utility and irrational "wanting" actually play this role in ordinary human lives and decisions seems to be an intriguing possibility that may deserve further consideration from psychologists who study decisions in action.

Acknowledgments

This chapter is based on an article for *Social Cognition*. Research described here was supported by grants from the NIH to KCB and to JWA (DA015188 and MH63649, DA017752), and writing of the original draft was supported by a fellowship from the John Simon Guggenheim Memorial Foundation. We are grateful to the editors for helpful comments on an earlier version.

References

Ainslie, G. (1992). *Picoeconomics.* Cambridge: Cambridge University Press.

Bargh, J. A., & Ferguson, M. J. (2000). Beyond behaviorism: On the automaticity of higher mental processes. *Psychological Bulletin, 126,* 925–945.

Bargh, J. A., Gollwitzer, P. M., Lee-Chai, A., Barndollar, K., & Trötschel, R. (2001). The automated will: Nonconscious activation and pursuit of behavioral goals. *Journal of Personality and Social Psychology, 81,* 1014–1027.

Bernheim, B. D., & Rangel, A. (2004). Addiction and cue-triggered decision processes. *American Economic Review, 94,* 1558–1590.

Berridge, K. C. (1999). Pleasure, pain, desire, and dread: Hidden core processes of emotion. In D. Kahneman, E. Diener, & N. Schwarz (Eds.), *Well-being: The foundations of hedonic psychology* (pp. 525–557). New York: Russell Sage Foundation.

Berridge, K. C. (2001). Reward learning: Reinforcement, incentives, and expectations. In D. L. Medin (Ed.), *The psychology of learning and motivation* (Vol. 40, pp. 223–278). New York: Academic Press.

Berridge, K. C. (2003a). Irrational pursuits: Hyperincentives from a visceral brain. In I. Brocas & J. Carrillo (Eds.), *Psychology and economics* (Vol. 1, pp. 14–40). Oxford: Oxford University Press.

Berridge, K. C. (2003b). Pleasures of the brain. *Brain and Cognition, 52,* 106–128.

Berridge, K. C. (2004). Motivation concepts in behavioral neuroscience. *Physiology and Behavior, 81,* 179–209.

Berridge, K. C. (2007). The debate over dopamine's role in reward: The case for incentive salience. *Psychopharmacology (Berl), 191*(3), 391–431.

Berridge, K. C., & Robinson, T. E. (1998). What is the role of dopamine in reward: Hedonic impact, reward learning, or incentive salience? *Brain Research Reviews, 28,* 309–369.

Berridge, K. C., & Valenstein, E. S. (1991). What psychological process mediates feeding evoked by electrical stimulation of the lateral hypothalamus? *Behavioral Neuroscience, 105,* 3–14.

Bindra, D. (1978). How adaptive behavior is produced: A perceptual-motivation alternative to response reinforcement. *Behavioral and Brain Sciences, 1,* 41–91.

Camerer, C. F., & Fehr, E. (2006). When does "economic man" dominate social behavior? *Science, 311,* 47–52.

Davidson, R. J., Jackson, D. C., & Kalin, N. H. (2000). Emotion, plasticity, context, and regulation: Perspectives from affective neuroscience. *Psychological Bulletin, 126*(6), 890–909.

Davidson, R. J., Shackman, A. J., & Maxwell, J. S. (2004). Asymmetries in face and brain related to emotion. *Trends in Cognitive Sciences, 8,* 389–391.

Dayan, P., & Balleine, B. W. (2002). Reward, motivation, and reinforcement learning. *Neuron, 36,* 285–298.

Dickinson, A., Smith, J., & Mirenowicz, J. (2000). Dissociation of Pavlovian and instrumental incentive learning under dopamine antagonists. *Behavioral Neuroscience, 114,* 468–483.

Dijksterhuis, A., Bos, M. W., Nordgren, L. F., & van Baaren, R. B. (2006). On making the right choice: The deliberation-without-attention effect. *Science, 311,* 1005–1007.

Gilbert, D. G., & Wilson, T. D. (2000). Miswanting: Some problems in forecasting future affective states. In Forgas, J. (Ed.), *Feeling and thinking: The role of affect in social cognition* (pp. 178–197). Cambridge: Cambridge University Press.

Heath, R. G. (1972). Pleasure and brain activity in man: Deep and surface electroencephalograms during orgasm. *Journal of Nervous and Mental Disease, 154,* 3–18.

Higgins, E. T. (2006). Value from hedonic experience and engagement. *Psychological Review, 113,* 439–460.

Hoebel, B. G. (1988). Neuroscience and motivation: pathways and peptides that define motivational systems. In R. C. Atkinson, R. J. Herrnstein, G. Lindzey, & R. D. Luce (Eds.), *Stevens' handbook of experimental psychology* (Vol. 1, pp. 547–626). New York: John Wiley & Sons.

Kahneman, D., Fredrickson, B. L., Schreiber, C. A., & Redelmeier, D. A. (1993). When more pain is preferred to less: Adding a better end. *Psychological Science, 4,* 401–405.

Kahneman, D., Wakker, P. P., & Sarin, R. (1997). Back to Bentham? Explorations of experienced utility. *Quarterly Journal of Economics, 112,* 375–405.

Kalivas, P. W., & Nakamura, M. (1999). Neural systems for behavioral activation and reward. *Current Opinion in Neurobiology, 9,* 223–227.

Kringelbach, M. L. (2004). Food for thought: Hedonic experience beyond homeostasis in the human brain. *Neuroscience, 126,* 807–819.

Loewenstein, G., & Schkade, D. (1999). Wouldn't it be nice? Predicting future feelings. In *Wellbeing: The foundations of hedonic psychology* (pp. 85–105). New York: Russell Sage Foundation.

Mahler, S. V., Smith, K. S. & Berridge, K. C. (2007). Endocannabinoid hedonic hotspot for sensory pleasure: Anandamide in nucleus accumbens shell enhances liking of a sweet reward. *Neuropsychopharmacology, 32*(11), 2267–2278.

McClure, S. M., Berns, G. S., & Montague, P. R. (2003). Temporal prediction errors in a passive learning task activate human striatum. *Neuron, 38,* 339–346.

McClure, S. M., Laibson, D. I., Loewenstein, G., & Cohen, J. D. (2004). Separate neural systems value immediate and delayed monetary rewards. *Science, 306*(5695), 503–507.

McFadden, D. (2005). The new science of pleasure (Frisch Lecture). *Econometric Society World Congress,* London. Retrieved July 17, 2008 from http://www.econ.berkeley.edu/wp/mcfadden0105/ScienceofPleasure.pdf

Meloy, T. S., & Southern, J. P. (2006). Neurally augmented sexual function in human females: A preliminary investigation. *Neuromodulation, 9,* 34–40.

Montague, P. R., Dayan, P., & Sejnowski, T. J. (1996). A framework for mesencephalic dopamine systems based on predictive Hebbian learning. *Journal of Neuroscience, 16,* 1936–1947.

Montague, P. R., Hyman, S. E., & Cohen, J. D. (2004). Computational roles for dopamine in behavioural control. *Nature, 431,* 760–767.

Morewedge, C. K., Gilbert, D. T., & Wilson, T. D. (2005). The least likely of times: How remembering the past biases forecasts of the future. *Psychological Science, 16,* 626–630.

O'Doherty, J. P., Dayan, P., Friston, K., Critchley, H., & Dolan, R. J. (2003). Temporal difference models and reward-related learning in the human brain. *Neuron, 38,* 329–337.

Olds, J., & Milner, P. (1954). Positive reinforcement produced by electrical stimulation of septal area and other regions of rat brain. *Journal of Comparative and Physiological Psychology, 47,* 419–427.

Oorschot, D. E. (1996). Total number of neurons in the neostriatal, pallidal, subthalamic, and substantia nigral nuclei of the rat basal ganglia: A stereological study using the cavalieri and optical disector methods. *Journal of Comparative Neurology, 366,* 580–599.

Peciña, S., & Berridge, K. C. (2000). Opioid eating site in accumbens shell mediates food intake and hedonic "liking": Map based on microinjection Fos plumes. *Brain Research, 863,* 71–86.

Peciña, S., & Berridge, K. C. (2005). Hedonic hot spot in nucleus accumbens shell: Where do mu-opioids cause increased hedonic impact of sweetness? *Journal of Neuroscience, 25,* 11777–11786.

Peciña, S., Smith, K. S., & Berridge, K. C. (2006). Hedonic hot spots in the brain. *Neuroscientist, 12,* 500–511.

Portenoy, R. K., Jarden, J. O., Sidtis, J. J., Lipton, R. B., Foley, K. M., & Rottenberg, D. A. (1986).

Compulsive thalamic self-stimulation: A case with metabolic, electrophysiologic and behavioral correlates. *Pain, 27,* 277–290.

Rescorla, R. A., & Wagner, A. R. (1972). A theory of Pavlovian conditioning: Variations in the effectiveness of reinforcement and non-reinforcement. In A. H. Black & W. F. Prokasy (Eds.), *Classical conditioning II: Current research and theory* (pp. 64–99). New York, Appleton-Century-Crofts.

Reynolds, S. M., & Berridge, K. C. (2002). Positive and negative motivation in nucleus accumbens shell: Bivalent rostrocaudal gradients for GABA-elicited eating, taste "liking"/"disliking" reactions, place preference/avoidance, and fear. *Journal of Neuroscience, 22,* 7308–7320.

Robinson, T. E., & Berridge, K. C. (1993). The neural basis of drug craving: An incentive-sensitization theory of addiction. *Brain Research Reviews, 18,* 247–291.

Robinson, T. E., & Berridge, K. C. (2003). Addiction. *Annual Review of Psychology, 54,* 25–53.

Robinson, T. E., & Kolb, B. (2004). Structural plasticity associated with exposure to drugs of abuse. *47,* 33–46.

Schultz, W. (2002). Getting formal with dopamine and reward. *Neuron, 36,* 241–263.

Schultz, W. (2006). Behavioral theories and the neurophysiology of reward. *Annual Review of Psychology, 57,* 87–115.

Schultz, W., Dayan, P., & Montague, P. R. (1997). A neural substrate of prediction and reward. *Science, 275,* 1593–1599.

Shizgal, P. (1997). Neural basis of utility estimation. *Current Opinion in Neurobiology, 7,* 198–208.

Shizgal, P. (1999). On the neural computation of utility: Implications from studies of brain stimulation reward. In D. Kahneman, E. Diener, & N. Schwarz (Eds.), *Well-being: The foundations of hedonic psychology* (pp. 500–524). New York: Russell Sage Foundation.

Shizgal, P., Fulton, S., & Woodside, B. (2001). Brain reward circuitry and the regulation of energy balance. *International Journal of Obesity, 25,* S17–S21.

Smith, K. S., & Berridge, K. C. (2005). The ventral pallidum and hedonic reward: Neurochemical maps of sucrose "liking" and food intake. *Journal of Neuroscience, 25,* 8637–8649.

Tindell, A. J., Berridge, K. C., Zhang, J., Peciña, S., & Aldridge, J. W. (2005). Ventral pallidal neurons code incentive motivation: Amplification by mesolimbic sensitization and amphetamine. *European Journal of Neuroscience, 22,* 2617–2634.

Tindell, A. J., Smith, K. S., Peciña, S., Berridge, K. C., & Aldridge, J. W. (2006). Ventral pallidum firing codes hedonic reward: When a bad taste turns good. *Journal of Neurophysiology, 96,* 2399–2409.

Toates, F. (1986). *Motivational systems.* Cambridge: Cambridge University Press.

Vanderschuren, L. J., & Everitt, B. J. (2005). Behavioral and neural mechanisms of compulsive drug seeking. *European Journal of Pharmacology, 526,* 77–88.

Vezina, P. (2004). Sensitization of midbrain dopamine neuron reactivity and the self-administration of psychomotor stimulant drugs. *Neuroscience and Biobehavioral Reviews, 27,* 827–839.

Wilson, T. D., Lindsey, S., & Schooler, T. Y. (2000). A model of dual attitudes. *Psychological Review, 107,* 101–126.

Winkielman, P., & Berridge, K. C. (2004). Unconscious emotion. *Current Directions in Psychological Science, 13,* 120–123.

Wyvell, C. L., & Berridge, K. C. (2000). Intra-accumbens amphetamine increases the conditioned incentive salience of sucrose reward: Enhancement of reward "wanting" without enhanced "liking" or response reinforcement. *Journal of Neuroscience, 20,* 8122–8130.

Wyvell, C. L., & Berridge, K. C. (2001). Incentive-sensitization by previous amphetamine exposure: Increased cue-triggered "wanting" for sucrose reward. *Journal of Neuroscience, 21,* 7831–7840.

Zahm, D. S. (2000). An integrative neuroanatomical perspective on some subcortical substrates of adaptive responding with emphasis on the nucleus accumbens. *Neuroscience and Biobehavioral Reviews, 24,* 85–105.

Zajonc, R. B. (2000). Feeling and thinking: Closing the debate over the independence of affect. In J. P. Forgas (Ed.), *Feeling and thinking: The role of affect in social cognition* (pp. 31–58). New York: Cambridge University Press.

On the Neural Implementation of Optimal Decisions

Patrick Simen, Philip Holmes, *and* Jonathan D. Cohen

Abstract

This chapter presents research on mathematical analyses and neural network models of simple forms of decision making. It focuses specifically on two-alternative forced-choice (2AFC) tasks. It is shown how the Ornstein Uhlenbeck process (a modest generalization of a drift-diffusion process) emerges from a mutually inhibiting leaky accumulator model of 2AFC decision making, and how time-dependent changes of gain in the accumulators can overcome varying signal-to-noise ratios to yield an optimal decision procedure. How such gain changes within a trial could be achieved via transient release of norepinephrine by neurons in the locus coeruleus is discussed. Finally, a model of reward driven feedback control of threshold height is described that adapts to changing response-to-stimulus intervals over the course of multiple trials, thereby accounting for observed adjustments of speed-accuracy tradeoff by human subjects in similar conditions.

Keywords: two-alternative forced choice, diffusion model, Ornstein-Uhlenbeck process, decision making

Introduction: Optimal Decisions

Here we summarize work carried out in our group over the past 5 years involving mathematical analyses and neural network computational models of simple forms of decision making. We focus on decisions involving a choice between two prespecified alternatives—often referred to as two-alternative forced choice (2AFC) decision making—because these lend themselves readily to analysis and because they allow us to examine mechanisms and the principles by which they operate that we believe are fundamental to an understanding of more complex forms of decision making. In particular, we are guided by the notion that computably optimal strategies provide limits to and may even guide human and animal decision making behavior. This notion provides a formally rigorous foundation on which to build more precise theories of cognitive control than have previously appeared in the literature. Within an optimality framework, cognitive control can be defined as the mechanisms responsible for adjusting decision parameters in order to optimize performance.

To identify and analyze optimal decision-making processes, we draw on mathematical methods and modeling approaches that make use of stochastic differential equations (SDEs), dynamical systems, and signal processing theory, and we relate these optimal processes to behavioral and neurobiological findings. We start by describing the drift diffusion (DD) model for identification of a noisy stimulus drawn at random from a pair of options in a standard 2AFC task. We derive optimal operating conditions, presuming that certain DD parameters that describe cortical function may be adjusted to suit the stimuli and task at hand. This allows computation of a universal, parameter-free speed–accuracy trade-off, that we compare with behavioral data.

We show how the Ornstein–Uhlenbeck process (a modest generalization of DD) emerges from a mutually inhibited leaky accumulator model of decision making and indicate how time-dependent gain changes in the accumulators can overcome varying signal-to-noise ratios, yielding an optimal decision procedure. We then briefly describe how such gain changes and related threshold changes within a trial (i.e., within the process of making a single 2AFC decision) can be achieved by transient release of the neurotransmitter norepinephrine via spiking noradrenergic neurons in the locus coeruleus (LC). We show that our optimal gain schedules compare well with direct recordings of LC activity. Finally, we describe a model of reward-driven feedback control of threshold height that adapts to changing task conditions over the course of multiple trials (i.e., trial-to-trial updates that correspond to observations of human performance in response to such changes in the environment).

The DD Process

The DD process can be described by the following SDE:

$$dx = \pm a \, dt + \sigma \, dW, \text{ with thresholds } \pm z.$$
$$(1)$$

Here σ is a constant that multiplies the time-dependent standard deviation of a Wiener (Brownian motion) process $W(t)$; a and $-a$ denote the drift rates corresponding to the two stimuli. Models like Equation 1 have been used since the 1960s to model human reaction time and error statistics in the 2AFC and other tasks (Laming, 1968). Not only is it the continuum limit of the sequential probability ratio test (SPRT), known to be the optimal decision maker for 2AFC tasks with accumulating noisy data (Lehmann, 1959; Wald, 1947), but its threshold-crossing behavior closely matches human behavioral data (Ratcliff, 1978; Ratcliff, Van Zandt, & McKoon, 1999). Moreover, direct neural recordings from oculomotor brain areas of monkeys performing choice tasks have recently shown that firing rates of groups of neurons selective for the response corresponding to the chosen alternative rise toward a threshold that signals the onset of motor response in a manner that seems to match sample DD paths (Ratcliff, Cherian, & Segraves, 2003; Roitman & Shadlen, 2002; Schall, 2001). Equation 1 can also be derived from "high-level" leaky competing accumulator (artificial neural network) models of neural function, as described in the next section.

In Equation 1, a is the mean growth rate of the log likelihood ratio, and $x(t)$ its accumulated value. If the stimuli are presented with equal frequency, sample paths are started at $x(0) = 0$, and a response is recorded when $x(t)$ first exceeds $+z$ or falls below $-z$, thus defining the *reaction time* (RT) on that trial. For drift $+a$, crossing $+z$ denotes correct responses and crossing $-z$ errors and vice versa. First passage time distributions yielding expected RTs (denoted $\langle RT \rangle$, with angle brackets denoting expectation) and expected error rates ($\langle ER \rangle$) are readily computed for Equation 1 from the backward Kolmogorov or

Fokker–Planck equation associated with it (Gardiner, 1985):

$$\langle RT \rangle = \frac{z}{a} \tanh\left(\frac{az}{\sigma^2}\right) \; ; \quad \langle ER \rangle = \frac{1}{1 + \exp\left(\frac{2az}{\sigma^2}\right)}. \quad (2)$$

For fixed signal-to-noise ratio (SNR) a/σ, as z increases, $\langle ER \rangle$ decreases but at the expense of longer RTs. This *speed–accuracy trade-off* is well known in psychology (Laming, 1968). However, as suggested by Gold and Shadlen (2002), one can explicitly compute thresholds that maximize the expected *reward rate* (RR):

$$\langle RR \rangle = \frac{1 - \langle ER \rangle}{\langle RT \rangle + D + D_{pen} \cdot \langle ER \rangle} ; \quad (3)$$

Here the numerator represents the expected proportion of correct responses, and the denominator is the expected time between responses: the sum of expected RT, an experimenter-imposed response-to-next-stimulus interval (RSI) with mean D, and possibly an additional penalty delay D_{pen} incurred by errors. (In applying this formula to data gathered from human or animal subjects, one must further subdivide RT into the "decision time" that represents information processing and an "overhead time" due to visual processing and motor response latencies [Bogacz, Brown, Moehlis, Holmes, & Cohen, 2006]. The latter tends to remain fixed for a given subject, and may be combined with D.) We assume for simplicity that correct responses are rewarded with one unit of reward, while errors are not rewarded; however, these assumptions can be loosened without changing our basic results.

Substituting Equation 2 into Equation 3 gives

$$\langle RR \rangle = \left[\frac{z}{a} + D + \left(D + D_{pen} - \frac{z}{a}\right)\exp\left(-\frac{2az}{\sigma^2}\right)\right]^{-1}. \quad (4)$$

Of the original DD parameters in Equations 2 and 3, only the two ratios $z/a \stackrel{\text{def}}{=} \tilde{z}$ (= threshold normalized by signal strength) and $(a/\sigma)^2 \stackrel{\text{def}}{=} \tilde{a}$ (= squared SNR) appear in Equation 4. Regarding $\tilde{a}, D > 0$, and $D_{pen} \geq 0$ as fixed and differentiating with respect to $\tilde{z}$, one finds that the unique maximum of $\langle RR \rangle$ as a function of threshold for fixed SNR and delays occurs when the following condition holds:

$$\exp(2\tilde{a}\tilde{z}) - 1 = 2\tilde{a}(D + D_{pen} - \tilde{z}); \quad (5)$$

Note that only the total delay $D_{tot} = D + D_{pen}$ appears in this expression. Increases in D shift the $\langle RR \rangle$ curve (Equation 3) downward and its maximum to the right, and increases in SNR move the maximum up. For $\tilde{z} = 0$ (no integration: guessing at random) we have $\langle RR \rangle = 1/(2D + D_{pen})$, and when SNR = 0 (no information in the stimulus), the curve degenerates to the function $\langle RR \rangle = 1/[2(z/c)^2 + 2D + D_{pen}]$ with maximum at $z = 0$. Examples appear in Figure 25.5.

We may solve for $\tilde{z}$ and $\tilde{a}$ in terms of $\langle RT \rangle$ and $\langle ER \rangle$ from Equation 2 to obtain

$$\tilde{z} = \frac{\langle RT \rangle}{1 - 2\langle ER \rangle} \quad \text{and} \quad \tilde{a} = \frac{1 - 2\langle ER \rangle}{2\langle RT \rangle}\log\left(\frac{1 - \langle ER \rangle}{\langle ER \rangle}\right), \quad (6)$$

and substituting Equation 6 into Equation 5 yields the speed–accuracy trade-off that corresponds to maximizing $\langle RR \rangle$:

$$\frac{\langle RT \rangle}{D_{tot}} = \left[\frac{1}{\langle ER \rangle \log\left(\frac{1-\langle ER \rangle}{\langle ER \rangle}\right)} + \frac{1}{1 - 2\langle ER \rangle}\right]^{-1}. \quad (7)$$

This *optimal performance curve* (OPC) uniquely relates the normalized reaction time ($\langle RT \rangle/[D_{tot}]$) to $\langle ER \rangle$: no other parameters appear. Hence, data collected for different subjects (who may exhibit differing SNRs, even when viewing the same stimuli) and for differing RSIs D and penalty delays D_{pen} can be pooled and compared with the theory. See Bogacz et al. (2006) for details.

Figure 25.1 shows the OPC of Equation 7 as a bold curve. The form of this curve may be understood by noting that the left-hand end, where both error rates and normalized reaction times are low, corresponds to high SNRs (decisions are quick and accurate), while at the right-hand end, the SNR approaches zero, and the optimum strategy is to guess without spending time to examine the stimulus, also giving a small reaction time. In between, the curve describes the optimal speed–accuracy compromise, reaching its maximum at ER ≈ 0.18.

Figure 25.1 also shows a histogram of behavioral data compiled from 80 human subjects, indicating that those who score in the top 30% overall on a series of tests with several delays and SNRs follow the optimal curve remarkably closely. More detailed

data analysis (Bogacz, 2004–2006; Bogacz et al., 2006; Ratcliff et al., 1999; Simen, Contreras, Buck, Hu, Holmes, & Cohen, in review) reveals that in each block of trials for which stimulus recognition difficulty (~SNR) and RSI are held constant, most subjects rapidly adjust their thresholds in the direction of the optimal value after the beginning of a block of trials. However, some—especially the lowest-scoring 10%—display suboptimal behavior, with significantly longer reaction times and correspondingly lower ERs. Previous studies have shown that humans often appear to favor accuracy over reward (Bohil & Maddox, 2003; Maddox & Bohil, 1998; Myung & Busemeyer, 1989), and alternative objective functions have been proposed to account for this observation.

For example, one can propose a modified reward rate, weighted toward accuracy by additionally penalizing errors, as suggested by the proposal that human subjects experience a competition between reward

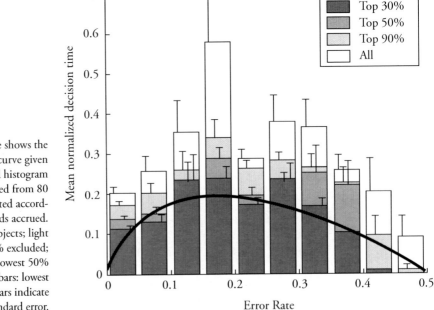

Fig. 25.1 Thick curve shows the optimal performance curve given by Equation 7, and histogram bars show data collected from 80 human subjects, sorted according to total rewards accrued. White bars: all subjects; light gray bars: lowest 10% excluded; medium gray bars: lowest 50% excluded; dark gray bars: lowest 70% excluded. Error bars indicate standard error.

and accuracy (COBRA) (Bohil & Maddox, 2003; Maddox & Bohil, 1998):

$$\text{RA} = \langle \text{RR} \rangle - \frac{q}{D_{\text{tot}}} \langle \text{ER} \rangle; \qquad (8)$$

Here the factor q specifies the additional weight placed on accuracy, and the characteristic time D_{tot} is included in the second factor so that the units of both terms in RA are consistent. Maximizing this function as previously, we obtain a family of OPCs parameterized by q:

$$\frac{\langle \text{RT} \rangle}{D_{\text{tot}}} = \frac{\mathcal{E} - 2q - \sqrt{\mathcal{E}^2 - 4q(\mathcal{E} + 1)}}{2q}, \quad (9)$$

$$\text{where} \quad \mathcal{E} = \left[\frac{1}{\langle \text{ER} \rangle \log \left(\frac{1 - \langle \text{ER} \rangle}{\langle \text{ER} \rangle} \right)} + \frac{1}{1 - 2\langle \text{ER} \rangle} \right]$$

$$(10)$$

is the reciprocal of the OPC formula (7). The weight q must satisfy

$$q \leq \min \left\{ \frac{\mathcal{E}^2}{4(\mathcal{E} + 1)} \right\} \approx 1.096, \quad (11)$$

or the normalized reaction time predicted by Equation 9 will be a complex number (Zacksenhouse, Holmes, & Bogacz, in preparation). However, if Equation 11 holds, then the curve (Equation 9) peaks at ER ≈ 0.18 like the OPC.

If rewards are monetary, one can also postulate a situation in which errors are rewarded (albeit less lavishly than correct responses) or penalized by subtraction of previous winnings:

$$\langle \text{RR}_{\text{m}} \rangle = \frac{(1 - \langle \text{ER} \rangle) - q\langle \text{ER} \rangle}{\langle \text{RT} \rangle + D_{\text{tot}}}. \quad (12)$$

This leads to the following OPC family:

$$\frac{\langle \text{RT} \rangle}{D_{\text{tot}}} = (1 + q) \left[\frac{\frac{1}{\langle \text{ER} \rangle} - \frac{q}{1 - \langle \text{ER} \rangle}}{\log \left(\frac{1 - \langle \text{ER} \rangle}{\langle \text{ER} \rangle} \right)} + \frac{1 - q}{1 - 2\langle \text{ER} \rangle} \right]^{-1}.$$

$$(13)$$

Both Equation 9 and Equation 13 reduce to Equation 7 for $q = 0$, as expected. Figure 25.2 shows an example of the second family (Equation 13). In this case, the maxima move rightward with increasing q.

These objective functions both include a weight parameter q, which will typically be subject-dependent since different people may place a greater or lesser weight on accuracy even if they understand that a specific balance is implied, as in Equation 12. Values of q should therefore be fitted to individuals or subgroups of subjects, and the theory becomes descriptive rather than prescriptive. We are currently assessing such theories against our original behavioral data (Bogacz et al., 2006) and carrying out additional experiments. However, in Figure 25.2, we show that an average weight (= 0.62) may be assigned to the entire group to provide a better overall fit than the optimal curve in Figure 25.1.

Note that while increased emphasis on accuracy produces (predictably) an overall increase in decision times, the shape of the curve does not match the empirical data; in particular, the peak occurs at higher error rates than is observed empirically. This suggests that an emphasis on accuracy may not provide a full account of deviations from optimality observed in human performance. Indeed, an alternative is that errors in the estimation of time, reward, or both could explain failures to achieve optimality and, in particular, the apparently more conservative behavior that many subjects seem to exhibit. For example, it has recently been shown that performance of the lower-scoring 70% of subjects is better matched by an "information gap" theory (Ben-Haim, 2006) that assumes that they maximize performance while allowing for uncertainty in delay estimation (Zacksenhouse et al., in preparation). A model that assumes that subjects are unable to accurately integrate reward feedback from the

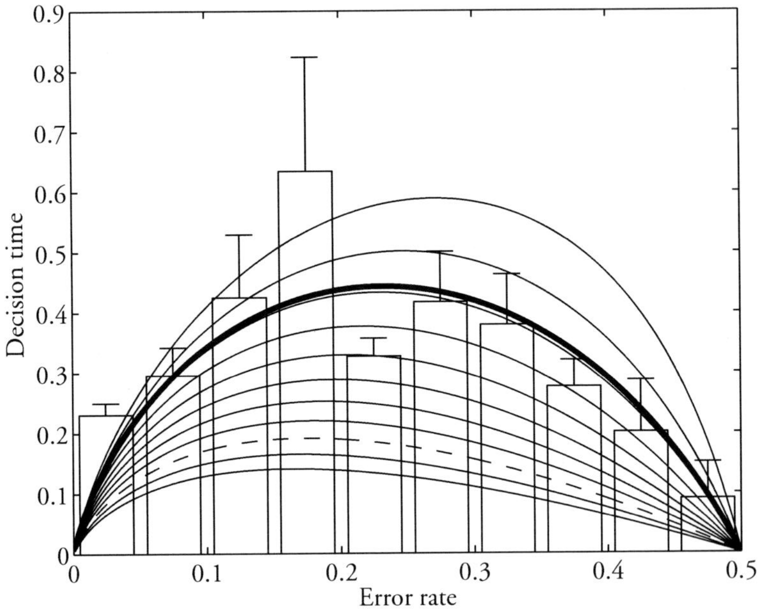

Fig. 25.2 Optimal performance curves of Equation 13 for the modified reward rate function $\langle RR_m \rangle$ of Equation 12 with q varied in steps of 0.1 between -0.2 (lowest curve) and 0.8 (highest curve). The dashed curve corresponds to $q = 0$ (Equation 7) and the bold solid curve to $q = 0.62$: the best fit to *all* the subjects in the study (white bars). Error bars indicate standard error.

environment can provide a similar account. Specifically, if subjects compute continuous, online estimates of reward rate that involve a time-discounted average of rewards earned in the recent past (see the section "Threshold Adaptation by Reward-Driven Feedback Control"), then errors in this estimation process (including errors in accurately reflecting the duration of elapsed time between rewards) could produce overestimates of the optimal threshold setting, which would appear as an emphasis on accuracy. In the remainder of this chapter, we describe models that adjust thresholds and are subject to suboptimality for this reason.

Leaky Accumulator Models and Optimal Gain Schedules

We first take a step down from the "high-level" DD process (Equation 1) toward more biophysically realistic models of neural activity. As shown in Bogacz et al. (2006), Equation 1 can be derived in suitable limits from artificial neural network (connectionist [Brown et al., 2005; Grossberg, 1988;

Rumelhart & McClelland, 1986; Usher & McClelland, 2001]) and firing rate models that in turn may be derived from biophysically detailed, spiking, ionic current equations (Keener & Sneyd, 1998) describing single cell activity (Abbott, 1991, 1994; Amit & Tsodyks, 1991; Ermentrout, 1994, 1998).

The leaky accumulator firing rate model for decision making in 2AFC may be written as a coupled pair of SDEs (Usher & McClelland, 2001):

$$dy_1 = \left[-\alpha y_1 + f_{g(t)}\left(-\beta y_2 + a_1(t) \right) \right] dt + g(t)\sigma(t)dW_1 , \quad (14)$$

$$dy_2 = \left[-\alpha y_2 + f_{g(t)}\left(-\beta y_1 + a_2(t) \right) \right] dt + g(t)\sigma(t)dW_2 , \quad (15)$$

where W_j are independent Weiner processes and the function $f_{g(t)}$ relating firing rate to inputs is typically sigmoidal:

$$f_{g(t)}(x) = \frac{1}{1 + \exp\left(-4g(t)\left(x - b \right) \right)} , \quad (16)$$

or piecewise-linear, being bounded above (by 1) and below (by 0) to represent biophysical limits on firing rates. The accumulator states $y_j(t)$ represent short-term average firing rates of groups of "decision" neurons that are selectively responsive to the two stimuli (e.g., neurons in the lateral intraparietal area [LIP]; Ratcliff et al., 2003; Roitman & Shadlen, 2002). In Equation 16, we allow time-varying stimuli $a_j(t)$, noise level $\sigma(t)$, and gain $g(t)$ (the maximum slope of $f_{g(t)}$) (cf. Grossberg, 1988; Usher & McClelland, 2001).

If decay (leak) α and/or inhibition β are large, then Equations 14 to 15 have a one-dimensional stochastic slow manifold (Arnold, 1998) that attracts solutions in a probabilistic sense. Starting from baseline, after a relatively brief initial transient rise in firing rates of both accumulators, their states approach a curve in the (y_1, y_2)-phase plane. We may approximate the dynamics of the process on this curve by linearizing Equation 16 at the point of maximum slope in the sigmoid and subtracting Equation 15 from Equation 14 to yield a scalar Ornstein–Uhlenbeck (OU) process (Gardiner, 1985) for the difference $x = y_1 - y_2$ in firing rates:

$$dx = [\lambda x + g(t)a]dt + g(t)\sigma dW . \quad (17)$$

Here $\lambda = g(t)\beta - \alpha$ and $a = a_1 - a_2$ and if g is constant and the network is *balanced* in that leak rate equals inhibition ($\lambda = 0$), Equation 17 reduces to the DD SDE (Equation 1) with $a = a_1 - a_2$. Hence, a balanced firing rate model with constant SNR closely approximates the optimal DD decision maker (Bogacz et al., 2006; Brown et al., 2005) (see Figure 25.3). We note that multiunit accumulator models have been developed to describe $N > 2$-alternative choices and that optimality analyses can also be done for them (they lead to multidimensional DD processes) (McMillen & Holmes, 2006). The use of linear theory, which enables analytical results such as

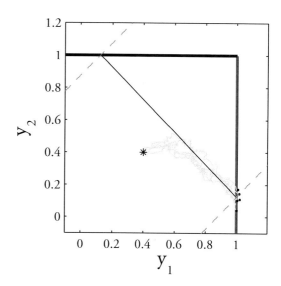

Fig. 25.3 Typical sample paths in the linearized leaky accumulator model illustrating convergence to an attracting line. The thick lines are the thresholds $y_i = \theta$, the thin solid line is the attracting line, the dashed lines are the thresholds for the DD process x, the star is the initial condition, and dots are the final states following threshold crossing. Parameter values are $g(t) \equiv 1$, $\alpha = \beta = 4$, $a_1 = 5$, $a_2 = 4$, $\theta = 1$, and $\sigma = 0.1$. Adapted from McMillen and Holmes (2006).

derivation of Equation 17 and the explicit formulae outlined in the previous section, may be (partially) justified by appealing to the arguments of Cohen, Dunbar, and McClelland (1990), who observe that cortical circuits are likely to adjust biases (b in Equation 16) to operate in their most sensitive central ranges with $x \approx b$, where $df_g/dx \approx gx$. For an introduction to the mathematical analysis of phase-plane pictures such as Figure 25.3 and neural network models in general, see Ermentrout (1998).

The SPRT optimality theory of the previous section assumes that the two distributions from which samples are drawn are stationary and hence that a and σ are constant in the DD process (Equation 1). In practice, stimuli may vary on fast time scales so that one is faced with decoding a signal that waxes and wanes during the decision process. In Brown et al. (2005), we address this problem of varying SNR and, using the linearized one-dimensional OU

SDE (Equation 17) with time-dependent drift $a(t)$ and noise strength $\sigma(t)$, we develop general expressions for optimal multiplicative gain schedules $g(t)$. Essentially, these are solutions to an inverse problem that balance the accumulators and turn Equation 17 into a constant coefficient DD process by implementing the matched filter strategy of signal processing (Papoulis, 1977).

Before giving an example, we briefly review a biophysical mechanism for gain adjustments of the type envisaged previously and in Servan-Schreiber, Printz, and Cohen (1990). It is known that the neurotransmitter norepinephrine (NE) has a modulatory influence on cortical circuits in the sense that response magnitudes (spike counts) evoked by the same stimulus depend on NE levels (Berridge & Waterhouse, 1990). Servan-Schreiber and colleagues have proposed that this can be simulated by assuming that NE release modulates the gain parameter of the logistic function relating firing rate (or probability) to net afferent, as described by Equation 16. Recordings from awake, behaving monkeys (Aston-Jones, Rajkowski, Kubiak, & Alexinsky, 1994; Clayton, Rajkowski, Cohen, & Aston-Jones, 2004) have revealed not only that the *locus coeruleus* (LC) maintains steady NE levels but also that coherent firing of LC cells following salient stimuli can release pulses of NE on the time scale of a few hundred milliseconds, consistent with speeding decisions and responses.

Direct recordings in monkeys reveal that the LC displays two operational modes: a "tonic" state in which baseline firing in the absence of external stimuli is relatively rapid and transient responses to stimuli relatively small; and a "phasic" state in which baseline rates are lower but transient responses significantly larger. Tonic modes are associated with poor performance and phasic modes with good performance (Usher, Cohen, Servan-Schreiber, Rajkowski, & Aston-Jones, 1999). See the recent review article by Aston-Jones and Cohen (2005) for further details and references. This has led to the proposition that, while average levels of NE are important in tuning cortical circuits, transient dynamics also play a major role: mathematical models based on ionic current models of spiking neurons have been proposed and analyzed in support of this (Brown et al., 2004; Usher et al., 1999), and recent findings using pupillometry as a proxy for LC activity have provided convergent support from studies of human decision making (Gilzenrat, 2006). Thus, a mechanism for gain changes not only is in place but also is known to operate on time scales appropriate for decision making.

We may therefore compute optimal gains $\bar{g}(t)$ for specific stimuli and, using a linear model of norepinephrine release as a function of LC firing rate $LC(t)$,

$$\tau_{NE}\,\dot{g}(t) = k_{LC}\,LC(t) - g(t)\,, \quad (18)$$

insert $\bar{g}(t)$ in Equation 18 and invert it to find the optimal firing rate:

$$\overline{LC}(t) = \frac{1}{k_{LC}}\left(\tau_{NE}\,\dot{\bar{g}}(t) + \bar{g}(t)\right). \quad (19)$$

Doing this, we find that the transient rates thus predicted are qualitatively similar to experimental peristimulus time history (PSTH) records of LC spikes, as shown in Figure 25.4. This lends further support to the hypothesis that LC activity, triggered by the arrival of salient stimuli in cortical decision areas, can tune those areas (as well as motor areas) to improve accuracy and speed responses (Aston-Jones & Cohen, 2005).

Gain changes can also lead to threshold changes. If the final processing step in a cortical circuit is an integrator with a fixed threshold and variable gain, then gain increases in the integrator cause more rapid accumulation, thus effectively lowering the threshold. Gain decreases have the complementary effect of raising thresholds. Similar

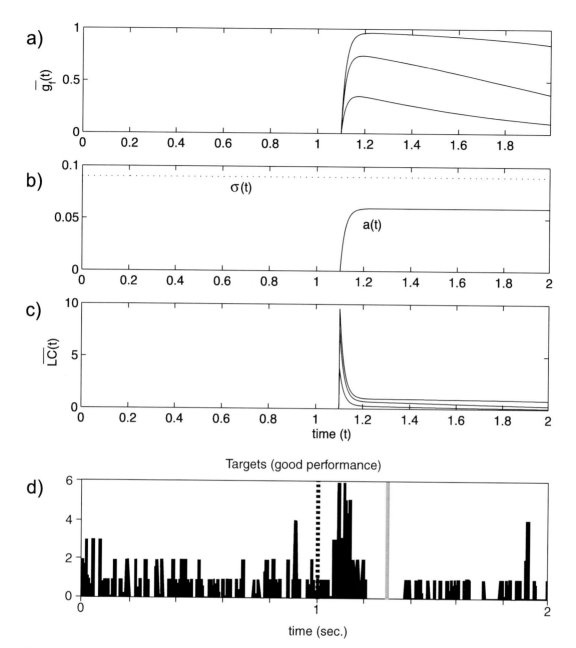

Fig. 25.4 Comparison of optimal gain theory with empirical data for a target detection task. (a) Optimal gain schedules for the firing rate model, with a processing time lag of 0.1 seconds following sensory cue (at time = 1 second) and signal that rises from 0 with constant noise, as shown in (b). (c) The corresponding optimal time course of LC firing rate. (d) Histogram of LC firing rates recorded in monkey during good performance. Adapted from Usher, Cohen, Servan-Schreiber, Rajkowski, and Aston-Jones (1999).

effects can be achieved by changing the bias b in the logistic function (Equation 16), as noted in the next section.

We have now seen how an optimal decision maker, the drift diffusion process, emerges as an approximate reduction of a two-unit leaky accumulator model, how threshold adjustment in such a model can optimize a speed–accuracy trade-off, and how the LC provides one mechanism for threshold adjustment within trials. It remains to describe how subjects might update their thresholds over the course of an experiment in which conditions change.

Threshold Adaptation by Reward-Driven Feedback Control

Equation 5 characterizes optimal performance by specifying the threshold $\tilde{z}$ for evidence accumulation as an implicit function of task conditions, $\tilde{a}$ and D_{tot}, which are assumed to remain constant for a block of trials. This equation is not explicitly soluble, but its solution is unique and can be estimated numerically with arbitrary accuracy (Bogacz et al., 2006); moreover, one can use Equations 5 and 6 to obtain an expression for the optimal threshold in terms of expected reaction time, error rate, and the total delay:

$$\tilde{z} = D_{tot} - \frac{\langle RT \rangle}{\langle ER \rangle \log \left(\frac{1 - \langle ER \rangle}{\langle ER \rangle} \right)} . \quad (20)$$

When conditions change, as in an experiment in which a block with $D = 1$ second is followed by one with $D = 2$ seconds, then $\tilde{z}$ must change if performance is to remain optimal. Experimental data (Bogacz, 2004–2006; Simen et al., in review), averaged over many subjects, suggests that this can occur rapidly, within three to five trials following the change. In modulating their speed–accuracy trade-offs, it is unlikely that subjects would utilize an expression such as Equation 20, but here we describe a simple model of threshold adaptation (Simen, Cohen, & Holmes, 2006) based on a running estimate of reward rate that can achieve near-optimal values of $\tilde{z}$ over a range of task conditions D_{tot} and that seems plausible. We regard the SNR parameter $\tilde{a} = (a/\sigma)^2$ as essentially constant for a given subject and focus on the effect of experimentally manipulated adjustments of RSI.

Our adaptation algorithm maximizes expected reward rate (approximately) by reducing thresholds in proportion to increased reward feedback from the environment. This algorithm results in rapid gradient ascent of the function $\langle RR \rangle$ plot-

ted against $\tilde{z}$, for fixed $\tilde{a}$. Figure 25.5 shows a plot of $\langle RR \rangle$ versus $\tilde{z}$ for three different values of D: 0.5 second, 1 second, and 2 seconds (for simplicity here, we set $D_{pen} = 0$). The peaks of these three functions shift rightward, and their values decrease as D grows. The dashed curve traces the envelope of $\langle RR \rangle$ maxima as D varies continuously, demonstrating that while it is a nonlinear function of $\tilde{z}$, it may be approximated over the range $0.5 \leq D \leq 2$ by a straight line. It is this geometric fact about the $\langle RR \rangle$ curves corresponding to different values of D that allows our algorithm to converge more quickly (in this problem) than more general hill-climbing and other stochastic gradient ascent methods and to do so with a minimum of computational operations.

An ideal threshold adaptation algorithm would instantly respond to a change in D by setting $\tilde{z}$ so that Equation 5 is satisfied. However, this approach would require online numerical computation or the retrieval of stored numerical solutions, $\tilde{z}$, for a range of $\tilde{a}$ and D values, as well as requiring subjects to recognize instantaneously the change in D. A more plausible approach would make minimal assumptions about the knowledge available to the subject and would require minimal computational complexity. First, it seems reasonable to assume that subjects do not have knowledge of the full range of functions relating $\langle RR \rangle$ to $\tilde{z}$ for different values of D (e.g., see Figure 25.5). Here we propose a simple approximation that may address this issue. Second, given that subjects must estimate $\langle RR \rangle$ online (i.e., based on recent experience), it seems reasonable to assume that some form of local averaging is used. Here we describe a simple mechanism that can accomplish this, using the type of neural network model discussed in the previous section in Equations 14 to 16.

First we describe the algorithm as a discrete-time, iterated map. Suppose one

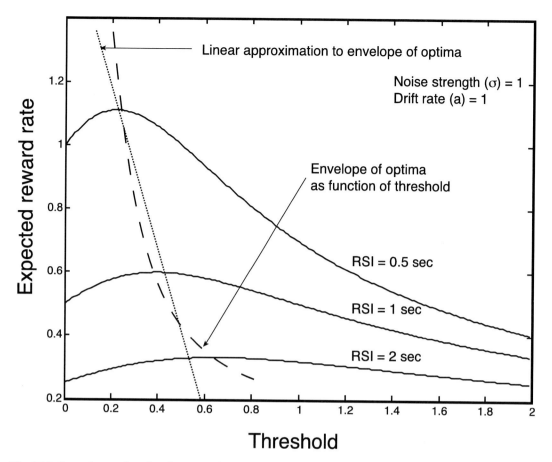

Fig. 25.5 Reward rates plotted as functions of normalized threshold $= \tilde{z}/a$ for RSIs $D = 0.5$, 1.0, and 2.0 (top to bottom), with $\tilde{a} = a/\sigma = 1$. The dashed line indicates the envelope of $\langle RR \rangle$ maxima, and the solid line is an affine approximation to it.

starts with some arbitrary threshold value, T_1, as in Figure 25.6 (left). The dark $\langle RR \rangle$ curve of Equation 3 specifies the expected reward rate at T_1, so one expects the first trial to yield RR_1, which may then be mapped into a new threshold, T_2, by an affine transformation:

$$\mathrm{RR} = \frac{z_{\max} - z}{w} \quad \text{or} \quad z = z_{\max} - w \cdot \mathrm{RR} \tag{21}$$

(the straight line with negative slope). In drawing the horizontal leftward arrow, we have assumed that an accurate estimate of $\langle RR \rangle$ is available; clearly, this may not be so after only one trial performed with a given value of $\tilde{z}$.

However, this poses no serious problem for the algorithm, as we demonstrate.

This process is repeated in order to compute RR_2 and thereby T_3: Figure 25.6 (right). Successive updates from the resulting iterated map can be traced by a staircase or "cobweb diagram" (Jordan & Smith, 1999), as in Figure 25.6. Given the unimodal shape of the expected reward rate function and the slope of the transformation, rapid convergence to the intersection of the line and the curve occurs. This occurs regardless of inaccurate $\langle RR \rangle$ estimates at any given step of the iteration: noisy estimates produce a cobweb in which the corners of stair steps are offset from the $\langle RR \rangle$ curve, but such cobwebs still tend to converge to the

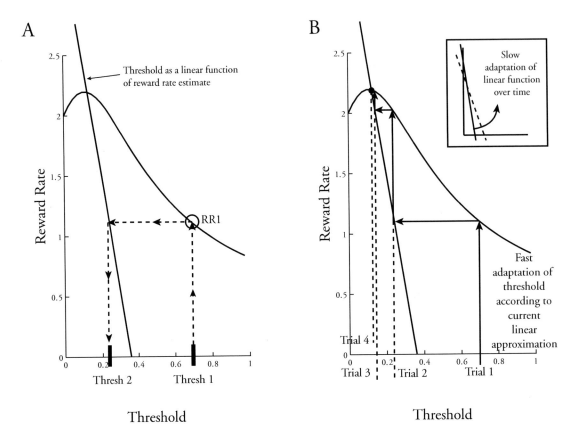

Fig. 25.6 The procedure for updating thresholds based on reward rate estimate, showing a single step (left) and multiple steps (right) with an indication of how the affine function might be updated on a longer time scale (inset).

intersection of the $\langle RR \rangle$ curve and the affine function, as the reader can verify. The intersection is therefore a global attractor for both the iterated map and the continuous system it approximates.

Obviously, to obtain near-optimal performance, the affine function must be placed so as to intersect the expected reward rate curve near its apex. This can be achieved for a range of reward rate curves corresponding to a range of D values by choosing the affine transformation to approximate the envelope of the optima (Figure 25.5). We assume that the slope or weight w and intercept z_{max} on which the algorithm depends is itself learned on a slower time scale by standard reinforcement learning mechanisms (Kushner & Yin, 1997; Sutton & Barto, 1998). We do not address this here.

A continuous time system that realizes this procedure may be written as a pair

of stochastic differential equations with conditions for threshold crossing and decision variable resetting as follows:

$$dx = A\, dt + c_1\, dW \quad \text{if } \mathrm{RSI}(t) = 0 \quad (22)$$

$$x = 0 \text{ if } \mathrm{RSI}(t) = 1 \quad (23)$$

$$dr = \frac{1}{k} \cdot (-r(t) + R(t))\, dt + c_2\, dW \quad (24)$$

$$z(t) = \max(0, z_{max} - w \cdot r(t)) \quad (25)$$

$$R(t) = \begin{cases} \delta(t - t') & \text{if reward present at time } t' \\ 0 & \text{otherwise} \end{cases} \quad (26)$$

$$\tau = \text{time of last threshold crossing} \quad (27)$$

$$\mathrm{RSI}(t) = \begin{cases} 1 & \text{if } |x| \geq z \text{ or } t - \tau < \mathrm{RSI}_{max} \\ 0 & \text{otherwise} \end{cases} \quad (28)$$

Here x in Equations 22 and 23 is the decision variable in the DD model, r in Equation 24 is the running estimate of reward rate, and z in Equation 25 is the threshold. When a stimulus is present, the variable RSI is 0 (Equation 28), and the first passage of the decision variable x beyond the threshold value z is taken as the time of decision, τ, (Equation 27). At this point, RSI is set to 1, Equation 28 specifies the response–stimulus interval $\mathrm{RSI}_{\max}$ for the next trial, and the decision variable $x(t)$ is reset to 0.[1] If the response was correct, Equations 24 and 26 state that a Dirac-delta impulse of reward is integrated by the reward rate estimator; at all other times, the current reward rate estimate r decays exponentially, providing an estimate of the recent reward rate. The threshold z is determined entirely by the reward rate estimate r via the linear function of Equation 25.

This system can be implemented in a neural network of the type discussed in the previous section. First, reward rate must be estimated as in Equation 24. This can be done by a unit with input $s(t)$, self-excitatory feedback of weight $k - 1$, and activation function slope:

$$\dot{y}(t) = -y(t) + \frac{1}{k}\left(s(t) + (k-1)y(t)\right)$$
$$= \frac{1}{k}\left(s(t) - y(t)\right). \tag{29}$$

As shown in the previous section, the decision variable can be approximately represented by differencing the firing rates of two competing neural populations that each accumulate evidence for one of the two possible stimuli. Figure 25.3 shows that thresholds applied to the single decision variable are approximately equivalent to absolute thresholds applied to the firing rates of each population, without

regard to the firing rate of its competitor, because of the clustering of solutions near a one-dimensional attracting manifold. Moreover, as noted at the end of the previous section, a threshold is effectively a step function applied to the level of accumulated evidence in the decision variable. In order to reduce or increase thresholds, gains may be changed, or extra positive or negative bias input can be applied to the threshold function, thereby reducing or increasing the amount of evidence necessary for the sum of the decision variable and the additional bias to exceed threshold. The neural network implementation of the algorithm uses the reward rate estimate r, weighted by a connection strength equal to w in the affine function already discussed (Equation 21), as the quantity by which to reduce the decision threshold from its maximum ($z_{\max}$).

By adding such a single unit that estimates reward rate and two units that act as threshold detectors to each of the accumulators in Equations 14 to 15, we arrive at a neural mechanism that adapts quickly to changes in task conditions D and so achieves near-optimal performance across a range of conditions. Figure 25.7 shows some representative results from such a model started with arbitrary initial data and run through a switch from RSI of $D = 0.5$ to $D = 2.0$ seconds at 42 seconds. Note the reduction of initially high thresholds to an asymptotic value, accompanied by increase in RR, followed by threshold increase and asymptote to a higher value for higher RSI. The RR is consequently reduced since reaction times become longer (bottom panel) and the average trial time increases significantly. For this simulation, the parameter values were as follows: $A = 1.5$, $k = 8$, $w = 0.15$, and $z_{\max} = 0.2$, with noise strengths $c_1 = 0.1$ and $c_2 = 0.01$.

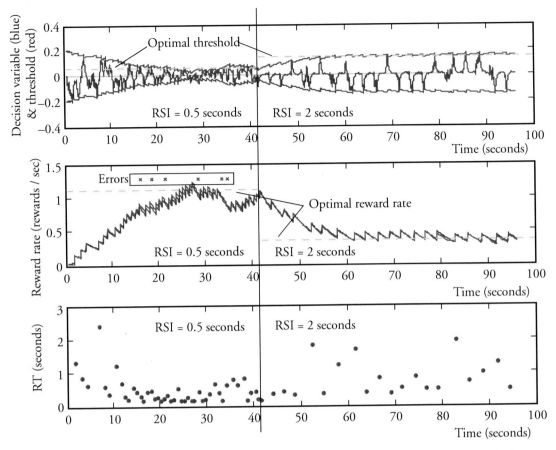

Fig. 25.7 Numerical simulations of the continuous time computational model of Equations 22 to 28. Panels from top to bottom, respectively, show thresholds as envelopes with DD solutions inside and optimal thresholds dashed; running reward rate estimate with errors indicated by *x*'s and optimal reward rates dashed; and reaction times. Parameter values are noted in text.

Summary

We have reviewed some recent work in modeling neural and behavioral responses to stimuli in simple decision tasks, focusing on provably optimal strategies based on the drift-diffusion process that predict specific speed–accuracy trade-offs.

Behavioral experiments indicate that while some human subjects do produce near-optimal performance over a range of task conditions, others do not. We show that this can be accounted for by supposing that they are effectively optimizing a different objective function (in this case weighted for accuracy), although it detracts from overall rewards by slowing down per-formance. This makes the prescriptive optimal theory descriptive.

We then show how time-dependent gain schedules can be found for systems with variable signal-to-noise ratios and recall how nor-epinephrine levels can effectively adjust gain and decision thresholds. We end by describing a simple algorithm that updates thresholds based on estimates of reward rates, and we illustrate results from a computational simulation of a continuous time version of it. This model identifies potential mechanistic bases for the suboptimality observed in human performance (such as poor estimates of rewards or inability to learn the relationship between thresholds and reward rate optima).

In general, this work contributes to the development of a formally rigorous foundation for understanding the mechanisms underlying simple forms of decision making in the human brain and their ability to adapt to changes in the environment. Ongoing work is now beginning to build on this theoretical foundation to address more complex forms of decision making that correspond more closely to real-world circumstances, including a multiplicity of choices and uncertainty in the timing and/or location of their appearance.

Acknowledgments

This work was supported by DoE grant DE-FG02-95ER25238 and PHS grants MH58480 and MH62196 (Cognitive and Neural Mechanisms of Conflict and Control, Silvio M. Conte Center). Parts of this work were first reported in Holmes et al. (2005), Simen et al. (2006), and Bogacz et al. (2006).

Note

1. This unrealistic assumption implies discontinuous resets of the decision variable, but it can be relaxed without loss of generality by introducing a refractory period and replacing Equation 22 by a stable, rapidly decaying Ornstein–Uhlenbeck process during the RSI.

References

Abbott, L. F. (1991). Firing-rate models for neural populations. In O. Benhar, C. Bosio, P. Del Giudice, & E. Tabat (Eds.), *Neural networks: From biology to high-energy physics* (pp. 179–196). Pisa, Italy: ETS Editrice.

Abbott, L. F. (1994). Decoding neuronal firing and modeling neural networks. *Quarterly Review of Biophysics, 64,* 353–430.

Amit, D. J., & Tsodyks, M. V. (1991). Quantitative study of attractor neural networks retrieving at low spike rates: I. Substrate-spikes, rates and neuronal gain. *Network: Computation in Neural Systems, 2,* 259–273.

Arnold, L. (1998). *Random dynamical systems.* Heidelberg, Germany: Springer Verlag.

Aston Jones, G., & Cohen, J. D. (2005). An integrative theory of locus coeruleus-norepinephrine function: Adaptive gain and optimal performance. *Annual Review of Neuroscience, 28,* 403–450.

Aston-Jones, G., Rajkowski, J., Kubiak, P., & Alexinsky, T. (1994). Locus coeruleus neurons in the monkey are selectively activated by attended stimuli in a vigilance task. *Journal of Neuroscience, 14,* 4467–4480.

Ben-Haim, Y. (2006). *Information gap decision theory: Decisions under severe uncertainty* (2nd ed.). New York: Academic Press.

Berridge, C. W., & Waterhouse, B. D. (1990). The locus coeruleus-noradrenergic system: Modulation of behavioral state and state dependent cognitive processes. *Brain Research Reviews, 42,* 892–895.

Bogacz, R. (2004–2006). Experimental work in progress.

Bogacz, R., Brown, E., Moehlis, J., Holmes, P., & Cohen, J. D. (2006). The physics of optimal decision making: A formal analysis of models of performance in two-alternative forced choice tasks. *Psychological Review, 113,* 700–765.

Bohil, C. J., & Maddox, W. T. (2003). On the generality of optimal versus objective classifier feedback effects on decision criterion learning in perceptual categorization. *Memory and Cognition, 31,* 181–198.

Brown, E., Gao, J., Holmes, P., Bogacz, R., Gilzenrat, M., & Cohen, J. D. (2005). Simple neural networks that optimize decisions. *International Journal of Bifurcation and Chaos, 15,* 803–826.

Brown, E., Moehlis, J., Holmes, P., Clayton, E., Rajkowski, J., & Aston-Jones, G. (2004). The influence of spike rate and stimulus duration on brainstem noradrenergic neurons. *Journal of Comparative Neuroscience, 17,* 13–29.

Clayton, E., Rajkowski, J., Cohen, J. D., & Aston-Jones, G. (2004). Phasic activation of monkey locus coeruleus neurons by simple decisions in a forced choice task. *Journal of Neuroscience, 24,* 9914–9920.

Cohen, J. D., Dunbar, K., & McClelland, J. L. (1990). On the control of automatic processes: A parallel distributed processing model of the Stroop effect. *Psychological Review, 97,* 332–361.

Ermentrout, G. B. (1994). Reduction of conductance-based models with slow synapses to neural nets. *Neural Computation, 6,* 679–695.

Ermentrout, G. B. (1998). Neural networks as spatio-temporal pattern-forming systems. *Reports on Progress in Physics, 64,* 353–430.

Gardiner, C. W. (1985). *Handbook of stochastic methods* (2nd ed.). New York: Springer-Verlag.

Gilzenrat, M. (2006). *The role of the locus coeruleus in cognitive control: Pupillometric measures and computational mechanisms.* Unpublished Ph.D. dissertation, Princeton University.

Gold, J. I., & Shadlen, M. N. (2002). Banburismus and the brain: Decoding the relationship between sensory stimuli, decisions and reward. *Neuron, 36,* 299–308.

Grossberg, S. (1988). Nonlinear neural networks: Principles, mechanisms, and architectures. *Neural Networks, 1,* 17–61.

Holmes, P., Brown, E., Moehlis, J., Bogacz, R., Gao, J., Aston-Jones, G., et al. (2005). Optimal decisions: From neural spikes, through stochastic differential equations, to behavior. *IEICE Transactions on Fundamentals on Electronics, Communications and Computer Sciences, 88,* 2496–2503.

Jordan, D. W., & Smith, P. (1999). *Nonlinear ordinary differential equations* (3rd ed.). New York: Oxford University Press.

Keener, J., & Sneyd, J. (1998). *Mathematical physiology.* New York: Springer-Verlag.

Kushner, H. J., & Yin, G. G. (1997). *Stochastic approximation algorithms and applications.* New York: Springer-Verlag.

Laming, D. R. J. (1968). *Information theory of choice-reaction times.* New York: Academic Press.

Lehmann, E. L. (1959). *Testing statistical hypotheses.* New York: Wiley.

Maddox, W. T., & Bohil, C. J. (1998). Base-rate and payoff effects in multidimensional perceptual categorization. *Journal of Experimental Psychology, 24,* 1459–1482.

McMillen, T., & Holmes, P. (2006). The dynamics of choice among multiple alternatives. *Journal of Mathematical Psychology, 50,* 30–57.

Myung, J., & Busemeyer, J. R. (1989). Criterion learning in a deferred decision-making task. *American Journal of Psychology, 102,* 1–16.

Papoulis, A. (1977). *Signal analysis.* New York: McGraw-Hill.

Ratcliff, R. (1978). A theory of memory retrieval. *Psychological Review, 85,* 59–108.

Ratcliff, R., Cherian, A., & Segraves, M. A. (2003). A comparison of macaque behavior and superior colliculus neuronal activity to predictions from models of two choice decisions. *Journal of Neurophysiology, 90,* 1392–1407.

Ratcliff, R., Van Zandt, T., & McKoon, G. (1999). Connectionist and diffusion models of reaction time. *Psychological Review, 106,* 261–300.

Roitman, J. D., & Shadlen, M. N. (2002). Response of neurons in the lateral intraparietal area during a combined visual discrimination reaction time task. *Journal of Neuroscience, 22,* 9475–9489.

Rumelhart, D. E., & McClelland, J. L. (Eds.). (1986). *Parallel distributed processing: Explorations in the microstructure of cognition.* Cambridge, MA: MIT Press.

Schall, J. D. (2001). Neural basis of deciding, choosing and acting. *Nature Neuroscience, 2,* 33–42.

Servan-Schreiber, D., Printz, H., & Cohen, J. D. (1990). A network model of catecholamine effects: Gain, signal-to-noise ratio, and behavior. *Science, 249,* 892–895.

Simen, P., Cohen, J. D., & Holmes, P. (2006). Rapid decision threshold modulation by reward rate in a neural network. *Neural Networks, 19,* 1013–1026.

Simen, P., Contreras, D., Buck, C., Hu, P., Holmes, P., & Cohen, J. D. *Reward rate optimization in two-alternative decision making: Empirical tests of theoretical predictions.* Manuscript in review.

Sutton, R. S., & Barto, A. G. (1998). *Reinforcement learning: An introduction.* Cambridge, MA: MIT Press.

Usher, M., Cohen, J. D., Servan-Schreiber, D., Rajkowski, J., & Aston-Jones, G. (1999). The role of locus coeruleus in the regulation of cognitive performance. *Science, 283,* 549–554.

Usher, M., & McClelland, J. L. (2001). On the time course of perceptual choice: The leaky competing accumulator model. *Psychological Review, 108,* 550–592.

Wald, A. (1947). *Sequential analysis.* New York: Wiley.

Zacksenhouse, M., Holmes, P., & Bogacz, R. *Robust versus optimal strategies for two-alternative forced choice tasks.* Manuscript in preparation.

26 Nonconscious Goal Pursuit and the Effortful Control of Behavior

Ran R. Hassin, Henk Aarts, Baruch Eitam, Ruud Custers, *and* Tali Kleiman

> We haven't really solved the problem of consciousness until that executive is itself broken down into subcomponents that are themselves clearly just unconscious underlaborers which themselves work (compete, interfere, dawdle, . . .) without supervision.
>
> —(*Dennett, 2001,* p. 228)

Abstract

This chapter begins with a discussion of existing literature on automatic, nonconscious goal pursuit. It then presents the adaptiveness paradox: on the one hand, in order to be effective, nonconscious goal pursuit must be adaptive. On the other hand, nonconscious, automatic processes are widely believed to rely on existing networks of associations and are hence thought to be inflexible. Three new hypotheses are proposed to resolve the paradox, because at their core lies the contention that working memory (WM) is involved in nonconscious goal pursuit. It is argued that given the nature of WM its involvement in nonconscious goal pursuits allows them to be flexible. A series of studies that focus on one particular type of automatic processes—nonconscious goal pursuit—is reviewed.

Keywords: adaptiveness paradox, working memory, automatic process, nonconscious goal pursuit

A significant proportion of human behavior is determined by nonconscious goal pursuits. This assertion is easily derived from two well-established and highly consensual observations about human nature. First, much of human behavior is purposeful, or goal directed. Our goals range from very trivial (e.g., to make a cup of coffee) and a little less so (e.g., to get to work) through more complex (e.g., to write an interesting chapter) to extremely difficult ones (e.g., to be a good parent). It is not completely unlikely that goals direct behavior at virtually every moment of our lives. Second, our consciousness is very—but very—limited in its processing resources. Memorize simple cooking instructions, count the number of knives you put on the table, or just think a simple thought—and

your conscious capacity drops substantially. In fact, even reading *this* trivial sentence is likely to consume much of your conscious processing resources. This grave limitation on conscious processing suggests that a big chunk of the mental processes related to goal pursuits have to occur outside of conscious awareness. Considered in tandem, then, these two observations imply that much of our behavior is determined by nonconscious goal pursuit and hence that the dynamics of nonconscious goal(s) pursuit are important determinants of the psychology of action.

We begin this chapter by discussing the existing literature on automatic, nonconscious goal pursuit. We then present the adaptiveness paradox: On the one hand, we argue, in order to be effective, nonconscious goal pursuit must be adaptive. On the other hand, nonconscious, automatic processes are widely believed to rely on existing networks of associations and are hence thought to be inflexible. We then propose three new hypotheses. These help to resolve the paradox because at their core lies the contention that working memory (WM), broadly defined, is involved in nonconscious goal pursuit. Given the nature of WM, we argue, its involvement in nonconscious goal pursuits allows them to be flexible.

We review a series of studies that support our predictions. The studies focus on one particular type of automatic processes—nonconscious goal pursuit. The resolution that we offer to the adaptiveness paradox—that is, the involvement of WM in automatic processes—is more general, though. Thus, we also review exciting advances in neighboring literatures. We conclude by examining the implications of the proposed framework to our understanding of the functions of the frontal lobes.

Introduction and Background

Traditionally, goal pursuit was considered to be a conscious and effortful process, one that requires (conscious) intention and can be stopped at (conscious) will. In other words, goal pursuit was considered to be a controlled process (cf. Ajzen, 1991; Bandura, 1986; Deci & Ryan, 1985; Locke & Latham, 1990). The intuition that underlies the traditional view is very appealing: Anyone who has ever attempted to pursue nontrivial goals would probably agree that goal pursuit often seems to be an effortful, conscious process.

This state of affairs has recently changed. Following Bargh's original idea (Bargh, 1990) and first empirical findings (Chartrand & Bargh, 1996), the past decade has witnessed a boost of empirical demonstrations of nonconscious goal pursuit

(e.g., Aarts & Hassin, 2005; Bargh, Gollwitzer, Lee-Chai, Barndollar, & Trötschel, 2001; Fishbach, Friedman, & Kruglanski, 2003; Fitzsimons & Bargh, 2003; Hassin, Bargh, & Zimerman, in press; Kruglanski et al., 2002; Moskowitz, Gollwitzer, Wasel, & Schaal, 1999; Shah, 2003). In light of this research, it seems safe to conclude that we now have solid empirical support for the idea that goals can be activated and pursued nonconsciously and unintentionally (for recent reviews, see Ferguson, Hassin, & Bargh, 2007; see Chapter 17).

Two definitional notes are in order before we continue. First, we define "goal" as a desired state (e.g., behavior or outcome) that the individual believes (consciously or nonconsciously) she knows how to produce. Hence, a mental representation of a goal is a mental representation of a desired state (cf. Aarts & Hassin, 2005; Austin & Vancouver, 1996; Kruglanski, 1996; Shallice & Burgess, 1998). While this formulation applies to goals in general—from low-level motor goals (e.g., to lift a finger; cf. Chapter 2) to high-level personal goals (e.g., to win someone's affection)—our work focuses on and applies to the latter.

Second, throughout this chapter we use the notion of habit. We use "habit" in a lay way to denote a routinized set of actions (broadly defined to include thought, emotion, motivation, and behavior) that may occur nonconsciously and unintentionally, specifically in the contexts in which these routines frequently occur.

Mechanisms for Nonconscious Pursuit of Habitual Goals

So how are goals pursued nonconsciously? Most of the work on nonconscious goal pursuit examined the pursuit of habitual goals in what might be thought of as relatively habitual contexts. Goal pursuit in these cases seems to depend on associative networks that include contexts, goals that are regularly pursued in these contexts, and means that one usually uses to attain these goals (Bargh, 1990; Kruglanski et al., 2002; see Chapter 21). These networks are shaped by one's history, and they allow for goal pursuit via spreading of activation (see Chapter 9). Thus, for example, the *context* of meeting an attractive colleague may instigate the *goal* of intimacy, which may bring about a certain way of talking that has proved in the past to be an effective *means* for attaining this goal. This chain of events (i.e., a context activates a goal that activates certain means) may occur outside of awareness, without a conscious decision, and sometimes even despite one's conscious intentions.

The nature of the representations that take part in these processes is yet to be determined. While earlier work—which is echoed in the previous paragraph—suggests that these are amodal, abstract, and semantic (Bargh, 1990; Kruglanski et al., 2002), recent work leans toward more modal, concrete, and embodied representations (Bargh, 2006).

Going Beyond Habits

The worlds we live in—be it the physical, the mental, or the social—are dynamic to their core. This characteristic suggests that even when we engage in habitual procedures, we may (frequently) confront novel circumstances.[1] Take courting as an example. On the one hand, courting obviously involves habitual procedures—from tone of speech through body gestures to preferred topics of conversation. Yet it seems quite obvious that in order for it to be effective, courting needs to be tailored to the specific courtee and the specific situation. So while one may habitually use humor during courtship, the specifics vary—from person to person and from context to context—and the possible variation seems

to be large. So large, in fact, that a finite set of previously used humor strategies would not seem to suffice for future goal pursuits.

This simple example suggests that in order to be effective even habitual courting procedures should enable us to confront novel circumstances and produce novel sets of behaviors. More generally, it illustrates the idea that habitual goal pursuits should allow for quick, "online," flexible adaptation to novel circumstances (otherwise, there will not be a second date).

At this point it may seem as if we are arguing that habits—and habitual goal pursuits in particular—are *always* underspecified. In other words, it may seem as if we are arguing that habits can never orchestrate behavior without further, context specific refinement. Note that while this strong claim may indeed be correct, it is not necessary for the argument we are making here. For the current purposes, the milder claim—under certain circumstances some habits are underspecified—suffices. Given the dynamic nature of the world, it seems to us that there is little doubt, if any, regarding the veracity of the latter claim.

So how do we go beyond preexisting routines in nonconscious goal pursuit? The traditional answer would be that we do not: Nonconscious goal pursuit, like every other automatic process, is limited to circumstances in which preexisting routines could be successfully applied. If they cannot be successfully applied, then nonconscious goal pursuit is bound to fail, and conscious processes would be called to the fore.

While tempting, this suggestion is psychologically improbable. Given the scarcity of conscious mental resources on the one hand (Kaheneman, 1973) and the dynamic nature of the worlds we inhabit on the other, it seems that we should be able to go beyond existing routines, that is, reveal quick flexibility, even during nonconscious goal pursuit.

The Adaptiveness Paradox

To explore the possibility that non-conscious goal pursuit may be flexible, Hassin, Bargh, & Zimerman (in press) examined the effect of goal priming on performance in the Wisconsin Card Sorting Test (WCST). The WCST was originally developed to assess abstract reasoning and the ability to shift cognitive strategies in response to changing environmental contingencies (Berg, 1948; Heaton, Chelune, Talley, Kay, & Curtiss, 1993). In this test, participants are asked to sort cards to one of four piles. Unbeknownst to the participants (at least at first), the cards can be sorted according to one of three rules: color, shape, or number. Participants are given feedback about the accuracy of each sorting ("right" versus "wrong") but never about the sorting rule itself. The crucial feature of the WCST is that after 10 consecutive correct sortings, the sorting rule changes without a warning. Participants have to adapt to this new environment until it, too, changes (after 10 correct sortings). This goes on until two decks of cards are sorted.

The WCST is particularly suitable for examining flexibility because it (intentionally) captures the essence of flexible adaptation to changing environments (e.g., Berg, 1948; Demakis, 2003). The logic is simple: Physical and social environments suggest behavioral rules that, if followed, lead to better survival. Environmental changes often entail changes in these rules, and in these cases better survival may depend on rapid adaptation to the new rules. The structure of the WCST reflects this logic: The rule that governs sorting changes without a prior warning, and participants have to look for a new rule and then follow it—without recourse to the previous one. Flexibility is measured here as the inverse of perseveration or, more concretely, by the number of perseverative errors. Thus, for example, if the sorting rule had just changed from color to number, color-congruent sortings would count as perseverative errors.

In this set of studies, participants were either primed with a goal or not, and they then went on to do the WCST. In the first two studies, participants who were primed with an achievement goal revealed more flexibility than control participants. Crucially, a thorough debriefing revealed that participants were unaware of the fact that they had been primed with a goal. Similarly, their goal commitment did not differ from that of control participants. In a third study, we directly primed the goal of becoming flexible and found similar effects: Primed participants more easily adapted to changes in their environment.

In conclusion, then, data from these three studies suggest that nonconscious goal pursuit results in increased cognitive flexibility as it is measured by the WCST. In other words, if one treats one's current sorting rule as one's (admittedly new) habit, then these studies show that primed goals enhance our capacity for overcoming habits, exactly when this adaptability is needed: Immediately after a crucial change in the environment.

Similar data were obtained in two related sets of studies. In the first we used goal priming procedures to examine participants' flexibility in attribution tasks. The results replicated those of the WCST studies: Primed participants were more flexible than controls (Hassin, in press). In the second set of studies we examined whether nonconscious goal pursuit can enhance adaptation to novel environments. More specifically, we examined whether achievement priming can result in improved implicit learning. The results yielded an unequivocal positive answer: Participants who had been primed with an achievement goal showed improved adaptation to new environments (Eitam, Hassin, & Schul, 2008).

This, then, may be thought of as the adaptiveness paradox: Automatic, nonconscious processes are held to be inflexible in the sense that they are limited to preexisting routines that are associated with them. We have argued, however, that in order to be truly beneficial, nonconscious goal pursuit should allow for rapid flexibility. And as we have just seen, automatic, nonconscious goal pursuits reveal exactly this kind of flexibility. In the following sections, we attempt to resolve this paradox by suggesting a mechanism that allows for rapid flexibility in nonconscious goal pursuit.

Beyond Networks of Goals and Means

The results briefly described previously reveal that nonconscious goal pursuit is not confined to routinized processes. To account for results of this sort and for nonhabitual nonconscious processes more generally, we propose the following principles:

1. Whenever a goal is activated beyond a threshold, it enters a WM, and some capacity is allocated to it.[2] This capacity may be thought of in terms of mental resources, processing time of a central processor (see Pashler, 1998), or, more generally, any component essential for processing of which there are limited quantities at any given point in time (cf. Navon, 1984).

2. Assuming that the goal is allocated sufficient capacity, then if only one applicable network of goals, means, and relevant knowledge (henceforth schema) for goal pursuit is readily accessible, the goal would be pursued in the situation via this schema. In most cases this is likely to be the habitual schema, but noise or (temporary) biases may bring about the selection of other schemas.

If, however, more than one existing schema is readily accessible, then schema selection is guided by principles reminiscent of those suggested by Norman and Shallice in their pioneering work on contention scheduling in action control (Norman & Shallice, 1986; Shallice & Burgess, 1993). (A more thorough discussion of these principles is presented in the last section of this chapter).

Finally, if no existing schema is readily accessible or in cases where schema selection proves to be difficult, the goal is maintained (cf. Goschke & Kuhl, 1993; Marsh, Hicks, & Bink, 1998; Zeigarnik, 1938), waiting for further developments. These may include, among other processes, the construction of a new schema, the selection of a schema that is justified by a change in the circumstances, or the haphazard selection of a schema for reasons that will be currently summarized as "noise." Alternatively, the goal may simply decay.

3. Once a schema (old or new) has been selected, goal pursuit is launched, and progress monitoring begins via a feedback loop.

Before we go on, we wish to elaborate on three points. First, as we described previously, models of nonconscious goal pursuit focused on habitual goal pursuit, that is, goals that are consistently pursued in certain contexts via habitual means (Bargh, 1990; Kruglanski, 1996). As far as the pursuit of habitual goals under habitual circumstances is concerned, our hypotheses are similar to those of these models: Principle 2 stipulates that activation of a goal of this kind is likely to lead to goal pursuit via its habitual schema.

Even under these circumstances, though, our predictions diverge from those of previous models. To mention a few of these differences: The current framework explicitly allows for a selection of nonhabitual courses of action; it stipulates involvement of WM in nonconscious goal pursuit, and it allows (but does not require) nonconscious monitoring and feedback processing. These differences may allow for more flexible and adaptive goal pursuits.

Second, the proposed principles apply to goal pursuits that are automatic in the following senses. First, conscious intention is not a prerequisite for any of the processes described previously (e.g., goal priming may unintentionally lead to allocation of capacity to this goal). Second, conscious awareness is not a prerequisite for these processes either (e.g., one does not have to be aware of the primed goal or its operation). Third, some aspects of these processes may be ballistic (e.g., one may not be able to stop the monitoring process, or one may fail to stop goal pursuit itself). Ex hypothesis, however, some of these processes are effortful; that is, they require mental resources. In our view, this does not render the processes described herein "controlled" or "not automatic" (for similar views, see Bargh, 1989, 1994; Hassin, 2008; Kahneman & Treisman, 1984; Wegner & Bargh, 1998).

Third, our account assumes that WM can operate outside of conscious awareness. While this may be a controversial supposition (e.g., Baars & Franklin, 2003; Baddeley, 1993; Cowan, 1999; O'Reilly, Braver, & Cohen, 1999), some of us have recently argued for it, marshaling both behavioral and functional magnetic resonance imaging evidence (Hassin, 2005; Hassin, Bargh, Engell, & McCulluch, 2007).

Working Memory

Given WM's hypothesized role in nonconscious goal pursuit, we turn now to a brief review of relevant aspects of the WM literature. For a long time, WM has attracted the attention of psychologists and neuroscientists who are interested in how people acquire knowledge, reason, solve problems, make decisions, achieve cognitive control, and, of special interest for the current concerns, pursue goals (Baddeley & Logie, 1999; Dudai, 2004; P. Shah & Miyake, 1999). A review of models of WM—its components, functions, and brain instantiations—is beyond the scope of this chapter (but see Miyake & Shah, 1999). However, as an inspection of these models and the tasks used to examine them reveals, there is a consensus regarding the functions of WM that is matched by a general agreement regarding its characteristics (e.g., Daneman & Carpenter, 1980; O'Reilly et al., 1999; Smith & Jonides, 1999; see Hassin, 2005, p. 209; Turner & Engle, 1989). These include (a) active maintenance of ordered information for relatively short periods of time, (b) context-relevant updating of information, and (c) *goal-relevant* computations involving active representations and rapid biasing of task-relevant cognitions and behaviors *in the service of currently held goals* (Hassin, 2005; O'Reilly et al., 1999). The latter functions include attending and inhibiting, scheduling, monitoring, and planning (cf. Smith & Jonides, 1999).

The cognitive literature assumes that WM is central for goal pursuit and then goes on to examine the operation and interaction of its components. To the best of our knowledge, however, it did not experimentally investigate WM's role in goal pursuit by introducing various goals and examining their effects (but, for a discussion of goal neglect, see Duncan, 1995; Duncan, Emslie, & Williams, 1996). Evidence from related literatures in neuropsychology, however, suggests that damage to brain tissues related to WM results in specific impairments to goal pursuit (cf. Baddeley, Della Salla, Papagno, & Spinnler, 1997; Damasio, 1994; Luria, 1966; Norman & Shallice, 1986; Shallice, 1982).

Alan Baddeley, one of the forefathers of the concept of WM and of one of the most influential models of WM (Baddeley

& Hitch, 1974), has recently added a new component to his WM model—the episodic buffer (Baddeley, 2000, 2003). This new buffer serves as an interface between a range of systems, including long-term memory, and as such it "provides not only a mechanism for modelling the environment, but also for creating new cognitive representations, which in turn might facilitate problem solving" (Baddeley, 2000, p. 421). A component of this kind seems to be exactly what successful goal pursuit requires: It allows episodic representations of the environment, interaction with long-term memory, and the construction of new cognitive representations.

To sum up, WM is a multicomponent cognitive structure with storage capacity and executive functions. It allows for flexible, context-sensitive representations of the environment as well as for the creation of new cognitive representations. These and other WM functions are instrumental for goal pursuit, and hence impairment in brain structures that are related to WM is associated with decreased capacity for goal pursuit.

Testing the Proposed Principles
Set I: Effort

We have recently completed an empirical examination of the first principle (Hassin, Aarts, Eitam, & Custers, 2005). To examine whether primed goals enter WM and are then assigned some capacity, participants in these studies were primed with a goal, and they then engaged in a WM task that was clearly novel to them.

Consider, first, a participant who is primed with a goal that may be applied (cf. Aarts, Gollwitzer, & Hassin, 2004; Higgins, 1996) to a WM task and who then goes on to engage in such a task. According to the first principle, on priming (and given that a threshold is passed), the goal enters WM, and some of its capacity is allocated

to it. Then, when the task is introduced, it too is allocated resources. Nonprimed (control) participants, on the other hand, enjoy only resources that are assigned to the task, meaning that they should fare worse than participants in the experimental condition.[3]

Consider, next, a participant who is primed with a goal that is inapplicable to a laboratory WM task (e.g., going out) and then goes on to engage in such a task. Again, the first two assumptions entail that the goal enters WM and that a proportion of its available resources are allocated to it. Since, ex hypothesis, the goal is inapplicable to the task, this allocated capacity cannot be used for the task.[4]

These, then, were our two hypotheses: Priming of an applicable goal should result in improved performance on a following WM task, and priming of an inapplicable goal should bring about reduced performance.

Results from five studies supported these predictions. In the first study, participants had either been primed with an applicable goal (achievement) or not, and they then engaged in one of the best-known WM tasks, the OSPAN (Turner & Engle, 1989). The OSPAN is a dual task that consists of correctly solving equations while memorizing lists of words. The results showed that the control and the experimental conditions achieved the same WM span, but participants in the priming condition achieved it in a significantly shorter time. These findings suggest that the dual-task performance of primed participants was better than that of the control group and thus that they devoted more resources to the experimental tasks.

To further examine the effect of goal priming on WM capacity, we ran another study in which we used the automated versions of the OSPAN and the conceptually similar reading span (RSPAN). In this experiment, achievement priming led to a significant increase in WM's capacity both on the OSPAN and on the RSPAN. In the third study, priming of an applicable goal was followed by a WM inhibition paradigm developed by Jonides and colleagues (Jonides, Smith, Marshuetz, Koeppe, & Reuter-Lorenz, 1998, study 2). The results of this study showed that primed participants were significantly better at inhibiting prepotent responses—an effortful, resource-demanding behavior. Together, the results from these studies support the first hypothesis developed previously.

Next, two studies examined the effect of priming of nonapplicable goals (e.g., to have fun) on performance in the inhibition paradigm mentioned previously. Supporting the second hypothesis, both studies documented decrease in performance following priming. That is, participants who had been primed with an inapplicable goal were significantly worse than their control counterparts at inhibiting prepotent responses. Together, the evidence from these five studies strongly supports the first principle.

Related findings were recently reported by Shah and Kruglanski (2002), who showed that priming of a goal that participants perceived as applicable to their task led them to invest more time and to do better on it (the two variables were strongly correlated). Taken together, then, these results mean that priming of an applicable goal led participants to invest more resources in the experimental task.

Yet there is a qualitative difference between these findings and the ones we discussed previously: We showed that goal priming leads to an increase/decrease of resources invested in a task *per unit of time;* that is, we documented changes in the online availability of resources. Shah and Kruglanski (2002; cf. Bargh et al., 2001), however, examined the *total amount* of resources invested in a task, which may also

be a function of the time spent in the task (and hence do not necessarily reflect the online availability of resources).

In a sense, then, their findings and ours are complimentary: It may well be the case that task, personality, and motivational factors determine which alternative we follow—whether we increase resource spending per unit of time (i.e., increase WM's capacity), increase the total quantity of resources spent on the task, both, or none.

Set II: Conflict

Very minor modifications to the principles presented previously allow the proposed framework to handle the nonconscious interaction of multiple goals. Simply, instead of describing the activation of one goal (and its later assignment to WM), they may describe the activation of multiple goals and their allocation to WM. These modifications do not require any changes in the nature of the proposed framework.

Note, then, that when two goals are in conflict, hence rendering relevant decisions more difficult, the goals are maintained until further developments help resolve or downplay the conflict. Thus, this principle makes a very simple prediction regarding nonconscious goal conflict: It should lead to longer decision times.

In a study that was designed to examine this prediction, we (Hassin & Kleiman, 2008) looked at participants' behavior in a commons resource dilemma (cf. Bargh et al., 2001). In this task, participants played fishermen, and they had been led to believe that they would be playing against another participant. On each "season" (i.e., trial), participants "caught" a certain number of fish, and their task was to decide how many fish they would throw back to the lake (and how many they would keep to themselves).

The conflict, like in every commons resource dilemma, is this: On the one hand, participants' competitive urges (and, ex-hypothesis, survival needs) lead them to keep to themselves as many fish as they can. In other words, participants' personal goal is to compete. On the other hand, if both fishermen behave too egotistically, then the fish population would be wiped out, thus causing a societal disaster. In other words, the high-level goal in this game is to cooperate. These two goals are, of course, in direct conflict—given a scale (of how many fish to return to the lake), they "pull" the response to opposite directions. Furthermore, given that this conflict is between a higher-level and a lower-level goal, we deem that it is a self-control conflict.

Prior to engaging in this commons resource dilemma, half of our participants were primed with a cooperation goal. Given the structure and nature of the task, we expected that this priming would result in increased conflict, that is, in more difficult decisions. Hence, by assumption 3c, priming should lead to increased decision times. And indeed, these were the results we obtained. First, replicating Bargh et al.'s (2001) results, participants who were primed with a cooperation goal cooperated more than control participants. In other words, they returned more fish to the lake. Crucially, primed participants' decision times were significantly longer than those of control participants, supporting the proposed principles.

During the game, there were a few occasions in which a message appeared on the screen, warning participants that the fish population is at risk. Interestingly, decision times following the warnings were longer for both groups, probably reflecting, among other things, an increase in the *conscious conflict* between the personal goal of competing and the higher goal of cooperating. Note that even in these trials, the decision times of participants in the primed condition were

longer than those of the control condition, implying that conscious conflict and non-conscious conflict may operate at the same time (cf. the additive effects of conscious and nonconscious goals in Bargh et al., 2001).

A second study in this series examined another implication of the proposed principles. Note that these principles imply that, at least under certain circumstances, noise should affect decisions under goal conflict more than decisions in which there is no goal conflict. The rationale is simple. Goal conflict is likely to result in close-call decisions. These, by their very nature, increase the probability that small differences—noise included—would tip the scales.

In this study, participants engaged in 120 trials of the commons resource dilemma described previously. Prior to each trial, participants engaged in another task in which they were asked to decide whether a number that appeared on the screen was odd or even. These numbers were meant to serve as irrelevant anchors (cf. Tversky & Kahneman, 1974). Crucially, on some trials the numbers were relatively big (9, 10, or 11), whereas on others they were relatively small (1, 2, or 3). Since, from participants' point of view, the two tasks were completely unrelated, these numerical anchors could be viewed as noise.

Recall that according to the prediction we developed previously, goal conflict may result in an increased effect of noise on decisions. Hence, the proposed principles predict that nonconscious goal conflict should enhance the use of anchors in this paradigm. And indeed, these were the results we obtained: Primed participants returned more fish to the lake in the high-anchor trials than in the low-anchor trials, while no such effect was found for the control group. Here, like in the first study in this set, a thorough debriefing revealed no differences between the groups in goal commitment or awareness of a conflict.

Set III: Monitoring

Although we have not yet started to systematically address the last principle, a set of recent studies provides preliminary support for the idea that nonconscious goal pursuit involves monitoring, discrepancy detection, and cognitive processes related to discrepancy reduction.

Generally, previous research failed to examine the question of monitoring during nonconscious goal pursuit for one of two reasons. First, studies that manipulated discrepancy (Fein & Spencer, 1997; Koole, Smeets, van Knippenberg, & Dijksterhuis, 1999; Moskowitz, 2002) usually manipulated it explicitly, hence leading to conscious awareness of the goal itself. Second, studies that manipulated goal accessibility usually did so in contexts in which goal discrepancy is inherent, that is, environments in which one's relevant goal is yet to be achieved (see Custers & Aarts, 2005). This possible confound makes it hard to determine whether the resulting behavior resulted from "simple" goal priming or whether it involved a reaction to detected discrepancy.

Recently, we conducted a line of experiments that examined how goal accessibility and discrepancy detection lead to the activation of means for goal achievement (Custers & Aarts, 2005). The goal that we used in these studies was that of looking well groomed, a goal that typically needs to be maintained over time and, according to pilot testing, was highly desirable to our participants. Accessibility was either measured as an individual difference (study 1) or manipulated (study 2). Discrepancy was manipulated via descriptions of either discrepant (e.g., "The shoes you put on look dirty") or control (e.g., "The shoes you put on have laces") situations.

To test the effect of discrepancy detection, we employed a probe-recognition paradigm (Hassin, Aarts, & Ferguson, 2005;

McKoon & Ratcliff, 1986; Uleman, Hon, Roman, & Moskowitz, 1996). In this paradigm, sentences that appear on the screen are immediately followed by probe words. Participants' task is to indicate, as quickly as possible, whether the probe appeared in the preceding sentence. Probes that are rendered more accessible during the reading of a sentence—without actually appearing in it—should lead to longer response times (versus control words). This is the case because while the correct response to these probes is negative, their heightened accessibility suggests a positive response.

In our studies, the scenarios were either goal discrepant (e.g., "The shirt you button up looks wrinkled") or control (e.g., "The shirt you button up is blue"). Both types of sentences were followed by a probe word that represented an action that may reduce discrepancy (e.g., "ironing"). And thus, if discrepancy detection leads to the automatic activation of appropriate means for goal achievement, probes that appear after goal-discrepant scenarios should take longer to react to than probes that appear after control sentences.

The first study looked at individual differences between people who are chronic well-groomers and people who are not. The results showed that, for chronic well-groomers, response times for probes that were preceded by a goal-discrepant scenario were longer than for those that were preceded by a control scenario. This effect was not present for people who did not frequently pursue the goal. These results suggest that perceived discrepancy may automatically facilitate access to discrepancy-reducing actions. Importantly, the differences between chronics and nonchronics suggest that this effect of discrepancy requires an active goal—but not necessarily a conscious one.

In a subsequent experiment, we experimentally manipulated the goal by way of subliminal priming. Thus, just before the onset of the goal-discrepant sentences, two (Dutch) synonyms for "well groomed" were flashed several times for 20 milliseconds in the fixation point (cf. Wigboldus, Dijksterhuis, & van Knippenberg, 2003). The results indicated that subliminal priming had the same effect as the chronic goal—it facilitated access to representations of instrumental actions (cf. Bargh, Lombardi, & Higgins, 1988; Higgins, Bargh, & Lombardi, 1985).

Together, these studies suggest that people can automatically react to goal-discrepant situations with the spontaneous activation of means for goal achievement. Note that this spontaneous activation of means occurs only if the goal is accessible. Furthermore, this effect occurs even when the goal is nonconsciously primed. This pattern suggests that enhanced accessibility of goals—whether conscious or not—leads people to monitor their environment for discrepancies. These findings, then, lend support to the idea that nonconscious goal pursuit may involve monitoring.

Summary

To sum up, three new sets of studies support our predictions regarding nonconscious goal pursuit. The first set showed that priming of applicable goals led to improved performance on resource-demanding WM tasks and therefore to an improvement in WM capacity. Priming of inapplicable goals, however, led to decreased performance on these tasks. The second set of studies demonstrated that nonconscious goal conflict leads to an increase in decision times. Furthermore, the second study in this set showed that nonconscious goal conflict increases the effect of irrelevant information on decisions. Finally, the studies described in the previous section suggest that nonconscious goal pursuit may lead to monitoring and discrepancy detection.

Nonconscious Thought

At the outset of this chapter, we argued that WM—and executive functions more generally—is involved in nonconscious goal pursuit and endows the latter the flexibility that is often a prerequisite for their effectiveness. We also argued that the basic notion of executive involvement in nonconscious processes may shed new light on neighboring literatures on complex nonconscious high-level cognitive processes. In this section, we explore one such example, that of nonconscious thought. In the following section, we discuss another example, the literature on controlled behavior, and the frontal lobes.

Recently, Dijksterhuis and his colleagues presented and tested a theory of unconscious thought (Dijksterhuis, 2004; Dijksterhuis, Bos, Nordgren, & van Baaren, 2006; Dijksterhuis & Nordgren, 2006). This theory holds that unconscious thought is an effortless (i.e., occurs without conscious attention) yet time-consuming process whose capacity to integrate and weigh information—even in high-level processes such as judgments and decision making—is much larger than that of conscious thought.

To examine unconscious thought Dijksterhuis (e.g., 2004) developed the following paradigm. Participants are first presented with decision-related information and then pursue one of three routes. In the immediate decision condition, participants make their decision immediately after they were exposed to the information. In the conscious thought condition, participants are asked to think about their decision for a certain amount of time, and they then indicate their choice. Participants in the third and crucial group—the unconscious thought condition—are given the same amount of time as participants in the conscious thought condition, but instead of thinking about their choice, they engage in an effortful task that does not allow for much conscious thought.

The general finding in this paradigm is that in complex decisions participants in the unconscious thought condition fare better than participants in the conscious thought condition. In other words, unconscious thought processes seem to be better at using multiple units of information to form a decision.

The theory's postulation that unconscious thought processes are effortless suggests that they do not involve WM-like executive functions. On the other hand, the theory's postulation that unconscious thought is time consuming does suggest a limited-resource process, if only in the sense of having to process information somewhat serially (otherwise, why would the process be time consuming?). Given that limited resources are usually associated with controlled processes (in social psychology) and with WM and executive processes (in the cognitive sciences more generally), it seems that unconscious thought may help itself to nonconsciously using (nonconscious) executive processes.

This is, admittedly, a speculative account of some of the possible cognitive mechanisms that underlie nonconscious thought. It opens, however, exciting routes for an improved understanding of executive processes on the one hand and of nonconscious thought on the other.

Nonconscious Goal Pursuit and the Frontal Lobes

In the previous sections, we discussed the proposed principles in the context of the social psychological literature on automatic goal pursuit and the cognitive literature regarding WM. In this section, we would like to discuss them in the context of the work of Shallice and his colleagues on action control and frontal lobe patients.

The Norman–Shallice Model

Norman and Shallice's (1986; Shallice, 1982, 2002) work suggests that two complementary processes operate in the selection and control of action. One, contention scheduling, handles well-learned sequences of behaviors, whereas the other, the supervisory attentional system (SAS), allows for conscious, willful control of behavior. While the model does not explicitly focus on goal pursuit, this seems to be mainly a terminological issue. A closer examination reveals that its founders hold the belief that their model of action control is intimately associated with goal pursuit (Cooper & Shallice, 2000; Shallice, 1972; Shallice & Burgess, 1998).

Norman and Shallice (1986) assumed that well-learned, routine, action sequences are represented in schemas and that these schemas may be activated by appropriate cues (either internal or external). When only one schema is activated, this schema controls behavior. When multiple schemas are activated, a selection process—which they termed contention scheduling—selects the one with the highest level of activation (the activation level of a schema is determined by the cues and context as well as by processes of lateral activation and inhibition). In cases where schema selection is difficult or conflictual (e.g., when one attempts to overcome temptations) or in cases where no schema is available to control behavior (especially in novel tasks or those that involve planning), the SAS comes into play. The SAS provides *attentional, conscious* control over behavior by changing the activation levels of different schemas, thus creating novel and adaptive sequences of behaviors.

This conceptualization of the division of labor between contention scheduling and the SAS is reminiscent of the class of models that we today refer to as dual-process models (Chaiken & Trope, 1999; Chapter 5).

There is one route of action control that is, grossly speaking, automatic (nonconscious, effortless, unintentional, and ballistic), and it accounts for routinized behaviors. The other route of action control is controlled (it requires attention and conscious intention), and it accounts for nonroutinized behavior. Note that, in the Norman–Shallice model, the latter route is implemented by way of modulation: The SAS modulates activation and inhibition levels—it does not have a more direct way of affecting behavior.

Evidence supporting this model comes mainly from neuropsychology. Assuming that the SAS is a frontal component, whereas contention scheduling is not, these researchers hypothesized a dissociation between performance on routine (automatic) tasks and on nonroutine ones. Specifically, they hypothesized that frontal patients—who, ex hypothesis, should have difficulties with the SAS—should show decreased performance on nonhabitual tasks but not on habitual ones. Patterns of this sort had been previously reported in the literature (e.g., Luria, 1966), and novel studies with frontal patients corroborate the hypothesis (e.g., Shallice, 1982; Shallice & Burgess, 1993).

While some of this model's principles are similar to the ones we propose here, there are numerous differences between the two frameworks. Among these are the treatment of abstract goals, the role of resources in nonconscious goal pursuit, the role of WM in nonconscious goal pursuit, the nonconscious coping with goal conflict, and so on. In the next section we focus on one difference that we deem as important—the role of the supervisory attentional system.

Nonconscious Goal Pursuit and the SAS

Note that the current principles have no SAS equivalent; they contain no necessarily

conscious, effortful executive processes per se. If we follow the logic of Norman and Shallice's (1986) model, then, our principles should only apply to routine, automatic behaviors. In fact, this logic is not unique to the Norman–Shallice model. Quite to the contrary—the equation "no executive = only automatic" seems to reflect the general perception of automatic and controlled processes in experimental psychology.

Yet we emphasized that the current principles apply not only to routinized goal pursuits but also to goal pursuits in novel, nonroutinized circumstances. Furthermore, we contended that they also encompass conflictual situations. These hypotheses were confirmed in two separate sets of studies. The studies that examined the effects of goal priming on cognitive flexibility, or adaptation to novel environments (see the section "The Adaptiveness Paradox"), supported the former assertion; the studies that examined nonconscious goal conflict supported the latter (see the section "Set II: Conflict").

So how do automatic goal pursuits get along without the necessarily conscious, effortful executive processes per se? Some of the feats of the SAS, we argue, may be achieved through nonconscious resource allocation. This allocation is bound to affect goals' activation levels—thus achieving one of the most central aspects of SAS.[5] It is important to note here that we do not suggest that SAS—or, more generally, conscious, effortful executive processes—are superfluous in the determination of human action. We do propose, however, that they are necessary neither in novel situations nor in conflictual ones.

Nonconscious Goal Pursuit and the Frontal Lobe Syndrome

Recall that the work of Shallice and his colleagues (Norman & Shallice, 1986;

Shallice, 1982; Shallice & Burgess, 1993) established a dissociation between routine and nonroutine action: Frontal lobe patients seem to be impaired on the latter but not on the former. At present we do not know whether the nonconscious resource-allocating process is implemented by a frontal component of the brain or not. Either way, its existence allows us to make novel predictions, and in the following paragraphs we explore a small subset of them.

First, assume that the nonconscious resource-allocating processes described in this chapter are not based in the frontal lobes or that they are frontal but subserved by neural networks that are not involved in conscious, effortful executive processes (after all, the frontal lobes make for a big portion of our brain). In this case we could make the prediction that patients with frontal syndrome should have some preserved ability to pursue goals in novel and conflictual situations. These patients, furthermore, should be affected by goal priming, maybe even more so than control participants, whose behavior may be concurrently controlled by conscious, effortful executive processes. Finally, patients with damage to this specific area may suffer from deficiencies in nonconscious—but not conscious—goal pursuit.

The second possibility is that these functions and those of more conscious, effortful executive processes are implemented by the same neural networks and operate on the same principles. In other words, the main difference between conscious and nonconscious executive processes lies in their phenomenology (how this phenomenology implemented in the brain is beyond the scope of the current discussion). This alternative has interesting consequences too. First, it implies that frontal patients should have difficulties not only with nonroutine action but also with some types of routine actions. More specifically, they may reveal deficiencies even in (certain kinds of) habitual goal pursuits. Second, it suggests that full-blown, effortful executive processes may be nonconscious. While this suggestion seems to be in conflict with the present Zeitgeist, it has received some empirical and theoretical support (Hassin, 2005; Hassin, Bargh, & Zimerman, in press; Hassin et al., 2007). Further evidence supporting this suggestion was recently published by Naccache et al. (2005), who studied a patient showing a dissociation between the operation of executive attention and the conscious feeling of effort.

Conclusion

Since much of human action is goal oriented, understanding goal pursuit promises to shed much light on the psychology of action. This chapter began with a rejection of the idea that goal pursuit is necessarily conscious and effortful (Bargh, 1990) and went on to present new principles for nonconscious goal pursuit. The current framework goes beyond previous models and findings by suggesting that nonconscious goal pursuit is not limited to existing networks of contexts, goals, and means. Rather, we argued, nonconscious goal pursuit may make use of WM and executive processes. More generally, we suggest that the involvement of WM and executive functions in nonconscious, automatic processes may help us resolve what we termed the adaptiveness paradox by proposing mechanisms that allow nonconscious, automatic processes quick adaptability.

Acknowledgments

The research reviewed in this paper was supported by ISF grants (#846/03 and 1035/07) to the first author, and NWO VIDI-grant 452-02-047 to the second author. Correspondence should be sent to Ran Hassin at ran.hassin@huji.ac.il.

Notes

1. A thorough discussion of the meaning of "new" or "novel" is beyond the scope of this chapter. In some sense, nothing is ever truly new, and in another, nothing is ever truly known, or "old." We use "new" and "novel" in a lay way that builds on shared common sense.

2. Note, furthermore, that the current principles refer to goals that enter "a working memory" and not "working memory." Recall that at any given point in time, WM may be engaged in the pursuit of multiple goals. The current notation follows from our belief that it may be theoretically advantageous to treat the processes related to each goal separately.

3. To put it more formally, assume that WM's available resources just before priming takes place are R_i, that the available postpriming resources are R_k (where $R_k < R_i$ due to the allocation of resources to the primed goal), and that, for simplicity's sake, WM assigns an initial proportion P of its available resources to *every* goal that is assigned to it. In the experimental situation described previously, the resources allocated to the task goal are P of R_i without prior priming and P of R_k following priming. The primed goal is always assigned P of R_i resources. Thus, without prior priming, the task proceeds with $P*R_i$ resources. With priming, however, it enjoys $P*R_i + P*R_k$ (assuming that the upper limit of resources was not reached). Priming of applicable goals, then, should result in the investment of more resources, thus leading to improved performance on WM tasks.

4. In the notation introduced previously, the task proceeds with $P*R_i$ resources when no prior priming occurs, whereas following priming it enjoys $P*R_k$. Since $R_k < R_i$, priming of an inapplicable goal would lead to decrease in performance (relative to a nonprimed control group).

5. In their original chapter, Norman and Shallice (1986) recognize the role of motivation in the determination of a schema's activation levels. Yet what they mean by "motivation" must be different than what we mean by "goal" because for them it is a "relatively slow acting system, working primarily to bias the operation of the horizontal thread structures toward the long term goals of the organism" (p. 7).

References

Aarts, H., Gollwitzer, P., & Hassin, R. R. (2004). Goal contagion: Perceiving is for pursuing. *Journal of Personality and Social Psychology, 87,* 23–37.

Aarts, H., & Hassin, R. R. (2005). Automatic goal inference and contagion: On pursuing goals one perceives in other people's behavior. In J. P. Forgas, D. W. Kipling, & W. Von Hipple (Eds.), *Social motivation: Conscious and unconscious processes* (pp. 153–167). New York: Psychology Press.

Ajzen, I. (1991). The theory of planned behavior. *Organizational Behavior and Human Decision Processes, 50,* 179–211.

Austin, J. T., & Vancouver, J. B. (1996). Goal constructs in psychology: Structure, process, and content. *Psychological Bulletin, 120,* 338–375.

Baars, B. J., & Franklin, S. (2003). How conscious experience and working memory interact. *Trends in Cognitive Science, 7,* 166–172.

Baddeley, A. D. (1993). Working memory and conscious awareness. In A. Collins & S. Gathercole (Eds.), *Theories of memory* (pp. 11–28). Hillsdale, NJ: Lawrence Erlbaum Associates.

Baddeley, A. D. (2000). The episodic buffer: A new component of working memory? *Trends in Cognitive Sciences, 4,* 417–423.

Baddeley, A. D. (2003). Working memory: Looking back and looking forward. *Nature Reviews Neuroscience, 4,* 829–839.

Baddeley, A. D., Della Salla, S., Papagno, C., & Spinnler, H. (1997). Dual task performance in dysexecutive and nondysexecutive patients with a frontal lesion. *Neuropsychology, 11,* 187–194.

Baddeley, A. D., & Hitch, G. (1974). Working memory. In G. Bower (Ed.), *The psychology of learning and motivation: Advances in research and theory* (Vol. 8, pp. 47–89). New York: Academic Press.

Baddeley, A. D., & Logie, R. H. (1999). Working memory: The multiple-component model. In A. Miyake & P. Shah (Eds.), *Models of working memory: Mechanisms of active maintenance and executive control* (pp. 28–61). New York: Cambridge University Press.

Bandura, A. (1986). *Social foundations of thought and action: A social cognitive theory.* Upper Saddle River, NJ: Prentice Hall.

Bargh, J. A. (1989). Conditional automaticity: Varieties of automatic influence in social perception and cognition. In J. Uleman & J. A. Bargh (Eds.), *Unintended thought* (pp. 3–51). New York: Guilford Press.

Bargh, J. A. (1990). Auto-motives: Preconscious determinants of social interaction. In E. T. Higgins & R. M. Sorrentino (Eds.), *Handbook of motivation and cognition: Foundations of social behavior,* (Vol. 2, pp. 93–130). New York: Guilford Press.

Bargh, J. A. (1994). The four horsemen of automaticity: Awareness, intention, efficiency, and control in social cognition. In R. J. Wyer & T. K. Srull (Eds.), *Handbook of social cognition* (pp. 1–40). Hillsdale, NJ: Lawrence Erlbaum Associates.

Bargh, J. A. (2006). Agenda 2006: What have we been priming all these years? On the development, mechanisms, and ecology of nonconscious social behavior. *European Journal of Social Psychology, 36,* 147–168.

Bargh, J. A., Gollwitzer, P., Lee-Chai, A., Barndollar, K., & Trötschel, R. (2001). The automated will: Nonconscious activation and pursuit of behavioral goals. *Journal of Personality and Social Psychology, 81,* 1014–1027.

Bargh, J. A., Lombardi, W. J., & Higgins, E. T. (1988). Automaticity of chronically accessible constructs in person x situation effects on person perception: It's just a matter of time. *Journal of Personality and Social Psychology, 55*, 599–605.

Berg, E. A. (1948). A simple objective test for measuring flexibility in thinking. *Journal of General Psychology, 39*, 15–22.

Chaiken, S., & Trope, Y. (1999). *Dual process theories in social psychology.* New York: Guilford Press.

Chartrand, T. L., & Bargh, J. A. (1996). Automatic activation of impression formation and memorization goals: Nonconscious goal priming reproduces effects of explicit task instructions. *Journal of Personality and Social Psychology, 71*, 464–478.

Cooper, R. & Shallice, T. (2000). Contention scheduling and the control of routine activities. *Cognitive Neuropsychology, 17*, 297–338.

Cowan, N. (1999). An embedded-processes model of working memory. In A. Miyake & P. Shah (Eds.), *Models of working memory: Mechanisms of active maintenance and executive control.* New York: Cambridge University Press.

Custers, R., & Aarts, H. (2005). Beyond priming effects: The role of positive affect and discrepancies in implicit processes of motivation and goal pursuit. In M. Hewstone & W. Stroebe (Eds.), *European review of social psychology* (Vol. 16, pp. 257–300). Hove: Psychology Press/Taylor & Francis.

Damasio, A. D. (1994). *Descartes' error: Emotion, reason, and the human brain.* New York: Grosset/Putnam.

Daneman, M., & Carpenter, P. (1980). Individual differences in working memory and reading. *Journal of Verbal Learning and Verbal Behavior, 19*, 450–466.

Deci, E. L., & Ryan, R. M. (1985). The general causality orientations scale: Self-determination in personality. *Journal of Research in Personality, 19*, 109–134.

Demakis, G. J. (2003). A meta-analytic review of the sensitivity of the Wisconsin Card Sorting Test to frontal and lateralized frontal brain damage. *Neuropsychology, 17*(2), 255–264.

Dennett, D. (2001). Are we explaining consciousness yet? *Cognition, 79*(1–2), 221.

Dijksterhuis, A. (2004). Think different: The merits of unconscious thought in preference development and decision making. *Journal of Personality and Social Psychology, 87*, 586–598.

Dijksterhuis, A., Bos, M. W., Nordgren, L. F., & van Baaren, R. B. (2006). On making the right choice: The deliberation-without-attention effect. *Science, 311*, 1005–1007.

Dijksterhuis, A., & Nordgren, L. F. (2006). A theory of unconscious thought. *Perspectives on Psychological Science, 1*, 95–109.

Dudai, Y. (2004). *Memory From A to Z: Keywords, concepts and beyond.* New York: Oxford University Press.

Duncan, J. (1995). Attention, intelligence, and the frontal lobes. In M. Gazzaniga (Ed.), *The cognitive neurosciences* (pp. 721–733). Cambridge, MA: The MIT Press.

Duncan, J., Emslie, H., & Williams, P. (1996). Intelligence and the frontal lobes: The organization of goal directed behavior. *Cognitive Psychology, 30*, 257–303.

Eitam, B., Hassin, R. R., & Schul, Y. (2008). Nonconscious goal pursuit in novel environments: The case of implicit learning. *Psychological Science, 19*, 261–267.

Fein, S., & Spencer, S. J. (1997). Prejudice as self-image maintenance: Affirming the self through derogating others. *Journal of Personality and Social Psychology, 73*, 31–44.

Ferguson, M. J., Hassin, R. R., & Bargh, J. A. (2007). Implicit Motivation. In J. Y. Shah & W. Wood (Eds.), *Handbook of motivation.* New York: Guilford Press.

Fishbach, A., Friedman, R. S., & Kruglanski, A. W. (2003). Leading us not unto temptation: Momentary allurements elicit overriding goal activation. *Journal of Personality and Social Psychology, 84*, 296–309.

Fitzsimons, G., & Bargh, J. A. (2003). Thinking of you: Nonconscious pursuit of interpersonal goals associated with relationship partners. *Journal of Personality and Social Psychology, 84*, 148–164.

Goschke, T., & Kuhl, J. (1993). Representation of intentions: Persisting activation in memory. *Journal of Experimental Psychology: Learning, Memory, and Cognition, 19*, 1211–1226.

Hassin, R. R. (2005). Nonconscious control and implicit working memory. In R. R. Hassin, J. S. Uleman, & J. A. Bargh (Eds.), *The new unconscious* (pp. 196–225). New York: Oxford University Press.

Hassin, R. R. (2008). *Beyond the automatic-controlled dichotomy in social cognition: A functional perspective.* Manuscript in preparation.

Hassin, R. R. (in press). Being open minded without knowing why: Evidence from non-conscious goal pursuit. *Social Cognition.*

Hassin, R. R., Aarts, H., Eitam, B., & Custers, R. (2005). *Goals at work: Automatic goal pursuit and working memory.* Manuscript in preparation.

Hassin, R. R., Aarts, H., & Ferguson, M. J. (2005). Automatic goal inferences. *Journal of Experimental Social Psychology, 41,* 129–140.

Hassin, R. R., Bargh, J. A., & Zimerman, S. (in press). Automatic and flexible: The case of nonconscious goal pursuit. *Social Cognition.*

Hassin, R. R., Bargh, J. A., Engell, A., & McCulluch, K. C. (2007). *Implicit working memory.* Manuscript in preparation.

Hassin, R. R. & Kleiman, T. (2008). *Non-conscious goal conflicts.* Manuscript in preparation.

Heaton, R. K., Chelune, G. J., Talley, J. L., Kay, G. G., & Curtiss, G. (1993). *Wisconsin Card Sorting test manual (revised and expanded).* Lutz, FL: PAR.

Higgins, E. T. (1996). Knowledge activation: Accessibility, applicability, and salience. In A. W. Kruglanski & E. T. Higgins (Eds.), *Social psychology: Handbook of basic principles* (pp. 133–168). New York: Guilford Press.

Higgins, E. T., Bargh, J. A., & Lombardi, W. J. (1985). Nature of priming effects on categorization. *Journal of Experimental Psychology: Learning, Memory, and Cognition, 11,* 59–69.

Jonides, J., Smith, E. E., Marshuetz, C., Koeppe, R. A., & Reuter-Lorenz, P. A. (1998). Inhibition in verbal working memory revealed by brain activation. *Proceedings of the National Academy of Sciences of the United States of America, 95,* 8410–8413.

Kahneman, D. (1973). *Attention and Effort.* Englewoods Cliff, NJ: Prentice-Hall.

Kahneman, D., & Treisman, A. (1984). Changing views of attention and automaticity. In R. Parasuraman & D. Davies (Eds.), *Varieties of attention* (pp. 29–61). New York: Academic Press.

Koole, S. L., Smeets, K., van Knippenberg, A., & Dijksterhuis, A. (1999). The cessation of rumination through self-affirmation. *Journal of Personality and Social Psychology, 77,* 111–125.

Kruglanski, A. W. (1996). Goals as knowledge structures. In P. M. Gollwitzer & J. A. Bargh (Eds.), *The psychology of action: Linking cognition and motivation to behavior* (pp. 599–618). New York: Guilford Press.

Kruglanski, A. W., Shah, J. Y., Fisbach, A., Friedman, R. S., Chun, W. Y., & Sleeth-Keppler, D. (2002). A theory of goal systems. In M. P. Zanna (Ed.), *Advances in experimental social psychology* (pp. 331–378). San Diego, CA: Academic Press.

Locke, E. A., & Latham, G. P. (1990). *A theory of goal setting and task performance.* Upper Saddle River, NJ: Prentice Hall.

Luria, A. R. (1966). *Higher cortical functions in man.* London: Tavistock.

Marsh, R. L., Hicks, J. L., & Bink, M. L. (1998). Activation of completed, uncompleted and partially completed intentions. *Journal of Experimental Psychology: Learning, Memory, and Cognition, 24,* 350–361.

McKoon, G., & Ratcliff, R. (1986). Inferences about predictable events. *Journal of Experimental Psychology: Learning, Memory, and Cognition, 12,* 82–91.

Miyake, A., & Shah, P. (1999). *Models of working memory: Mechanisms of active maintenance and executive control.* New York: Cambridge University Press.

Moskowitz, G. B. (2002). Preconscious effects of temporary goals on attention. *Journal of Experimental Social Psychology, 38,* 397–404.

Moskowitz, G. B., Gollwitzer, P., Wasel, W., & Schaal, B. (1999). Preconscious control of stereotype activation through chronic egalitarian goals. *Journal of Personality and Social Psychology, 77,* 167–184.

Naccache, L., Dehaene, S., Cohen, L., Habert, M., Guichart-Gomez, E., Galanaud, D., et al. (2005). Effortless control: Executive attention and conscious feeling of mental effort are dissociable. *Neuropsychologia, 43,* 1318–1328.

Navon, D. (1984). Resources—A theoretical soup stone? *Psychological Review, 91,* 216–234.

Norman, D. A., & Shallice, T. (1986). Attention to action: Willed and automatic control of behavior. In J. R. Davidson, G. E. Schwartz, & D. Shapiro (Eds.), *Consciousness and self regulation: Advances in research and theory* (Vol. 4, pp. 1–18). New York: Plenum Press.

O'Reilly, R., Braver, T., & Cohen, J. D. (1999). A biologically based computational model of working memory. In A. Miyake & P. Shah (Eds.), *Models of working memory: Mechanisms of active maintenance and executive control* (pp. 375–411). New York: Cambridge University Press.

Pashler, H. E. (1998). *The psychology of attention.* Cambridge, MA: MIT Press.

Shah, J. Y. (2003). Automatic for the people: How representations of significant others implicitly affect goal pursuit. *Journal of Personality and Social Psychology, 84,* 661–681.

Shah, J. Y., & Kruglanski, A. W. (2002). Priming against your will: How accessible alternatives affect goal pursuit. *Journal of Experimental Social Psychology, 38,* 368–383.

Shah, P., & Miyake, A. (1999). Toward unified theories of working memory: Emerging general consensus, unresolved theoretical issues, and future research directions. In A. Miyake & P. Shah (Eds.), *Models of working memory: Mechanisms of active maintenance and executive control* (pp. 442–482). New York: Oxford University Press.

Shallice, T. (1972). Dual functions of consciousness. *Psychological Review, 79,* 383–393.

Shallice, T. (1982). Specific impairments of planning. *Philosophical Transactions of the Royal Society of London, 298,* 199–209.

Shallice, T. (2002). Fractionation of the supervisory system. In D. T. Stuss & R. T. Knight (Eds.), *Principles of the frontal lobe function* (pp. 261–277). Oxford: Oxford University Press.

Shallice, T., & Burgess, P. (1993). Supervisory control of action and thought selection. In A. D. Baddeley & L. Weiskrantz (Eds.), *Attention: Selection awareness and control* (pp. 171–187). Oxford: Oxford University Press.

Shallice, T., & Burgess, P. W. (1998). The domain of supervisory processes and the temporal organization of behaviour. In A. C. Roberts, T. W. Robbins, & L. Weiskrantz (Eds.), *The prefrontal cortex: Executive and cognitive functions* (pp. 22–35). New York: Oxford University Press.

Smith, E. E., & Jonides, J. (1999). Storage and executive processes in the frontal lobes. *Science, 283,* 1657–1661.

Turner, M. L., & Engle, R. W. (1989). Is working memory capacity task dependent? *Journal of Memory and Language, 2,* 127–154.

Tversky, A., & Kahneman, D. (1974). Judgment under uncertainty: Heuristics and biases. *Science, 185,* 1124–1131.

Uleman, J. S., Hon, A., Roman, R. J., & Moskowitz, G. B. (1996). On-line evidence for spontaneous trait inferences at encoding. *Personality and Social Psychology Bulletin, 22,* 377–394.

Wegner, D. M., & Bargh, J. A. (1998). Control and automaticity in social life. In D. Gilbert & S. Fiske (Eds.), *The handbook of social psychology* (Vol. 1, pp. 446–496). New York: McGraw-Hill.

Wigboldus, D. H. J., Dijksterhuis, A., & van Knippenberg, A. (2003). When stereotypes get in the way: Stereotypes obstruct stereotype-inconsistent trait inferences. *Journal of Personality and Social Psychology, 84,* 470–484.

Zeigarnik, B. (1938). On finished and unfinished tasks. In W. D. Ellis (Ed.), *A source book of gestalt psychology* (pp. 300–314). New York: Harcourt Brace & World.

PART 7

Phenomenal and Metacognitive Components of Action

Elbow Grease: When Action Feels Like Work

Jesse Preston *and* Daniel M. Wegner

Abstract

This chapter examines the experience of effort across different domains of exertion: physical exertion, mental concentration, and self-regulation. Despite the differences among these kinds of effort, in general, the feeling of self-mustered energy is the same no matter how it is applied. Rather than a specific sensation germane to a particular source, effort is a general cognitive feeling of work that applies to different kinds of intentional activity. The sensation of effort provides a constant monitor on energy expenditure and is fundamental in the production and judgment of personal action. Important information about task difficulty is given by subjective feelings of effort during an action—allowing one to predict the probability of success and to adjust the intensity of effort to an appropriate level of difficulty. In the cognitive domain, feelings of mental difficulty can affect judgments of familiarity, diagnosticity, confidence, and the like, depending on the mental activity and the salient features.

Keywords: effort, human action, energy, physical exertion, mental concentration, self-regulation

Human action is fueled by the exertion of the person in action. Just as cars run on gas and toy bunnies run on batteries, agents run on effort. Effort is easily recognizable all around us. We can see it in others when they strain and sweat and grimace as they work; we can see it in ourselves each time we raise a hand or walk up a hill or scrub potatoes for dinner. Our ease in perceiving effort brings up key questions about how such effort perception and experience is related to the actual expenditure of energy that occurs in our minds and bodies. This chapter examines a variety of the manifestations of effort that have appeared in psychological research and theory, with the goal of understanding how the *experience*

of effort is involved in the psychology of human action.

The Experience of Effort

Why would the experience of effort be important? Some might say that the human experience of effort, the mere sensation of elbow grease, is quite beside the point: A physicist could suggest that effort should be understood as the actual expenditure of energy—defined by Newton as a physical variable (*work,* the acceleration of a mass over a distance). Many psychologists have been equally dismissive of self-reports of effort, focusing instead on "real" effort, for example, how mental or physical tasks can be differentially disrupted by concurrent task demands and so seem to require different degrees of attentional or cognitive resources. Effort in action has been studied in the same way one might study a physical system—by examining what taxes the system to see how much "effort" the system requires.

Yet despite the attempts to ignore it or set it aside, the experience of effort continues to surface in psychology in various ways. Lay theories of action see effort as a causal force in action that is internal to the actor and under personal control (Heider, 1958). Actions carried out with vigor are perceived to be more motivated (Malle & Knobe, 1997) and ultimately are expected to be more successful (Kruger, Wirtz, Van Boven, & Altermatt, 2004). Beliefs about the exertion of effort have influences on the person's effort expenditure as well (e.g., Dweck & Leggett, 1988). The experience of effort seems to have a variety of psychological influences quite apart from any role as an indicator of the expenditure of energy occurring in the underlying mental and physical systems. The experience seems to have a life of its own.

The experience of effort is the particular feeling of that energy being exerted, or the phenomenal experience of effort (Block, 1995; Morsella, 2005; Nagel, 1974). In Nagel's (1974) terms, there is "something it is like" to exert effort. Imagine yourself pulling on a rope in a tug of war, running to catch a bus, or trying to conduct regression analyses in your head. Exertion is accompanied by a sensation of strain and labor, a feeling that intensifies the harder a person tries. But unlike the strain felt from some external force (like having one's arm pulled), effort feels mustered from within. It taps one's personal strength and at the same time demands that the person continue to draw on that energy.

The phenomenal experience of effort during action influences both the production and the judgment of action as it occurs. More broadly, the experience of exertion is connected to the concept of willpower that establishes the agent as a personal force behind action. To the person in action, subjective feelings of exertion serve as an authorship indicator for attributions of personal responsibility (Wegner & Sparrow, 2004). That is, effort felt during movement indicates that it is the self who is responsible for that action. In what follows, we review the literature on the interplay of effort experience and action and then conclude with recent studies from our laboratory indicating that misattributions of effort can lead people to take personal responsibility for actions performed by another.

Sources of Effort

Feelings of effort are experienced during *physical exertion* (e.g., lifting weights), *mental concentration* (e.g., studying statistics), and *self-restraint* (e.g., dieting). Although sometimes the sensation can feel localized, like the straining of particular muscles, the sense of effort can also surface as a nonspecific feeling of labor and difficulty that is transferable between different channels of exertion. The effort mustered in these activities is directed toward very different ends, but similar feelings of intensity and self-applied energy is common to all effortful pursuits. To examine the sources of the experience of effort, it is helpful to review how effort is sensed in physical, mental, and self-regulatory pursuits.

Physical Exertion

The kind of effort people are most familiar with is physical exertion—the muscular effort put into labor. Just where the feeling comes from—whether from a centrally generated muscle sense or from sensory feedback from peripheral cues—was the subject of hot debate among early psychologists (James, 1890/1983; Sherrington, 1900). The dispute appeared to reach some resolution with evidence that both efferent (brain to body) and afferent (body to brain) pathways leave a trace of action detailing the expected bodily sensation, such as feelings of muscular movement or shifting joints (Gandevia, 1987; Jeannerod, 1997). However the perception of *force* in action appears to be cued by a centrally generated impulse sent along efferent pathways (e.g., Gandevia & McCloskey, 1976) that is sometimes called *corollary discharge* (Sperry, 1950) or *efference copy* (von Holst, 1954). Greater efferent activity generally results in greater feelings of effort during the activity. For example, effort feels more intense as a handgrip is squeezed harder, as measured by actual tension on the handgrip (Stevens & Cain, 1970), and numerous replications have shown that the perception of effort correlates with overall cardiovascular output in a predictable formula (e.g., Borg, 1982; Gearhart, Becque, Palm, & Hutchins, 2005). Perceived effort increases with the actual difficulty of a task, such as resistance level on a treadmill (Rejeski, 1981) and the strength of gravity (Ross & Reschke, 1982). If efferent activity is increased artificially (e.g., by shortening the muscle, changing the joint angle), perceived effort intensifies even if the absolute force and difficulty remain constant (Cafarelli & Bigland-Ritchie, 1979; Gordon, Huxley, & Julian, 1966). In contrast, movement that is initiated involuntarily (through tendon taps, muscle vibration, or transcranial magnetic stimulation) feels completely effortless (Goodwin, McCloskey, & Matthews, 1972). And if capacity is completely extinguished so that efferent activity is not possible (e.g., in paralysis),

then no effort is felt even when intentionally trying to move (Rode, Rossetti, & Boisson, 1996).

Although effort is often associated with feelings of difficulty, the sensation of effort seems separable from both pain and pleasure—particularly when the effort is minimal. At low levels of exertion, sense of effort may amount to little more than the mere perception of bodily movement. Once inertia is overcome, a little bit of exercise can be energizing. It gets the blood rushing and prepares one for new challenges. Cases of clinical depression are often marked by lack of activity and energy, but getting depressed persons to increase activity can alleviate depressive symptoms, and even small amounts of exercise have been shown to boost mood (Dunn & McAuley, 2000). As more energy is expended the sensation of effort intensifies both in instantaneous force production (Nussbaum & Lang, 2005) and in continued exertion over time (Stevens & Cain, 1970).

Mental Concentration

The intensity of effort is generally expressed in physical metaphors (e.g., muscle power, sweat, or "elbow grease") that conjure images of manual labor. However, the experience of effort also extends to cognitive activities such as decision making, problem solving, and paying attention (Kahneman, 1973). Engaging in these activities requires deliberate concentration, channeling cognitive resources away from other matters to the task at hand. Like physical acts, mental acts vary in their difficulty and the amount of effort required for success. It is much easier to listen to a George Carlin comedy routine than to the Queen's address to the Commonwealth or to read an article in *Reader's Digest* than the original text of *The Odyssey*. The concentration mustered in these activities has an intensive active aspect that differs from mere consciousness, akin to the intensity felt in muscular exertion.

Mental ease is sometimes associated with the perceived fluency of thought. Some thoughts may appear and reappear in consciousness with such frequency that they seem to require no effort at all (Wegner, 1989). A slow steady rate of cognition, however, feels turgid and mentally difficult (Jacoby & Dallas, 1981; Schwarz et al., 1991). In an early test of the availability heuristic, Tversky and Kahneman (1973) found that people estimate there are more words that begin with the letter "t" than have "t" as the third letter (though the opposite is true) simply because it is much easier to generate examples. Schwarz et al. (1991) expanded on this general finding to show that it is not the content of thoughts that impacts these judgments but the experience of mental ease in generating the thoughts. In one study, participants who listed many instances when they acted with either low or high self-assurance rated themselves as lower on the target trait than those who listed only a few. Even though they had more examples of behavior available, listing 12 instances of any behavior is difficult, so people given this arduous task concluded that the trait was not particularly self-descriptive.

The experience of ease of thinking can also influence mood, even leading to experiences of elation, self-confidence, and grandiosity. Pronin and Wegner (2006) asked participants to read a series of mood-induction statements, either all positive (e.g., "I'm feeling better all the time") or all negative (e.g., "I'm down in the dumps today"). The statements indeed had the effect initially observed by Velten (1968)—the positive statements enhanced good mood, whereas the negative statements induced bad mood. However, when participants were prompted by the computer to read their statements rapidly (as compared to another group who read them slowly), there was an independent influence of reading pace on mood. Those participants who read statements quickly, whether the statements were positive or negative, reported more positive mood as well as increased energy and indications of the confidence, self-perceived creativity, and grandiosity often associated with mania.

There are no sensory nerves in the brain, so there can be no true proprioception for thought as there is for physical activity. However, the intensive aspect of mental effort is accompanied by physical arousal (Berlyne, 1960), increased cortisol (Fibiger & Singer, 1989), and cardiovascular response (Van Roon, Mulder, Veldman, & Mulder, 1995), just as is found in physical exertion. Perhaps the most common physical indicator of both kinds of effort is the contraction of the corrugator muscle, the key muscle involved in scrunching the eyebrows down toward the nose as one frowns. Cacioppo, Petty, and Morris (1985) have observed that cognitive effort experienced by participants is often accompanied by a visible or invisible activation of the forehead muscle. Consistent with a growing literature on social embodiment effects demonstrating a bidirectional association between emotional expression and affective experience (e.g., Cacioppo, Priester, & Bernston, 1993; Epley & Gilovich, 2001; for a review, see Barsalou, Niedenthal, Barbey, & Ruppert, 2003), recent research has found that adopting a furrowed brow can elicit feelings of mental effort.

In an update of the study on mental ease by Schwarz et al. (1991), participants listed instances in which they felt either low or high self-assurance while they either smiled or furrowed their brow (Stepper & Strack, 1993). As expected, the brow furrowers identified less with the trait than those who had been smiling during the task. Notably, the effect worked only for subjects who could successfully maintain the furrowed brow and not for participants who could not hold the expression. In another study, furrowing the brow was found to impact judgments of familiarity and attributions of fame (Strack & Neumann, 2000). Ordinarily, exposure to nonfamous names has a sleeper effect: At a second viewing of names, the familiarity resulting from initial exposure is falsely credited to the person's celebrity (Jacoby, Kelley, Brown, & Jasechko, 1989). However, false attributions of fame declined if people were induced to furrow their brow at the second viewing. The furrowed expression suggested feelings of doubt and difficulty in remembering the name, countering the feelings of familiarity from the initial exposure (Strack & Neumann, 2000).

Self-Restraint

Effort can also be felt when inhibiting action, if one is otherwise inclined to act. Dieters, newly reformed smokers, and other miscellaneous addicts must exercise deliberate restraint to keep from indulging in their favorite vices (Baumeister, Heatherton, & Tice, 1994). When a bad habit is given up for good, the difficulty of self-regulation is compounded by the fact that the overall goal can never be fully completed. Alcoholics who overcome their addiction still consider themselves to be alcoholics years after they have given up drinking because they believe relapse remains a constant possibility. Attempts to delay gratification temporarily can be extremely difficult and taxing on the individual, especially when under stress or when resisting "hot" impulses that have a strong hedonic attraction (Metcalfe & Mischel, 1999). Just like other forms of effort, the capacity for continued self-regulation is limited. Exhibiting self-control in the face of temptation can make continued resistance more difficult, and indulgence in other vices more likely

in the future (Baumeister, Bratslavsky, Muraven, & Tice, 1998). Periods of intense resistance can negatively impact performance on other cognitive tasks, such as reading comprehension and analytical ability (Schmeichel, Vohs, & Baumeister, 2003). Acts of both self-control and problem solving have a cognitive component, but, notably, self-control tasks have also been shown to impact performance on physical actions. Persistence at squeezing a handgrip, for example, deteriorates more rapidly if people are asked to simultaneously inhibit emotional responses to an emotionally arousing film (Baumeister et al., 1998; Martijn, Tenbült, Merckelbach, Dreezens, & de Vries, 2002). Although in this case one must inhibit rather than initiate action, doing so is difficult and tiring, and the energy to regulate behavior depletes over time just as physical effort does.

One Effort to Rule Them All

Physical exertion, mental concentration, and self-restraint are activities directed toward different goals and manifest themselves in very different forms. What these activities share, however, is the experience of effort exerted toward achieving the goal. Whether a person spends the day grading exams or digging graves, the work feels difficult and grueling, and the feeling intensifies as greater personal force is applied. The feeling of effort is more than a mere sense of movement, as though it were the body's own speedometer or gas gauge. Rather, effort is a general feeling of labor and personal strength common to all deliberate activity. Whereas muscular force and sweat characterize the bodily feelings associated with physical exertion, the experience of effort is probably best characterized as a cognitive feeling (Schwarz & Clore, 1996) that commonly accompanies labor of all kinds.

Similar to the way specific emotions can arise from nonspecific arousal (Schacter

& Singer, 1962), nonspecific feelings of effort must be interpreted in the context of the action being performed. Effort felt during exercise therefore feels like physical exertion, and effort felt during a statistics lecture feels like concentration. The nonspecific quality of effort has two important implications for how effort is experienced by the individual. First, effort can be easily misinterpreted. An exam written in messy handwriting might wind up with a poorer grade than the same work in clear writing simply because the reader would have to exert that much extra effort just to make sense of the answer. Second, effort is transmutable, or easily transferred between different channels of exertion.

Physical effort can interfere with performance on mental activities (e.g., Wegner, Ansfield, & Pilloff, 1998). Efforts at physical self-regulation deplete mental resources (Vohs et al., 2008) just as efforts at mental self-regulation deplete physical strength (Muraven, Tice, & Baumeister, 1998). Baumeister and colleagues suggest that a single fluid energy source (that they identify as the executive control, or self) fuels all these activities, and this is why engaging in different effortful activities is mutually exhausting (e.g., Baumeister et al., 1998). In addition to their shared origins, these activities also share a common phenomenal experience. If a person were to perform two difficult tasks simultaneously (e.g., grading exams while digging graves), it might be difficult to tell where feelings of effort were coming from and which of the tasks was creating more difficulty.

The Value of Effort Experience

The fact that effort exertion is accompanied by a phenomenal experience raises the question, Why do we feel effort? What does the experience of effort do for us? Life would certainly be more pleasant if no effort was ever felt—imagine the work you could do if you never got tired or felt any difficulty. Some have argued that phenomenal experiences like effort or even consciousness itself do not require an explanation, that they are merely epiphenomenal to other biological activity (e.g., Kinsbourne, 1996; Pinker, 1997). Others, meanwhile, say that the production costs involved in creating the phenomenal experience requires that its existence be justified by some useful function. For example, Morsella (2005; Chapter 30) has recently suggested that effort represents one type of conscious conflict—like pain—where one need must be chosen over another, and this conscious conflict ultimately serves a self-regulatory function. But whether effort is functional or epiphenomenal, the experience of effort does provide (at least) three important benefits to the actor. First, effort provides direct feedback about task difficulty, allowing the actor to adjust exertion appropriately. Second, feelings of effort prompt conservation of energy when it becomes necessary, as the levels of personal strength deteriorate over time. Third, effort is an indicator of personal authorship for action, contributing to the feeling of conscious will.

Judgments of Difficulty

An important benefit to sensations of effort during labor is that it provides important information about task difficulty. This can be used to predict the probability of success in a task and to adjust the intensity of effort to an appropriate level match difficulty. Discrepancies between the effort felt in an action and the actual force can inform an individual of impaired motor function (Burgess & Jones, 1997). Increased feelings of effort in action can result in some distorted perceptions related to the action. For example, people overestimate the weight of objects when they are fatigued compared to when energy levels are high (McCloskey, Ebeling, & Goodwin, 1974).

Just as in physical acts, the difficulty associated with cognitive activities can help to regulate the amount of effort and attention given to the particular cognitive task. One might turn down the car radio while searching for a street address or elect to spend more time reading notes for an advanced string theory course than for Basket Weaving 101. Feeling of mental effort can also impact judgments about the subject of thought itself (Schwarz, 2002; Schwarz & Clore, 1996). For instance, in the mental ease study by Schwarz et al. (1991) discussed earlier, people thought a trait was less self-descriptive if they had to think of many instances they acted in a way consistent with that trait compared to just a few. The difficulty experienced coming up with many examples was interpreted as having to do with the topic rather than the task.

Depending on the particular subject of thought and context, difficulty can be construed in different ways (Unklebach, 2006). If you find yourself having to exert intense effort to pay attention to a colloquium talk, you could attribute the effort to an unconvincing argument, difficult statistical analyses, or to the speaker's coarse accent.

There are times, however, when difficulty results in distortions of the action produced. For instance, in *effort justification,* people seek to reconcile the amount of effort exerted toward some goal and the value of the outcome (Aronson & Mills, 1959). As in general dissonance theory (Festinger, 1957), people are motivated to see internal consistency between their thoughts and actions. For example, fraternities that employ hazing rituals usually arouse more love and loyalty from their members than clubs that do not require such a harsh initiation (Aronson & Mills, 1959). The effort put into gaining membership does not detract from the value of the goal; rather, it only makes it seem more worthwhile. By the same token, doing a favor for someone can actually increase liking for that person (Jecker & Landy, 1969) or a potential love interest who "plays hard to get" might seem more attractive (Roberson & Wright, 1994). People generally expect that effort will lead to successful actions, so people might inflate the success of an outcome to be consistent with the exertion of effort (Kruger et al., 2004; Preston & Wegner, 2005).

Another example of distortions caused by effort is the altered perceptions of inclines during difficult physical tasks. When carrying a heavy load, the inclines of hills appear steeper than when without extra weight (Bhalla & Proffitt, 1999; Proffitt, 2006). The authors account for these distorted perceptions by the increased effort required to perform the task successfully. Mismatches between difficulty and force can result in unsuccessful action. This is true when not enough energy is put into a difficult task and also if one puts too much energy into an easy task. For example, imagine you are walking up a staircase, but at the very last step you are distracted and do not notice when the plateau has been reached. Expecting another step to come, you raise your leg with unnecessary height and force—only to find yourself doing something like a John Cleese silly walk as the anticipated resistance melts into unexpected ease. Proffitt and colleagues argue that the perception of incline is exaggerated under fatigue or weight load because this illusion maintains proper relation to physiological capacity (Bhalla & Proffitt, 1999). Walking uphill requires more energy from a person than walking on flat surfaces both in the size and the force of the gait. If a person must walk uphill with a backpack full of groceries, the energy required is even greater than usual. Although the reported incline changes as a function of fatigue and load, actual action toward the incline does not. That is, people may distort how they see the incline but manage to adjust their walking steps to the appropriate size. The distorted perceptions of the incline under high load or fatigue might help one to adjust action to the appropriate level of force.

Feelings of mental effort have been shown to influence judgments of diagnosticity (Schwarz et al., 1991), confidence (Alter, Oppenheimer, Epley, & Eyre, 2007), truth (Reber & Schwarz, 1999), familiarity (Jacoby & Dallas, 1981), stimulus clarity (Whittlesea, Jacoby, & Girard, 1990), and event frequency (Tversky & Kahneman, 1973). For instance, in the *revelation effect,* judgments of familiarity increase for words that are revealed one letter at a time rather than presented intact (e.g., LeCompte, 1995). But, interestingly, the revelation effect works even if the item being judged is different than the one that is revealed—for example, if participants solve an unrelated anagram, such as RAINDROP, before judging the familiarity of another word, such as VINEYARD (Westerman & Greene, 1996). The mere activity before judgment increases feelings of recognition and familiarity and does not depend on the relevance of that activity to the actual target of judgment. This suggests the revelation effect results from an increase in *conceptual fluency* rather than perceptual fluency (Westerman & Greene, 1996). It was not so much that people's vision clarified in the task but rather that they felt clarified when they were making the judgment.

Conservation of Energy

Unfortunately, effort is a limited resource (Chapter 23). We cannot keep going and going like the Energizer bunny because it would eventually lead to collapse or death. A second advantage to having a feeling of effort is that it allows us to monitor energy expenditure and then to conserve energy when necessary. Prolonged exertion is tiring,

and mustering the strength to act becomes less invigorating and more uncomfortable as one goes on. Running the second mile in a marathon is a breeze compared to running the 23rd mile later on, even though actual physical output and pace have both slowed down considerably (Garcin & Billat, 2001). When muscles are fatigued, people tend to overestimate the weight of objects because it takes more energy to move those objects (e.g., McCloskey et al., 1974). The increased effort felt as one tires is associated with actual detriments in muscle capacity—fatigue increases directly with reduced strength in relation to task difficulty (Jones & Hunter, 1983). Feelings of fatigue may signal to a person that the capacity to continue action has depleted (Burgess & Jones, 1997) and can prompt one to restrict spending either by deteriorating the strength of action over time or by ceasing action altogether. After a rest, energy supplies are restocked, and one can continue in a task rejuvenated.

One of the principal determinants of withholding exertion is the agent's own perceived efficacy—beliefs about personal ability to perform action (Bandura, 1986). Quite reasonably, people prefer to put their energy toward tasks that are expected to succeed but are reluctant to waste effort by pursuing goals that are impossible. Effort is usually enjoyable if it is in favorable relation to the outcome, that is, if the exertion is not too hard and success is likely (Atkinson & Feather, 1966). Experiences with repeated failure reinforce an apparent noncontingency between effort and outcome, which can ultimately extinguish effort altogether (Abramson, Seligman, & Teasedale, 1978). A further reason to conserve energy supplies is to save some energy to devote to other (more important) tasks that might arise unexpectedly. Goals that are of high importance or desirability tend to be pursued more heartily than those of minimal importance (Lynch, 2005)—for example, the pursuit of romantic partners is generally more vigorous than the search for a really great tie clip. The most important goals (biological drives like sex and food) seem to have an energizing effect on the actor so that it seems to take less energy than the same effort directed toward an unimportant goal. The experience of effort, in other words, is valuable as a guide toward the adaptive expenditure of effort.

Sensation of Authorship

A third advantage of the experience of effort is that it provides a marker for identifying one's own actions (Wegner, 2002). In a mechanistic sense, effort is the energy that produces action. But the ultimate source of power seems to come from within the self, or willpower (Metcalfe & Mischel, 1999). Attributions of personal responsibility may have both a cold, cognitive component (hmm, that seems like something I'd do) and a "hot," affective component (that was me, alright!). But for the most part, conscious will is experienced as an authorship emotion rather than a reasoned deduction. People judge themselves to have caused action because they have the strong feeling of personal causation. When the veridicality of the will is challenged, people defend their free will with arguments that they "just know" when they have caused an action or similar justifications like they *feel it in their bones* or *know it in their gut*. The sensation of effort during action helps produces the feeling of will as the action takes place. Applying one's personal strength requires deliberate attention and control, usually overriding other competing behavioral responses. As effort increases, the exertion feels more willfully forced by the agent. Effortlessness in action, on the other hand, is characteristic of automaticity, as the easiest actions require little control or conscious supervision (Bargh, 1994). In

this sense, the experience of effort during action contributes to the development of a sense of self as author when none might exist if actions were never experienced as effortful or consciously willed (Wegner, 2005).

Studies of passivity experiences in schizophrenia have suggested that feelings of effort exertion are crucial in distinguishing the acting self from the acting other (e.g., Daprati et al., 1997; Frith, Blakemore, & Wolpert, 2000). Passivity experiences are a common symptom in schizophrenia when a patient lacks the appropriate feelings of will for own actions. Although patients with schizophrenia are equally able to exert energy as normal controls (van Beilen, van Zomeren, van den Bosch, Withaar, & Bouma, 2005), they may not properly sense the exertion, so when the action is initiated, they do not feel responsible. This is supported by evidence that schizophrenic patients who suffer from delusions of control show little memory of their previous movements. When identifying a drawing they had previously made without visual feedback, they showed much poorer accuracy than normal controls, suggesting they had no memory for the feeling of drawing. Similarly, reports of verbal hallucinations (i.e., hearing voices) in schizophrenia may also result from failed sensory feedback (Hoffman, 1986). The voices heard can often be traced to the patient's own speech—voices are no longer heard when patients undertake a maneuver to prevent subvocalization (Bick & Kinsbourne, 1987). As in cases of motor illusions, the voice is not recognized as self-produced and is attributed instead to some external source (Silbersweig, Stern, Frith, & Cahill, 1995).

In mental activities, the effortlessness of creative bursts can carry with it the sense that it is *happening to* a person rather than *authored by* the person (Csikszentmihalyi, Abuhamdeh, & Nakamura, 2005), as though the artist is the medium for an external source of inspiration. In some cases the ease of creativity leads the artist to make attributions to supernatural or divine influence—such as the nine Muses of ancient Greek mythology. Instances of insight are often characterized by the suddenness of the idea in mind, feeling like a flash of knowledge that occurs from nowhere (e.g., Metcalfe & Weibe, 1987; Schooler & Melcher, 1995). Across such experiences, the thinkers often report as much surprise at the occurrence of the idea as they do to the details of the idea itself. The abrupt nature of insight means that it comes with no foreshadowing or means of prediction (Bowden, 1997). When the solution does arrive, it typically feels completely unwilled by the thinker and is attributed solely to unconscious processes (Schooler & Melcher, 1995). Ironically, the greatest mental achievements a person ever has might feel completely alien, not a product of the person's own earnest labors.

Misattributions of Effort in Action: The Case of Inadvertent Plagiarism

If an idea is reached through careful reasoning and concentration, flowing directly from the thoughts that precede it, it feels controlled and intentional. If, on the other hand, a solution comes into the mind that is discordant with prior mental activity, it is unclear to the thinker how she arrived at the idea. The hard work put into the action emphasizes feelings of authorship. Key in the experience is the point that effort is released—the moment of realization when the solution is found or idea is discovered. When one is truly generating an idea or solution, mental effort should be high as one grapples with the problem and low when the effort is released as the idea comes into mind. The point of idea realization represents a shift from difficult thought to fluid thought. However, these feelings of effort

can sometimes falsely indicate authorship, just as physical effort can sometimes distort other judgments of an action's success (Aronson & Mills, 1959) or the perception of the environment (Proffitt, 2006). When people are trying to solve problems together, effort experiences can be the basis for unintended plagiarism. Two people working on the same problem might have the same high–low effort shift when a problem is solved regardless of who actually did the solving. Consequently, people might be more likely to take credit for their partners' solutions if they also exerted effort working on the problem before it was solved.

We recently investigated the effect of effort cues on plagiarism by having pairs of people take turns in an anagram task as they exerted effort on an unrelated activity, such as squeezing a handgrip (Preston & Wegner, 2007). One partner would try to solve an anagram problem that appeared on a computer screen, followed by the presentation of the anagram solution on-screen. After each anagram, partners switched turns, and the other person tried to solve the next anagram. As participants worked on these anagrams, the effort exerted by both partners varied between high or low during the appearance of both the problem and its solution. Thus, the presentation of each anagram problem and its solution was associated with one of four different effort patterns: (a) low effort during problem, low effort during solution; (b) low effort during problem, high effort during solution; (c) high effort during problem, low effort during solution; and (d) high effort during problem, high effort during solution. The high–low effort pattern most closely resembles the sequence of real effort experienced when one generates a solution. Effort is released just as the answer is presented, much like the experience of discovery after a period of intense thought. Other patterns of effort—for example, low effort during the problem phase followed by high effort when idea is produced—should lead to less plagiarism because they do not resemble the sequence of exertion associated with feelings of authorship. As compared to other patterns of effort, we predicted that the experience of a shift from high to low exertion would be misattributed as feelings of responsibility for the thought process, misleading people to feel they had produced ideas they had not.

In one study, we manipulated font clarity to induce feelings of mental effort, which in previous studies has affected perceived mental ease (Jacoby, Baker, & Brooks, 1989). The fonts of both the problems and solutions changed between black lettering (low effort to read) and pale yellow lettering (high effort to read). On a given trial, an anagram problem would appear on the screen to both partners as one partner tried to solve it. After the player indicated if he or she knew the correct answer, the solution appeared on the screen, and both players wrote down the word on a piece of paper. Later, a surprise memory test was given for all words in the anagram task and some new words. Participants were asked to identify whether the word was new (i.e., not on the anagram task), presented on their partner's turn, or presented on their own turn. Plagiarisms were defined as instances when a participant falsely recalled both that (a) a partners' anagram had been on one's own turn and (b) the anagram was successfully solved in time. As predicted, plagiarism was more prevalent for words that appeared in the high–low effort sequence compared to the other effort patterns (see Figure 27.1). Plagiarism increased only if effort was felt during the problem phase and dissipated as the solution appeared—the pattern that occurs when one truly generates an idea. Notably, the magnitude of this effect was moderated by the perceived difficulty of the yellow font. Plagiarism was amplified in the high–low effort pattern among participants who rated the yellow font as highly difficult, but the effect did not emerge for those who rated the yellow font as relatively easy to read. This is consistent with our hypothesis: Greater effort felt during the problem should be interpreted as harder work in trying to solve the anagram.

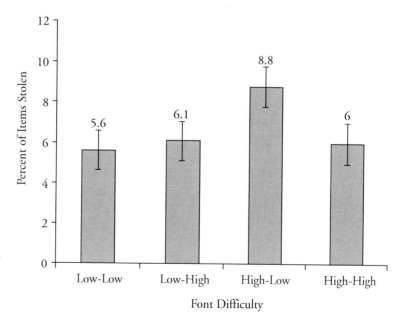

Fig. 27.1 Percentage of plagiarism by font difficulty (in Preston & Wegner, 2007, experiment 2).

A second plagiarism study specifically addressed the problem of the generality of effort. Recall our earlier suggestion that because effort is a nonspecific feeling of labor, it is easily misinterpreted and transmutable between different channels of sensation. In this second study, we had people solve anagrams with a partner as they exerted effort in a physical task. Participants were asked to squeeze a handgrip with their nondominant hand whenever a red dot appeared in the bottom right corner of the screen. Instances of plagiarism were highest when participants squeezed during the anagram and released the grip just as the answer was presented as compared to the other three patterns. Replicating the results of the font study, inflated plagiarism was only found when the effort dissipated as the solution appeared, just like the feeling of effort experienced in genuine idea generation. But also important is the fact that mental authorship was cued by physical actions, that is, squeezing the handgrip. Effort experienced in one domain was misattributed to activity in another domain despite the fact the two entail very different kinds of work. Not only does this suggest that the experience of effort is malleable, but also there is a crossover between physical and mental agency. Rather than separate systems of attribution, there may be an authorship processing mechanism that accepts as input the experience of effort from both physical and mental actions.

The results of these two studies fit in with a long line of research on the perception of psychological states by observation of internal physiological states (e.g., James, 1890-1983; Schachter, 1964). In such research, misattributions result when the true source is unclear, but the misattributed cue is salient. Such mistakes might be less likely, however, if the true source were to become salient. When Schachter and Singer (1962) warned participants that an epinephrine shot could lead to increased feelings of arousal, participants did not report the usual heightened euphoria or anger but remained in a relatively neutral mood. Zillman, Katcher, and Milavsky (1972) found in studies of "excitation transfer" that residual arousal from exercise could be misinterpreted as emotional reactivity. For example, after cycling on a stationary bike, people responded more aggressively to provocation. Excitation transfer happened only if the exercise had already been stopped for a while. People fail to account for lingering physical impact of exercise on arousal, but immediately after the cessation of exercise the source of arousal is clear.

To pursue these ideas, a third plagiarism study was conducted. In line with the findings of Zillman, we predicted that an admonition to attend to effort cues would reduce the incidents of plagiarism. We replicated the anagram task using the font clarity manipulation but added a reminder condition that directed participants' attention to the font difficulty. Immediately following each anagram trial, people in this condition were asked to report the font color of both the problem and the solution. Any enhanced feeling of authorship they felt as a result of the high–low effort pattern could be discounted at this time, preventing the inflation in plagiarism normally associated with this effort pattern. As predicted, there was an interaction between the font pattern and reminder condition on levels of plagiarism. In the control condition, people plagiarized more often in the high–low pattern, replicating our previous results. However, this was not the case for those participants who were reminded of the font color after each trial. These people showed no differences in plagiarism, and if anything there was a trend to decrease plagiarism for the high–low effort items. When participants' attention was directed to the font color as the explanation of their feelings of effort, they discounted the inflated feelings of difficulty elicited by reading the yellow lettering and, by doing so, avoided plagiarizing in the high–low effort pattern. Plagiarism did not disappear completely, but it dropped to the same levels of plagiarism observed in the low–high effort pattern.

In these studies, plagiarism increased when a person experienced a period of mental exertion and release that coincided with the generation of a mental action by an external source. People remembered having solved their partner's anagrams if they had been induced to exert irrelevant effort during the problem phase and then to relax that effort at the moment the solution was presented. Inadvertent plagiarism was not affected when people had experienced effort in some other sequence relative to the idea, such as a sudden onset of effort at the presentation of the solution or a constant level of high effort. Just as in physical action, authorship for thoughts is indicated by an effortful process that precedes the thought.

The sense of effort is only one kind of many authorship indicators that gives rise to a feeling of conscious will for action, along with other cues like foreknowledge of the act, or a desire for outcome (Wegner & Sparrow, 2004). But unlike mental states such as intentions and plans, which may be easily forgotten, the sensation of effort is often vivid and memorable to the actor. In this sense, the experience of effort may be a particularly important source of "authorship emotion"—the feeling one gets on doing something that one indeed performed the action (Wegner, 2002). Perhaps in defense of free will, people should add that they *know it in their muscles* and *feel it in their furrowed brows* to their list of reasons to believe in their own roles as the causes of their actions. With so many actions prompted by unconscious processing, the self can sometimes be misplaced among automaticities.

But the effort mustered to perform the action emphasizes the person's role as an intentional actor and resurrects the self as the primary controller of action—or at least so it would seem to the actor.

The Virtue of Effort

With attributions of responsibility for action also come the implications of moral responsibility. An agent who exerts herself in an action seems purposive and strong willed, and it is the agent's determination rather than ability that seems responsible for the end result. Unlike other causes of success—natural ability, low difficulty of a task, or just good luck—an agent is given personal credit for the amount of effort put into a task (Weiner & Kukla, 1970), and the degree of effort is strongly linked to perceptions of a person's character (Graham & Brown, 1988; Nicholls, 1976). Self-regulation is associated with its own moral virtues—for example, delay of gratification, obedience to moral restrictions, and long-term planning all require a person to control action and restrain impulses.

Lack of effort, however, is often looked on with disgust and considered to be lazy and even shameful. Consider the recent scandal surrounding Rafael Palmeiro, who in the summer of 2005 became the fourth player in Major League Baseball to reach 500 home runs and 3,000 hits. Not long after he reached the tremendous milestone (hit number 3,018), he tested positive for steroids and was suspended from play. When he returned from suspension to his first home game, he was greeted by booing fans at the stadium, holding up signs that read "Welcome Back Cheater." The resistance to artificial enhancers is partly because it is seen as unfair, making the playing field uneven between those who do and do not take risky substances.

A similar attitude exists in the general population toward the development and use of "smart drugs" that enhance mental function (Rose, 2002; Riis, Simmons, & Goodwin, in press). Gazzaniga (2005) notes that people are wary of smart drugs because it seems like cheating: "If, somehow, someone gets ahead through hard work, that's okay . . . But popping a pill and mastering information after having read it only once seems unfair" (p. 73). An additional reason for the aversion to smart drugs, we suspect, lies in the concern that the burgeoning intelligence would not really be one's true mind. By taking these medications, a person dissolves personal control in exchange for ease.

Yet there is some inconsistency in how we decide what we can do to improve our own performance. Health food stores are stocked full of various supplements and vitamins designed to enhance muscle bulk and improve energy. Late night television is teeming with ads for new devices and contraptions sold with the promise of making exercise virtually effortless. In a busy day, a person may neglect to eat his cereal, drink his juice, or even take his vitamin supplement—but rarely do people forget their caffeine fix. Shortcuts to success like steroids or smart drugs are condemned because the success they reap seems unnatural and less than genuine. But at the same time, people condone other shortcuts they view as enhancers of success, unlocking potential that was always present but not realized. The dividing line seems to fall on whether the drug is the direct cause of performance—making success in the task effortless—or an enhancer of performance that improves the efficiency of the effort. As long as success requires hard work, then enhancement is not dishonorable.

Conclusion

Effort encompasses two interrelated components: It is the energy that is used to propel an agent and the feeling of difficulty and labor experienced during exertion. In this chapter, we reviewed the experience of effort across different domains of exertion: physical exertion, mental concentration, and self-regulation. There are differences among these kinds of effort, but in general the feeling of self-mustered energy is the same no matter how it is applied. Rather than a specific sensation germane to a particular source, effort is a general cognitive feeling of work that applies to different kinds of intentional activity. The sensation of effort provides a constant monitor on energy expenditure and is fundamental in the production and judgment of personal action. Important information about task difficulty is given by subjective feelings of effort during an action—allowing one to predict the probability of success and to adjust the intensity of effort to an appropriate level of difficulty. In the cognitive domain, feelings of mental difficulty can affect judgments of familiarity, diagnosticity, confidence, and the like, depending on the mental activity and the salient features. Feelings of effort are also used to monitor reserves of energy. Prolonged exertion drains resources and prompts the actor to conserve energy by restricting output, at least until energy supplies are replenished. Finally, the feeling of effort serves as an authorship indicator in feelings of conscious will for action. The experience of effort contributes to the important task of accounting for who does what in social life, helping us to determine what we have done and what has been done by others. Effort is not just a drain on personal resources but also drain on the person, not merely an exertion of power but also an exertion of willpower.

Acknowledgments

Preparation of this chapter was facilitated by funding from NIMH grant MH 49127 and from SSHRC of Canada.

References

Abramson, L. Y., Seligman, M. E., & Teasdale, J. D. (1978). Learned helplessness in humans: Critique and reformulation. *Journal of Abnormal Psychology, 87*(1), 49–74.

Alter, A., Oppenheimer, D., Epley, N., & Eyre, R. (2007). Overcoming intuition: Metacognitive difficulty activates analytical thought. *Journal of Experimental Psychology: General, 136,* 569–576.

Aronson, E., & Mills, J. (1959). The effect of severity of initiation on liking for a group. *Journal of Abnormal and Social Psychology, 59,* 177–181.

Atkinson, J. W., & Feather, N. T. (1966). *A theory of achievement motivation.* New York: Wiley.

Bandura, A. (1986). The explanatory and predictive scope of self-efficacy theory. *Journal of Social & Clinical Psychology. Special Issue: Self-Efficacy Theory in Contemporary Psychology, 4*(3), 359–373.

Bargh, J. A. (1994). The four horsemen of automaticity: Awareness, intention, efficiency, and control in social cognition. In R. S. Wyer Jr. & T. K. Srull (Eds.), *Handbook of social cognition* (2nd ed. (pp. 1–40)). Hillsdale, NJ: Lawrence Erlbaum Associates.

Barsalou, L. W., Niedenthal, P., Barbey, A. K., & Ruppert, J. A. (2003). Social embodiment. In B. Ross (Ed.), *The psychology of learning and motivation* (Vol. 43, pp. 43–92). San Diego, CA: Academic Press.

Baumeister, R. F., Bratslavsky, E., Muraven, M., & Tice, D. M. (1998). Ego depletion: Is the active self a limited resource? *Journal of Personality and Social Psychology, 74,* 1252–1265.

Baumeister, R. F., Heatherton T. F., & Tice, D. M. (1994). *Losing control: How and why people fail at self-regulation.* San Diego, CA: Academic Press.

Berlyne, D. E., (1960). *Conflict, arousal, and curiosity.* New York: McGraw-Hill.

Bhalla, M., & Proffitt, D. R. (1999). Visual-motor recalibration in geographical slant perception. *Journal of Experimental Psychology: Human Perception and Performance, 25,* 1076–1096.

Bick, P. A., & Kinsbourne, M. (1987). Auditory hallucinations and subvocal speech in schizophrenic patients. *American Journal of Psychiatry, 144,* 222–225.

Block, N. (1995). On a confusion about a function of consciousness. *Behavioral and Brain Sciences, 18,* 227–287.

Borg, G. (1982). Psychophysical bases of perceived exertion. *Medicine and Science in Sports and Exercise, 14,* 377–381.

Bowden, E. M. (1997). The effect of reportable and unreportable hints on anagram solution and the aha! experience. *Consciousness and Cognition: An International Journal, 6*(4), 545–573.

Burgess, P. R., & Jones, L. F. (1997). Perceptions of effort and heaviness during fatigue and during size-weight illusion. *Somatosensory and Motor Research, 14,* 189–202.

Cacioppo, J. T., Petty, R. E., & Morris, K. J. (1985). Semantic, evaluative, and self-referent processing: Memory, cognitive effort, and somatovisceral activity. *Psychophysiology, 22,* 371–384.

Cacioppo, J. T., Priester, J. R., & Bernston, G. G. (1993). Rudimentary determination of attitudes II: Arm flexion and extension have differential effects on attitudes. *Journal of Personality and Social Psychology, 65,* 5–17.

Cafarelli, E. W., & Bigland-Ritchie, B. (1979). Sensation of static force in muscles of different length. *Experimental Neurology, 65,* 511–525.

Csikszentmihalyi, M., Abuhamdeh, S., & Nakamura, J. (2005). Flow. In A. J. Elliot & C. S. Dweck (Eds.), *Handbook of competence and motivation* (pp. 598–608). New York: Guilford Press.

Daprati, E., Franck, N., Georgieff, N., Proust, J., Pacherie, E., Dalery, J., et al. (1997). Looking for the agent: An investigation into consciousness of action and self-consciousness in schizophrenic patients. *Cognition, 65*(1), 71–86.

Dunn, E. C., & McAuley, E. (2000). Affective responses to exercise bouts of varying intensities. *Journal of Social Behavior and Personality, 15,* 201–214.

Dweck, C. S., & Leggett, E. L. (1988). A social cognitive approach to motivation and personality. *Psychological Review, 95,* 256–273.

Epley, N., & Gilovich, T. (2001). Putting adjustment back in the anchoring and adjustment heuristic: Divergent processing of self-generated and experimenter-provided anchors. *Psychological Science, 12,* 391–396.

Festinger, L. (1957). *A theory of cognitive dissonance.* Stanford, CA: Stanford University Press.

Fibiger, W., & Singer, G. (1989). Biochemical assessment and differentiation of mental and physical effort. *Work and Stress, 3,* 237–247.

Frith, C. D., Blakemore, S., & Wolpert, D. M. (2000). Abnormalities in the awareness and control of action. *Philosophical Transactions of the Royal Society of London, 355,* 1771–1788.

Gandevia, S. C. (1987). Roles for perceived voluntary motor commands in motor control. *Trends in Neuroscience, 15,* 81–85.

Gandevia, S. C., & McCloskey, D. I. (1976). Perceived heaviness of lifted objects and effects of sensory inputs from related, non-lifting parts. *Brain Research, 109*(2), 399–401.

Garcin, M., & Billat, V. (2001). Perceived exertion scales attest to both intensity and exercise duration. *Perceptual and Motor Skills, 93,* 661–671.

Gazzaniga, M. (2005). *The ethical brain.* New York: Dana Press.

Gearhart, R. F., Becque, M. D., Palm, C. M., & Hutchins, M. D. (2005). Rating perceived exertion during short duration, very high intensity cycle exercise. *Perceptual and Motor Skills, 100,* 767–773.

Goodwin, G. M., McCloskey, D. I., & Matthews, P. B.C. (1972). The contribution of muscle afferents to kinaesthesia shown by vibration induced illusions of movement and the effects of paralyzing joint afferents. *Brain, 95,* 705–748.

Gordon, A. M., Huxley, A. F., & Julian, F. J. (1966). The variation in isometric tension with sarcomere length in vertebrate muscle fibres. *Journal of Physiology, 184,* 170–192.

Graham, S., & Brown, J. D. (1988). Attributional mediators of evaluation, expectancy, and affect: A response time analysis. *Journal of Personality & Social Psychology, 55,* 873–881.

Heider, F. (1958). *The psychology of interpersonal relations.* New York: Wiley.

Hoffman, R. E. (1986).Verbal hallucinations and language production processes in schizophrenia. *Behavioral and Brain Sciences, 9,* 503–548.

Jacoby, L. L., Baker, J. G., & Brooks, L. R. (1989). Episodic effects on picture identification: Implications for theories of concept learning and theories of memory. *Journal of Experimental Psychology: Learning, Memory, and Cognition, 15,* 275–281.

Jacoby, L. L., & Dallas, M. (1981). On the relationship between autobiographical memory and perceptual learning. *Journal of Experimental Psychology: General, 100,* 306–340.

Jacoby, L. L., Kelley, C., Brown, J., & Jasechko, J. (1989). Becoming famous overnight: Limits on the ability to avoid unconscious influences of the past. *Journal of Personality and Social Psychology, 56,* 326–338.

James, W. (1983) *The principles of psychology.* Cambridge, MA: Harvard University Press. Original work published 1890)

Jeannerod, M. (1997). *The cognitive neuroscience of action.* Oxford: Blackwell.

Jecker, J., & Landy, D. (1969). Liking a person as a function of doing him a favour. *Human Relations, 22,* 371–378.

Jones, L. A., & Hunter, I. W. (1983). Effect of fatigue on force sensation. *Experimental Neurology, 81,* 640–650.

Kahneman, D. (1973). *Attention and effort.* Englewood Cliffs, NJ: Prentice Hall.

Kinsbourne, M. (1996). What qualifies a representation for a role in consciousness? In J. D. Cohen & J. W. Schooler (Eds.), *Scientific approaches to consciousness* (pp. 335–355). Hillsdale, NJ: Lawrence Erlbaum Associates.

Kruger, J., Wirtz, D., Van Boven, L., & Altermatt, T. W. (2004). The effort heuristic. *Journal of Experimental Social Psychology, 40,* 91–98.

LeCompte, D. C. (1995). Recollective experience in the revelation effect: Separating the contributions of recollection and familiarity. *Memory and Cognition, 23,* 324–334.

Lynch, J. G. (2005). The effort effects of prizes in the second half of tournaments. *Journal of Economic Behavior & Organization, 57,* 115–129.

Malle, B. F., & Knobe, J. (1997). The folk concept of intentionality. *Journal of Experimental Social Psychology, 33,* 101–121.

Martijn, C., Tenbült, P., Merckelbach, H., Dreezens, E., & de Vries, N. K. (2002). Getting a grip on ourselves: Challenging expectancies about loss of energy after self-control. *Social Cognition, 20*(6), 441–460.

McCloskey, D. I., Ebeling, P., & Goodwin, G. M. (1974). Estimation of weights and tensions and apparent involvement of a "sense of effort." *Experimental Neurology, 42,* 220–232.

Metcalfe, J., & Mischel, W. (1999). A hot/cool-system analysis of delay of gratification: Dynamics of willpower. *Psychological Review, 106,* 3–19.

Metcalfe, J., & Wiebe, D. (1987). Intuition in insight and noninsight problem solving. *Memory and Cognition, 15,* 238–246.

Morsella, E. (2005). The function of phenomenal states: Supramodular interaction theory. *Psychological Review, 112,* 1000–1021.

Muraven, M., Tice, D. M., & Baumeister, R. F. (1998). Self-control as a limited resource: Regulatory depletion patterns. *Journal of Personality and Social Psychology, 74,* 774–789.

Nagel, T. (1974). What is it like to be a bat? *Philosophical Review, 83,* 435–450.

Nicholls, J. G. (1976). Effort is virtuous, but it's better to have ability: Evaluative responses to perceptions of effort and ability. *Journal of Research in Personality, 10,* 306–315.

Nussbaum, M. A., & Lang, A. (2005). Relationships between static load acceptability, ratings of perceived exertion, and biomechanical demands. *International Journal of Industrial Ergonomics, 35,* 547–557.

Pinker, S. (1997). *How the mind works.* New York: Norton.

Preston, J., & Wegner, D. M. (2005). Ideal agency: The perception of self as an origin of action. In A. Tesser, J. V. Wood, & D. A. Stapel (Eds.), *On building, defending and regulating the self: A psychological perspective* (pp. 103–125). New York: Psychology Press.

Preston, J., & Wegner, D. M. (2007). The eureka error: Inadvertent plagiarism by misattributions of effort. *Journal of Personality and Social Psychology, 92,* 576–587.

Proffitt, D. R. (2006). Embodied perception and the economy of action. *Perspectives on Psychological Science, 1,* 110–122.

Pronin, E., & Wegner, D. M. (2006). Manic thinking: Independent effects of thought speed and thought content on mood. *Psychological Science, 9,* 807–813.

Reber, R., & Schwarz, N. (1999). Effects of perceptual fluency on judgments of truth. *Consciousness and Cognition: An International Journal, 8*(3), 338–342.

Rejeski, W. J. (1981). The perception of exertion: A social psychophysiological integration. *Journal of Sport Psychology, 3,* 305–320.

Riis, J., Simmons, J. P., & Goodwin, G. P. (in press). Preferences for enhancement pharmaceuticals: The reluctance to enhance fundamental traits. *Journal of Consumer Research.*

Roberson, B. F., & Wright, R. A. (1994). Difficulty as a determinant of interpersonal appeal: A social-motivational application of energization theory. *Basic and Applied Social Psychology, 15,* 373–388.

Rode, G., Rossetti, Y., & Boisson, D. (1996). Inverse relationship between sensation of effort and muscular force during recovery from pure motor hemiplegia: A single-case study. *Neuropsychologia, 34,* 87–95.

Rose, S. P. R. (2002). "Smart drugs": Do they work? Are they ethical? Will they be legal? *Neuroscience, 3,* 975–979.

Ross, H. E., & Reschke, M. F. (1982). Mass estimation and discrimination during brief periods of zero gravity. *Perception and Psychophysics, 31,* 429–436.

Schachter, S. (1964). The interaction of cognitive and physiological determinants of emotional state. In L. Berkowitz (Ed.), *Advances in social psychology* (Vol. 1, pp. 49–80). New York: Academic Press.

Schachter, S., & Singer, J. E. (1962). Cognitive, social, and physiological determinants of emotional states. *Psychological Review, 69,* 379–399.

Schmeichel, B. J., Vohs, K. D., & Baumeister, R. F. (2003). Intellectual performance and ego depletion: Role of the self in logical reasoning and other information processing. *Journal of Personality and Social Psychology, 85,* 33–46.

Schooler, J. W., & Melcher, J. (1995). The ineffability of insight. In S. M. Smith, & T. B. Ward (Eds.), *The creative cognition approach* (pp. 97–133). Bradford-MIT Press: Cambridge, MA.

Schwarz, N. (2002). Feelings as information: Moods influence judgments and processing strategies. In T. Gilovich, D. Griffin, & D. Kahneman (Eds.), *Heuristics and biases: The psychology of intuitive judgment.* (pp. 534–547). New York: Cambridge University Press.

Schwarz, N., Bless, H., Strack, F., Klumpp, G., Rittenauer-Schatka, H., & Simons, A. (1991). Ease of retrieval as information: Another look at the availability heuristic. *Journal of Personality and Social Psychology, 61,* 195–202.

Schwarz, N., & Clore, G. L. (1996). *Feelings and phenomenal experiences.* New York: Guilford Press.

Sherrington, C. S. (1900). *The muscular sense.* In E. A. Shäfer (Ed.), *Textbook of physiology* (Vol. 2, pp. 1002–1025). Edinburgh: Pentland.

Silbersweig, D. A., Stern, E., Frith, C., & Cahill, C. (1995). A functional neuroanatomy of hallucinations in schizophrenia. *Nature, 378*(6553), 176–179.

Sperry, R. W. (1950). Neural basis of the spontaneous optokinetic response produced by visual neural inversion. *Journal of Comparative Physiological Psychology, 45,* 482–489.

Stepper, S., & Strack, F. (1993). Proprioceptive determinants of emotional and nonemotional feelings. *Journal of Personality and Social Psychology, 64,* 211–220.

Stevens, J. C., & Cain, W. S. (1970). Effort in isometric muscular contractions related to force level and duration. *Perception and Psychophysics, 8,* 240–244.

Strack, F., & Neumann, R. (2000). Furrowing the brow may undermine perceived fame: The role of facial feedback in judgments of celebrity. *Personality and Social Psychology Bulletin, 26,* 762–768.

Tversky, A., & Kahneman, D. (1973). Availability: A heuristic for judging frequency and probability. *Cognitive Psychology, 5,* 207–232.

Unklebach, C. (2006). Learned interpretation of cognitive fluency. *Psychological Science, 17*, 339–345.

van Beilen, M., van Zomeren, E. H., van den Bosch, R. J., Withaar, F. K., & Bouma, A. (2005). Measuring the executive functions in schizophrenia: The voluntary allocation of effort. *Journal of Psychiatric Research, 39*, 585–593.

Van Roon, A. M., Mulder, L. J. M., Veldman, J. B. P., & Mulder, G. (1995). Beat-to-beat blood-pressure measurements applied in studies on mental workload. *Homeostasis, 36*, 3316–3324.

Velten, J. E. (1968). A laboratory task for the induction of mood states. *Behaviour Research and Therapy, 6*, 473–482.

Vohs, K. D., Baumeister, R. F., Twenge, J. M., Schmeichel, B. J., Tice, D. M., & Crocker, J. (2008). *Decision fatigue exhausts self-regulatory resources.* Manuscript in preparation.

von Holst, E. (1954). Relations between the central nervous system and the peripheral organs. *British Journal of Animal Behavior, 2*, 89–94.

Wegner, D. M. (1989). *White bears and other unwanted thoughts: Suppression, obsession, and the psychology of mental control.* New York: Viking/Penguin.

Wegner, D. M. (2002). *The illusion of conscious will.* Cambridge, MA: MIT Press.

Wegner, D. M. (2005). Who is the controller of controlled processes? In R. Hassin, J. S. Uleman, & J. A. Bargh (Eds.), *The new unconscious* (pp. 19–36). New York: Oxford University Press.

Wegner, D. M., Ansfield, M., & Pilloff, D. (1998). The putt and the pendulum: Ironic effects of the mental control of action. *Psychological Science, 9*, 196–199.

Wegner, D. M., & Sparrow, B. (2004). Authorship processing. In M. Gazzaniga (Ed.), *The cognitive neurosciences* (3rd ed., pp. 1201–1209). Cambridge, MA: MIT Press.

Weiner, B., & Kukla, A. (1970). An attribution analysis of achievement motivation. *Journal of Personality and Social Psychology, 15*, 1–20.

Westerman, D. L., & Greene, R. L. (1996). On the generality of the revelation effect. *Journal of Experimental Psychology: Learning, Memory, and Cognition, 22*, 1147–1153.

Whittlesea, B. W. A., Jacoby, L. L., & Girard, K. (1990). Illusions of immediate memory: Evidence of an attributional basis for feelings of familiarity and perceptual quality. *Journal of Memory and Language, 29*, 716–732.

Zillman, D., Katcher, A. H., & Milavsky, B. (1972). Excitation transfer from physical exercise to subsequent aggressive behavior. *Journal of Experimental Social Psychology, 8*, 247–259.

CHAPTER 28

Consciousness as a Troubleshooting Device? The Role of Consciousness in Goal Pursuit

Karin C.A. Bongers *and* Ap Dijksterhuis

Abstract

This chapter focuses on the role of consciousness in goal-directed behavior. It begins by reviewing evidence that goals can be activated outside awareness and run to completion without the person being aware. It then reviews literature concerning evaluation processes in conscious goal pursuit and explores whether people are indeed able to detect success and failure to attain unconsciously activated goals. It is argued that failure renders goal-related constructs highly accessible. In turn, this heightened accessibility of goal-related constructs can ultimately lead to conscious awareness of the goal. Evidence is presented that supports the idea that people start to think consciously about unconsciously activated goals when progress is problematic. The chapter ends with a discussion of whether conscious goal-related thoughts serve a regulatory function.

Keywords: goal-directed behavior, success, failure, unconscious goal pursuit

Imagine you are presenting your work at a major conference and your presentation meets with disaster. Your laptop crashes, your jokes fall flat, and a lot of people attending your presentation start to yawn. At some point, some of them even fall asleep. Immediately after this horrible fiasco, thoughts about the goal you actually pursued, the goal of making an excellent, lasting impression on your colleagues spontaneously keeps popping into consciousness. Moreover, you feel foolish, devastated even, and your self-esteem is tragically low. During the remainder of the day, thoughts about your failure keep intruding consciousness. The evening drinks only help a little bit.

As illustrated here, failure to attain your goals can have an impact on conscious

thoughts, feelings, and self-esteem. In this chapter, we focus on the role of consciousness in goal-directed behavior. Although recent research has shown that goals can be activated outside awareness and even run to completion without any conscious intervention (e.g., Bargh, Gollwitzer, Lee-Chai, Barndollar, & Trötschel, 2001), there is no denying that we are often consciously aware of our goals. We are sometimes aware of the fact that we want to achieve, that we want to be honest, or, indeed, that we want to make a good impression at a major conference. This is an interesting conundrum: On the one hand, we are faced with the observation that goal pursuit does not need consciousness (at least under some circumstances); on the other hand, we know that we are frequently aware of our goals. The question we want to address in this chapter is when and why we are aware of our goals? We argue that one cause of becoming consciously aware of goals is failure in goal-attainment. That is, we propose that especially when people fail to attain their goals, they will start to think consciously about these goals, as illustrated in the opening example.

This idea is in line with ideas proposed by others (Atkinson & Birch, 1970; Lewin, 1936; Mandler, 1975; McClelland, Atkinson, Clark, & Lowell, 1953; Morsella, 2005; Shiffrin & Schneider, 1977). Mandler (1975), for example, already argued that structures that are normally not represented in consciousness might be brought into consciousness when they are defective in their particular function. For example, if one key is stuck when typing a letter, then particular representations of that action may intrude consciousness. More recently, Morsella (2005; Chapter 30) introduced a framework that suggested that we become aware of our actions when there is conflict among different (unconscious) response systems. For example, normally you are not aware of your air intake or the blinking of your eyes. However, if for some reason this air intake or blinking is obstructed (i.e., when there is conflict), you become aware of your breathing or blinking.

Before answering the central question about when goals intrude consciousness, we first briefly review evidence that goals can be activated outside awareness and run to completion without the person being aware. Subsequently, we review literature concerning evaluation processes in conscious goal pursuit and explore whether people are indeed able to detect success and failure to attain unconsciously activated goals. We present some research conducted in our own laboratory investigating the consequences of success and failure to attain unconsciously activated goals. We argue, in line with other research, that failure renders goal-related constructs highly accessible. In turn, we propose that this heightened accessibility of goal-related constructs can ultimately lead to conscious awareness of the goal. We present research from our own laboratory that supports our idea that people start to think consciously about unconsciously activated goals when progress is problematic. We end this chapter by speculating about whether such conscious goal-related thoughts serve a regulatory function.

Unconscious Goal Pursuit

Today, the notion that goals can be activated by situational cues outside awareness and guide behavior unconsciously is widely accepted. Converging evidence has shown that the entire process from goal activation to goal completion can ensue without conscious awareness (e.g., Bargh, 1990; Bargh et al., 2001; Chartrand & Bargh, 1996; Fishbach, Friedman, & Kruglanski, 2003; for reviews, see Custers & Aarts, 2005a; Dijksterhuis, Chartrand, & Aarts, 2007). For instance, priming participants with the goal to achieve led to a better performance on an intellectual task relative to participants not primed with that goal (Bargh et al., 2001). Moreover, participants who were unobtrusively exposed to citrus-scented all-purpose cleaner kept their environment more clean during an experiment in which they had to eat than participants who were not exposed to the cleaner (Holland, Hendriks, & Aarts, 2005).

Furthermore, it has been shown that the representation of significant others can induce goal-directed behavior (Fitzsimons & Bargh, 2003; Shah, 2003). Activating the representation of a close friend led to more helping behavior (Fitzsimons & Bargh, 2003), and priming participants with their father increased achievement. Shah (2003), for example, subliminally primed participants with words related to father or neutral words. Participants were then given an anagram task that was introduced as an important measure of analytic reasoning. After the anagram task, participants were asked to indicate how close they were with their father and whether their father valued the task goal (i.e., achievement). The findings showed that especially participants who were close to their father and perceived their father as wanting them to do well on the task were more committed to the task, were more persistent in the task, and performed better on the task (Shah, 2003).

Aarts, Gollwitzer, and Hassin (2004) recently demonstrated "goal contagion," the tendency for people to engage in unconscious goal pursuit merely because other people in their environment are doing so. For example, in one experiment (Aarts et al., 2004, experiment 2), male participants were asked to read a short story in which the goal of seeking casual sex was primed, whereas other male participants were not primed with that goal. Subsequently, the tendency to help the experimenter, who was either male or female, was measured. The findings indicated that participants who were primed with the goal of seeking casual sex were more inclined to help the female experimenter than participants who were not primed with that goal, whereas no such differences were found when the experimenter was male.

Many authors have argued that goals that are frequently chosen consciously can over time develop the capacity of becoming unconsciously activated (e.g., Bargh, 1990; Bargh et al., 2001; Custers, 2006; Kruglanski, 1996; Shah, Kruglanski, & Friedman, 2003). When goals are consistently and repeatedly activated in a specific situation, such goals can be activated automatically whenever the person encounters that same situation (Aarts & Dijksterhuis, 2000, 2003; Shiffrin & Dumais, 1981; Wegner & Bargh, 1998). For example, after consistently and repeatedly choosing the goal to be polite whenever you visit your parents-in-law, merely seeing your parents-in-law will unconsciously activate the goal of being polite.

Despite considerable research concerning the effects of unconsciously activated goals on behavior and cognition, very little research has been done to examine the effects of failure to attain such unconsciously activated goals (but see Chartrand, 1999; Riketta & Dauenheimer, 2003). We all know that goal setting does not always lead to successful goal pursuit. As illustrated in our opening example, especially when people fail to attain their goals, they start to think about these goals. But how do people know whether they succeed or fail if they are pursuing unconsciously activated goals? We propose that in order to know whether performed actions are in line with (unconsciously) activated goals, goal-directed behavior has to be monitored.

Goal-Discrepancy Detection

We have all had the experience that setting a goal for ourselves does not always lead to attainment. Attempts to quit smoking, for example, very often remain attempts. So how do we know whether the selected actions are in accordance with our chosen goals? To make sure that the actions we are performing are indeed in line with the intended goals, we compare our behavior and its effects with the goal we pursue (e.g., Carver & Scheier, 1981, 1998; Powers, 1973; Scheier & Carver, 1988; Wiener, 1948).

Many self-regulation theories have proposed some kind of feedback control (e.g., Carver & Scheier, 1981, 1998; Miller, Galanter, & Pribram, 1960; Powers, 1973; Wiener, 1948; Chapter 15). For example,

Miller et al. (1960) described a feedback loop in their test-operate-test-exit model. According to this model, once a goal (or standard) is activated, the present behavior is tested against the standard (test phase). If discrepancies are detected between the goal and the present behavior, behavior has to be stopped, changed, or even reversed (operate phase). Subsequently, the altered behavior and its effects are tested against the standard (test phase). This feedback loop continues to operate until discrepancies are no longer detected. If no discrepancies are detected between the present behavior and the goal (indicating that the goal was attained), no further actions are necessary, and the feedback loop is discontinued (exit phase). Feedback control works like the system we all have at home to control our heating: a thermostat. A thermostat checks the temperature and compares it to a set standard. When the temperature is below the standard, it activates the heating system. If the desired temperature is reached, the heating system is deactivated.

Discrepancy detection has effects on feelings. If people detect discrepancies between their current and their desired states a negative evaluation will follow, resulting in a negative mood (e.g., Bandura, 1997; Carver & Scheier, 1981, 1990; Frijda, 1988). For example, when intending to go to the gym twice a week, finding out after 2 weeks that you did not visit the gym even once will likely lead to feelings of sadness and perhaps guilt. However, when no discrepancies are observed, a positive evaluation ensues, resulting in a positive mood.

Depending on the perceived self-relevance of goals, successful or problematic goal pursuit may also affect self-esteem (e.g., Crocker, Sommers, & Luthanen, 2002; Crocker & Wolfe, 2001; Wolfe & Crocker, 2002). For example, Crocker and colleagues (Crocker, Karpinski, Quinn, & Chase, 2003; Crocker et al., 2002) showed that the more self-relevant academic performance is for students, the greater the fluctuations in self-esteem in response to positive and negative academic events will be. They (Crocker et al., 2002) assessed self-esteem of college seniors applying to graduate programs several times during 2 months. During this period, students were likely to receive acceptance letters as well as rejection letters from graduate programs. The findings showed that the more self-relevant academic performance was for the student, the greater was the impact of the letters on self-esteem.

To recap, people evaluate their progress toward their intended goals. Because people evaluate their goal-directed behavior, self-esteem (and sometimes mood) are affected by success and failure. Although the evidence reported thus far pertained to conscious goals, we argue that goals that are activated outside awareness will be monitored as well. That is, we propose that people will implicitly evaluate their progress toward goal-attainment and hence that self-esteem (and mood) are affected by success and failure on unconscious goals as well. Next we review supporting evidence for such an "implicit monitoring" process.

Implicit Monitoring

In line with our reasoning, Moskowitz, Li, and Kirk (2004) also proposed that unconsciously activated goals are monitored. According to their implicit volition model, people are very likely to evaluate or monitor their progress toward their goals regardless of whether a goal is activated consciously or unconsciously. When discrepancies are detected between the current level of goal attainment and the desired state, some tension arises, instigating different kinds of goal operations, such as adjusting current behavior or inhibiting competing goals.

In the literature on thought suppression, such a monitoring process has been proposed as well (Wegner, 1994, 1997; Wegner & Wenzlaff, 1996). It has been argued that while intentionally suppressing a certain thought from entering consciousness, an (ironic) monitoring process remains active in the background to search for mental contents that signal the failure to achieve the desired state. Concretely, when people are asked not to think about a white bear, they indeed try to consciously avoid thoughts of a white bear. Meanwhile, a monitoring process starts to search for information that may signal failure: thoughts about a white bear (e.g., Wegner & Erber, 1992). Although the goal to suppress thoughts in the thought suppression literature is activated consciously, the monitoring process is assumed to be unconscious.

Other support for implicit monitoring processes can be found in neurocognitive research (e.g., Angel, 1976; J. R. Higgins & Angel, 1970; Rabbitt, 1966; Rabbitt & Rodgers, 1977; Ridderinkhof, van den Wildenberg, Segalowitz, & Carter, 2004). It has been suggested that largely overlapping brain areas, clustering in the rostral cingulate zone, are involved in monitoring by searching for unfavorable outcomes and response errors (Ridderinkhof, Ullperger, Crone, & Nieuwenhuis, 2004). These brain areas signal that goals may not be achieved or that rewards may not be obtained (Ridderinkhof, van den Wildenberg et al., 2004). An error detection system appears to compare a representation of the response actually made against a representation of the appropriate response (Bernstein, Scheffers, & Coles, 1995; Scheffers & Coles, 2000). Recent studies of event-related potentials have shown a negative potential (i.e., error-related negativity [ERN]) when participants make errors in a choice-reaction-time paradigm. This ERN reaches a peak about 150 milliseconds after the onset of the erroneous response (e.g., Dehaene, Posner, & Tucker, 1994; Falkenstein, Hohnsbein,

Hoormann, & Blanke, 1990; Gehring, Goss, Coles, Meyer, & Donchin, 1993). Moreover, the degree of mismatch between the two representations (or the degree of error detected by the system) is reflected in the amplitude of the ERN (e.g., Bernstein et al., 1995; Scheffers & Coles, 2000).

Assuming that people indeed monitor their unconsciously activated goals, consequences of success and failure for mood and for self-esteem can be expected to be the same for unconsciously activated goals and consciously chosen goals. After all, changes in self-esteem are caused by people's ability to detect failures and successes. When goal progress is successful, no discrepancies are detected, resulting in a better mood and higher self-esteem, whereas when goal progress is problematic, discrepancies are detected, resulting in a worse mood and lower self-esteem.

Recently, Chartrand (1999; Chartrand & Bargh, 2002) started to explore the effects of success and failure to attain unconsciously activated goals on mood. In one of her experiments, participants were given either a difficult or an easy anagram task after being primed with the goal to achieve or not. Participants primed with the goal to achieve were in a worse mood after performing the difficult anagram task than after performing the easy anagram task. For participants not primed with that goal, no such differences were found (but see Bongers, Dijksterhuis, & Spears, 2008a). Chartrand (1999; Chartrand & Bargh, 2002) called the resulting moods "mystery moods." Participants were, depending on conditions, in a good or bad mood without knowing the origins of these moods.

Furthermore, Riketta and Dauenheimer (2003) investigated the effects of anticipated success on mood and self-esteem. Participants were primed with a knowledge-seeking goal or not. Before measuring mood and self-esteem, half the participants were told that they would receive a personality test with feedback on their results, thereby anticipating to satisfy their goal. However, the other half of the participants received this announcement after mood and self-esteem were measured. The findings showed that, when mood and self-esteem were measured after the announcement, participants primed with the knowledge-seeking goal were in a better mood and reported higher self-esteem than participants not primed with that goal. However, when mood and self-esteem were measured before the announcement, no such differences were found.

Because Riketta and Dauenheimer (2003) investigated only anticipated successful goal pursuit, claims about a monitoring process may be somewhat bold. That is, participants were not yet pursuing the goal. However, their findings are difficult to explain without assuming a monitoring process. Why would mood and especially self-esteem increase by an announcement suggesting an opportunity to fulfill a goal if someone does not monitor their (unconscious) goal pursuit? Some kind of evaluative process (is the goal going to be attained or not?) starts to operate after a goal is activated. And this process will search the environment for cues that will promote goal pursuit, in this case the announcement, or will search for cues that signal failures to attain activated goals.

To investigate whether actual success and failure to attain unconsciously activated goals will affect self-esteem similarly as success and failure on consciously chosen goals, we (Bongers et al., 2008a) conducted several experiments in our own laboratory. The design of these experiments is comparable to the design used by Chartrand (1999; Chartrand & Bargh, 2002). However, we measured self-esteem rather than mood. In one of our experiments (Bongers et al., 2008a, experiment 1), we primed participants with an achievement goal or

not using a scrambled sentences task (Srull & Wyer, 1980). Subsequently, they were given either 10 difficult (failure condition) or 10 easy (success condition) items of the Raven Progressive Matrices Test[1] (Raven, 1941). Subsequently, self-esteem was measured with the state self-esteem scale (Heatherton & Polivy, 1991). Three types of self-esteem were distinguished: performance self-esteem, social self-esteem, and appearance self-esteem. If people indeed evaluate their behavior, one may expect the strongest effects on the type of self-esteem that is closest to the domain of succeeding or failing. Therefore, we expected that success and failure to attain an unconsciously activated achievement goal would affect mainly performance self-esteem and perhaps social self-esteem but not appearance self-esteem. The findings indeed demonstrated that participants primed with an achievement goal reported higher self-esteem after the easy test than after the difficult test, whereas no such differences were found for participants not primed with that goal. Moreover, these effects emerged only for performance self-esteem and social self-esteem but not for appearance self-esteem.

To recapitulate, although goals are activated outside awareness, people monitor their goal-directed behavior, and hence people are able to detect successes and failures. We already argued that especially when people fail to attain their goals, they will start to think consciously about these goals. In other words, when failures are detected, thoughts about the goal will spontaneously pop into consciousness. In the next section, we review theories concerning intrusive thoughts to shed more light on the kind of thoughts that are most likely to enter consciousness spontaneously.

Motivated Conscious Thoughts

According to Klinger (1975), conscious thoughts can be divided into two categories:

operant thoughts and respondent thoughts. Operant thoughts are a function of a person's current concerns. These thoughts are related to a person's current activity, are intentionally directed toward task completion, and are under a person's control, such as conscious thoughts about all-purpose cleaner while housekeeping. Respondent thoughts, on the other hand, are thoughts that are not related to a person's current activity, that enter consciousness unintentionally, and that shift attention away from the person's current activity. For instance, conscious thoughts about an argument with your best friend while housekeeping are respondent thoughts. These respondent thoughts, also called intrusive thoughts, are the ones that are important here.

Respondent or intrusive thoughts are mostly motivationally driven, although there are exceptions (Beckmann, 1998). Some intrusive thoughts have no motivational source (Martin & Tesser, 1989, 1996), as one thought may simply activate another thought by association. For example, thinking about a book you are reading may activate thoughts about the library, which may activate thoughts about the university, and so on. Another example of intrusive thoughts that are not always motivational is daydreaming (Singer, 1966, 1975). Although the content of daydreaming is usually positive, it shifts attention away from the person's current activity. Intrusive thoughts without a motivational source are not very vigorous and will extinguish over time. Conversely, motivationally driven intrusions are more persistent and powerful. In general, these intrusions concern incomplete intentions or frustrated goals. Such incomplete intentions instigate conscious thoughts about these unattained goals, such as thinking about your disastrous presentation (e.g., Beckmann, 1998; Klinger, 1996; Martin & Tesser, 1996). Intrusive thoughts will enter consciousness unintentionally, even without the necessity of cues in the environment, and then interfere with what one is currently doing (Chapter 5). In addition, these thoughts are likely to keep intruding consciousness until the goal is either attained or abandoned (Beckmann, 1998; Klinger, 1996, 1999; Lyubomirsky & Nolen-Hoeksema, 1995; Martin & Tesser, 1989, 1996; Mikulincer, 1996).

Although the actual experience of the thought is considered to be conscious, the underlying mechanism is unconscious (Martin & Tesser, 1996). It is assumed that these conscious thoughts might be caused by heightened accessibility of goal-related concepts (see Rholes & Pryor, 1982; Williams, 1993). In the next section, we explore whether goal-related concepts are indeed more accessible after goal activation and whether these goal-related concepts remain highly accessible when goal progress is problematic.

Accessibility

Goals can be seen as mental representations like semantic concepts or stereotypes (Bargh, 1990; Kruglanski, 1996), and they are mentally represented as desired states in a hierarchically ordered knowledge structure. Such hierarchical knowledge structure includes desired states, actions, and means to reach the desired states (Aarts & Dijksterhuis, 2000; Aarts et al., 2004; Bargh & Gollwitzer, 1994; Carver & Scheier, 1998; Custers & Aarts, 2005b; Dijksterhuis et al., 2007; Gollwitzer & Moskowitz, 1996). A major difference between mental representations of goals and other mental constructs is that goal representations have a motivational content. Whereas non-motivational priming effects are known to decrease in strength over time (e.g., Dijksterhuis & Bargh, 2001; E. T. Higgins, Bargh, & Lombardi, 1985), goal-priming effects are known to be able to increase in strength over time until the goal is attained (e.g., Atkinson & Birch, 1970; Bargh et al., 2001; Chartrand & Bargh, 1996). It has been suggested that the increase in strength over time is due to enhanced accessibility of goal-related concepts (e.g., Goschke & Kuhl, 1993; Marsh, Hicks, & Bink, 1998).

There is ample evidence that active goals are characterized by enhanced accessibility of goal-related constructs (e.g., Goschke & Kuhl, 1993; E. T. Higgins & King, 1981; Kuhl & Kazén-Saad, 1988). Classic work of Anderson and Pichert (1978) has shown that information becomes accessible if a related schema is invoked. For example, in experiment 2 (Anderson & Pichert, 1978), participants were asked to take either a burglar perspective or a home-buyer perspective and were then asked to read a story about two boys playing hooky from school. The story contained some points of interest to a burglar and some points of interest to a home buyer. The data demonstrated that depending on the goal (or perspective) that is active, information becomes accessible and is more likely to be recalled.

Furthermore, Aarts, Dijksterhuis, and De Vries (2001) showed that thirsty people were faster in responding to drinking-related items in a lexical decision task and had better memory for these items in a surprise free recall task relative to nonthirsty people. This indicates that thirst increases the accessibility of drinking-related items and heightens the perceptual readiness for environmental stimuli instrumental in the goal of reducing thirst.

Förster, Liberman, and Higgins (2005) also showed that active goals enhance the accessibility of goal-related constructs (Chapter 9). Interestingly, after goal attainment, these constructs are inhibited, rendering them less accessible than before attainment and even less accessible than before goal activation. However, when goals

are not attained, goal-related constructs remain highly accessible. Thus, active goals enhance accessibility of goal-related constructs, and these constructs will remain accessible as long as people are motivated to attain these goals.

Furthermore, research of Kawada, Oettingen, Gollwitzer, and Bargh (2004) on implicit goal projection (ascribing one's own goals onto others) supports the idea that goal-related constructs are more accessible after failure than after success. Implicit goal projection results from heightened accessibility of goal-related constructs. Therefore, highly accessible concepts are more likely to be projected than less accessible concepts. It was hypothesized that people would project more after failure than after success. That is, after goal-pursuit failure, goals will remain highly accessible and hence will be more likely to be projected. However, after goal-pursuit success, goals will be less accessible or not accessible anymore and hence are not likely to be projected.

In one of their studies, Kawada et al. (2004, experiment 3) primed one-third of the participants subliminally with a goal to compete, one-third was given an explicit goal to compete, and another one-third was given no goal. Then participants performed an intermediate task on which they could compete. Participants were told that the computers were connected via the network, and they were made to believe that they would be playing with a (fictitious) partner. Half the participants were told that they outperformed the partner (success feedback), and the other half were told that the partner outperformed them (failure feedback). Then participants were given an opportunity to project their goal. Participants were asked to predict how many competitive moves the fictional characters would make when engaged in a prisoner's dilemma game. The results showed that participants who were subliminally primed with a goal to compete and participants who were given an explicit goal to compete projected their competition goal only after failure and not after success feedback. That is, these participants ascribed more competitive moves to the partner after failure than after success feedback. Participants who did not have a competition goal did not project that goal, neither after success nor after failure.

We argue that heightened accessibility of goal-related constructs after failure is the stepping-stone to becoming consciously aware of the goal. When people are motivated to attain a goal toward which progress is problematic, a monitoring process detects discrepancies between the current state and the desired states, making goal-related concepts highly accessible and therefore making these goals susceptible to enter consciousness.

The classic Zeigarnik effect (Zeigarnik, 1938) is reminiscent of this idea. In a typical empirical demonstration, participants were asked to work on a series of tasks until each task was completed. However, during some of the tasks, participants were interrupted, and hence they were not able to complete them. Afterward they were asked to recall the tasks they had worked on. The findings showed that unfinished tasks were recalled twice as often as finished ones. Thus, interrupted tasks remained highly accessible and therefore were more likely to be (consciously) remembered, suggesting that these interrupted tasks are more likely to intrude consciousness.

In addition, Martin (1986) showed that participants who were interrupted during a priming task continued to think about the primed concepts during a subsequent impression-formation task and hence interpreted the target person in terms of the primed concepts. However, participants who were not interrupted during a priming task did not engender thought preservation and hence did not interpret the target person in terms of the primed concepts.

The well-known "white bear" experiments by Wegner and colleagues (e.g., Wegner, 1994; Wegner & Erber, 1992; Wegner, Schneider, Carter, & White, 1987) also suggest that concepts that are highly accessible are more likely to intrude consciousness. Participants who were asked not to think about a white bear during an initial phase (suppression condition) thought more about white bears afterward than participants who were allowed to think about a white bear during the initial phase (no suppression condition). Hence, for participants in the suppression condition, a monitoring process starts to search for failures not to think about white bears, that is, for mental contents about white bears. It is assumed that the mental representation of white bears, therefore, becomes highly accessible and hence that participants in the suppression conditions start to think more about white bears after the initial phase than participants in the no-suppression condition.

In sum, failure leads to increasing accessibility of goal-related constructs (see Förster et al., 2005; Kawada et al., 2004). Therefore, it is likely that for people who fail, goals will enter consciousness. We present evidence for that idea in the next section.

Consciousness in Goal Pursuit

In several studies, we (Bongers, Dijksterhuis, & Spears, 2008b) investigated whether people would start to think consciously about unconsciously activated goals when they are frustrated in their goal pursuit. In one of our experiments (Bongers et al., 2008b, experiment 1), participants were subliminally primed with a goal to achieve or not in a lexical decision task. To manipulate failure and success, participants were given a Dutch version[2] of the

Remote Associates Test (Mednick, 1962) that was either difficult or easy. While performing the Remote Associates Test, participants were asked to say everything they were thinking out loud regardless of the relation to the task. The findings indicated that participants who failed to attain their unconsciously activated achievement goal reported more conscious goal-related thoughts than participants in all other three conditions. These findings demonstrate that even when people are not aware of the goals they are pursuing, they will start to think consciously about unconsciously activated goals. Because participants reported these conscious goal-related thoughts without receiving any cues or hints to do so in the think-aloud protocol, we can conclude that people start to think consciously about unconsciously activated goals spontaneously when goal pursuit is problematic. We have replicated these findings several times, also within a different goal domain. All experiments demonstrated that people who are not aware of the goals they are pursuing spontaneously started to think consciously about these goals when progress was problematic.

Given that we become conscious of our goals in the face of failure, it is interesting to explore whether consciousness of a goal serves a regulatory function. Does it, or is conscious awareness merely an irrelevant epiphenomenon or perhaps even detrimental for goal pursuit? In the next section, we tentatively try to unravel these questions.

Consequences of Conscious Awareness

Most people will intuitively answer the previously stated questions by saying that consciousness serves to correct for failures. For instance, imagine you are at a conference and during the morning session some of your colleagues are staring at you and start to chuckle. After a while, you find out that you are wearing your shirt inside out. This discovery will lead to conscious thoughts about your goal to look respectable, and you will immediately change matters in order to look normal. However, things are not always that simple. Imagine, for example, that you receive a rejection letter for a paper you have worked on for several months. This rejection will lead to conscious thoughts about your achievement goal. However, it may not immediately stimulate you to proceed and rewrite your paper.

It is highly likely that it depends on many different factors whether conscious awareness of goals is helpful. There are a number of differences between the two examples described previously. For example, changing your shirt is very easy to do and will cost little effort, whereas rewriting your paper may be very difficult and time consuming. Furthermore, it is more likely that you will reach your goal to look respectable after changing your shirt than attaining your achievement goal after rewriting your paper since your paper may still be rejected afterward.

As illustrated previously, the motivation to still attain your goals may depend on the difficulty of the task, the effort it takes to engage in goal-directed behavior, and the likelihood of attaining the goal. These factors may therefore moderate the effects of consciousness of a goal on goal pursuit. If expectancies of goal attainment are high and the task is easy, people are often still motivated to attain the goal leading to renewed effort, whereas if expectancies of goal attainment are low and the task is difficult, people are often more likely to disengage from the goal and reduce effort or even quit trying (Carver & Scheier, 1998; Klinger, 1975; Wright, 1996; Wrosch, Scheier, Miller, Schulz, & Carver, 2003).

Another important factor that can potentially moderate the effects of consciousness of a goal on goal-pursuit concerns the cognitive resources it takes to think about your goal after failure. That is, conscious thoughts concerning goal-pursuit failure may use up cognitive resources that are needed for engaging in goal-directed behavior (Kuhl, 1981; Martin & Tesser, 1996). For instance, consciously thinking about the goal to achieve during a difficult exam may in itself take up resources that could better be used for the exam itself. Indeed, several studies in research on desire showed that intrusive desire-related thoughts use up considerable cognitive resources and that they impair performance on other tasks that compete for these resources (e.g., Cepeda-Benito & Tiffany, 1996; Sayette & Hufford, 1994). For example, exposure to an imagery script that was intended to elicit an urge to smoke subsequently impaired the accuracy of reading comprehension for smokers but not for nonsmokers (Zwaan & Truitt, 1998).

Similarly, Rude, Zentner, and Morrow (1993) showed that people who were given negative feedback about their intelligence were faster at recognizing words related to intelligence compared to people who were given positive feedback, whereas no differences were found for words unrelated to intelligence. Moreover, people who were given negative feedback showed lower reading comprehension than people who were given positive feedback. These findings indicate that higher accessibility of intelligence, evoking intrusions into consciousness, impaired performance on a second task.

To sum up, on the one hand, one may hypothesize that consciously thinking about a goal after failure may be beneficial for subsequent goal pursuit. Again, discovering that you are wearing your shirt inside out will motivate you immediately to redress the situation (literally) in order to attain your goal to look respectable. On the other hand, when it takes a lot of effort to engage in goal-directed behavior and the likelihood of attaining the goal is low, one may hypothesize that consciously thinking about a goal after failure may be detrimental for subsequent goal pursuit. Furthermore, when consciously thinking about goal-pursuit failure uses up cognitive capacity that is needed for goal-directed behavior, it may be detrimental as well.

Besides, it may be that conscious awareness of failure to attain a goal lowers expectancies for future performance and hence will lead to reduced effort toward goal attainment or even disengagement from that goal. In accordance with this reasoning, Chartrand (1999; Chartrand & Bargh, 2002) indeed demonstrated that people who failed to attain an unconsciously activated achievement goal in an initial language task believed that they would do worse at an immediate language task, resulting in a worse performance in a subsequent language task than people who succeeded in attaining their goal.

Recently, we (Bongers, Dijksterhuis, & Spears, 2006) conducted an experiment to investigate the effects of conscious thoughts concerning an unconsciously activated achievement goal on perseverance. Participants were subliminally primed with the goal to achieve or not in a lexical decision task. Subsequently, participants were asked to find all the identical pairs of cards in a memory game (Bongers et al., 2006) within the time given. To manipulate success and failure, participants were given a maximum time of either 3 minutes (which was too short to complete it) or 12 minutes (which was more than enough time to complete it), respectively. After a break of 2 minutes, conscious goal-related thoughts were measured with a sentence completion test. They were asked to complete a number of sentences (i.e., I . . . and I wished . . .)

with the first thing that came to mind. Finally, participants were given a word-search puzzle and were asked to find the 10 words that were presented next to the puzzle. In fact, only 5 of the 10 given words were indeed hidden in the puzzle. Participants could quit the puzzle when they thought that they could not find any more words. The time participants used to find the words was taken as motivation to achieve.

The results replicated earlier findings in that participants who failed to attain their unconsciously activated achievement goal reported more conscious goal-related thoughts than participants in all other three conditions. Furthermore, the analyses showed that participants who performed the 3-minute memory game (failure condition) quit the word-search puzzle earlier when primed with the goal to achieve than participants not primed with the goal to achieve. There were no such differences for participants who performed the 12-minute memory game (success condition). These findings indicate that consciously thinking about an achievement goal in the face of failure is not always functional for subsequent goal pursuit. This is also supported by the negative correlation we found between the conscious goal-related thoughts and the time participants spend at the word-search puzzle for participants who were primed with the goal to achieve. The more participants engaged in conscious goal-related thoughts, the less motivated they were in achieving at the word-search puzzle. No correlation was found for participants not primed with the goal to achieve. These findings were also replicated in another experiment (see Bongers et al., 2006).

Conclusions

In this chapter, we focused on the role of consciousness in goal-directed behavior. Various researchers have shown that goals can be activated outside awareness and then guide behavior unconsciously. As there is no denying that we are often aware of the goals we are pursuing, we have to deal with an interesting paradox. On the one hand, we are faced with the observation that goal pursuit does not need consciousness; on the other hand, we observe frequent conscious awareness of our goals. The question we addressed in this chapter was why and when we become aware of the goals we are pursuing.

We argued that when failures to attain a goal are detected, goal-related concepts will become highly accessible. This heightened accessibility of goal-related concepts will lead to conscious awareness of the goal. In various experiments from our own laboratory, we compared people who failed to attain their unconsciously activated goal with people who succeeded in attaining their unconsciously activated goal and to people who did not have an activated goal. We demonstrated that people who failed to attain their goals started to think about them. Simply stated, we become aware of goals when the going gets tough.

Notes

1. Items on the original Raven test are ranked by difficulty such that the first item is the easiest and the last the most difficult (Raven, 1941). For the easy condition, the first 10 items of the original Raven tests were selected, and for the difficult condition, the last 10 items were selected.

2. We conducted a pilot test with a Dutch translation and extension of the Remote Associates Test. Participants were asked to solve 30 randomly presented associations consisting of three words. After each association, they were asked to indicate how difficult that association was. Based on these findings, 10 difficult and 10 easy associations were selected for this experiment.

References

Aarts, H., & Dijksterhuis, A. (2000). Habits as knowledge structures: Automaticity in goal-directed behavior. *Journal of Personality and Social Psychology, 78,* 53–63.

Aarts, H., & Dijksterhuis, A. (2003). The silence of the library: Environment, situational norm, and social behavior. *Journal of Personality and Social Psychology, 84,* 18–28.

Aarts, H., Dijksterhuis, A., & De Vries, P. (2001). On the psychology of drinking: Being thirsty and perceptually ready. *British Journal of Psychology, 92,* 631.

Aarts, H., Gollwitzer, P. M., & Hassin, R. R. (2004). Goal contagion: Perceiving is for pursuing. *Journal of Personality and Social Psychology, 87,* 23–37.

Anderson, R. C., & Pichert, J. W. (1978). Recall of previously unrecallable information following a shift in perspective. *Journal of Verbal Learning and Verbal Behavior, 17,* 1–12.

Angel, R. W. (1976). Efference copy in the control of movement. *Neurology, 26,* 1164–1168.

Atkinson, J. W., & Birch, D. (1970). *The dynamics of action.* Oxford: Wiley.

Bandura, A. (1997). *Self-efficacy: The exercise of control.* New York: Freeman.

Bargh, J. A. (1990). Auto motives: Preconscious determinants of social interaction. In R. M. Sorrentino & E. T. Higgins (Eds.), *Handbook of motivation and cognition: Foundations of social behavior* (Vol. 2, pp. 93–130). New York: Guilford Press.

Bargh, J. A., & Gollwitzer, P. M. (1994). Environmental control of goal-directed action: Automatic and strategic contingencies between situations and behavior. In W. D. Spaulding (Ed.), *Integrative views of motivation, cognition and emotion* (Vol. 41, pp. 71–124). Lincoln: University of Nebraska Press.

Bargh, J. A., Gollwitzer, P. M., Lee-Chai, A., Barndollar, K., & Trötschel, R. (2001). The automated will: Nonconscious activation and pursuit of behavioral goals. *Journal of Personality and Social Psychology, 81,* 1014–1027.

Beckmann, J. (1998). Intrusive thoughts, rumination, and incomplete intentions. In M. Kofta, G. Weary, & G. Sedek (Eds.), *Personal control in action: Cognitive and motivational mechanisms* (pp. 259–278). New York: Plenum Press.

Bernstein, P. S., Scheffers, M. K., & Coles, M. G. H. (1995). "Where did I go wrong?" A psychophysiological analysis of error detection. *Journal of Experimental Psychology: Human Perception and Performance, 21,* 1312–1322.

Bongers, K. C. A., Dijksterhuis, A., Spears, R. (2006). *Is consciously thinking always helpful? The regulatory functions of consciousness in goal-pursuit.* Unpublished manuscript.

Bongers, K. C. A., Dijksterhuis, A., & Spears, R. (2008a). *Self-esteem regulation after success and failure to attain unconsciously activated goals.* Manuscript submitted for publication.

Bongers, K. C. A., Dijksterhuis, A., & Spears, R. (2008b). *On the role of consciousness in goal-pursuit.* Manuscript submitted for publication.

Carver, S. C., & Scheier, M. F. (1981). *Attention and self-regulation: A control theory approach to human behavior.* New York: Springer-Verlag.

Carver, S. C., & Scheier, M. F. (1990). Principles of self-regulation: Action and emotion. In E. T. Higgins & R. M. Sorrentino (Eds.), *Handbook of motivation and cognition: Foundations of social behavior* (Vol. 2, pp. 3–52). New York: Guilford Press.

Carver, S. C., & Scheier, M. F. (1998). *On the self-regulation of behavior.* New York: Cambridge University Press.

Cepeda-Benito, A., & Tiffany, S. T. (1996). The use of a dual-task procedure for the assessment of cognitive effort associated with cigarette craving. *Psychopharmacology, 127,* 155–163.

Chartrand, T. L. (1999). *Mystery moods and perplexing performance: Consequences of succeeding and failing at a nonconscious goal.* Unpublished doctoral dissertation, New York University.

Chartrand, T. L., & Bargh, J. A. (1996). Automatic activation of impression formation and memorization goals: Nonconscious goal priming reproduces effects of explicit task instructions. *Journal of Personality and Social Psychology, 71,* 464–478.

Chartrand, T. J., & Bargh, J. A. (2002). Nonconscious motivations: Their activation, operation, and consequences. In D. A. Stapel & A. Tesser (Eds.), *Self and motivation: Emerging psychological perspectives* (pp. 13–41). Washington, DC: American Psychological Association.

Crocker, J., Karpinski, A., Quinn, D. M., & Chase, S. K. (2003). When grades determine self-worth: Consequences of contingent self worth for male and female engineering and psychology majors. *Journal of Personality and Social Psychology, 85,* 507–516.

Crocker, J., Sommers, S. R., & Luhtanen, R. K. (2002). Hopes dashed and dreams fulfilled: Contingencies of self-worth and graduate school admissions. *Personality and Social Psychology Bulletin, 28,* 1275–1286.

Crocker, J., & Wolfe, C. T. (2001). Contingencies of self-worth. *Psychological Review, 108,* 593–623.

Custers, R. (2006). *On the underlying mechanisms of nonconscious goal pursuit.* Unpublished doctoral dissertation, Utrecht University, Utrecht.

Custers, R., & Aarts, H. (2005a). Beyond priming effects: The role of positive affect and discrepancies in implicit processes of motivation and goal pursuit. In W. Stroebe & M. Hewstone (Eds.), *European review of social psychology* (Vol. 16, pp. 257–300). Hove: Psychology Press.

Custers, R., & Aarts, H. (2005b). Positive affect as implicit motivator: On the nonconscious operation of behavioral goals. *Journal of Personality and Social Psychology, 89,* 129–142.

Dehaene, S., Posner, M. I., & Tucker, D. M. (1994). Localization of a neural system for error detection and compensation. *Psychological Science, 5,* 303–305.

Dijksterhuis, A., & Bargh, J. A. (2001). The perception-behavior expressway: Automatic effects of social perception on social behavior. In M. P. Zanna (Ed.), *Advances in experimental social psychology* (Vol. 33, pp. 1–40). San Diego, CA: Academic Press.

Dijksterhuis, A., Chartrand, T. L., & Aarts, H. (2007). Effects of priming and perception on social behavior and goal pursuit. In J. A. Bargh (Ed.), *Social psychology and the unconscious: The automaticity of higher mental processes* (pp. 51–131). Philadelphia: Psychology Press.

Falkenstein, M., Hohnsbein, J., Hoormann, J., & Blanke, L. (1990). Effects of errors in choice reaction tasks on the ERP under focused and divided attention. In C. H. M. Brunia, A. W. K. Gaillard, & A. Kok (Eds.), *Psychophysiological brain research* (pp. 192–195). Tilburg: Tilburg University Press.

Fishbach, A., Friedman, R. S., & Kruglanski, A. W. (2003). Leading us not unto temptation: Momentary allurements elicit overriding goal activation. *Journal of Personality and Social Psychology, 84,* 296–309.

Fitzsimons, G. M., & Bargh, J. A. (2003). Thinking of you: Nonconscious pursuit of interpersonal goals associated with relationship partners. *Journal of Personality and Social Psychology, 84,* 148–163.

Förster, J., Liberman, N., & Higgins, E. T. (2005). Accessibility from active and fulfilled goals. *Journal of Experimental Social Psychology, 41,* 220–239.

Frijda, N. H. (1988). The laws of emotion. *American Psychologist, 43,* 349–358.

Gehring, W. J., Goss, B., Coles, M. G. H., Meyer, D. E., & Donchin, E. (1993). A neural system for error-detection and compensation. *Psychological Science, 4,* 385–390.

Gollwitzer, P. M., & Moskowitz, G. B. (1996). Goal effects on action and cognition. In E. T. Higgins & A. W. Kruglanski (Eds.), *Social psychology:*

Handbook of basic principles (pp. 361–399). New York: Guilford Press.

Goschke, T., & Kuhl, J. (1993). Representation of intentions: Persisting activation in memory. *Journal of Experimental Psychology: Learning, Memory, and Cognition, 19,* 1211–1226.

Heatherton, T. F., & Polivy, J. (1991). Development and validation of a scale for measuring state self-esteem. *Journal of Personality and Social Psychology, 60,* 895–910.

Higgins, E. T., Bargh, J. A., & Lombardi, W. J. (1985). Nature of priming effects on categorization. *Journal of Experimental Psychology: Learning, Memory, and Cognition, 11,* 59–69.

Higgins, E. T., & King, G. (1981). Accessibility of social constructs: Information processing consequences of individual and contextual variability. In N. Cantor & J. Kihlstrom (Eds.), *Personality, cognition, and social interaction* (pp. 69–121). Hillsdale, NJ: Lawrence Erlbaum Associates.

Higgins, J. R., & Angel, R. W. (1970) Correction of tracking errors without sensory feedback. *Journal of Experimental Psychology, 84,* 412–416.

Holland, R. W., Hendriks, M., & Aarts, H. (2005). Smells like clean spirit: Nonconscious effects of scent on cognition and behavior. *Psychological Science, 16,* 689–693.

Kawada, C. L. K., Oettingen, G., Gollwitzer, P. M., & Bargh, J. A. (2004). The projection of implicit and explicit goals. *Journal of Personality and Social Psychology, 86,* 545–559.

Klinger, E. (1975). Consequences of commitment to and disengagement from incentives. *Psychological Review, 82,* 1–25.

Klinger, E. (1996). The contents of thoughts: Interference as the downside of adaptive normal mechanisms in thought flow. In I. G. Sarason, G. R. Pierce, & B. R. Sarason (Eds.), *Cognitive interference: Theories, methods, and findings* (pp. 3–23). Mahwah, NJ: Lawrence Erlbaum Associates.

Klinger, E. (1999). Thought flow: Properties and mechanisms underlying shifts in content. In J. A. Singer & P. Salovey (Eds.), *At play in the fields of consciousness* (pp. 29–50). Mahwah, NJ: Lawrence Erlbaum Associates.

Kruglanski, A. W. (1996). Goals as knowledge structures. In J. A. Bargh & P. M. Gollwitzer (Eds.), *The psychology of action: Linking cognition and motivation to behavior* (pp. 599–618). New York: Guilford Press.

Kuhl, J. (1981). Motivational and functional help-lessness: The moderating effect of state versus action orientation. *Journal of Personality and Social Psychology, 40,* 155–170.

Kuhl, J., & Kazén-Saad, M. (1988). A motivational approach to volition: Activation and de-activation of memory representations related to uncompleted intentions. In V. Hamilton, G. H. Bower, & N. H. Frijda (Eds.), *Cognitive perspectives on emotion and motivation* (pp. 63–85). New York: Kluwer Academic/Plenum.

Lewin, K. (1936). *Principles of topological psychology.* New York: McGraw-Hill.

Lyubomirsky, S., & Nolen-Hoeksema, S. (1995). Effects of self-focused rumination on negative thinking and interpersonal problem solving. *Journal of Personality and Social Psychology, 69,* 176–190.

Mandler, G. (1975). *Mind and emotion.* New York: Wiley.

Marsh, R. L., Hicks, J. L., & Bink, M. L. (1998). Activation of completed, uncompleted, and partially completed intentions. *Journal of Experimental Psychology: Learning, Memory, and Cognition, 24,* 350–361.

Martin, L. L. (1986). Set/reset: Use and disuse of concepts in impression formation. *Journal of Personality and Social Psychology, 51,* 493–504.

Martin, L. L., & Tesser, A. (1989). Toward a motivational and structural theory of ruminative thought. In J. A. Bargh & J. S. Uleman (Eds.), *Unintended thought* (pp. 306–326). New York: Guilford Press.

Martin, L. L., & Tesser, A. (1996). Some ruminative thoughts. In R. S. Wyer (Ed.), *Ruminative thoughts* (pp. 1–47). Hillsdale, NJ: Lawrence Erlbaum Associates.

McClelland, D. C., Atkinson, J. W., Clark, R. A., & Lowell, E. L. (1953). *The achievement motive.* New York: Appleton-Century-Crofts.

Mednick, S. A. (1962). The associative basis of the creative process. *Psychological Review, 69,* 220–232.

Mikulincer, M. (1996). Mental rumination and learned helplessness: Cognitive shifts during helplessness training and their behavioral consequences. In I. G. Sarason, G. R. Pierce, & B. R. Sarason (Eds.), *Cognitive interference: Theories, methods, and findings* (pp. 191–209). Hillsdale, NJ: Lawrence Erlbaum Associates.

Miller, G. A., Gallanter, E., & Pribram, K. H. (1960). *Plans and the structure of behavior.* New York: Holt, Rinehart and Winston.

Morsella, E. (2005). The function of phenomenal states: Supramodular interaction theory. *Psychological Review, 112,* 1000–1021.

Moskowitz, G. B., Li, P., & Kirk, E. R. (2004). The implicit volition model: On the preconscious regulation of temporarily adopted goals. In M. P. Zanna (Ed.), *Advances in experimental social psychology* (Vol. 36, pp. 317–413). San Diego, CA: Elsevier/Academic Press.

Powers, W. T. (1973). *Behavior: The control of perception.* Chicago: Aldine Atherton.

Rabbitt, P. M. A. (1966). Errors and error correction in choice-response tasks. *Journal of Experimental Psychology, 71,* 264–272.

Rabbitt, P., & Rodgers, B. (1977). What does a man do after he makes an error? An analysis of response programming. *Quarterly Journal of Experimental Psychology, 29,* 727–743.

Raven, J. C. (1941). Standardization of progressive matrices, 1938. *British Journal of Medical Psychology, 19,* 137–150.

Rholes, W. S., & Pryor, J. B. (1982). Cognitive accessibility and causal attributions. *Personality and Social Psychology Bulletin, 8,* 719–727.

Ridderinkhof, K. R., Ullperger, M., Crone, A. E., & Nieuwenhuis, S. (2004). Role of the medial frontal cortex in cognitive control. *Science, 306,* 443–447.

Ridderinkhof, K. R., van den Wildenberg, W. P. M., Segalowitz, S. J., & Carter, C. S. (2004). Neurocognitive mechanisms of cognitive control: The role of prefrontal cortex in action selection, response inhibition, performance, monitoring, and reward-based learning. *Brain and Cognition, 56,* 129–140.

Riketta, M., & Dauenheimer, D. (2003). Anticipated success at unconscious goal pursuit: Consequences for mood, self-esteem, and the evaluation of a goal-relevant task. *Motivation and Emotion, 27,* 327–338.

Rude, S., Zentner, M., & Morrow, D. (1993, August). *Building a model of attention regulation relevant to depressive memory impairments.* Paper presented at the annual convention of the American Psychological Society, Montreal.

Sayette, M. A., & Hufford, M. R. (1994). Effects of cue exposure and deprivation on cognitive resources in smokers. *Journal of Abnormal Psychology, 103,* 812–818.

Scheffers, M. K., & Coles, M. G. H. (2000). Performance monitoring in a confusing world: Error-related brain activity, judgments of response accuracy, and types of errors. *Journal of*

Experimental Psychology: Human Perception and Performance, 1, 141–151.

Scheier, M. F., & Carver, C. S. (1988). A model of behavioral self-regulation: Translating intention into action. In L. Berkowitz (Ed.), *Advances in experimental social psychology: Vol. 21. Social psychological studies of the self: Perspectives and programs* (pp. 303–346). San Diego, CA: Academic Press.

Shah, J. (2003). Automatic for the people: How representations of significant others implicitly affect goal pursuit. *Journal of Personality and Social Psychology, 84,* 661–681.

Shah, J. Y., Kruglanski, A. W., & Friedman, R. S. (2003). Goal systems theory: Integrating the cognitive and motivational aspects of self-regulation. In S. J. Spencer, S. Fein, M. P. Zanna, & M. A. Olson (Eds.), *Motivated social perception: The Ontario symposium, Vol. 9* (pp. 247–275). Mahwah, NJ: Lawrence Erlbaum Associates.

Shiffrin, R. M., & Dumais, S. T. (1981). The development of automatism. In J. R. Anderson (Ed.), *Cognitive skills and their acquisition* (pp. 111–140). Hillsdale, NJ: Lawrence Erlbaum Associates.

Shiffrin, R. M., & Schneider, W. (1977). Controlled and automatic human information processing: II. Perceptual learning, automatic attending, and general theory. *Psychological Review, 84,* 127–190.

Singer, J. L. (1966). *Daydreaming.* New York: Random House.

Singer, J. L. (1975). Navigating the stream of consciousness: Research in daydreaming and relate inner experience. *American Psychologist, 30,* 727–738.

Srull, T. K., & Wyer, R. S. (1980). Category accessibility and social perception: Some implications for the study of person memory and interpersonal judgments. *Journal of Personality and Social Psychology, 38,* 841–856.

Wegner, D. M. (1994). Ironic processes of mental control. *Psychological Review, 101,* 34–52.

Wegner, D. M. (1997). When the antidote is the poison: Ironic mental control processes. *Psychological Science, 8,* 148–150.

Wegner, D. M., & Bargh, J. A. (1998). Control and automaticity in social life. In S. T. Fiske & D. T. Gilbert, (Eds.), *The handbook of social psychology* (pp. 446–496). New York: McGraw-Hill.

Wegner, D. M., & Erber, R. (1992). The hyperaccessibility of suppressed thoughts. *Journal of Personality and Social Psychology, 63,* 903–912.

Wegner, D. M., Schneider, D. J., Carter, S. R., & White, T. L. (1987). Paradoxical effects of thought suppression. *Journal of Personality and Social Psychology, 53,* 5–13.

Wegner, D. M., & Wenzlaff, R. M. (1996). Mental control. In E. T. Higgins & A. W. Kruglanski (Eds.), *Social psychology: Handbook of basic principles* (pp. 466–492). New York: Guilford Press.

Wiener, N. (1948). *Cybernetics; or control and communication in the animal and the machine.* Oxford: Wiley.

Williams, C. W. (1993). The effect of priming causal dimensional categories on social judgments. *Social Cognition, 11,* 223–242.

Wolfe, C. T., & Crocker, J. (2002). What does the self want? A contingencies of self-worth perspective on motivation. In S. S. Z. Kunda (Ed.), *The Ontario Symposium: Goals and motivated cognition* (pp. 147–170). Hillsdale, NJ: Lawrence Erlbaum Associates.

Wright, R. A. (1996). Brehm's theory of motivation as a model of effort and cardiovascular response. In J. A. Bargh & P. M. Gollwitzer (Eds.), *The psychology of action: Linking cognition and motivation to behavior* (pp. 424–453). New York: Guilford Press.

Wrosch, C., Scheier, M. F., Miller, G. E., Schulz, R., & Carver, S. C. (2003). Adaptive self-regulation of unattainable goals: Goal disengagement, goal reengagement, and subjective well-being. *Personality and Social Psychology Bulletin, 29,* 1494–1508.

Zeigarnik, B. (1938). On finished and unfinished tasks. In W. D. Ellis (Ed.), *A source book of gestalt psychology* (pp. 300–314). New York: Harcourt Brace & World. (Reprinted and condensed from *Psychologische Forschung, 9,* 1927, 1–85.)

Zwaan, R. A., & Truitt, T. P. (1998). Smoking urges affect language processing. *Experimental and Clinical Psychopharmacology, 6,* 325–330.

Living on the Edge: Shifting Between Nonconscious and Conscious Goal Pursuit

Peter M. Gollwitzer, Elizabeth J. Parks-Stamm, *and* Gabriele Oettingen

Abstract

This chapter discusses recent research exploring how shifts between conscious, controlled processing and automaticity affect goal pursuit. It begins by reviewing past approaches to nonconscious goal pursuit, including the search for both similarities between conscious and nonconscious goal pursuit and differences between the two. It then addresses the consequences of shifting between conscious and nonconscious goal striving, and the question of whether people can strategically shift from effortful, controlled goal striving to automaticity through forming implementation intentions.

Keywords: goal-directed behavior, controlled processing, automaticty, nonconcious goal pursuit, goal striving

This chapter discusses recent research exploring how shifting between conscious, controlled processing, and automaticity affect goal pursuit. First, we review past approaches to nonconscious goal pursuit, including both the search for similarities between conscious and nonconscious goal pursuit and differences between the two. We next address the consequences of shifting between conscious and nonconscious goal striving. We start by addressing the shift from nonconscious goal pursuit to conscious awareness. What is the consequence of becoming aware of a behavior driven by a nonconscious goal pursuit? We then address the question of whether people can strategically plan to shift from effortful, controlled goal striving to automaticity through forming implementation

intentions. How is this achieved, and what are the consequences of this strategic shift to automatic goal striving?

Conscious Versus Nonconscious Goal Pursuit
The Origins of the Distinction Between Conscious and Nonconscious Goal Pursuit

The descriptions of successful goal pursuit have changed drastically in the history of psychology (Gollwitzer & Moskowitz, 1996; Oettingen & Gollwitzer, 2001). *Behaviorists* (e.g., Skinner, 1953) defined goal striving objectively, from the perspective of the researcher rather than from the perspective of the actor. Accordingly, they focused on the observable features of goal striving; effective goal striving was defined as being associated with persistence (striving until the goal is reached), appropriateness (when one path to the goals is blocked, an alternative path to the same goal is taken), and searching (restlessness in the presence of good opportunities to meet the goal). Facilitating goal attainment according to this tradition involved shaping behavior related to these features by using classic and instrumental conditioning principles.

Cognitive social learning theorists (e.g., Bandura, 1977; Heckhausen, 1977; Mischel, 1973), on the other hand, focused on the internal subjective goal of the individual as the reference point for goal striving. Successful goal striving now required conscious involvement in goal pursuit, committing to proper goals, and effectively guiding their implementation. From this perspective, strong goal commitments are assumed to be formed when the given goal is both desirable and feasible (Ajzen, 1985; Chapter 5); thus, the person should first consult his or her needs and motives to determine the desirability of the potential goal (Brunstein, Schultheiss, & Graessmann, 1998) and then reflect on his or her own relevant skills, talents, and competencies, as well as facilitating or hindering external influences, to compute the likelihood that goal-related outcomes may actually be obtained. This type of reflection should require conscious processing.

Recent research shows that even the mode of thought with which these issues are approached (e.g., mentally contrasting the desired future with the obstacles of present reality versus only dreaming about a positive future or only dwelling on the negative reality) makes a difference; high-feasibility beliefs are translated into strong goal commitments most effectively when one mentally contrasts the desired future with obstacles of present reality (Oettingen, Pak, & Schnetter, 2001). Recent research also shows that it matters how the desired goal

state is framed. Conceptualizing one's goals in terms of promoting positive outcomes as opposed to preventing negative outcomes (promotion versus prevention goals; Higgins, 1997), acquiring competence as opposed to demonstrating the possession of competence (learning versus performance goals; Dweck, 1999), and attaining external as opposed to internal rewards (extrinsic versus intrinsic goals; Ryan & Deci, 2000) affect goal attainment; promotion, learning, and intrinsic conceptualizations are commonly associated with better outcomes than prevention, performance, and extrinsic conceptualizations. Even the degree of precision with which the desired outcome is spelled out (e.g., the time frame and standards of quantity and quality for its completion) affects a person's chances to reach the desired goal. Goals with a proximal as compared to a more distal time frame (or deadline) are more likely achieved, and it is the goals with specific rather than "do your best" standards that lead to better performances (Locke & Latham, 2002).

But goal attainment cannot be secured solely by forming strong goal commitments and framing the goals at hand in an appropriate manner (Gollwitzer, 1990, 2006). There is the second issue of implementing a chosen goal, meaning that people need to successfully tackle a series of implementational issues. There are four problems that stand out for goal implementation: getting started with goal pursuit, staying on track, calling a halt, and not overextending oneself (Gollwitzer & Sheeran, 2006). Getting started with goal pursuit is often difficult because we are busy with other things and thus fail to detect, attend to, and remember to use good opportunities to act toward the chosen goal. Even if the presence of a good opportunity is detected, we are often too slow to seize it in time and thus fail to initiate goal-directed behaviors. Once we do get started with goal-directed actions, we face the problem of staying on track. Persevering becomes difficult when distractions mount (particularly very tempting distractions; Mischel, Shoda, & Rodriguez, 1989; Chapter 23), when forced disruptions demand the resumption of goal-directed activity (Gollwitzer & Liu, 1995; Mahler, 1933), and when increases in the difficulty of the task demand more effort expenditure (Wright, 1996). Moreover, successful goal implementation requires that we call a halt to using a chosen means or route to goal attainment if this means (or route) lacks instrumentality (Kruglanski, 1996), and it demands disengagement from goal pursuit altogether if the originally desired goal turns into something unattractive or unfeasible (Klinger, 1977). Finally, goals cannot be implemented successfully if we overextend ourselves when striving for the goal at hand. People commonly hold more than one goal, and exceeding one's limitations in the pursuit of the goal at hand can be a disadvantage with respect to the successful implementation of the other goals one is also holding (i.e., ego-depletion effect; Muraven & Baumeister, 2000). From the perspective of cognitive social learning theory, all these problems can be tackled by engaging in conscious self-regulatory thought. For instance, it has been observed that delay of gratification is enhanced when the rewards at issue are thought of in an abstract (as opposed to concrete) manner (Metcalfe & Mischel, 1999).

In most recent history, the psychology of goals has been enriched by the assertion that people's thoughts, feelings, and actions might be affected not only by conscious but also by nonconscious goal striving. In his auto-motive model, Bargh (1990) built on *automaticity* research of the 1970s and especially 1980s that demonstrated the automatic activation capability of social mental representations, such as trait concepts

(e.g., honest or aggressive), attitudes, and group stereotypes (reviews by Bargh, 1989; Brewer, 1988; Wegner & Bargh, 1998; Chapter 9). This research showed that frequently used mental representations will, over time, become active when relevant information is encountered in the environment. For stereotypes, relevant cues may include easily identifiable group features, such as skin color, gender, accent, and so on. For attitudes, an environmental trigger could be the mere presence of the attitude object in the environment (Fazio, 1986). For trait concepts, features of observed social behaviors corresponding to the trait in question could activate these representations (Uleman, Newman, & Moskowitz, 1996).

The principle underlying these cases of automatic process development was that automatic associations are formed between the representations of environmental features (such as attitude objects or common situations and settings) and other representations (such as evaluations or stereotypes, respectively) to the extent that they are consistently active in memory at the same time (Hebb, 1948; Chapter 20). If one repeatedly and consistently thinks of members of a particular social group in stereotypic ways, for instance, then eventually the stereotype would become active automatically in the presence of a member of that group (Bargh, 1989; Brewer, 1988). Under the assumption that goals, too, are represented mentally and become automatically activated by the same principles, goal representations should also be capable of automatic activation through contact with features of the contexts in which those goals have been pursued often and consistently in the past (Chapter 21). If, for a given individual, interaction with one's colleagues usually leads to competitive behavior, then the goal of competition should become automatically activated in the mere presence of a colleague.

In other words, a competition goal should become active even though the person may not intentionally and consciously choose to compete at that time and in that situation. The auto-motive model further asserts that once activated in this unconscious manner, the goal representation should then operate in the same way as when it is consciously and intentionally activated. That is, the model predicts that an automatically activated goal would have the same effects on thought, feelings, and behavior as when the person consciously pursues that same goal (i.e., as when the goal is activated by an act of conscious will).

First-Generation Research on Nonconscious Goal Pursuit: Searching for Similarities to Conscious Goal Pursuit

It is often implicitly assumed that successful goal pursuit necessitates conscious involvement. Sometimes this assumption is even expressed explicitly. For instance, Dehaene and Naccache (2001) suggest that consciousness is required for three important mental operations: the maintenance of information over time (i.e., beyond the immediate perception), the planning and enactment of novel strategies, and the generation of intentional, goal-directed behaviors. This claim raises the question of whether the theoretical derivations on which the auto-motive model rests are actually unfounded. Accordingly, first-generation experimental research on the auto-motive model focused on the following questions: Can we observe effects on thoughts, feelings, and behaviors by implicitly activated (primed) goals? And is automatic goal pursuit characterized by the same features as is conscious goal pursuit?

The aim of first-generation research on nonconscious goal pursuit was to document the similarities between conscious and nonconscious goal pursuit (summaries

by Chartrand, Dalton, & Cheng, 2007; Gollwitzer & Bargh, 2005). For example, based on an early study (Hamilton, Katz, & Leirer, 1980) showing that individuals with a conscious impression-formation goal recalled information in a more organized way than those with a memorization goal, Chartrand and Bargh (1996) primed participants with these processing goals through exposure to goal-related words within scrambled sentences. Again, they found that those primed with impression-formation goal-related words were more likely to organize these behaviors by categories than those primed with a memorization goal. Subsequent research has shown that nonconscious activation of other goals, including achievement goals (Bargh, Gollwitzer, Lee-Chai, Barndollar, & Trötschel, 2001, studies 1 and 2), egalitarian goals (Moskowitz, Gollwitzer, Wasel, & Schaal, 1999), interpersonal goals (Fitzsimons & Bargh, 2003), and the goals of significant others (Shah, 2003), results in the cognition and behavior expected from conscious goal pursuit.

In addition to behavioral outcomes, nonconsciously activated goals exhibit the motivational qualities traditionally considered to be characteristics of conscious goal striving (Gollwitzer, 1990; Lewin, 1951). Using paradigms designed to elucidate these classic goal characteristics, Bargh et al. (2001) found that the activation of nonconsciously activated goals increased in strength over time until acted on (study 3), produced persistence when obstacles were encountered (study 4), and brought about resumption of goal-directed behaviors following interruption (study 5). Thus, these studies suggest that nonconscious priming activates goals themselves, resulting in cognition, behavior, and goal-relevant motivational qualities in line with consciously set goals. Kawada, Oettingen, Gollwitzer, and Bargh (2004) even observed that the projection of one's own goals on others holds for conscious and nonconscious goals alike.

The activation of goals does not occur only through semantic primes in the laboratory; relevant goals can also be activated outside of awareness by objects and individuals in the environment. Significant others can activate the goals that they have for you (Shah, 2003), or they can activate the goals that you normally pursue when you encounter these individuals (Fitzsimons & Bargh, 2003). For example, Fitzsimons and Bargh (study 1) approached individuals waiting at the gate in an airport and asked them to answer a few questions about either a friend or a colleague. Activating the representation of a friend in this way activated the goals that participants normally pursue with these individuals (e.g., helping), leading to more offers to help the experimenter following the activation of a friend than a colleague. Other individuals can also nonconsciously activate goals through a process known as "goal contagion." Aarts, Gollwitzer, and Hassin (2004) demonstrated that a goal can be nonconsciously activated merely through the presence of others enacting a behavior that implies that goal (Chapter 26). However, goal contagion took place only when the goal was contextually and socially appropriate. This research illustrates that goals can be nonconsciously activated by the mere presence of others, a social trigger of a personal nonconscious goal pursuit.

In line with this approach of highlighting the similarities between conscious and nonconscious goal pursuit, Chartrand (1999) has suggested that the emotional consequences of success or failure at conscious and nonconscious goal pursuits do not differ either. Chartrand (1999, in Chartrand et al., 2007) primed participants with words related to an achievement goal (or neutral words) and then led them

to either succeed or fail in a subsequent task. Those who had been primed with the goal to achieve reported being in a better mood following success than those who had not been primed with a goal, whereas those who failed following goal priming reported being in a worse mood than those who had not been primed with a goal. This work demonstrates the similarities between the emotional consequences of completed conscious and nonconscious goal pursuit, with successful versus unsuccessful completion of nonconscious goal pursuits leading to the emotional consequences expected from conscious goal pursuits.

Second-Generation Research on Nonconscious Goal Pursuit: Potential Differences From Conscious Goal Pursuit

Although there is ample evidence now that there are many similarities between conscious and nonconscious goal pursuit, recent research has begun to investigate the differences between goal striving resulting from conscious versus nonconscious goal activation (Gollwitzer et al., 2006). The relative advantages of conscious versus nonconscious goal pursuit can be inferred by looking at theoretical approaches to conscious versus nonconscious mental operations in other fields. For instance, Dijksterhuis's unconscious thought theory (Dijksterhuis, 2004; Dijksterhuis & Nordgren, 2006) distinguishes between processes associated with conscious and nonconscious thought in decision making. This theory proposes a number of principles regarding conscious and nonconscious thought; we focus on two of these principles here that are most relevant to potential differences between conscious and nonconscious goal pursuit. The first, the capacity principle, proposes that whereas conscious thought is limited by capacity (i.e., conscious decision makers must focus on a limited numbers of features), unconscious thought may incorporate many more factors in a decision (Dijksterhuis & Nordgren, 2006).

THE CAPACITY ISSUE

The capacity principle is particularly relevant to goal striving because conscious self-regulation draws from a limited resource that can be depleted. Thus, conscious goal striving should be limited by capacity as well. Ego-depletion studies (Muraven & Baumeister, 2000) demonstrate that engaging in self-control with respect to a first task deleteriously affects performance on a subsequent task that also necessitates self-control to attain a good performance. The capacity principle therefore suggests that conscious goal striving should be hurt by being in a state of ego depletion more so than nonconscious goal striving, and striving consciously should lead to more ego depletion than striving nonconsciously. At least for the first conclusion there is some evidence. A recent study by Govorun and Payne (2006) looked at the effects of ego depletion on the automatic versus the controlled components of self-regulation. After performing an ego depletion task designed to drain self-regulatory resources, participants completed the weapon identification task, in which they had to identify whether an object was a weapon after seeing briefly presented black or white faces (Payne, 2001). Using the process dissociation procedure (Jacoby, 1991), Govorun and Payne found that ego depletion affected the controlled component of the response but did not affect automatic race bias in the subsequent weapon identification task. Although this does not directly address the hypothesis that nonconscious goal striving should be less affected by ego depletion than conscious goal striving, it does suggest that automatic self-regulatory processes are less affected by ego depletion than controlled processes. Further research

could expand on these findings, examining whether nonconscious goal striving is indeed less limited by capacity than conscious goal striving and whether nonconscious goal striving produces less ego depletion than conscious goal striving.

THE REFLECTIVE VERSUS REFLEXIVE CONTROL ISSUE

A second principle from Dijksterhuis's unconscious thought theory, the bottom-up-versus-top-down principle (Dijksterhuis & Nordgren, 2006), also sheds light on possible differences between conscious and nonconscious goal striving. In line with Sloman (1996), Dijksterhuis argues that conscious processing is hierarchical, and conscious thought is therefore more driven by broad concepts and schemas (Chapter 5). Nonconscious processing, on the other hand, integrates information in a summative fashion. It makes sense that nonconscious goal striving (i.e., striving without awareness of a goal) would work in much the same way. Whereas conscious striving is performed in reference to the conceived goal, nonconscious striving would presumably proceed in a more stimulus-driven, bottom-up manner. Gollwitzer, Parks-Stamm, and Oettingen (2008) found evidence for this assumption. In one study, a newly developed goal conflict paradigm was used. Participants performed a very simple classification task. They were asked to indicate by pressing a right or a left button whether a flashed stimulus (i.e., a string of letters) was presented either in the dark-colored area of the computer screen or in the light-colored area (both areas were equally large but intertwined). The classification task goals of being either accurate or fast were either induced outside of conscious awareness (i.e., the letter strings functioned as masks to the subliminally presented words of either "accurate" or "fast") or consciously set (i.e., assigned by the experimenter), resulting in four initial goal conditions. After more than 100 trials, a nonconscious goal of being either accurate or fast was then activated by subliminal priming in the participants of all four conditions while they performed a second set of more than 100 classification trials.

As participants' classification responses showed hardly any errors (i.e., the classification task indeed was easy to perform), their classification response times for the second set of trials were used as the dependent variable of classification performance. When both the first and the second goal activation occurred outside of awareness, the combination of the two goals followed a straightforward additive pattern such that the accurate–accurate combination led to the slowest classification responses, followed by the two conflict conditions (i.e., accurate–fast and fast–accurate), with the fast–fast goal condition resulting in the fastest responses. However, individuals who adopted the first goal explicitly (consciously) failed to show this same summative pattern. They instead evidenced a conflict pattern in response to the second nonconsciously activated goal. The two conflicting combinations (accurate–fast and fast–accurate) resulted in the slowest reaction times, and the two matching combinations (accurate–accurate and fast–fast) resulted in the fastest reaction times.

These findings illustrate that activating goals consciously versus nonconsciously can have a differential impact on subsequent cognitive processing. These findings suggest that conscious and nonconscious goal striving have different processing characteristics, with conscious goal striving resulting in reflective thought guided by the conscious awareness of the goal (or goals) at hand, leading to attempts to integrate conflicting behavioral tendencies, and non-

conscious goal striving resulting in more bottom-up reflexive processing that deals with conflicting behavioral tendencies in a summative manner.

Because conscious goal pursuit seems to be driven by top-down processes, with goal striving achieved with reference to the activated goal, Gollwitzer et al. (2008) also hypothesized and tested in a further study that awareness of one's goal should be beneficial to participants when flexibility is needed in terms of switching to a more appropriate means to the goal. Participants were first given a conscious or nonconscious goal to perform well (or no goal at all). They were then confronted with a series of "water jar" problems, a classic task to assess flexibility in problem solving (Luchins, 1942; Luchins & Luchins, 1994). These problems each involved three water jars labeled with volumes (jars A, B, and C); participants were asked to add or subtract the volume of each jar to come up with a given outcome volume (with the volumes changing for each trial). The first eight trials had the same solution (B − A − 2C), the next two trials (i.e., trials 9 and 10) could be solved either by the original formula or by a more simple solution (i.e., A − C or A + C, respectively), and the 11th trial could be solved only by the solution of A − C.

The findings indicated that in the first eight trials, participants in both the conscious and the nonconscious achievement goal conditions were faster to find the correct solution than the control group. Thus, both conscious and nonconscious goals were successful in improving task performance. In trial 9, where an easier solution was also possible (A − C), no differences between groups were observed, as only 8% of the participants discovered this new solution. However, when the results of trial 10 were analyzed, a significantly higher percentage of participants in the conscious goal condition discovered the possible easier solution (35%) as compared to the nonconscious goal condition (9%) and the control condition (9%). Finally, with respect to trial 11, where only the easier new solution was possible (A − C), all participants discovered this solution. Importantly, when we looked at how fast participants found this correct solution, those in the conscious goal group were significantly faster than both participants in the nonconscious goal group and those in the no-goal control group. These findings strongly suggest that being consciously aware of a goal is beneficial for switching means to attain the goal, either when easier means become available or when the old means no longer promote goal attainment. We argue that being consciously aware of the goal to perform well instigated a more intensive and/or effective search for alternative means as compared to being unaware of the high-performance goal.

DOES PERSONALITY MODERATE PERFORMANCE RESULTING FROM NONCONSCIOUS VERSUS CONSCIOUS GOAL STRIVING?

Whether conscious versus nonconscious goal striving facilitates performance may also depend on attributes of the individual. Parks-Stamm, Gollwitzer, and Oettingen (2008) looked at individual differences related to choking under pressure (i.e., test anxiety and reinvestment) in individuals pursuing performance goals activated consciously or nonconsciously. We hypothesized that these individual differences would predict costs for consciously adopted achievement goals, but not nonconsciously activated achievement goals. In a first study, for individuals high in test anxiety, conscious awareness of the goal to perform well was damaging to their performance in a memory test, whereas for those low in test anxiety, it was beneficial to performance (study 1). This finding suggests that

it may be more beneficial for those high in test anxiety to nonconsciously strive for performance goals, whereas those low in test anxiety may benefit from consciously adopting achievement goals.

In a second study, we tested the idea that *reinvestment,* an individual difference associated with the tendency to exert conscious control over skilled behaviors (Masters, Polman, & Hammond, 1993), would predict costs in typing speed when accuracy goals where consciously adopted but not when nonconsciously activated. The results obtained suggested that trait reinvestment was associated with costs in typing speed only when the accuracy goal was consciously adopted but not when nonconsciously activated. These two studies reported by Parks-Stamm, Gollwitzer, and Oettingen (2008) illustrate that person factors must be taken into account in order to make valid predictions about whether conscious or nonconscious goal striving is more effective for goal attainment.

Shifting Between Conscious and Nonconscious Goal Pursuit

The nature of the experimental designs used in research on nonconscious goal pursuit (i.e., nonconsciously priming goal constructs versus consciously adopting goals) has led researchers to examine these two forms of goal pursuit in isolation from or in opposition to each other. In reality, however, during goal pursuit individuals shift back and forth seamlessly between conscious and nonconscious processing. Dehaene and Naccache (2001) review evidence from functional magnetic resonance imaging research demonstrating that neural structures associated with conscious control engage and disengage from processing as they are (or are not) needed. For example, Raichle et al. (1994) found that prefrontal cortex and anterior cingulate activity (often present when conscious guidance is needed) "is present during initial task performance, vanishes after the task has become automatized, but immediately recovers when novel items are presented" (Dehaene & Naccache, 2001, p. 24). In addition, it seems that even if task (or goal) performance has not yet been habitualized, simply distracting a person with an unrelated activity after they have started to work on the focal goal (e.g., trying to select a car from a set of four cars that differ in attractiveness; Dijksterhuis, 2004; Dijksterhuis, Bos, Nordgren, & van Baaren, 2006) may lead goal-directed cognitions to depart from consciousness to return at a later point in time (e.g., when new information is discovered on the choice objects or one's own relevant values or competencies are considered). Given the possibility of shifting from nonconscious goal pursuit to conscious goal pursuit and the other way around, we discuss research on the consequences of these two shifts for goal pursuit—starting with the return of consciousness to nonconscious goal pursuit and then turning to the departure of consciousness from conscious goal pursuit.

Shifting From Nonconscious to Conscious Goal Pursuit: When Consciousness Returns

Under what circumstances does consciousness return to control nonconscious goal striving? Numerous explanations have been given to explain why consciousness returns to a previously unmonitored goal pursuit. The German psychologist Theodor Lipps (1851–1914) addressed this issue in his "Gesetz der psychischen Stauung" (Law of Psychological Blockage). He characterized goal striving as a stream of water that flows unaided until it encounters an obstacle (a *Stau*, or dam). When habitual and unmonitored behavior is blocked by the obstacle, consciousness emerges to interpret the behavior in

order to overcome the obstacle (for a summary, see Arievitch & Van der Veer, 2004). Thus, in this model, consciousness returns to interpret nonconscious goal-directed behavior when an obstacle is encountered; indeed, Lipps suggests that "it is only then that the person becomes consciously aware of what he or she is doing and can start to consciously pursue a goal" (Arievitch & Van der Veer, 2004, p. 158). That consciousness is summoned by obstacles to nonconscious goal striving makes sense given Gollwitzer et al.'s (2008) findings that conscious awareness of a goal seems to improve one's ability to switch to a more suitable means in goal pursuit (see above). Similarly, Bongers and Dijksterhuis (Chapter 28) argue that we become aware of our goals consciously when we experience failure in our goal striving. They report a number of studies in which failure causes conscious awareness of nonconsciously pursued goals. In addition, consciousness may return to goal pursuit when goals conflict, and higher-level processes are therefore needed to solve this conflict (Morsella, 2005; Chapter 30). Thus, consciousness appears to return when nonconscious goal striving is disrupted and consciousness is needed to overcome an obstacle or failure.

Consciousness can also return to nonconscious goal pursuit when one is consciously questioned about the purpose of goal-directed behaviors. Gazzaniga (2000) has demonstrated that consciousness returns to a goal pursuit initiated outside of awareness when an actor is questioned about what he or she is trying to accomplish, thereby engaging conscious interpretation through conscious questioning. We suggest this interpretation may be simple when the goal driving that behavior was originally adopted consciously (i.e., when a conscious goal pursuit recedes into nonconsciousness through automation). However, when the goal driving one's behavior is outside of awareness, this interpretation can be more difficult.

THE INTERPRETATION OF NONCONSCIOUS GOAL PURSUIT

We propose that consciousness may return to an ongoing nonconscious goal pursuit when an obstacle is encountered, disrupting automaticity and requiring an interpretation of one's behavior. When the goal is adopted consciously, the interpretation of one's goal-directed behavior is easily achieved. Individuals only have to remember their earlier conscious setting of the goal at hand; the interpretation of one's actions should be possible even if individuals have been distracted while acting on the goal (e.g., by the occurrence of irrelevant internal or external events). In their Rubicon model of action phases, Heckhausen and Gollwitzer (1987; Gollwitzer, 1990) have described interpretive efforts after goal striving as characteristic of the postactional evaluative phase of goal pursuit.

However, when goals have been activated nonconsciously, interpretation of one's goal-directed behavior should be more difficult. Interpretation does often occur even when the cause is not consciously accessible. It is widely accepted that many cognitive processes are outside of conscious awareness, and therefore individuals often cannot report accurately on higher mental processes in trying to explain their behavior (Nisbett & Wilson, 1977). Indeed, the dissonance literature is based on the idea that individuals are motivated to interpret their behavior and that they often erroneously assign internal attributions as the cause of their externally affected behavior, as they underestimate the power of the experimenter's influence on their behavior (for a discussion of how easily people are tricked into assuming free choice, see Wicklund & Brehm, 1976). Nisbett and Wilson (1977) report a number of studies where dissonance researchers asked their participants why they acted the way they did; participants gave false explanations for their behavior (e.g., when unable to sleep after taking what was said to be a relaxation pill, participants responded that they "usually found it easier to get to sleep later in the day"; p. 238). Thus, there is evidence that individuals form ad hoc causal theories to explain their behavior when the cause is not obvious. One fruitful source of such explanations is social norms.

Because social norms often provide a default explanation for behavior, acting in a way that violates social norms demands an explanation for one's behavior. When an explanation for one's behavior cannot be found, this triggers negative emotion and guilt. This response has been demonstrated by research on emotional responses to accidental harmdoing. When one causes harm accidentally, one is faced with an abrupt norm violation that has no salient explanation. For such an accidental act, justification as a guilt-reduction technique is not possible (McGraw, 1987), and thus the common consequence is the experience of negative affect. Relating this line of research to nonconscious goal pursuit, it follows that negative emotions should be more likely to result from norm-violating behaviors that are based on nonconsciously activated goals rather than conscious goals. With nonconscious goals, the actor faces a lack of reasons for his or her norm-violating actions, as they have occurred without conscious intent.

Accordingly, Oettingen, Grant, Smith, Skinner, and Gollwitzer (2006) have argued that when goals are not consciously adopted (i.e., are nonconsciously activated) and not explained by the situational context (i.e., are norm violating), actors will find themselves in an "explanatory vacuum" when attempting to interpret their own behavior, which in turn will lead to the experience of negative affect. In their study, participants had to work with a "fellow student" on interpreting pictures from the Thematic Apperception Test. Participants were asked to give feedback on the story offered by their presumed partner, which gave an unusual interpretation of a picture of a boy looking at a violin (i.e., "he's training to be a magician"). Before starting on this task, they were either consciously or nonconsciously compelled to form the goal to cooperate (a norm-conforming goal) or compete (a norm-violating goal). Following this goal-setting procedure, participants responded to the partner's unusual interpretation. Regardless of whether the goal to compete was consciously adopted or nonconsciously activated, the feedback given by participants with a norm-violating goal was rated as more combative.

Oettingen et al. (2006) then asked participants to report on their current emotions. When the activated goal was norm conforming (i.e., to be accommodating in the collaborative task), awareness of the goal did not affect participants' emotional response to their own behavior. Presumably, those with the nonconscious goal explained their behavior by taking cues from the environment and interpreting their behavior in line with the norms of the situation. However, participants pursuing the goal that caused them to act in a norm-violating way (i.e., to be confrontational in the collaborative task) reported more negative affect when the goal was activated nonconsciously than when it was set consciously. These participants whose norm-violating goal had been activated nonconsciously found themselves in an explanatory vacuum, unable either to link their behavior to a consciously set goal (because they were unaware of this goal activation) or to explain it by the norms of the situation. As suggested by McGraw (1987), those who were unable to justify their behavior based

on either their conscious goal or social norms felt more negative affect.

Further research has examined this explanatory vacuum notion. How can a goal-directed behavior be interpreted when the actual goal of that behavior is outside of conscious awareness, as in the case of nonconscious goal pursuit? In line with evidence from brain-damaged patients illustrating the reflex-like automatic interpretation of behavior, Parks-Stamm, Oettingen, and Gollwitzer (2008) hypothesized that providing participants with an unrelated (but reasonable) explanation for norm-violating behavior would eliminate the negative emotions associated with an explanatory vacuum. We created an experimental paradigm where participants completed two tasks. In the first task, participants were explicitly given the goal to be either fast or accurate. This goal to be fast or accurate (i.e., slow) was borne out in the completion of the first task. In the second task, participants were given the conscious or nonconscious goal to compete or cooperate in a task where competing required acting faster (i.e., a "compete" goal was achieved by scoring points more quickly) and cooperating required acting slower (i.e., a "cooperate" goal was achieved by sharing the points by acting more slowly). Thus, individuals who had a nonconscious goal to compete (i.e., the "explanatory vacuum" condition) had consciously adopted an earlier goal that either could explain this behavior (i.e., was applicable) or could not (i.e., was inapplicable).

Parks-Stamm, Oettingen, and Gollwitzer (2008) found that the negative affect associated with an explanatory vacuum was observed only for those who had a first conscious goal to be accurate (i.e., the first goal did not explain their fast, norm-violating behavior in the second task). Those whose competitive (norm-violating) behavior could be attributed to their earlier conscious goal to be *fast* felt as positive as those with either a conscious or a nonconscious norm-conforming goal. These findings suggest that when automatically activated behavior creates an explanatory need, other goals with congruent behavioral effects can reduce the explanatory vacuum and its associated negative affect.

In a further study on this issue, we examined whether conscious reflection about one's norm-violating behavior was necessary for participants to explain their behavior via this earlier applicable goal. Using just the explanatory vacuum condition (i.e., when a competitive goal was activated nonconsciously), we varied both whether the first goal explained the norm-deviant behavior (again using an earlier conscious goal to be either fast or accurate on a separate task) and whether participants were given time to reflect on the cause of their norm-violating behavior (driven by a nonconscious goal to compete in the second task). In the reflection condition, participants were asked a number of questions about their performance (e.g., What were you thinking about during the task? What were you trying to accomplish? Why?) before completing the self-report measures regarding their emotions. The no reflection participants immediately reported on their emotions at the completion of the second task. We found that providing a time for reflection had no effect on the reduction of the explanatory vacuum found when an earlier goal could explain the norm-violating behavior; whether participants were asked to reflect on their behavior or not, an earlier conscious goal to be fast effectively reduced the negative affect associated with an explanatory vacuum. This suggests that the attempt to reduce an explanatory vacuum when acting in a norm-violating way in response to a nonconsciously activated goal is automatic and reflex-like.

In a third study, Parks-Stamm et al. (2008) examined the behavioral consequences of successfully or unsuccessfully interpreting goal striving in an explanatory vacuum by examining lottery tickets shared with a partner, as well as the impact of individual differences on interpretation and tickets shared. Based on the findings of an earlier study suggesting that conscious reflection was not necessary for interpretation (see above), we expected Need for Cognition (NFC, Cacioppo, Petty, & Kao, 1984) would not interact with the applicability of the earlier goal to predict tickets shared. However, we expected the Preference for Consistency scale (PFC; Cialdini, Trost, & Newsom, 1995) would interact with the applicability of the earlier goal to predict interpretation (and tickets shared). In line with these predictions, we found that PFC was associated with greater sharing when participants first had an accuracy goal (as they were motivated to reduce the negative affect associated with an explanatory vacuum with an inapplicable earlier goal). We also found that PFC was associated with sharing less tickets when participants first had a speed goal, which could be used to explain their competitive behavior and thereby eliminated the motivation to help one's partner. NFC, on the other hand, did not interact with the first goal. These findings suggest that there are both individual differences associated with the interpretation of nonconsciously-activated goal-directed behavior and behavioral consequences of interpretation in an explanatory vacuum.

SUMMARY

Early work (e.g., Chartrand, 1999) suggested that the emotional consequences of conscious and nonconscious goal pursuit would not differ, and this is certainly true when it comes to emotions that are linked to goal attainment, such as feelings of pride after success and feelings of shame after failure. However, when goal-directed behavior that is triggered by nonconscious goal activation breaks norms, this creates an explanatory vacuum. This explanatory vacuum is associated with negative affect for those individuals who are unable to unearth a plausible explanation for their behavior. Thus, norm-breaking nonconscious goal pursuit can produce negative affect when conscious understanding of the resultant behavior is stymied by lack of goal awareness, particularly when an alternative explanation cannot be found. The presented explanatory vacuum research explores the return of consciousness to nonconscious goal pursuit. The departure of consciousness from conscious goal pursuit is the other shift that we are concerned with and that we turn to in the next section.

Shifting From Conscious to Nonconscious Goal Pursuit: The Departure of Consciousness

In principle, there are three types of shifts from conscious to nonconscious goal pursuit. The first is explicated in Dijksterhuis's experiments on nonconscious thought (Dijksterhuis, 2004; Dijksterhuis et al., 2006). The person who has consciously adopted a goal and started to act on it becomes distracted with an irrelevant activity and thus loses conscious sight of the goal and the ongoing striving for it. This shift has the positive consequence that complex information becomes more easily digested, and in turn the quality of complex decisions is improved.

The second type of shift from conscious to nonconscious goal pursuit is more effortful. William James (1842–1940) states, "If an act require for its execution a chain, *A, B, C, D, E, F, G,* etc . . . then in the first performances of the action the conscious will must choose each of these events from a number of wrong alternatives that tend to present themselves; but habit soon brings it about that each event calls up its own

appropriate successor without any alternative offering itself, and without any references to the conscious will, until at last the whole chain . . . rattles itself off as soon as A occurs" (James, 1890, p. 114). James saw the value of shifting from conscious to nonconscious acting in saving mental energy: "the more of the details of our daily life we can hand over to the effortless custody of automatism, the more our higher powers of mind will be set free for their own proper work" (p. 122). James's view that consciousness plays a role early in the process and then becomes less necessary has received a lot of theoretical and empirical attention by subsequent researchers. Bargh's (1990) automotive theory follows the logic of James's chain of successive events that eventually "rattle off" as soon as the first is encountered.

A third type of shift from conscious to nonconscious goal pursuit has been described by Gollwitzer (1993, 1999). He proposes that by making if–then plans (i.e., implementation intentions) that specify a critical situational cue (e.g., a good opportunity) in the "if" part and an instrumental goal-directed response (e.g., getting started on the goal) in the "then" part, a person can switch the conscious control of goal striving from a top-down (by the subjective goal) to a bottom-up (by situational stimuli) mode. Given that strong if–then links are formed in the person's mind, the execution of the goal-directed behavior is expected to acquire features of automaticity (i.e., immediacy, efficiency, and redundancy of conscious intent once the critical situation is encountered). Therefore, forming implementation intentions has been referred to as creating instant habits and the automaticity of action control by implementation intentions has been referred to as strategic automaticity. But what is the experimental evidence for these assumptions?

IF—THEN PLANS: IMMEDIACY AND EFFICIENCY OF ACTION CONTROL

Gollwitzer and Brandstätter (1997, study 3) demonstrated the immediacy of action initiation in a study where participants had been induced to form implementation intentions that specified viable opportunities for presenting counterarguments to a series of racist remarks made by a confederate. It was found that participants with implementation intentions initiated their counterargument more quickly than the participants who had formed the mere goal intention to counterargue. In further experiments (Brandstätter, Lengfelder, & Gollwitzer, 2001, studies 3 and 4), the efficiency of action initiation was explored. All participants formed the goal intention to press a button as fast as possible if numbers appeared on the computer screen but not if letters were presented (go/no-go task). Participants in the implementation intention condition also made the plan to press the response button particularly fast if the number 3 was presented. This go/no-go task was then embedded as a secondary task in a dual-task paradigm. Implementation intention participants showed a substantial increase in speed of responding to the number 3 compared to the control group regardless of whether the simultaneously demanded primary task (a memorization task in study 3 and a tracking task in study 4) was either easy or difficult to perform. This suggests that the immediacy of responding induced by implementation intentions is also efficient in the sense that it does not require much in the way of cognitive resources (i.e., can be performed even when dual tasks have to be performed at the same time). The following additional observations further support this claim: Response times to noncritical numbers in the implementation intention condition were the same as in the goal condition, response times to noncritical numbers in the implementation intention

condition did not differ between practice and test trials (after the implementation intention had been formed), and performance on the load task (a memory test in study 3 and tracking performance in study 4) was the same in the goal-only and the implementation intention conditions. A more recent study by Parks-Stamm, Gollwitzer, and Oettingen (2007) also demonstrated efficiency of action control by implementation intentions.

Parks-Stamm et al. (2007, study 2) examined the efficiency of implementation intentions by creating a task with both planned and unplanned means to a desired goal. In this task, participants' goal was to identify words starting with a D in an auditorily presented story and to type the number of letters of that word into the computer as quickly as possible. Thus, this was a task where executing the behavior specified in the "then" component of the implementation intention was particularly difficult. All participants were given the two most common words ("Danny" and "dragon"), and the number of letters in each word (five and six, respectively). However, only half the participants formed an implementation intention with this information (i.e., "If I hear the word 'Danny,' then I will immediately press the 5; if I hear the word 'dragon,' then I will immediately press the 6."), whereas the others only memorized the critical words and responses. We predicted that if implementation intentions were efficient, enacting the response specified in the "then" component of the implementation intention at a higher rate would require little cognitive capacity. The efficiency of the planned response would be shown if implementation intentions allowed participants to enact the planned response more than those with only a goal, but without a cost in the number of alternative means used to reach the goal (relative to the goal-only condition). This hypothesis was supported (see

Figure 29.1). Implementation intentions effectively facilitated the planned response but did not hamper the initiation of alternative, unplanned responses. This suggests that implementation intentions efficiently facilitate planned routes to the goal (i.e., without burdening cognitive resources) so that alternative goal-directed responses are not impaired.

But the immediacy and efficiency of action control by implementation intentions can be also tested by using a quite different angle. By (a) assuming that action control by implementation intentions is immediate and efficient and (b) adopting a simple racehorse model of action control, people can be expected to be in a position to break habitualized responses by forming implementation intentions (i.e., if–then plans that spell out a response that is contrary to the habitualized response to the critical situation). Such studies have been conducted successfully in the field (Holland, Aarts, & Langendam, 2006) but also in the laboratory (Cohen, Bayer, Jaudas, & Gollwitzer, 2008).

Holland et al. (2006) addressed whether implementation intentions could help break unwanted habits (and replace them with new wanted behaviors) in a field experiment in an institution. The goal of the researchers was to increase the use of recy-cling bins for plastic cups and paper and to reduce the bad habit of throwing out these recyclable items in personal wastebaskets. Participants were randomly assigned to one of six conditions: a no-treatment control condition, a control condition with a behavior report questionnaire, a facility condition where each participant received his or her own recycle bin, a combined facility and questionnaire condition, and two implementation intention conditions—one with a personal facility and one without. Recycling behavior was substantially improved in the facility as well as in the implementation intentions conditions in week 1 and week 2 and still 2 months after the manipulation. In addition, the correlation between past and future behavior was strong in the control conditions, whereas these correlations were nonsignificant and close to zero in the implementation intention conditions. Apparently, implementation intentions effectively broke old habits by facilitating new recycling behavior. This shows that even strongly habitualized behaviors can be replaced by new planned goal-directed behaviors via implementation intentions.

Cohen et al. (2008, study 2) explored the suppression of habits in a more controlled laboratory experiment using the

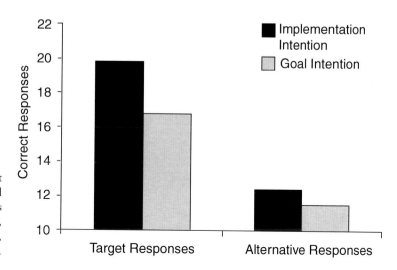

Fig. 29.1 Mean correct target and alternative responses by goal condition when letter counting is required for response initiation, based on Parks-Stamm, Gollwitzer, & Oettingen (2007, study 2).

Simon task. In this paradigm, participants are asked to respond to a nonspatial aspect of a stimulus (e.g., whether a tone is high or low) by pressing a left or right key and to ignore the location of the stimulus (e.g., if it is presented on the left or on the right side). The difficulty of this task is in ignoring the spatial location (left or right) of the tone in one's response (Simon & Berbaum, 1990). The cost in reaction time is seen when the location of the tone (e.g., right) and required key press (e.g., left) are incongruent. Cohen et al. (2008) found that implementation intentions eliminated the Simon effect for the stimulus that was specified in the implementation intention. Reaction times for the critical (planned) stimulus did not differ between the congruent and incongruent trials.

Automatic biases and stereotyping represent another habitualized pattern of thought and behavior that can be in opposition to one's goals. Although one may have the goal to be egalitarian, automatic stereotyping happens quickly and unintentionally; some attempts to control automatic stereotyping has even resulted in backfire effects (e.g., Payne, Lambert, & Jacoby, 2002). Extending earlier work by Gollwitzer and Schaal (1998), Stewart and Payne (in press) examined whether implementation intentions designed to counter automatic stereotypes (e.g., "when I see a black face, I will then think 'safe'") could reduce stereotyping toward a category of individuals (versus a single exemplar). They used the process dissociation procedure (Jacoby, 1991) to estimate whether the reduction in automatic stereotyping came about by reducing automatic stereotyping, increasing control, or a combination of these two processes. It was found that implementation intentions reduced stereotyping in a weapon identification task (studies 1 and 2) and an Implicit Association Test (IAT) (study 3) by reducing automatic effects of the stereotype (without

increasing conscious control). This reduction in automatic race bias held for even new members of the category (study 2). These studies suggest that implementation intentions are an efficient way to overcome automatic stereotyping.

REDUNDANCY OF CONSCIOUS INTENT

Research by Bayer, Achtziger, Gollwitzer, and Moskowitz (in press) has tested the hypothesis that—once the critical cue specified in the "if" part of an implementation intention is encountered—a conscious intention to perform the response specified in the "then" component of an if–then plan is not necessary to facilitate response initiation. This was done by presenting the critical cue specified in the "if" part subliminally and assessing whether such subliminal presentation still managed to facilitate response initiation. Study 1 showed that the subliminal presentation of a cue (in this case, the experimenter) increased the accessibility of words needed for the execution of their planned goal-directed behavior toward the experimenter (i.e., expressing a complaint about unfriendly behavior). In study 2, Bayer et al. investigated whether the subliminal presentation of the specified cue facilitated the actual performance of the planned action. Participants were asked to categorize geometrical target figures as either angular (e.g., triangles and squares) or round (e.g., circles and ovals). Participants in the implementation intention condition memorized the if–then plan: "If I see a triangle, then I will press the right key particularly fast!" Goal-intention participants were familiarized with the triangle shape by drawing it three times on a piece of paper. Then either the triangle or a neutral shape (i.e., the percent sign) was subliminally presented as a prime before the target figures (to be classified). The speed with which the target figures were categorized was the dependent variable of the study. It was found that the subliminal presentation of the triangle (i.e., the critical cue specified in the implementation intention) resulted in faster classification responses to congruent trials (i.e., the classification of the triangle and other angular figures) among the implementation-intention participants only. This suggests that the response specified in the implementation intention is initiated automatically on contact with the situational cue, even if one has not consciously processed this cue.

IMPLEMENTATION INTENTIONS IN THE BRAIN

In their gateway hypothesis of rostral prefrontal cortex (area 10) function, Burgess, Simons, Dumontheil, and Gilbert (2007; see also Burgess, Dumontheil, et al., 2007) suggest a distinction between action control that is primarily triggered by low-level stimulus input and action control that is guided primarily by higher-level goal representations. In a host of studies using different kinds of executive function tasks, they observed in a meta-analysis that stimulus-driven, bottom-up action control is associated with medial area 10 activity, whereas goal-driven, top-down action control is associated with lateral area 10 activity. Accordingly, Gilbert, Gollwitzer, Cohen, Oettingen, and Burgess (2008) postulated that action control by implementation intentions should by characterized by medial area 10 activity, whereas action control by mere goals should be associated with lateral area 10 activity.

To test this hypothesis, we used a prospective memory (PM) paradigm. Such PM tasks require participants to perform an ongoing task (e.g., a lexical decision task or a classification task) but remember to also perform an additional response (i.e., the PM response, e.g., pressing the space bar) whenever a particular stimulus

is presented within the ongoing task (e.g., a particular word or a particular constellation of the stimuli to be classified). In the Gilbert et al. (2007) study, each participant had to perform two different prospective memory tasks, one with a goal intention to perform the PM responses and the other with an implementation intention to perform these responses. As it turned out (see Figure 29.2), implementation intentions facilitated the performance of PM responses as compared to mere goal intentions, and this gain in performance did not lead to any additional costs in performing the ongoing task. Even more important, PM performance based on a goal intention was accompanied by greater lateral area 10 activity, whereas PM performances based on implementation intentions were associated with greater activity in the medial area 10. Moreover, the difference in brain activity associated with correctly responding to PM targets under goal versus implementation intentions correlated strongly and significantly with the behavioral difference as a consequence of acting on the basis of goal versus implementation intentions. The fact that acting on implementation intentions is associated with medial area 10 activity whereas acting on goal intentions is associated with lateral area 10 activity adds further support to our theory that by forming implementation intentions, people can switch from goal striving that is guided by conscious top-down control to direct, stimulus-triggered goal striving.

SUMMARY

There are at least three ways in which consciousness may depart from goal pursuit: distraction, habituation, and if–then planning. We have focused on this third approach and described research on the consequences of if–then planning. This research

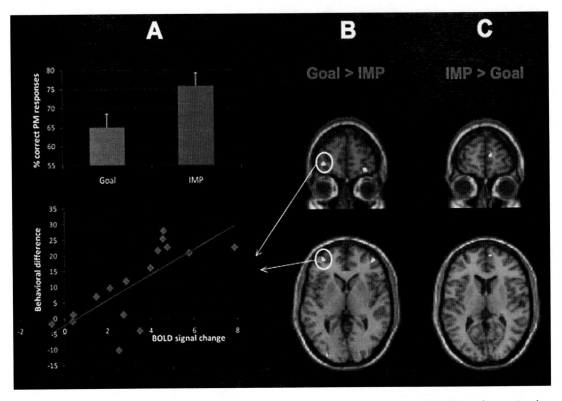

Fig. 29.2 Comparisons between the goal-intention ("Goal") and implementation-intention ("IMP") conditions. Panel A, top: Percentage of correctly detected prospective memory (PM) targets in the two conditions. Panel A, bottom: Correlation between the difference in BOLD signal in left lateral BA 10 elicited by correctly detected PM targets in the two conditions (horizontal axis) and the behavioral difference between the two conditions (vertical axis). Panel B: Brain regions showing greater target-related activity in the goal-intention condition compared with the implementation-intention condition, plotted on coronal ($y = 56$) and axial ($z = 2$) slices of a normalized T1-weighted scan. Panel C: Brain regions showing greater target-related activity during the implementation-intention condition compared with the goal-intention condition (plotted at $y = 60$ and $z = 10$).

shows that if–then plans that specify critical anticipated situations in the "if" part and instrumental goal-directed responses in the "then" part automate goal striving. The subjective goal and its respective top-down processes no longer control one's goal striving; rather, goal-directed action becomes immediate, efficient, and redundant of conscious intent (i.e., shows features of automaticity). That forming implementation intentions can indeed be used to switch from top-down to bottom-up control of goal-directed action is also supported by the observed changes in brain activity in the area 10 (i.e., from lateral area 10 activity to medial area 10 activity). This is not to say, however, that implementation intentions may not also be used to facilitate switching from reflexive to more reflective forms of action control. In a recent study on escalation of commitment, Henderson, Gollwitzer, and Oettingen (2007) showed that implementation intentions that specify a reflection response in their "then" part achieve the necessary switch from impulsive escalation of commitment (i.e., failing to disengage from a lost course of action) to taking a more reflective stance that prevents sunk cost behavior.

Conclusion

In this chapter, we have arrived at the view that conscious and nonconscious goal pursuit are two collaborative partners taking turns in working toward goal attainment. Whereas historically research has focused on conscious and nonconscious goal striving in comparison to each other—how are they alike? how are they different?—we have investigated when and with what consequences conscious and nonconscious goal pursuit come to the forefront. People are "living on the edge," shifting between conscious and nonconscious processes in their quest to effectively and efficiently reach their goals. We discussed shifting in both directions: when conscious awareness returns to automatic striving, and when automaticity replaces conscious, controlled striving. The shift from automatic goal striving to conscious awareness has intrigued psychologists for more than a century. In 1906, Lipps described consciousness returning to aid nonconscious goal pursuit when the flow (like a river) collided with an obstacle. In this chapter, we focused on our research examining the explanatory vacuum that emerges when consciousness cannot easily explain nonconsciously triggered goal pursuit by referring to relevant norms. Finally, we examined the planned shift to automaticity achieved through implementation intentions. By forming if–then plans that automate a goal-directed response to an anticipated cue, individuals may willingly shift from effortful, controlled processing to nonconscious goal striving.

References

Aarts, H., Gollwitzer, P. M., & Hassin, R. R. (2004). Goal contagion: Perceiving is for pursuing. *Journal of Personality and Social Psychology, 87,* 23–37.

Ajzen, I. (1985). From intentions to actions: A theory of planned behavior. In J. Kuhl & J. Beckman (Eds.), *Action-control: From cognition to behavior* (pp. 11–39). Heidelberg: Springer.

Arievitch, I. M., & Van der Veer, R. (2004). The role of nonautomatic processes in activity regulation: From Lipps to Galperin. *History of Psychology, 7,* 154–182.

Bandura, A. (1977). *Social learning theory.* Oxford: Prentice Hall.

Bargh, J. A. (1989). Conditional automaticity: Varieties of automatic influence in social perception and cognition. In J. S. Uleman & J. A. Bargh (Eds.), *Unintended thought* (pp. 3–51). New York: Guilford Press.

Bargh, J. A. (1990). Auto-motives: Preconscious determinants of social interactions. In E. T. Higgins & R. M. Sorrentino (Eds.), *Handbook of motivation and cognition* (Vol. 2, pp. 93–130). New York: Guilford Press.

Bargh, J. A., Gollwitzer, P. M., Lee-Chai, A., Barndollar, K., & Trötschel, R. (2001). The automated will: Nonconscious activation and pursuit of behavioral goals. *Journal of Personality and Social Psychology, 81,* 1014–1027.

Bayer, U. C., Achtziger, A., Gollwitzer, P. M., & Moskowitz, G. B. (in press). Strategic automaticity by implementation intentions: Action initiation without conscious intent. *Social Cognition.*

Brandstätter, V., Lengfelder, A., & Gollwitzer, P. M. (2001). Implementation intention and efficient action initiation. *Journal of Personality and Social Psychology, 81,* 946–960.

Brewer, M. B. (1988). A dual process model of impression formation. In T. K. Srull & R. S. Wyer Jr. (Eds.), *Advances in social cognition* (Vol. 1, pp. 1–36). Hillsdale, NJ: Lawrence Erlbaum Associates.

Brunstein, J. C., Schultheiss, O. C., & Graessman, R. (1998). Personal goals and emotional well-being: The moderating role of motive dispositions. *Journal of Personality and Social Psychology, 75,* 494–508.

Burgess, P. W., Dummontheil, I., Gilbert, S. J., Okuda, J., Schölvinck, M. L., & Simons, J. S. (2007). On the role of rostral prefrontal cortex (area 10) in prospective memory. In M. Kliegel, M. A. McDaniel, & G. O. Einstein (Eds.), *Prospective memory: Cognitive, neuroscience, developmental, and applied perspectives* (pp. 235–260). Mahwah, NJ: Lawrence Erlbaum Associates.

Burgess, P. W., Simons, J. S., Dumontheil, I., & Gilbert, S. J. (2007). The gateway hypothesis of rostral prefrontal cortex (area 10) function. In J. Duncan, L. Phillips, & P. McLeod (Eds.), *Measuring the mind: Speed, control, and age* (pp. 217–248). Oxford: Oxford University Press.

Cacioppo, J. T., Petty, R. E., & Kao, C. F. (1984). The elicent assessment of need for cognition. *Journal of Personality Assessment, 48,* 306–307.

Ciadini, R. B., Trost, M. R., & Newsom, J. T. (1995). Preference for consistency: The development of a valid measure and the discovery of surprising behavioral implications. *Journal of Personality and Social Psychology, 69,* 318–328.

Chartrand, T. L. (1999). *Mystery moods and perplexing performance: Consequences of succeeding and failing at a nonconscious goal.* Unpublished doctoral dissertation, New York University.

Chartrand, T. L., & Bargh, J. A. (1996). Automatic activation of impression formation and memorization goals: Nonconscious goal priming reproduces effects of explicit task instructions. *Journal of Personality and Social Psychology, 71,* 464–478.

Chartrand, T. L., Dalton, A. N., & Cheng, C. M. (2007). The antecedents and consequences of nonconscious goal pursuit. In J. Shah & W. Gardner (Eds.), *Handbook of motivation science* (pp. 342–355). New York: Guilford Press.

Cohen, A-L., Bayer, U. C., Jaudas, A., & Gollwitzer, P. M. (2008). Self-regulatory strategy and executive control: Implementation intentions modulate task switching and Simon Task performance. *Psychological Research, 72,* 12–26.

Dehaene, S., & Naccache, L. (2001). Towards a cognitive neuroscience of consciousness: Basic evidence and a workspace framework. *Cognition, 79,* 1–37.

Dijksterhuis, A. (2004). Think different: The merits of unconscious thought in preference development and decision making. *Journal of Personality and Social Psychology, 87,* 586–598.

Dijksterhuis, A., Bos, M. W., Nordgren, L. F., & van Baaren, R. B. (2006). On making the right choice: The deliberation-without-attention effect. *Science, 311,* 1005–1007.

Dijksterhuis, A., & Nordgren, L. F. (2006). A theory of unconscious thought. *Perspectives on Psychological Science, 1,* 95–109.

Dweck, C. S. (1999). *Self-theories: Their role in motivation, personality, and development.* Philadelphia: Psychology Press.

Fazio, R. H. (1986). How do attitudes guide behavior? In R. M. Sorrentino & E. T. Higgins (Eds.), *Handbook of motivation and cognition: Foundations of social behavior* (pp. 204–243). New York: Guilford Press.

Fitzsimons, G. M., & Bargh, J. A. (2003). Thinking of you: Nonconscious pursuit of interpersonal goals associated with relationship partners. *Journal of Personality and Social Psychology, 84,* 148–164.

Gazzaniga, M. S. (2000). Cerebral specialization and interhemispheric communication: Does the corpus collosum enable the human condition? *Brain, 123,* 1293–1326.

Gilbert, S. J., Gollwitzer, P. M., Cohen, A.-L., Oettingen, G., & Burgess, P. W. (2008). *Separable brain systems supporting realization of future goals versus if-then plans.* Manuscript submitted for publication.

Gollwitzer, P. M. (1990). Action phases and mind-sets. In R. M. Sorrentino & E. T. Higgins (Eds.), *Handbook of motivation and cognition* (Vol. 2, pp. 53–92). New York: Guilford Press.

Gollwitzer, P. M. (1993). Goal achievement: The role of intentions. *European Review of Social Psychology, 4,* 141–185.

Gollwitzer, P. M. (1999). Implementation intentions: Strong effects of simple plans. *American Psychologist, 54,* 493–503.

Gollwitzer, P. M. (2006). Successful goal pursuit. In Q. Jing, H. Zhang, & K. Zhang (Eds.), *Progress in psychological science around the world* (Vol. 1, pp. 143–159). Philadelphia: Psychology Press.

Gollwitzer, P. M., & Bargh, J. A. (2005). Automaticity in goal pursuit. In A. Elliot & C. Dweck (Eds.), *Handbook of competence and motivation* (pp. 624–646). New York: Guilford Press.

Gollwitzer, P. M., & Brandstätter, V. (1997). Implementation intentions and effective goal pursuit. *Journal of Personality and Social Psychology, 73,* 186–199.

Gollwitzer, P. M., & Liu, C. (1995). Wiederaufnahme [Resumption]. In J. Kuhl & H. Heckhausen (Eds.), *Enzyklopaedie der Psychologie: Teilband C/IV/4. Motivation, Volition und Handlung* (pp. 209–240). Goettingen: Hogrefe.

Gollwitzer, P. M., & Moskowitz, G. B. (1996). Goal effects on action and cognition. In E. T. Higgins & A. W. Kruglanski (Eds.), *Social psychology: Handbook of basic principles* (pp. 361–399). New York: Guilford Press.

Gollwitzer, P. M., Parks-Stamm, E.J., & Oettingen, G. (2006, January). *Differential consequences of implicit and explicit goals.* Paper presented at the annual meeting of the Society for Personality and Social Psychology, Palm Springs, CA.

Gollwitzer, P. M., Parks-Stamm, E. J., & Oettingen, G. (2008). *Conscious and nonconscious goal pursuit: Differences in terms of top-down vs. bottom-up processing.* Manuscript in preparation.

Gollwitzer, P. M., & Schaal, B. (1998). Meta-cognition in action: The importance of implementation intentions. *Personality and Social Psychology Review, 2,* 124–136.

Gollwitzer, P. M., & Sheeran, P. (2006). Implementation intentions and goal achievement: A meta-analysis of effects and processes. *Advances in Experimental Social Psychology, 38,* 69–119.

Govorun, O., & Payne, K. B. (2006). Ego-depletion and prejudice: Separating automatic and controlled processes. *Social Cognition, 24,* 111–136.

Hamilton, D. L., Katz, L. B., & Leirer, V. O. (1980). Organizational processes in impression formation. In R. Hastie, T. M. Ostrom, E. B. Ebbesen, R. S. Wyer, D. L. Hamilton, & D. E. Carlston (Eds.), *Person memory: The cognitive biases of social perception* (pp. 121–153). Hillsdale, NJ: Lawrence Erlbaum Associates.

Hebb, D. O. (1948). *Organization of behavior.* New York: Wiley.

Heckhausen, H. (1977). Achievement motivation and its constructs: A cognitive model. *Motivation and Emotion, 1,* 283–329.

Heckhausen, H., & Gollwitzer, P. M. (1987). Thought contents and cognitive functioning in motivational versus volitional states of mind. *Motivation and Emotion, 11,* 101–120.

Henderson, M. D., Gollwitzer, P. M., & Oettingen, G. (2007). Implementation intentions and disengagement from a failing course of action. *Journal of Behavioral Decision Making, 20,* 81–102.

Higgins, E. T. (1997). Beyond pleasure and pain. *American Psychologist, 52,* 1280–1300.

Holland, R. W., Aarts, H., & Langendam, D. (2006). Breaking and creating habits on the working floor: A field-experiment on the power of implementation intentions. *Journal of Experimental Social Psychology, 42,* 776–783.

Jacoby, L. L. (1991). A process dissociation framework: Separating automatic from intentional uses of memory. *Journal of Memory and Language, 20,* 513–541.

James, W. (1890). *The principles of psychology.* Oxford: Holt.

Kawada, C. L. K., Oettingen, G., Gollwitzer, P. M., & Bargh, J. A. (2004). The projection of implicit and explicit goals. *Journal of Personality and Social Psychology, 86,* 545–559.

Klinger, E. (1977). *Meaning and void: Inner experience and the incentives in people's lives.* Minneapolis: University of Minnesota Press.

Kruglanski, A. W. (1996). Motivated social cognition: Principles of the interface. In E. T. Higgins & A. W. Kruglanski (Eds.), *Social psychology: Handbook of basic principles* (pp. 493–520). New York: Guilford Press.

Lewin, K. (1951). *Field theory in social science: Selected theoretical papers.* New York: Harper & Row.

Locke, E. A., & Latham, G. P. (2002). Building a practically useful theory of goal setting and task motivation. *American Psychologist, 57,* 705–717.

Luchins, A. S. (1942). Mechanization in problem solving. *Psychological Monographs, 54.*

Luchins, A. S., & Luchins, E. H. (1994). The water jar experiments and Einstellung effects. Part II: Gestalt psychology and past experience. *Gestalt Theory, 16,* 205–270.

Mahler, W. (1933). Ersatzhandlungen verschiedenen Realitatsgrades. *Psychologische Forschung, 18,* 27–89.

Masters, R. S., Polman, R. C., & Hammond, N. V. (1993). "Reinvestment": A dimension of personality implicated in skill breakdown under pressure. *Personality and Individual Differences, 14,* 655–666.

McGraw, K. M. (1987). Guilt following transgression: An attribution of responsibility approach. *Journal of Personality and Social Psychology, 53,* 247–256.

Metcalfe, J., & Mischel, W. (1999). A hot/cool-system analysis of delay of gratification: Dynamics of willpower. *Psychological Review, 106,* 3–19.

Mischel, W. (1973). Toward a cognitive social learning reconceptualization of personality. *Psychological Review, 80,* 252–283.

Mischel, W., Shoda, Y., & Rodriguez, M. L. (1989). Delay of gratification in children. *Science, 244,* 933–938.

Morsella, E. (2005). The function of phenomenal states: Supramodular interaction theory. *Psychological Review, 112,* 1000–1021.

Moskowitz, G. B., Gollwitzer, P. M., Wasel, W., & Schaal, B. (1999). Preconscious control of stereotype activation through chronic egalitarian goals. *Journal of Personality and Social Psychology, 77,* 167–184.

Muraven, M., & Baumeister, R. F. (2000). Self-regulation and depletion of limited resources: Does self-control resemble a muscle? *Psychological Bulletin, 126,* 247–259.

Nisbett, R. E., & Wilson, T. D. (1977). Telling more than we can know: Verbal reports on mental processes. *Psychological Review, 84,* 231–259.

Oettingen, G., & Gollwitzer, P. M. (2001). Goal setting and goal striving. In A. Tesser & N. Schwarz (Eds.), *Blackwell handbook of social psychology: Intraindividual processes* (pp. 329–347). Oxford: Blackwell.

Oettingen, G. Grant, H., Smith, P. M., Skinner, M., & Gollwitzer, P. M. (2006). Nonconscious goal pursuit: Acting in an explanatory vacuum. *Journal of Experimental Social Psychology, 42,* 668–675.

Oettingen, G., Pak, H., & Schnetter, K. (2001). Self-regulation of goal-setting: Turning free fantasies about the future into binding goals.

Journal of Personality and Social Psychology, 80, 736–753.

Parks-Stamm, E. J., Gollwitzer, P. M., & Oettingen, G. (2007). Action control by implementation intentions: Effective cue detection and efficient response initiation. *Social Cognition, 25,* 248–266.

Parks-Stamm, E. J., Gollwitzer, P. M., & Oettingen, G. (2008). *Nonconscious goal activation: Protection from choking under pressure.* Manuscript in preparation.

Parks-Stamm, E. J., Oettingen, G., & Gollwitzer, P. M. (2008). *Making sense of one's actions in an explanatory vacuum: The interpretation of nonconscious goal striving* Manuscript submitted for publication.

Payne, B. K. (2001). Prejudice and perception: The role of automatic and controlled processes in misperceiving a weapon. *Journal of Personality and Social Psychology, 81,* 181–192.

Payne, B. K., Lambert, A. J., & Jacoby, L. L. (2002). Best laid plans: Effects of goals on accessibility bias and cognitive control in race-based misperceptions of weapons. *Journal of Experimental Social Psychology, 38,* 384–396.

Raichle, M. E., Fiez, J. A., Videen, T. O., Macloed, A. M., Pardo, J. V., Fox, P. T., et al. (1994). Practice-related changes in human brain functional anatomy during non-motor learning. *Cerebral Cortex, 4,* 8–26.

Ryan, R. M., & Deci, E. L. (2000). Self-determination theory and the facilitation of intrinsic motivation, social development, and well-being. *American Psychologist, 55,* 68–78.

Shah, J. Y. (2003). Automatic for the people: How representations of significant others implicitly affect goal pursuit. *Journal of Personality and Social Psychology, 84,* 661–681.

Simon, J. R., & Berbaum, K. (1990). Effect of conflicting cues on information processing: The "Stroop effect" vs. the "Simon effect." *Acta Psychologica, 73,* 159–170.

Skinner, B. F. (1953). *Science and human behavior.* Oxford: Macmillan.

Sloman, S. A. (1996). The empirical case for two systems of reasoning. *Psychological Bulletin, 119,* 3–22.

Stewart, B. D., & Payne, B. K. (in press). Bringing automatic stereotyping under control: Implementation intentions as an efficient means of thought control. *Personality and Social Psychology Bulletin.*

Uleman, J. S., Newman, L. S., & Moskowitz, G. B. (1996). People as flexible interpreters: Evidence and issues from spontaneous trait inferences. In M. P. Zanna (Ed.), *Advances in experimental social psychology* (Vol. 28, pp. 211–279). San Diego, CA: Academic Press.

Wegner, D. M., & Bargh, J. A. (1998). Control and automaticity in social life. In D. T. Gilbert, S. T. Fiske, & G. Lindzey (Eds.), *The handbook of social psychology* (Vol. 2, pp. 446–496). New York: McGraw-Hill.

Wicklund, R. A., & Brehm, J. W. (1976). *Perspectives on cognitive dissonance.* Oxford, England: Lawrence Erlbaum.

Wright, R. A. (1996). Brehm's theory of motivation as a model of effort and cardiovascular response. In P. M. Gollwitzer & J. A. Bargh (Eds.), *The psychology of action: Linking cognition and motivation to behavior* (pp. 424–453). New York: Guilford Press.

The Primary Function of Consciousness: Why Skeletal Muscles Are "Voluntary" Muscles

Ezequiel Morsella, Stephen C. Krieger, *and* John A. Bargh

Abstract

This chapter attempts to illuminate what consciousness *is* by examining why one is aware of some nervous system events (e.g., pain and the urge to breath or eat) but not others (e.g., intersensory interactions, peristalsis, and the pupillary reflex). It is argued that conscious states serve a basic and specific, nuts-and-boltsy function in the nervous system, one that is intimately related to the actions of, specifically, skeletal muscle.

Keywords: conscious state, skeletal muscle, awareness, nervous system

Although there is usually a sharp, intuitively obvious distinction between unconscious action and actions that are consciously intended, drawing a principled distinction between the two kinds of processes is less than straightforward. On close examination, unconscious processes prove to be no less complex, flexible, deliberative, controlling, or action-like than their conscious counterparts (see review in Bargh & Morsella, 2008). For example, as repeatedly illustrated in the chapters in this book, action plans can be activated, selected, and, in some cases, expressed without conscious mediation. Given what the nervous system can achieve without recourse to consciousness

(reviewed here), what, if anything, does the state of "being aware" contribute to human action? Would actions be limited in some way without it?

Answering this question depends on identifying the primary function of conscious states—those elusive phenomena falling under the rubrics of "phenomenal states," "qualia," "awareness," "sentience," or "subjective experience." These real, physical, but somewhat intangible phenomena have proven to be difficult to pin down. Faced with them, a scientist is comforted by Karl Popper's adage that *defining* something is the end product and not the beginning of scientific inquiry. For now, the best working definition has been put forth by the philosopher Thomas Nagel (1974), who proposed that an organism has conscious states if there is *something it is like* to be that organism—something it is like, for example, to be human and experience pain, breathlessness, or yellow afterimages.

Many regard the functional role of conscious states to be an unexplained, fundamental aspect of the human experience (Banks, 1995; Crick & Koch, 2003; Donald, 2001; Sherrington, 1906; Sperry, 1952):

The problem of consciousness occupies an analogous position for cognitive psychology as the problem of language behavior does for behaviorism, namely, an unsolved anomaly within the domain of the approach. (Shallice, 1972, p. 383)

In this final chapter,[1] we attempt to illuminate what consciousness *is* by examining why one is aware of some nervous system events (e.g., pain and the urge to breath or eat) but not others (e.g., intersensory interactions, peristalsis, and the pupillary reflex). Thereafter, we propose that conscious states serve a basic and specific, nuts-and-boltsy function in the nervous system, one that is intimately related to the actions of, specifically, skeletal muscle.

Acknowledging the Unacknowledgeable: Impenetrable Processes

Complex processes including the pupillary reflex, peristalsis, digestion, breathing, and other "vegetative" organismic actions occur deep beneath the horizon of consciousness. To one, these actions certainly do not *feel* like venerable forms of action, but they are actions nonetheless, at least from an objective point of view. It is important to appreciate that, to an intelligent nonhuman observer (e.g., an imaginary, extraterrestrial ethologist), events such as the pupillary reflex would be worthy of being "coded" and jotted down as actions on an observation log. To an observer that is agnostic regarding our internal states, the pupillary reflex would appear as action-like as the movements of a finger (Skinner, 1953).

From "input" to "output," the mediation of these highly complex actions is *consciously impenetrable*. For instance, under normal circumstances, one is unaware of whether the pupillary reflex or peristalsis is taking place. Knowledge of these actions comes only from some form of roundabout, scientific inquiry. For example, one can learn of the pupillary reflex from reading a textbook, observing others, or from carrying out an experiment using

one's reflection in still water. (Without the presence of others, the latter would be the only method by which one could have observed this action before the advent of mirrors.) Although profoundly unconscious (indeed, it can be elicited in comatose patients; Klein, 1984), the reflex is far from simple.[2] As with other "vegetative" actions, the more that is learned about it, the less unintelligent the action becomes.

One is conscious of several aspects of "voluntary" actions (e.g., their associated urges and perceptual products; Gray, 2004), but many of their component processes too are consciously impenetrable. For example, foraging and hunting are predicated on consciously impenetrable mechanisms, including the complex processes in motor control (Chapter 6; Rosenbaum, 2002) and low-level perceptual analyses (e.g., motion detection, color, and auditory analyses; Zeki & Bartels, 1999).

Regarding the sophistication of unconscious processing, one must also acknowledge the sheer cleverness of the fast motor acts displayed during a tennis match or a piano recital—in which the input → output arc unfolds too quickly to be mediated consciously (Gray, 1995, 2004; Lashley, 1951; Libet, 2004)—and appreciate the theoretical importance of basic neurological findings. It is well documented that behaviors of notable complexity can occur unconsciously in forms of coma, seizures, and persistent vegetative states, in which patients can behave as if awake but possess no consciousness (Klein, 1984; Laurey, 2005). In addition, without consciousness, licking, chewing, swallowing, and other consummatory behaviors can occur automatically once the incentive stimulus activates the appropriate receptors (Bindra, 1974; Kern, Jaredeh, Arndorfer, & Shaker, 2001). Following other kinds of brain injury in which a general awareness is spared, actions can be decoupled from consciousness, as in *blind sight* (Weiskrantz, 1997). In this condition, patients report to be blind but still exhibit visually guided behaviors (see also Goodale & Milner, 2004, and *blind smell;* Sobel et al., 1999).

In conclusion, there exists substantial evidence that the unconscious is not identifiably less flexible, complex, controlling, deliberative, or action-like than its counterpart (Bargh & Morsella, 2008). With this knowledge at hand, one reencounters the question, What does the state of "being aware" contribute to action?

The Integration Consensus

Regarding the primary function of conscious states, many hypotheses have been proposed (Block, 1995; Dickinson & Balleine, 2000; Hobson, 2000; Jack & Shallice, 2001; Mandler, 1998).[3] A recurring idea in recent theories is that these states somehow integrate neural activities and information-processing structures that would otherwise be independent. This notion, referred to as the *integration consensus* (Morsella, 2005), has now resurfaced in diverse areas of research. The idea is that conscious states allow diverse kinds of information to be gathered in some sort of global workspace (Baars, 2002; Merker, 2007). From this standpoint, the response to a painful stimulus (e.g., when carrying a hot plate of food) is consciously mediated because an adaptive response depends on taking several different kinds of information into account (e.g., the need for food and the extent of tissue damage; Morsella, 2005). Despite its complexity, such overarching considerations are not made for unconscious processes such as the pupillary reflex and peristalsis.

However, it has remained unclear exactly which kinds of information must be distributed and integrated in a conscious manner and which kinds can be distributed and integrated unconsciously. Obviously not all

kinds of information are capable of being distributed globally (e.g., neural activity related to vegetative functions, reflexes, unconscious motor programs, low-level perceptual analyses, and so on) and many kinds can be disseminated and combined with other kinds without conscious mediation, as in the case of intersensory processing. For example, the McGurk effect (McGurk & MacDonald, 1976) involves interactions between visual and auditory processes: An observer views a speaker mouthing "ba" while presented with the sound "ga." Surprisingly, the observer is unaware of any intersensory interaction, perceiving only "da." Similar consciously impenetrable interactions are exemplified in countless intersensory phenomena (see Morsella, 2005, app. A), including the popular ventriloquism effect, in which visual and auditory inputs regarding the source of a sound interact unconsciously (cf. Vroomen & de Gelder, 2003). At a minimum, these phenomena demonstrate that conscious states are unnecessary to integrate information from sources as diverse as the information from different modalities. Intersensory cross talk can occur without consciousness.

Hence, regarding the integration consensus, a critical issue remaining unaddressed pertains to which kinds of integration require consciousness and which kinds do not. *Supramodular interaction theory* (SIT; Morsella, 2005) addresses this issue by contrasting the task demands of the kinds of consciously impenetrable processes presented previously and consciously penetrable processes (for related paradigms, see Baars, 1988; Dulany, 1991; Jacoby, 1991; Jacoby, Yonelinas, & Jennings, 1997; for a criticism of this kind of paradigm, see O'Brien & Opie, 1999). This approach contrasts processes that are consciously available (e.g., aspects of pain and hunger) with those nervous processes that, as far as we know, are never consciously available (e.g., the mediation of reflexes and vegetative processes).

Unlike SIT, previous approaches have contrasted the task demands of the same cognitive process when it is novel and presumably consciously mediated (e.g., the first time driving or tying one's shoes) and when the process is overlearned, automatized, and presumably less consciously mediated (Logan, Taylor, & Etherton, 1999). By contrasting only penetrable and impenetrable processes, a benefit of SIT is that it diminishes the likelihood of conflating conscious and attentional processes, a recurring problem in accounts concerning the relationships among conscious, automatic, and unconscious processes (cf. Baars, 1997). There is substantial evidence that attention and consciousness are two distinct brain processes (see review in Koch & Tsuchiya, 2007). Assuming that consciously penetrable processes accomplish something that impenetrable processes cannot, the contrastive approach of SIT helps identify the primary contribution of consciousness.

Specifically, SIT addresses this issue by contrasting interactions that are consciously impenetrable (e.g., intersensory conflicts, peristalsis, and the pupillary reflex) with *conscious conflicts,* a dramatic class of conscious interactions between different information-processing systems. Conscious conflicts are a basic part of the human experience. For example, when one experiences the common event of holding one's breath underwater, withstanding pain, or suppressing consumatory, elimination, or sleep onset behaviors, one is simultaneously conscious of the inclinations to perform certain actions and of the inclinations to not do so. Unlike unconscious interactions (e.g., intersensory conflicts), the informational products from these diverse systems are consciously-penetrable.

SIT builds on the integration consensus by proposing that consciousness is required to integrate information *but* only certain kinds of information. Specifically, it is required to integrate information from specialized, high-level (and often multimodal) systems that are unique in that they may conflict with skeletal muscle plans, as described by the principle of *parallel responses into skeletal muscle* (PRISM). These *supramodular* systems are defined in terms of their "concerns" (e.g., bodily needs) rather than their sensory afference. In contrast, defining systems in terms of their sensory afference (e.g., auditory versus visual) has been the traditional approach to identifying mental faculties.

Supramodular Response Systems

Although operating in parallel, supramodular response systems may have different operating principles, concerns, and phylogenetic histories (Morsella, 2005). For example, in this framework, an *air-intake* system has the skeletal muscle tendencies of inhaling and yawning, a *tissue-damage* system has those of pain withdrawal and scratching, an *elimination system* has those of micturating and defecating, and a *food-intake* system has those of licking, chewing, swallowing, and other behaviors (e.g., the rooting and sucking reflexes) that can occur automatically following appropriate stimulation. For example, the food-intake system can influence skeletal muscle (henceforth "skeletomotor") action when confronted with the appropriate gustatory, olfactory, or even visual stimuli (Bindra, 1976). Thus, each system can influence skeletomotor action directly and unconsciously, but it is only through conscious states that they can influence action collectively, as during a conscious conflict (e.g., when carrying a scorching plate or holding one's breath) (Figure 30.1).

Consistent with classic experiments demonstrating that the instrumental competence needed for a task (e.g., navigating

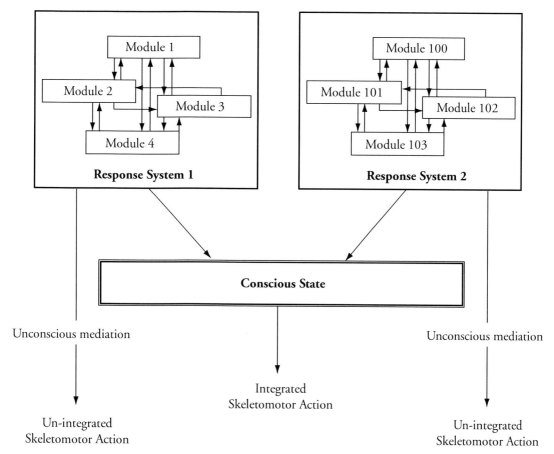

Fig. 30.1 Supramodular interaction theory: Fodorian modules operate within a few multimodal, supramodular response systems, each defined by its concern. Response system 1 may be the instrumental system, concerned with how the organism should physically interact with the world (e.g., to touch an object). Response system 2 may be an incentive system, concerned, for example, with whether the organism should approach or avoid a stimulus (e.g., withdraw limbs from scorching objects). Although the response systems can influence action directly (illustrated by the lateral arrows), only in virtue of conscious states can they can interact and influence action collectively, as when one carries a hot plate of food. Each system modulates a different aspect of conscious experience.

a maze) is predicated on forms of knowledge and goals that are different in nature from those of incentive learning (e.g., Tolman, 1948), Bindra (1974, 1978) proposed that, in addition to the kinds of *incentive systems* mentioned previously, there is a "cool" (Metcalfe & Mischel, 1999) multimodal, high-level system that is devoted to physically negotiating instrumental actions with the environment. It is involved with navigating through a space, approaching the location of objects, grabbing objects, pressing levers, manipulating objects, and other kinds of instrumental acts. From this perspective, the system treats and represents

all objects in the same manner regardless of the organism's motivational state (Bindra, 1974). Stimuli such as food and water are negotiated in roughly the same manner whether the organism is hungry, thirsty, or sated (Lorenz, 1963). Phenomenally, it is thus a "cool" (versus a "hot") system (Metcalfe & Mischel, 1999), for it is not hedonic or emotional in nature. Hence, it is proposed that, in addition to the need-related systems, there is a "cool," *instrumental response system* that has access to skeletal muscle and is capable of instrumental, vicarious, and latent learning. Its planned actions can be understood in terms of *ideomotor* principles

(Chapters 2 and 18); it enacts instrumental goals, which are subjectively experienced as *instrumental wants*.

Supramodular Conflict

These supramodular systems are unintelligent and inflexible in the sense that, without conscious states, they are incapable of taking information generated by other systems into account. For example, the tissue-damage system will protest damage even when the action engendering the damage is lifesaving. According to SIT, one can breathe unconsciously, but consciousness is required in order to suppress breathing. Similarly, one can unconsciously emit a pain-withdrawal response, but one cannot override such a response for food or water concerns without consciousness. Conflicts involving consummatory behavior form another class of conscious conflict. These occur, for example, when one is inclined to consume food, but for other reasons, one is inclined not to. In our evolutionary history, this may have occurred when a coveted food source was violently guarded by an animal (e.g., a fresh kill protected by a leopard) or located in a precarious environment (e.g., fishing crabs in ice-cold water). In modern times, the conflict is perhaps more common as the anguish arising from self-imposed food restrictions, as in fast-related dieting: One consciously desires food but has negative affect toward consuming it. To the detriment of extreme dieters, the negative affect is difficult (or impossible) to voluntarily quell. As in the tissue damage example, the nature or intensity of the affective state cannot be controlled (Öhman & Mineka, 2001), but the motor system can be controlled, to an extent. There is probably a threshold at which consummatory behavior also becomes quasi-reflexive (cf. Baker, Piper, McCarthy, Majeskie, & Fiore, 2004).

Similar classes of conflict involve air intake, water intake, sleep onset, temperature regulation, and various elimination behaviors. For example, if compelled to hold one's breath underwater, as when trapped under ice, one feels the urge to breathe (for not doing so leads to death) and the urge to refrain from doing so (for inhaling water leads to drowning). Although the urge to breathe is adaptive in most circumstances, the negative affect it elicits in this scenario can be fatal. One can readily imagine analogous conflicts involving the need for water (e.g., when the only water available is seawater or painfully cold), the need for sleep (e.g., when being hunted by a predator), and the needs related to various elimination behaviors.

PRISM

Figuratively speaking, it could be said that, in the nervous system, there are multiple systems trying to control the same "steering wheel," which is the skeletal muscle system. For example, expressing (or suppressing) inhaling, coughing, blinking, pruritus-induced scratching, pain withdrawal, licking, swallowing, micturating, and defecating all involve, specifically, skeletal muscle plans. Accordingly, regarding processes such as digestion, one is conscious of only those phases of the processes that require coordination with skeletomotor plans (e.g., chewing or micturating) and none of those that do not (e.g., peristalsis). Conversely, no skeletal muscle plans are directly involved in the actions of consciously impenetrable processes such as the pupillary reflex, peristalsis, stomach action, bronchial dilation, and vasoconstriction (which all involve smooth muscle) and the regulation of heart rate (which involves cardiac muscle).

Perhaps a more contemporary way to think about it is as follows. There are many quasi-independent computers in the brain, and each can do complicated things and influence overt action independently. Physical action could be construed as the activities and outputs of a computer printer.

Each computer can influence the printer, but in order for two computers to interact and influence the printer collectively, a wi-fi system may be required. Consciousness functions as such a wi-fi system to integrate the different systems in the brain and influence action collectively.

The PRISM acronym is conceptually related to the principle, for just as a prism can combine different colors to yield a single hue, conscious states cull simultaneously activated tendencies to yield adaptive skeletomotor action. PRISM is unique in its capacity to successfully differentiate conscious from unconscious processes a priori. The digestive system, which possesses both consciously controllable actions and involuntary actions, is perhaps most representative of the fact that consciousness is required only when cross talk is necessary. In general, the stomach does not need to know what the eyes or ears perceive, but other parts of the process of digestion certainly do, and it is only these parts that partake in this kind of information exchange.

Why Skeletal Muscles Are "Voluntary" Muscles

It has been known since at least the 19th century that, though often functioning unconsciously (as in the frequent actions of blinking, breathing, and postural shifting), skeletal muscle is the only effector that can be consciously controlled, but why this is so has never been addressed. SIT introduces a systematic reinterpretation of this age-old fact: *skeletomotor actions are at times "consciously mediated" because they are directed by multiple, encapsulated systems that, when in conflict, require conscious states to yield adaptive action.* Although identifying still higher-level systems is beyond the purview of SIT, PRISM correctly predicts that certain aspects of the expression (or suppression) of emotions (e.g., aggression, affection,

disgust, and so on), reproductive behaviors, parental care, and addiction-related behaviors should be coupled with conscious states (cf. Chapter 24), for the action tendencies of such processes may compromise skeletal muscle plans (of other systems) (Chapter 14).

The idea of "action-prone" systems above the level of the module is not new. Plato, Aristotle, and Freud have each divided up the psyche into sophisticated, supramodular agents (e.g., Freud's id, ego, and superego). These agents doggedly pursue their own agenda and can come into conflict with those of other agents—the id wants to eat cake, but the ego wants to lose weight. It is important to note that, in order for each agent to possess such knowledge about the present state of affairs (e.g., knowing that there is candy before one), each must receive conclusions from multiple information-processing structures.

SIT sheds some light on the nature of several disorders of consciousness. It explains why skeletomotor action will occur but will seem fragmented and irrational when consciousness is absent or impaired. Accordingly, the behaviors accompanying *blind sight* reflect a lack of interaction among different systems. Blind-sight patients can navigate through a space, but their behavior is not purposeful: When hungry, they cannot seek food. Seeking food, for example, requires the combined outputs of systems used to navigate through space and grab objects and a food-intake system (to desire and ingest food). In other disorders in which action seems to be decoupled from phenomenal states, behavior is often perceived as impulsive, situationally inappropriate, and irrational (Chan & Ross, 1997). For example, in alien hand syndrome (Bryon & Jedynak, 1972), anarchic hand syndrome (Marchetti & Della Sala, 1998), and utilization behavior syndrome (Lhermitte, 1983), brain damage causes hands and arms to function autonomously, carrying out relatively complex goal-directed behaviors (e.g., the manipulation of tools; Yamadori, 1997) that are maladaptive and, in some cases, at odds with a patient's reported intentions.

Consistent with this approach, automatic behaviors (e.g., reflexive pharyngeal swallowing) are believed to involve substantially fewer brain regions and systems than their intentional counterparts (e.g., volitional swallowing; Kern, Jaradeh, Arndorfer, & Shaker, 2001; Ortinski & Meador, 2004). Moreover, beyond cognitive operations, one will never be conscious of activities such as those regulating blood pressure and glucose levels in the blood because they do not require communication across systems in order to yield adaptive action.

Specifically, an action plan can be mediated unconsciously insofar as it may not potentially conflict with any skeletal muscle goal (e.g., of any response system). One would be aware (e.g., as in the form of a conscious "urge") of anything that could interfere with skeletal muscle plans. Moreover, without consciousness, it is impossible to perform an instrumental skeletomotor act for an incentive. Thus, traditional examples of operant conditioning such as pressing a lever to obtain food or avoid shock cannot occur unconsciously. Regardless of the consequences, it is impossible to suppress the behavioral tendencies (e.g., blinking, pain withdrawal; cf. Chapter 3) of any supramodular system, which is consistent with the fact that one is incapable of voluntarily asphyxiating oneself, for one can hold one's breath only while conscious (Tortora, 1994).

In summary, SIT addresses fundamental questions about the human nervous system: why some processes are conscious while others are not and why skeletal muscle is the only muscle that is controlled "voluntarily." Building on the integration consensus, the framework allows one to appreciate that not all kinds of integration involve consciousness and that conscious and unconscious processes may be distinguished by the nature of the effectors involved.

The evolutionary trend toward increased compartmentalization of function in the nervous system introduced various integrative solutions, including unconscious reflexes and neural convergence. Although integration across supramodular systems could conceivably occur without something like consciousness, such a solution was not selected in our evolutionary history. Instead, and for reasons that only the happenstance process of evolution could explain (Chapter 1), it is proposed that the physical state of consciousness was selected to solve this large-scale, cross-talk problem. From this mechanistic standpoint, explaining how humans function without invoking conscious states is analogous to explaining how radios work without implicating the electromagnetic spectrum. Using Marr's (1982) terminology, conscious states are the "implementational"-level solution to the "computational" problem of integrating the tendencies of multiple systems that are otherwise encapsulated. Thus, consciousness is a tool that is ultimately in the service of adaptive skeletomotor action.

Acknowledgments

Preparation of this chapter was supported by the National Institutes of Health (R01-MH60767). We acknowledge the advice of Robert Krauss, Andy Poehlman, and Lawrence Williams.

Notes

1. This chapter is based in large part on a theory that first appeared in *Psychological Review* (Morsella, 2005).

2. Controlled by both divisions of the autonomic nervous system, it responds in a highly adaptive manner to conditions as diverse as changes in light level, arousal, and point of focus. Regardless of light conditions, both pupils are always matched in diameter. When one eye is covered, the pupil of the other dilates; when it is then uncovered, the pupil of the other constricts.

3. For example, it has been hypothesized that phenomenal states play a role in voluntary behavior (Shepherd, 1994), language (Banks, 1995), "theory of mind" (Stuss & Anderson, 2004), the formation of the self (Greenwald & Pratkanis, 1984), cognitive homeostasis (Damasio, 1999), the monitoring of mental functions (Reisberg, 2001), semantic processing (Kouider & Dupoux, 2004), the interpretation of situations (Roser & Gazzaniga, 2004), and simulations of behavior and perception (Hesslow, 2002).

References

Baars, B. J. (1988). *A cognitive theory of consciousness.* Cambridge: Cambridge University Press.

Baars, B. J. (1997). Some essential differences between consciousness and attention, perception, and working memory. *Consciousness and Cognition, 6,* 363–371.

Baars, B. J. (2002). The conscious access hypothesis: Origins and recent evidence. *Trends in Cognitive Sciences, 6,* 47–52.

Baker, T. B., Piper, M. E., McCarthy, D. E., Majeskie, M. R., & Fiore, M. C. (2004). Addiction motivation reformulated: An affective processing model of negative reinforcement. *Psychological Review, 111,* 33–51.

Banks, W. P. (1995). Evidence for consciousness. *Consciousness and Cognition, 4,* 270–272.

Bargh, J. A., & Morsella, E. (2008). The unconscious mind. *Perspectives on Psychological Science, 3,* 73–79.

Bindra, D. (1974). A motivational view of learning, performance, and behavior modification. *Psychological Review, 81,* 199–213.

Bindra, D. (1976). *A theory of intelligent behavior.* New York: Wiley-Interscience.

Bindra, D. (1978). How adaptive behavior is produced: A perceptual-motivational alternative to response-reinforcement. *Behavioral and Brain Sciences, 1,* 41–91.

Block, N. (1995). On a confusion about a function of consciousness. *Behavioral and Brain Sciences, 18,* 227–287.

Bryon, S., & Jedynak, C. P. (1972). Troubles du transfert interhémisphérique: A propos de trois observations de tumeurs du corps calleux. Le signe de la main étrangère. *Revue Neurologique, 126,* 257–266.

Chan, J.-L., & Ross, E. D. (1997). Alien hand syndrome: Influence of neglect on the clinical presentation of frontal and callosal variants. *Cortex, 33,* 287–299.

Crick, F., & Koch, C. (2003). A framework for consciousness. *Nature Neuroscience, 6,* 1–8.

Damasio, A. R. (1999). *The feeling of what happens: Body and emotion in the making of consciousness.* New York: Harcourt Brace.

Dickinson, A., & Balleine, B. W. (2000). Causal cognition and goal-directed action. In C. Heyes & L. Huber (Eds.), *The evolution of cognition. Vienna series in theoretical biology* (pp. 185–204). Cambridge, MA: MIT Press.

Donald, M. (2001). *A mind so rare: The evolution of human consciousness.* New York: Norton.

Dulany, D. E. (1991). Conscious representation and thought systems. In R. S. Wyer & T. K. Srull (Eds.), *The content, structure, and operation of thought systems. Advances in social cognition* (Vol. 4, pp. 97–120). Hillsdale, NJ: Lawrence Erlbaum Associates.

Goodale, M., & Milner, D. (2004). *Sight unseen: An exploration of conscious and unconscious vision.* New York: Oxford University Press.

Gray, J. A. (1995). The contents of consciousness: A neuropsychological conjecture. *Behavioral and Brain Sciences, 18,* 659–676.

Gray, J. (2004). *Consciousness: Creeping up on the hard problem.* New York: Oxford University Press.

Greenwald, A. G., & Pratkanis, A. R. (1984). The self. In R. S. Wyer & T. K. Srull (Eds.), *Handbook of social cognition* (pp. 129–178). Hillsdale, NJ: Lawrence Erlbaum Associates.

Hesslow, G. (2002). Conscious thought as simulation of behavior and perception. *Trends in Cognitive Sciences, 6,* 242–247.

Hobson, J. A. (2000). *Consciousness.* New York: Scientific American Library.

Jack, A. I., & Shallice, T. (2001). Introspective physicalism as an approach to the science of consciousness. *Cognition, 79,* 161–196.

Jacoby, L. L. (1991). A process dissociation framework: Separating automatic from intentional uses of memory. *Journal of Memory and Language, 30,* 513–541.

Jacoby, L. L., Yonelinas, A. P., & Jennings, J. M. (1997). The relations between conscious and unconscious (automatic) influences: Toward showing independence. In J. D. Cohen & J. W. Schooler (Eds.), *Scientific approaches to consciousness* (pp. 13–47). Mahwah, NJ: Lawrence Erlbaum Associates.

Kern, M. K., Jaradeh, S., Arndorfer, R. C., & Shaker, R. (2001). Cerebral cortical representation of reflexive and volitional swallowing in humans. *American Journal of Physiology: Gastrointestinal and Liver Physiology, 280,* G354–G360.

Klein, D. B. (1984). *The concept of consciousness: A survey.* Lincoln: University of Nebraska Press.

Koch, C., & Tsuchiya, N. (2007). Attention and consciousness: Two distinct brain processes. *Trends in Cognitive Sciences, 11,* 16–22.

Kouider, S., & Dupoux, E. (2004). Partial awareness creates the "illusion" of subliminal semantic priming. *Psychological Science, 15,* 75–81.

Lashley, K. S. (1951). The problem of serial order in behavior. In L. A. Jeffress (Ed.), *Cerebral mechanisms in behavior: The Hixon symposium* (pp. 112–146). New York: Wiley.

Laurey, S. (2005). The neural correlate of (un)awareness: Lessons from the vegetative state. *Trends in Cognitive Sciences, 12,* 556–559.

Lhermitte, F. (1983). "Utilization behavior" and its relation to lesions of the frontal lobes. *Brain, 106,* 237–255.

Libet, B. (2004). *Mind time: The temporal factor in consciousness.* Cambridge, MA: Harvard University Press.

Logan, G. D., Taylor, S. E., & Etherton, J. L. (1999). Attention and automaticity: Toward a theoretical integration. *Psychological Research, 62,* 165–181.

Lorenz, K. (1963). *On aggression.* New York: Harcourt Brace & World.

Mandler, G. (1998). Consciousness and mind as philosophical problems and psychological issues. In J. Hochberg (Ed.), *Perception and cognition at century's end: Handbook of perception and cognition* (2nd ed., pp. 45–65). San Diego, CA: Academic Press.

Marchetti, C., & Della Sala, S. (1998). Disentangling the alien and anarchic hand. *Cognitive Neuropsychiatry, 3,* 191–207.

Marr, D. (1982). *Vision.* New York: Freeman.

McGurk, H., & MacDonald, J. (1976). Hearing lips and seeing voices. *Nature, 264,* 746–748.

Merker, B. (2007). Consciousness without a cerebral cortex: A challenge for neuroscience and medicine. *Behavioral and Brain Sciences, 30,* 63–134.

Metcalfe, J., & Mischel, W. (1999). A hot/cool-system analysis of delay of gratification: Dynamics of willpower. *Psychological Review, 106,* 3–19.

Morsella, E. (2005). The function of phenomenal states: Supramodular interaction theory. *Psychological Review, 112,* 1000–1021.

Nagel, T. (1974). What is it like to be a bat? *Philosophical Review, 83,* 435–450.

O'Brien, G., & Opie, J. (1999). A connectionist theory of phenomenal experience. *Behavioral and Brain Sciences, 22,* 127–196.

Öhman, A., & Mineka, S. (2001). Fears, phobias, and preparedness: Toward an evolved module of fear and fear learning. *Psychological Review, 108,* 483–522.

Ortinski, P., & Meador, K. J. (2004). Neuronal mechanisms of conscious awareness. *Neurological Review, 61,* 1017–1020.

Reisberg, D. (2001). *Cognition: Exploring the science of the mind,* 2nd ed. New York: Norton.

Rosenbaum, D. A. (2002). Motor control. In H. Pashler (Series Ed.) & S. Yantis (Vol. Ed.), *Stevens' handbook of experimental psychology: Vol. 1. Sensation and perception* (3rd ed., pp. 315–339). New York: Wiley.

Roser, M., & Gazzaniga, M. S. (2004). Automatic brains—Interpretive minds. *Current Directions in Psychological Science, 13,* 56–59.

Shallice, T. (1972). Dual functions of consciousness. *Psychological Review, 79,* 383–393.

Shepherd, G. M. (1994). *Neurobiology* (3rd ed.). New York: Oxford University Press.

Sherrington, C. S. (1906). *The integrative action of the nervous system.* New Haven, CT: Yale University Press.

Skinner, B. F. (1953). *Science and human behavior.* New York: Macmillan.

Sobel, N., Prabhakaran, V., Hartley C. A., Desmond J. E., Glover, G. H., Sullivan, E. V., et al. (1999). Blind smell: Brain activation induced by an undetected air-borne chemical. *Brain, 122,* 209–217.

Sperry, R. W. (1952). Neurology and the mind-brain problem. *American Scientist, 40,* 291–312.

Stuss, D. T., & Anderson, V. (2004). The frontal lobes and theory of mind: Developmental concepts from adult focal lesion research. *Brain and Cognition, 55,* 69–83.

Tolman, E. C. (1948). Cognitive maps in rats and men. *Psychological Review, 55,* 189–208.

Tortora, G. J. (1994). *Introduction to the human body: The essentials of anatomy and physiology,* 3rd ed. New York: HarperCollins.

Vroomen, J., & de Gelder, B. (2003). Visual motion influences the contingent auditory motion aftereffect. *Psychological Science, 14,* 357–361.

Weiskrantz, L. (1997). *Consciousness lost and found: A neuropsychological exploration.* New York: Oxford University Press.

Yamadori, A. (1997). Body awareness and its disorders. In M. Ito, Miyashita, Y., & E. T. Rolls (Eds.), *Cognition, computation, and consciousness* (pp. 169–176). Washington, DC: American Psychological Association.

Zeki, S., & Bartels, A. (1999). Toward a theory of visual consciousness. *Consciousness and Cognition, 8,* 225–259.

INDEX

setting of, 444
social norms for, negative feelings and, 614–16
theories of, 105
behavioral decisions, 104
as behavior determinant, 106–7
intending bridging of, 113–14
behavioral flexibility, 386, 391
balance/locomotion and, 400–401
conclusion on, 423–25
goal-directed action and, 399
perception and, 400
behaviorism, 2, 22n1
behavioral mimicry, 458, 461
behavioral preparedness, 108
behavioral responses, priming and, 261
behavioral withdrawal, 16
behavior control, by SAS, 560
behavior patterns, applications to
aggression, 501–2
existential threats, 502–3
helping, 502
impulses/appetites, 503
intelligence performance and, 500
interracial interactions, 503–4
intimate relationships and, 500–501
money, 504
Bernstein, Nicolai, 123
bimanual coordination, performance and, 43–44
binding, action control and, 382–91
actional phase of, 387–89
planning phase of, 384–87
postactional phase of, 389–91
summary on, 391
bipolar dimensions
as affect issues, 305–6
anger and, 305–6
self-discrepancy theory and, 305
Blake, William, 225
blindsight, 20, 628
behaviors accompanying, 632
body position, 121
action representation and, 381
future knowledge of
end-state comfort and, 126–29
evidence for, 125–30
study on, 126–28, 126f, 127f, 128f
infinite variations of, 122
bottom-up process, action control
and, 314
brain limbic hedonic hot spots, negative
aversive/positive hedonic reaction
to, 516f
brain matter, in children, 259–60
brain mechanisms
action control and, 320
of reward utility, 512–13
brain regions. See also motor cortex
activation of, 254, 260–61
apraxia and, 137, 137f, 151f
frontal lobes, nonconscious goal pursuit
and, 560
in human action, 8f, 22n11

hypothesized function/interconnections
of, 12f
imitation disorders and, 142–43
implementation intentions in, 621
IPL, 264f
lateral view of, 254f
motor planning and, 123–24
movement formula and, 138f–139f
oculomotor network in, 76f
pantomime and, 146
posterior-to-anterior stream and, 138f
brain stimulation
incentive salience and, 514
pleasure and, 514
Broca's Region (Grodzinsky/Amunts), 14
Burns, Robert, 434

C

Carlin, George, 572
carryover, 58–59
effect of, 387
procedural priming and, 175
cascade model, language production and,
14–15, 22n12
children
ASD and, 258, 262
brain matter in, 259–60
choice
equifinality effect and, intrasystemic
effects and, 357–58
self-regulation influence on, 494
Cleese, John, 576
coasting
affect issues and, 307–8
positive feelings, 307
multiple concerns and, 308–9
tendencies for, 308
COBRA. See competition between reward
and accuracy
code-occupation hypothesis, for action
plans, 385
cognition, 277, 298
action control and, 280–81
model for, 315
actions and, 226–30
for action v. as action, 242–43
control of, 427
task switching and, 431
cultural differences and, 341
disembodied activity of, 229
emotion and, 278, 290
mechanics of, action knowledge and,
36–37
motivation as, 351, 364–65
normal processing and, 226
perceptual-motor simulations
and, 226
cognitive approaches, 35
to action
cognitive mechanics, 36–37
task sets, 37
volitional dynamics, 37
to motion planning
dynamical systems, 123

feed-back theory, 123
neuroscience, 123–24
cognitive map, Tolman and, 122
cognitive neuroscience, 72
laboratory tests and, 73–75
cognitive performance, 225, 226
acting-out process and, 238–39
motivational variables influencing,
341–43, 345–46
self-construal and, 341
cognitive processing, 225, 328. See also
real-time cognitive processing
actions and, 226
measure/influence of, 237
memory and, 344
common coding, 39, 251–52
core assumption of, 252
communication, mimicry as, 471–72
competition between reward and accuracy
(COBRA), 536–37
compound-cue retrieval, task switching as,
433–34
conditional contingencies
of contextual processing, 344
unconditional contingencies v.,
344–45
conditioned stimulus (CS), 518
conditioning, 1, 11, 13
conflict
action plans and, 22n14
affinity-based/approach-approach,
18–19
conscious, 557, 629
goal paradigm of, 609
nonconscious goal pursuit and,
556–57
SEF and, 82
task and, 391
WM and, 556–57
implication of, 557
connectionist principles, 156
implicit learning and, 170
conscious conflict, 557, 629
conscious goal pursuit. See also
nonconscious goal pursuit
capacity issues of, 609
classification responses for, 610
conclusion on, 621–22
ego depletion and, 609
emotion and, 615–16
nonconscious goal pursuit shifting
between, 611–21
consciousness returns, 612–16
emotions and, 615–16
nonconscious goal pursuit v.
differences of, 608–11
distinction origins, 604–7
personality moderating, 611
similarities of, 607–8
reflective v. reflexive control issues of,
609–10
as top-down process, 610
consciousness
action plan and, 19–20

reflective system (*continued*)
impulsive system interactions with,
112–13
knowledge generation/transformation
by, 111–12
RIM and, 111–12
reinforcer devaluation insensitivity
phenomenon, 451
relationship. *See* intimate relationships
remembered utility, 509, 510
repeating sequence procedure, plans and,
435–36
RT increase of, 436
representational approach, to PFC
function, 198
representations. *See also* action
representations; distributed
representations; goal-based
representations; mental
representations; motor
representations; shared
representations
of actions, 22n3, 22n4
embodied *v.* classical approaches,
4–7, 22n7
ideomotor approaches, 3–4
by motor systems, 228
reprioritization
goals and, 310
negative feelings and, 309
Simon on, 309–10
resonance, action understanding and,
256–58
response, 72
to implementation intentions, 617–18,
618f
inhibition of, 383
laboratory tests and, 73–75
microaffordance and, 229
selection of, 98–99
response-effect compatibility, learning
and, 46
response-related components, of switch
costs, 57–58
response-related goals. *See* goal(s)
reverse engineering, 1, 22n2
challenge of, 2–3
reward utility, 509
brain mechanisms of, 512–13
of decisions
mismatch of, 511
rational *v.* irrational, 511–12
subtypes of, 510–12
RIM. *See* Reflective Impulsive Model
Robinson, Terry, 522
rostral anterior cingulate cortex (rACC),
292
RSPAN. *See* reading span
RT. *See* reaction time

S

saccade neurons
eye movement and, 230–31, 234–36
firing rate of, 78f

SAS. *See* supervisory attentional system
satisficing, constraint hierarchy and, 131
SC. *See* superior colliculus
scope insensitive manner, decision-making
and, 283–84
SCRs. *See* skin conductance responses
SDEs. *See* stochastic differential equations
second-order constraints. *See* speech
constraints
SECs. *See* structured event complexes
SEF. *See* supplementary eye fields
self-construal
cognitive performance and, 341
cultural variations of, 342
explorations of, 343–45
fear of isolation and, 342
independent, 341
self-control, 299
aggression and, 501–2
depletion effects and, 492
empowering, 497–500
long-term interventions for, 499–500
short-term boots of, 498–99
impulse/restraint and, 319–20
appetites/sexual behavior, 503
money and, 504
muscle analogy for, 499
relationship importance of, 500–501
self-regulation and, 489
self-discrepancy theory, bipolar dimension
evidence and, 305
self-monitoring, of social lives/mimicry,
464–65
self-perception theory, attitudes and, 111
self-regulation, 298–99, 328, 571
benefits of, 490–91
choice influenced by, 494
difficulty of, 575
efforts for, 313f, 575, 576
evaluation patterns and, 362
feedback control and, 590–91
interracial interactions and, 503–4
items and, 330
laboratory studies on, 491
limited resource and, 491–92
main spheres of, 491
nonconscious forms of, 489
nonsocial impact of, 469–71
priority management in
automatic affect function prevention
and, 311
depression feelings and, 312–14
effort for, 313f
negative feelings and, 309
positive feelings and, 309–11
self-control and, 489
semantic constructs, 173
behavior priming and, 179
goal gradients and, 182
hierarchy of, 186
semantic priming, 174, 188–89n1
goal activation *v.,* 179
sense of agency, 250, 251, 263
acknowledgement of, 264

sensorimotor units
action representation and, 374–75, 379
perceptual/motor component of, 374
sensory-motor experience, perception
and, 227
sensory-motor routines, judgments and, 228
serial models, language production and, 15
Shah, J. Y., 556
shared representations
action imitation and, 261
conclusion on, 268–69
importance of, 250
of perception-behavior link, 474
social interaction and, 256
Simon effect
implementation intentions and, 619
LRPs and, 378
mapping and, 378
SRC and, 215
Simon, Herbert, 131, 309–10
SIT. *See* supramodular interaction theory
skeletal muscle, 626
as action-prone system, 632
consciousness and, 632–33
as voluntary muscles, 632–33
skill development, constraint hierarchy
and, 132
skin conductance responses (SCRs), 287
Skinner, B. F.
instrumental learning and, 122
on mental representation, 122
social behavior, 104
dual-process model of, 109
theory of planned action and, 106
theory of reasoned action and, 106
social-cognitive approach, 350
social interaction
motor representations in, 250
shared representations and, 256
social lives, 458
distinctiveness/assimilation and, 463–64
ostracism and, 464
self-monitoring of, 464–65
social mirroring
action imitation and, 258–64
intentional imitation, 259–64
conclusion on, 268–69
social neuroscience approach, to mimicry
empathy and, 476–78
perspective taking and, 478–79
social norms, for behaviors, negative
feelings and, 614–16
social psychology
motivation theories and, 350–52
persuasion models and, 351
two-mode models in, action control
and, 315
spatial attraction, hand movements and,
233, 234f
spatial reasoning tasks, acting-out process
for, 238
speech constraints
between consonants/adjacent vowels,
160–61, 161f

Printed in the USA/Agawam, MA
August 11, 2015

621309.049